Examination & Board Review

Pharmacology

fourth edition

a **LANGE medical book**

Examination & Board Review

Pharmacology

fourth edition

Bertram G. Katzung, MD, PhD
Professor of Pharmacology
Department of Pharmacology
University of California, San Francisco

Anthony J. Trevor, PhD
Professor of Pharmacology and Toxicology
Department of Pharmacology
University of California, San Francisco

APPLETON & LANGE
Norwalk, Connecticut

96 97 98 / 10 9 8 7 6 5 4 3

Prentice Hall International (UK) Limited, *London*
Prentice Hall of Australia Pty. Limited, *Sydney*
Prentice Hall Canada, Inc., *Toronto*
Prentice Hall Hispanoamericana, S.A., *Mexico*
Prentice Hall of India Private Limited, *New Delhi*
Prentice Hall of Japan, Inc., *Tokyo*
Simon & Schuster Asia Pte. Ltd., *Singapore*
Editora Prentice Hall do Brasil Ltda., *Rio de Janeiro*
Prentice Hall, *Englewood Cliffs, New Jersey*

ISBN 0-8385-8067-X
ISSN 1063-8636

Acquisitions Editor: John Dolan
Production Editor: Chris Langan
Art Coordinator: Becky Hainz Baxter
Illustrator: Linda F. Harris

ISBN 0-8385-8067-X
90000
9 780838 580677

PRINTED IN THE UNITED STATES OF AMERICA

Contents

VIII. CHEMOTHERAPEUTIC DRUGS

IX. TOXICOLOGY

X. SPECIAL TOPICS

Preface

This book is designed to help students review Pharmacology and to prepare for regular course exams and board exams. The fourth edition of this book has been extensively revised to make such preparation as efficient as possible. Many new tables and figures have been added and color has been used to further clarify difficult concepts. As with earlier editions, the most rigorous standards of accuracy and currency have been maintained, in keeping with the book's status as companion to the textbook *Basic & Clinical Pharmacology.*

Several strategies are employed to make reviewing effective and efficient:

First, the book breaks Pharmacology down into the topics used in most courses and textbooks, rather than combining them into larger, unwieldy groups. Major introductory chapters (eg, autonomic pharmacology and CNS pharmacology) are included, so that students can integrate their review of pharmacology with a review of physiology and biochemistry. This chapter-based approach also encourages students to use the Review in conjunction with their course notes or with a larger text.

Second, each unit explicitly lists a set of objectives, providing students with a checklist against which they can challenge themselves as they progress through the book.

Third, each chapter provides an expanded but still concise review of the core subject matter. The determination of what is core is based on a careful analysis of the content of actual board examinations over the past several years as well as the content of major medical school courses. Tables of definitions and figures illustrating the major subdivisions of drugs within each group are provided.

Fourth, a table of important drug names is provided in every chapter dealing with specific drug groups. Recognition of drug names is an important part of board exams. We make the process more efficient by distinguishing between those drugs important as prototypes, those recognized as major variants on the prototypes, and those that should simply be recognized as belonging to a particular drug group.

Fifth, each chapter ends with practice questions followed by a list of answers and explanations. Because each area of pharmacology is represented by a separate chapter, students are assured of having practice questions in every important area. Questions that require analysis of graphic or tabular data are included. Appendices II and III comprise two complete examinations, each covering the entire field of Pharmacology. In keeping with the format adopted for the United States Medical Licensure Examination (USMLE), the questions are of the "A" (single best answer) and "B" (matching, including *extended* matching) types. Many of the questions are set in the "clinical vignette" format currently favored on many examinations. More than 1000 questions, with answers, are provided in this book.

Sixth, Appendix I provides a list of key drugs that appear frequently in board exam questions with concise keyword descriptions. This unique learning aid provides an efficient "flashcard" list of the topics most likely to appear on an examination.

The book provides several additional sections of value to the student preparing for a board exam: (1) a set of 16 case histories, with questions and answers, providing additional review and testing of the student's preparation for questions about clinical pharmacology; and (2) a short appendix on test strategies, which summarizes time-saving devices for approaching specific types of questions used on most "objective" exams.

It is recommended that this book be used with a regular text. *Basic & Clinical Pharmacology* (Appleton & Lange, 1995) follows the chapter sequence used here. However, this Review is designed to complement any standard medical pharmacology text. A student completing this review will greatly improve his or her chance of performing well on examinations and will have an excellent command of the area of Pharmacology.

Because it was developed in parallel with the textbook *Basic & Clinical Pharmacology,* the Review represents the authors' interpretations of chapters written by contributors to that text. We are very grateful to these contributors, to our other faculty colleagues, and to our students—who have taught us most of what we know about teaching.

Suggestions and criticisms regarding this study guide should be mailed to us at the following address:

> Pharmacology Department, Box 0450
> University of California
> San Francisco, CA 94143-0450, USA
>
> Bertram G. Katzung, MD, PhD
> Anthony J. Trevor, PhD
> San Francisco
> March 1995

Part 1: Basic Principles

Introduction

1

OBJECTIVES

You should be able to:

- Predict the relative ease of permeation of a weak acid or base from a knowledge of its pK_a and the pH of the medium.
- List and discuss the common routes of drug administration and excretion.
- Draw graphs of the blood level versus time for drugs subject to zero-order elimination and for drugs subject to first-order elimination.

Learn the definitions that follow.

Table 1–1. Definitions.

Term	Definition
Pharmacology	The study of the interaction of chemicals with living systems
Drugs	Substances that act on living systems at the chemical (molecular) level
Drug receptors	The molecular components of the body with which a drug interacts to bring about its effect
Medical pharmacology	The study of drugs used for the diagnosis, prevention, and treatment of disease
Toxicology	The study of the undesirable effects of chemical agents on living systems; considered an area of pharmacology. In addition to the adverse effects of therapeutic agents on individuals, toxicology also deals with the actions of industrial pollutants, natural organic and inorganic poisons, and other chemicals on species and ecosystems
Pharmacodynamics	Refers to the actions of a drug on the body, including receptor interactions, dose-response phenomena, and mechanisms of therapeutic and toxic action
Pharmacokinetics	Refers to the actions of the body on the drug, including absorption, distribution, metabolism, and excretion. **Elimination** of a drug may be achieved by metabolism or by excretion. **Biodisposition** is a term sometimes used to describe the processes of metabolism and excretion

CONCEPTS

A. **The Nature of Drugs:**
   1. **Size and molecular weight (MW):** Drugs in common use vary in size from MW 7 (lithium) to over MW 50,000 (thrombolytic enzymes). The majority of drugs, however, lie between MW 100 and 1000.
   2. **Drug-receptor bonds:** Drugs bind to receptors with a variety of chemical bonds. These include very strong covalent bonds (which usually result in irreversible action), somewhat weaker electrostatic bonds, eg, between a cation and an anion, and much weaker interactions such as hydrogen, van der Waals, and hydrophobic bonds.

B. The Movement of Drugs in the Body: In order to reach its receptors and bring about a biologic effect, a drug molecule must travel from the site of administration (eg, the gastrointestinal tract) to the site of action (eg, the brain).

    1. Permeation: Permeation refers to the movement of drug molecules within the biologic environment. Permeation involves several processes, of which the following are the most important:

        a. Aqueous diffusion: Aqueous diffusion is the simple movement of molecules through the watery extracellular and intracellular spaces. The membranes of most capillaries have small aqueous pores that permit the aqueous diffusion of molecules up to the size of small proteins. This is a passive process governed by Fick's Law (see below).

        b. Lipid diffusion: Lipid diffusion is the solution in, and movement through, membranes and other lipid structures. Like aqueous diffusion, this is a passive process governed by Fick's Law (see below).

        c. Transport by special carriers: Transport of drugs across barriers may occur by carrier mechanisms that transport similar endogenous substances, eg, the secretory and re-absorptive carriers for weak acids located in the renal tubule. Unlike aqueous and lipid diffusion, carrier transport is not governed by Fick's law and is capacity limited. Selective inhibitors, which exist for some of these carriers, may have clinical value, eg, probenecid, which inhibits transport of uric acid, penicillin, and other weak acids.

        d. Endocytosis, pinocytosis: Endocytosis occurs through binding to specialized components of the membrane, with subsequent internalization by infolding of that area of the membrane. The contents of the vesicle are subsequently released into the cytoplasm of the cell. Endocytosis permits very large or very lipid-insoluble chemicals to enter cells. For example, large molecules such as peptides may enter cells by this mechanism. Smaller, polar, substances such as vitamin B_{12} and iron combine with special proteins (B_{12} with intrinsic factor and iron with transferrin), and the complexes enter cells by this mechanism. Exocytosis is the reverse process, ie, the expulsion of membrane-encapsulated material from cells.

    2. Fick's Law of Diffusion: Fick's Law predicts the rate of movement of molecules across a barrier; the concentration gradient and permeability coefficient for the drug, and the area and thickness of the barrier membrane are used to compute the rate, as follows:

$$\textbf{Rate} = (\textbf{C}_1 - \textbf{C}_2) \times \frac{\textbf{Permeability Coefficient}}{\textbf{Thickness}} \times \textbf{Area} \qquad \textbf{(1)}$$

This relationship demonstrates that a faster rate of drug absorption occurs from organs with large surface areas, eg, the small intestine, than organs with small areas, eg, the stomach; also, drug absorption is faster from organs with thin membrane barriers, eg, the lung, than from those with thick barriers, eg, skin.

    3. Water and lipid solubility of drugs:

        a. Aqueous diffusion: The aqueous solubility of a drug is often a function of the electrostatic charge (degree of ionization, polarity) of the molecule, because water molecules behave as dipoles and are attracted to charged drug molecules, forming an aqueous shell around them. Conversely, the lipid solubility of a molecule is inversely proportionate to its charge.

        b. Lipid diffusion: A large number of drugs are weak bases or weak acids. The pH of the medium determines the fraction of molecules charged (ionized) if the molecule is a weak acid or base. If the pK_a of the drug and the pH of the medium are known, the fraction of ionized molecules can be predicted by means of the Henderson–Hasselbalch equation:

$$\log\left(\frac{\textbf{Protonated form}}{\textbf{Unprotonated form}}\right) = \textbf{pK}_a - \textbf{pH} \qquad \textbf{(2)}$$

"Protonated" means *associated with a proton* (a hydrogen ion); this form of the equation applies to both acids and bases.

        c. Ionization of weak acids and bases: Weak bases are ionized—and therefore more polar and more water-soluble—when they are protonated; weak acids are not ionized—and so less water-soluble—when they are protonated.

The following equations summarize these points:

$$RNH_3^+ \quad \rightleftharpoons \quad RNH_2 \quad + \quad H^+$$

RNH$_3^+$ $\rightleftharpoons$	**RNH$_2$** +	**H$^+$**
protonated weak base (charged, more water-soluble)	unprotonated weak base (uncharged, more lipid-soluble)	proton

(3)

RCOOH $\rightleftharpoons$	**RCOO$^-$** +	**H$^+$**
protonated weak acid (uncharged, more lipid-soluble)	unprotonated weak acid (charged, more water-soluble)	proton

(4)

The Henderson–Hasselbalch relationship is clinically important when it is necessary to accelerate the excretion of drugs by the kidney, eg, in the case of an overdose. Most drugs are freely filtered at the glomerulus, but sufficiently lipid soluble drugs can be reabsorbed from the tubular urine. When a patient takes an overdose of a weak acid drug, its excretion may be accelerated by alkalinizing the urine, eg, by giving bicarbonate. This is because a weak acid dissociates to its charged, polar, form in alkaline solution and this form can not readily diffuse from the renal tubule back into the blood. Conversely, excretion of weak bases is accelerated by acidifying the urine, eg, by administering ammonium chloride, see Figure 1–1.

C. Absorption of Drugs:
    1. Routes of administration: Drugs usually enter the body at sites remote from the target tissue or organ, and thus require transport by the circulation to the intended site of action. To enter the bloodstream, a drug must be absorbed from its site of administration (unless the drug has been injected directly into the bloodstream). The rate and efficiency of absorption differ depending on a drug's route of administration. Common routes of administration and some of their features include the following:
        a. Oral (swallowed): The oral route offers maximum convenience but may be slower and less complete than parenteral routes. Ingested drugs are subject to the **first-pass ef-**

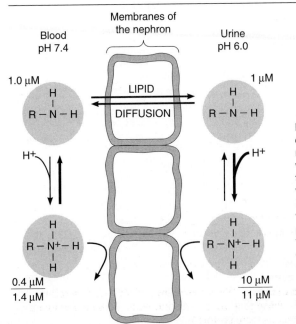

Figure 1–1. "Trapping" is a method for accelerating excretion of drugs. Because the unionized form diffuses readily across the lipid barriers of the nephron, this form will equilibrate, ie, it may reach equal concentrations in the blood and urine; the ionized form will not. Protonation will occur within the blood and the urine according to the Henderson–Hasselbalch equation. Pyrimethamine, a weak base of pK$_a$ 7.0, is used in this example. At blood pH, only 0.4 µM of the protonated species will be present for each 1.0 µM of the unprotonated form. The total concentration in the blood will thus be 1.4 µM/L for each micromol of the unprotonated drug. In the urine at pH 6.0, 10 µM of the nondiffusible ionized form will be present for each 1.0 µM of the unprotonated, diffusible form. Therefore, the total urine concentration (11 µM/L) may be almost 8 times higher than the blood concentration.

fect, in which metabolism of a significant amount of the agent occurs in the gut wall and the liver before the drug reaches the systemic circulation.

   b. **Buccal (in the pouch between gums and cheek):**   The buccal route permits direct absorption into the systemic venous circulation, bypassing the hepatic portal circuit and first-pass metabolism. This process may be fast or slow depending on the physical formulation of the product.

   c. **Sublingual (under the tongue):**   The sublingual route offers the same features as the buccal route.

   d. **Rectal (suppository):**   The rectal route offers partial escape from the first-pass effect (though not as complete as the sublingual route). Larger amounts of drug may be administered this way than by the buccal or sublingual route. Some drugs administered rectally may cause significant irritation.

   e. **Intramuscular:**   Absorption from an intramuscular injection is often (but not always) faster and more complete than with oral administration. Large volumes (eg, more than 5 mL in each buttock) may be given.

   f. **Subcutaneous:**   The subcutaneous route offers slower absorption than the intramuscular route. Large volumes are not feasible.

   g. **Inhalation:**   In the case of respiratory diseases, the inhalation route offers delivery closest to the target tissue. This route often provides rapid absorption because of the large alveolar surface area available.

   h. **Topical:**   The topical route includes application to the skin or mucous membrane of the eye, nose, throat, airway, or vagina for *local* effect. The rate of absorption varies with the area of application and the drug formulation, but is usually slower than any of the routes listed above.

   i. **Transdermal:**   The transdermal route involves application to the skin for *systemic* effect. Absorption usually occurs very slowly, but the first-pass effect is avoided.

   j. **Intravenous:**   The intravenous route offers instantaneous and complete absorption (by definition, bioavailability is 100%). This route is potentially more dangerous, however, because of the high blood levels that may be produced.

D. Distribution of Drugs:

   1. **Determinants of distribution:**   The distribution of drugs to the various tissues depends upon the following:

      a. **Size of the organ:**   The size of the organ determines the concentration gradient between blood and the organ. For example, skeletal muscle can take up a large amount of drug because the concentration in the muscle tissue remains low (and the blood–tissue gradient high) even after relatively large amounts of drug have been transferred; this occurs because skeletal muscle is a very large organ. In contrast, because the brain is smaller, distribution of a smaller amount of drug into it will raise the tissue concentration and eliminate the blood–tissue concentration gradient, preventing further uptake of drug.

      b. **Blood flow:**   Blood flow to the tissue is important in the *rate* of uptake, although blood flow may not affect the steady-state amount of drug in the tissue. As a result, well-perfused tissues (eg, brain, heart, kidneys, splanchnic organs) will often achieve high tissue concentrations sooner than poorly perfused tissues (eg, adipose, bone). If the drug is rapidly eliminated, the concentration in poorly perfused tissues may never rise significantly.

      c. **Solubility:**   The solubility of a drug in tissue influences the concentration of the drug in the extracellular fluid surrounding the blood vessels. If the drug is very soluble in the cells, the concentration in the perivascular extracellular space will be lower and diffusion from the vessel into the extravascular tissue space will be facilitated. For example, some organs (including the brain) have a high lipid content and thus dissolve a high concentration of lipid-soluble agents. As a result, a very lipid soluble anesthetic will transfer out of the blood and into the brain tissue more rapidly and to a greater extent than a drug with low lipid solubility.

      d. **Binding:**   Binding of a drug to macromolecules in the blood or a tissue compartment will tend to increase the drug's concentration in that compartment. For example, warfarin is strongly bound to plasma albumin, which restricts warfarin's diffusion out of

Table 1–2. Average values for some physical volumes within the adult human body.

Compartment	Volume (L/kg body weight)
Plasma	0.04
Blood	0.08
Extracellular water	0.2
Total body water	0.6
Fat	0.2–0.35

the vascular compartment. Conversely, chloroquine is strongly bound to tissue proteins, which results in a marked reduction in the plasma concentration of chloroquine.

    2. Apparent volume of distribution: The apparent volume of distribution (Vd) is an important pharmacokinetic parameter that reflects the above determinants of drug distribution in the body. Vd relates the amount of drug in the body to the concentration in the plasma. See Chapter 3.

E. Metabolism of Drugs: Metabolism of a drug sometimes terminates its action, but other effects of metabolism are also important. Some drugs, when given orally, are metabolized before they enter the systemic circulation. This is called **first-pass** metabolism. Other drugs are administered as inactive **pro-drugs** and must be metabolized to active agents. Some drugs are not metabolized at all; their action must be terminated by excretion.

    1. Drug metabolism as a mechanism of termination of drug action: The action of many drugs (eg, local anesthetics, phenothiazines) is terminated before they are excreted because they are metabolized to biologically inactive derivatives.

    2. Drug metabolism as a mechanism of drug activation: Some **pro-drugs** (eg, levodopa, methyldopa, parathion) are inactive as administered and must be metabolized in the body to become active. Many drugs are active as administered and have active metabolites as well, eg, many benzodiazepines.

    3. Drug elimination without metabolism: Some drugs (eg, lithium, penicillin G) are not modified by the body; they continue to act until they are excreted.

F. Elimination of Drugs: Along with the dosage, the rate of elimination (disappearance of the active molecule from the bloodstream or body) determines the duration of action for most drugs. Therefore, knowledge of the time course of concentration in plasma is important in predicting the intensity and duration of effect for most drugs. *Note:* Drug *elimination* is not the same as drug *excretion:* a drug may be eliminated by metabolism long before the modified molecules are excreted from the body. Conversely, for drugs with active metabolites (eg, diazepam), elimination of the parent molecule by metabolism is not synonymous with termination of action. For drugs that are not metabolized, excretion is the mode of elimination. A small number of drugs combine irreversibly with their receptors, so that disappearance from the bloodstream is not equivalent to cessation of drug action: these drugs may have a very prolonged action. For example, phenoxybenzamine, an irreversible inhibitor of alpha adrenoceptors, is eliminated from the bloodstream in an hour or less after administration. The drug's action, however, lasts for 48 hours.

    1. First-order elimination: First order implies that the rate of elimination is proportionate to the concentration, ie, the higher the concentration, the greater the amount of drug eliminated per unit time. The result is that the drug's concentration in plasma decreases exponentially with time (Figure 1–2, left). Drugs with first-order elimination have a characteristic **half-life of elimination** that is constant, regardless of the amount of drug in the body. The concentration of such a drug in the blood will decrease by 50% for every half-life. Most drugs in clinical use demonstrate first-order kinetics.

    2. Zero-order elimination: Zero order implies elimination at a constant rate regardless of concentration (Figure 1–2, right panel). A few drugs saturate their elimination mechanisms even at low concentrations. As a result, the drug's concentration in plasma decreases in a linear fashion over time. This is typical of ethanol (over most of its plasma concentration range), and of phenytoin and aspirin at high therapeutic or toxic concentrations.

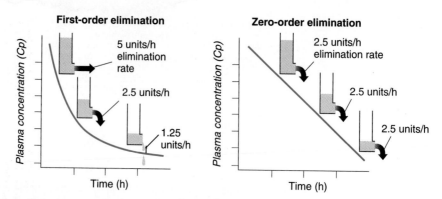

Figure 1–2. Comparison of first-order and zero-order elimination. In drugs with first-order kinetics (left panel) rate of elimination is proportionate to concentration; in the case of zero-order elimination (right panel), the rate is constant and independent of concentration.

G. **Pharmacokinetic Models:**
1. **Multicompartment distribution:**   After absorption, many drugs undergo an early distribution phase, followed by a slower elimination phase. Mathematically, this behavior can be modeled by means of a "two compartment model" as shown in Figure 1–3. (Note that each phase is associated with a characteristic half-life: $t_{1/2\alpha}$ for the first phase, $t_{1/2\beta}$ for the second.)
2. **Single compartment distribution:**   A few drugs may behave as if they are distributed to only one compartment (eg, if they are restricted to the vascular compartment). Others have more complex distributions that require more than two compartments for accurate modeling.

QUESTIONS

DIRECTIONS: Each of the numbered items or incomplete statements in this section is followed by answers or by completions of the sentence. Select the ONE lettered answer or completion that is BEST in each case.

1. All of the following are mechanisms of drug permeation EXCEPT
    (A)   Aqueous diffusion
    (B)   Aqueous hydrolysis
    (C)   Lipid diffusion
    (D)   Pinocytosis or endocytosis
    (E)   Special carrier transport
2. Johnny is an active three-year-old who has just ingested a large overdose of promethazine, an antihistaminic drug. Promethazine is a weak base with a pK_a of 9.1. In the treatment of this overdose of the promethazine,
    (A)   Urinary excretion would be accelerated by administration of NH_4Cl
    (B)   Urinary excretion would be accelerated by giving $NaHCO_3$
    (C)   More of the drug would be ionized at blood pH than at stomach pH
    (D)   Absorption of the drug would be faster from the stomach than from the small intestine
    (E)   Hemodialysis is the only effective therapy for overdose
3. All of the following statements about routes of drug administration are correct EXCEPT
    (A)   Blood levels often rise faster after intramuscular injection than after oral dosing
    (B)   The "first-pass" effect is the result of metabolism of a drug after administration and before it enters the systemic circulation
    (C)   Administration of antiasthmatic drugs by inhaled aerosol is usually associated with more adverse effects than is administration of these drugs by mouth

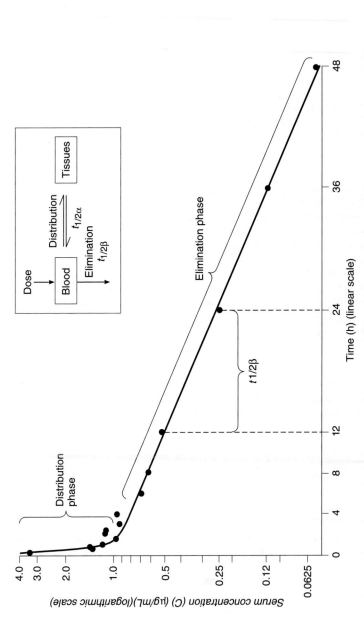

Figure 1–3. Serum concentration-time curve after administration of chlordiazepoxide as an intravenous bolus to a 75 kg patient. The experimental data are plotted on a semilogarithmic scale as filled circles. If the drug follows two-compartment kinetics, the initial curvilinear portion of the data represents the distribution phase, with drug moving into the tissues. The linear portion of the curve represents drug elimination. The elimination half-life ($t_{1/2\beta}$) can be extracted graphically as shown, by measuring the time between any two plasma concentration points that differ by two-fold. See Chapter 3 for additional details. (Modified and reproduced, with permission, from Greenblatt DJ, Koch-Weser J: Drug therapy: Clinical pharmacokinetics. N Engl J Med 1975;293:702.)

(D) Bioavailability of most drugs is less with rectal (suppository) administration than with intravenous administration

(E) Administration of a drug by transdermal patch is often slower, but is associated with less first-pass metabolism than oral administration

4. Aspirin is a weak organic acid with a pK_a of 3.5. What percentage of a given dose will be in the lipid-soluble form at a stomach pH of 2.5?
   (A) About 1%
   (B) About 10%
   (C) About 50%
   (D) About 90%
   (E) About 99%

5. If the plasma concentration of a drug declines with "first-order kinetics," this means that
   (A) There is only one metabolic path for drug disposition
   (B) The half-life is the same regardless of plasma concentration
   (C) The drug is largely metabolized in the liver after oral administration and has low bioavailability
   (D) The rate of elimination is proportionate to the rate of administration at all times
   (E) The drug is not distributed outside the vascular system

6. Regarding termination of action,
   (A) Drugs must be excreted from the body to terminate their action
   (B) Metabolism of drugs always increases their water solubility
   (C) Metabolism of drugs always abolishes their pharmacologic activity
   (D) Hepatic metabolism and renal excretion are the two most important mechanisms involved
   (E) Distribution of a drug out of the bloodstream terminates the drug's effects

7. Distribution of drugs to specific tissues
   (A) Is independent of blood flow to the organ
   (B) Is independent of the solubility of the drug in that tissue
   (C) Depends on the unbound drug concentration gradient between blood and the tissue
   (D) Is increased for drugs that are strongly bound to plasma proteins
   (E) Has no effect on the half-life of the drug

8. Pilocarpine is a weak base of pK_a 6.9. Which of the following statements is FALSE?
   (A) After parenteral administration, the concentration of pilocarpine in the aqueous humor (pH 7.8) will be lower than the concentration in the duodenum (pH 5.5)
   (B) When administered as eye drops, absorption into the eye will be faster if the drops are alkaline (pH 8.0) than if they are acidic (pH 5.0)
   (C) Excretion in the urine will be faster if urine pH is alkaline (pH 8.0) than if the urine pH is acidic (pH 5.8)
   (D) The proportion of pilocarpine in the protonated form will be approximately 90% at pH 5.9
   (E) The proportion of pilocarpine in the more lipid soluble form will be approximately 99% at pH 8.9

DIRECTIONS: These items consist of lettered headings followed by a numbered phrase or question. Select the ONE lettered heading that is most closely associated with the phrase or question.

Items 9–10:
   (A) Weak acid with pK_a of 5.5
   (B) Weak base with pK_a of 3.5
   (C) Weak acid with pK_a of 7.5
   (D) Weak base with pK_a of 6.5

9. Excretion will be most significantly accelerated by acidification of the urine

10. The drug that fits the graph at the right:

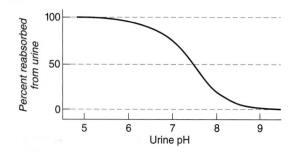

Items 11–14:
- **(A)** Distribution
- **(B)** Elimination
- **(C)** Endocytosis
- **(D)** First-pass effect
- **(E)** First-order kinetics
- **(F)** Lipid solubility
- **(G)** Permeation
- **(H)** Pharmacodynamics
- **(I)** Pharmacokinetics
- **(J)** Protonation
- **(K)** Volume of distribution
- **(L)** Zero-order kinetics

11. Properties that characterize the effects of a drug on the body
12. Properties that describe the effects of the body on a drug
13. Process by which the amount of active drug in the body is reduced after absorption into the systemic circulation
14. Process by which drug in the body is reduced after administration but before entering the systemic circulation

ANSWERS

1. Hydrolysis has nothing to do with the mechanisms of permeation; rather, hydrolysis is one mechanism of drug metabolism. The answer is **(B)**.

2. Questions that deal with acid-base (Henderson–Hasselbalch) manipulations are common. Since absorption involves permeation across lipid membranes, we can treat an overdose by decreasing absorption from the gut and reabsorption from the tubular urine by making the drug *less lipid-soluble*. Ionization attracts water molecules and decreases lipid solubility. Promethazine is a weak base—which means that it will be more ionized (protonated) at acid pH than at a basic pH. Choice **(C)** suggests that the drug would be more ionized at pH 7.4 than at pH 2: clearly wrong. **(D)** says (in effect) that the more ionized form will be absorbed faster and that is wrong. **(A)** and **(B)** are opposites, since NH_4Cl is an acidifying salt and sodium bicarbonate an alkalinizing one. From the point of view of test strategy, opposites always deserve careful attention and, in this case, permit us to exclude **(E)**, a distracter. Since an acid environment favors ionization of a weak base, we should give NH_4Cl. The answer is **(A)**.

3. **(A)**, **(B)**, **(D)**, and **(E)** are correct. **(C)** is wrong: delivering the drug directly to the target organ usually reduces adverse effects, because the total dose is lower and the concentration reaching other organs is lower. The answer is **(C)**.

4. Aspirin is an acid, so it will be more ionized at more basic pH and less ionized at acidic pH. The Henderson–Hasselbalch equation predicts that the ratio will change from 50/50 at the pH equal to the pK_a to 10/1 (protonated/unprotonated) at 1 pH unit more acidic than the pK_a. For acids, the protonated form is the nonionized, more lipid-soluble form. The answer is **(D)**.

5. See **Definitions** on the first page of this unit. First-order means that the elimination is proportionate to the concentration perfusing the organ of elimination. The result is that a plot of the logarithm of the plasma concentration on the vertical axis versus time on the horizontal axis is a straight line. The half-life is a constant. The rate of elimination is proportionate to the rate of administration only at steady state. (Zero-order elimination means that a constant number of moles or grams are eliminated per unit of time, regardless of plasma concentration. The half-life will then be concentration-dependent and is not a useful variable. Ethanol is the most common drug with zero-order elimination.) The answer is **(B)**.

6. Note the "trigger" words (must, always) in choices **(A)**, **(B)**, and **(C)**. All drugs that affect tissues other than circulating blood act outside of the "bloodstream." The answer is **(D)**.

7. Fairly straightforward. There are no trigger words to give the answer away, but it can be deduced without much trouble. Given the list of determinants of drug distribution, choice **(C)** is correct.

8. More Henderson–Hasselbalch concepts. Weak bases are more protonated in an acidic environment because more protons (hydrogen ions) are available. In the protonated state, weak bases

are ionized, polar, and less lipid soluble. Therefore, less pilocarpine will be lipid soluble and able to diffuse out of the duodenum (pH 5.5) than into the eye (pH 7.8). By the same reasoning, the drug will diffuse faster if the eyedrops are alkaline than if they are acidic. Less drug will diffuse back into the body from the urine if the urine pH is acidic than if it is alkaline so excretion will be faster in acidic urine. The answer is (**C**).

9. Since acceleration of excretion requires an increase in the ionized fraction in the urine, the basic drugs, which become more ionized in an acid environment, are the ones to be considered here. How much would their excretion be affected by the degree of urinary acidification that is achievable (ie, within the physiologic range of pH 5.5 to 8)? Clearly, a basic drug with a pK_a much lower than this range will not be significantly ionized: The drug of pK_a 3.5 will go from 1 part in 316,000 ionized at pH 8 to 1 part in 100 ionized at pH 5.5—ie, less than 1% change in the total nonionized fraction. In contrast, the basic drug of pK_a 6.5 is about 3% ionized, 97% nonionized at pH 8 but changes to 10% nonionized, 90% ionized at pH 5.5. The answer is (**D**).

10. The graph illustrates decreased reabsorption as the urine pH increases, suggesting that the fraction ionized (and therefore less lipid soluble) is greater at higher pH. This is characteristic of weak acids. The pH at which 50% of the drug is reabsorbed (about 7.5) is probably close to the pH at which 50% of the drug is ionized, ie, the pK_a. The answer is **C**.

11. More definitions. Pharmacodynamics is the term given to the properties of drug action on the body. The answer is (**H**).

12. Pharmacokinetics is the general term that describes all the actions of the body on the drug. The answer is (**I**).

13. The amount of active drug is reduced by excretion and metabolism, processes that are included in the term elimination. The answer is (**B**).

14. The first-pass effect is the term given to elimination of a drug before it enters the systemic circulation, ie, on its first pass through the liver. The answer is (**D**).

2

Pharmacodynamics

OBJECTIVES

You should be able to:

- Specify whether an antagonist is competitive or irreversible based on its effect on the dose-response curve of the agonist.
- Compare the efficacy and potency of drugs on the basis of their dose-response curves.
- Predict the effect of a partial agonist on a system in the presence and in the absence of a full agonist.
- Name two proteins in blood that have important inert drug binding sites.
- Predict the effect of adding drug B when a barely subtoxic dose of drug A is present, if drug A and drug B both bind to the same inert binding sites.
- Give examples of partial agonists, competitive and irreversible pharmacologic antagonists, and physiologic and chemical antagonists.
- Name the coupling and effector proteins activated by the beta-adrenoceptor.
- Name four methods by which drug-receptor signals bring about their biologic effects.

Learn the definitions that follow.

Table 2–1. Pharmacodynamic definitions.

Term	Definition
Receptor	Component of the biologic system with which a drug interacts to bring about a change in function of the system
Inert binding site	Component of the biologic system with which a drug interacts without changing any function
Receptor site	Specific region of the receptor molecule at which the drug binds
Agonist	A drug that activates its receptor upon binding
Effector	Component of the biologic system that accomplishes the biologic effect after being activated by the receptor; often a channel or enzyme
Pharmacologic antagonist	A drug that binds to its receptor without activating it
Competitive antagonist	A pharmacologic antagonist that can be overcome by increasing the dose of agonist
Irreversible antagonist	A pharmacologic antagonist that cannot be overcome by increasing the dose of agonist
Physiologic antagonist	A drug that counters the effect of another by binding to a different receptor and causing opposing effects
Chemical antagonist	A drug that counters the effects of another by binding the drug and preventing its action
Partial agonist	A drug that binds to its receptor but only partially activates it
Graded dose-response curve	A graph of the incrementing responses to incrementing doses of a drug
Quantal dose-response curve	A graph of the fraction of a population that shows a specified response to incrementing doses of a drug
EC50	In graded dose-response curves, the concentration or dose that produces 50% of the maximum possible response; in quantal dose-response curves, the dose that causes the specified response in 50% of the population
K_d	The concentration of drug that results in binding to 50% of the receptors
Efficacy	The maximum effect a drug can bring about at any dose
Potency	The dose or concentration required to bring about some fraction of a drug's maximum effect
Spare receptor	Receptors that do not have to bind drug in order for the maximum effect to be produced; ie, K_d greater than the EC50

PHARMACODYNAMIC CONCEPTS

A. Receptors: Receptors are the specific molecular components of a biologic system with which drugs interact to produce changes in the function of the system. Receptors must be selective in their ligand-binding characteristics (so as to respond to the proper chemical signal and not to meaningless ones). Receptors also must be modified as a result of binding an agonist molecule (to bring about the functional change). Many receptors have been identified, purified, chemically characterized, and cloned. The majority of the receptors characterized to date are proteins; a few are other macromolecules such as DNA. The *receptor site* or *recognition site* for a drug is the specific region of the macromolecule that has a high and selective affinity for the drug molecule. The interaction of a drug with its receptor is the fundamental event that initiates the action of the drug.

B. Effectors: Effectors are molecules that translate the drug-receptor interaction into a change in cellular activity. The best examples of effectors are enzymes such as adenylyl cyclase. Some receptors are also effectors, ie, a single molecule may incorporate both the drug binding site and the effector mechanism, eg, the tyrosine kinase effector of the insulin receptor.

C. Graded Dose-Response Relationships: When the response of a particular receptor-effector system (which can be an in vitro system, an animal, or a patient) is measured against increasing concentrations of a drug, the graph of the response versus the drug concentration or dose is called a graded dose-response curve (Figure 2–1A). Plotting the same data on semiloga-

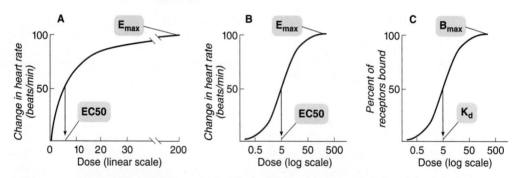

Figure 2–1. Graded dose-response and dose-binding graphs. **A.** Relation between drug dose or concentration and drug effect. When the dose axis is linear, a hyperbolic curve is commonly obtained. **B.** Same data, logarithmic dose axis. The dose or concentration at which effect is half-maximal is denoted EC50. **C.** If the percentage of receptors that bind drug is plotted against drug concentration, a similar curve is obtained, and the concentration at which 50% of the receptors are bound is denoted K_d.

rithmic axes often results in a sigmoid curve, simplifying the mathematical manipulation of these dose-response curves (Figure 2–1B). A similar plot can be made of the fraction of receptors that bind a drug, versus the drug's concentration (Figure 2–1C). The maximal efficacy, EC50, and K_d parameters are derived from these data (see below).

D. Quantal Dose-Response Relationships: When the minimum dose required to produce a specified response is determined in each member of a population, the quantal dose-response relationship is defined (Figure 2–2). When plotted as the fraction of the population that responds at each dose level versus the log of the dose administered, a cumulative quantal dose-response curve, usually sigmoid in shape, is obtained. The median effective (ED50), median toxic (TD50), and median lethal doses (LD50) are extracted from experiments carried out in this manner.

E. Spare Receptors: Spare receptors are said to exist if the maximum drug response is obtained at less than saturation (complete occupation) of the receptors. In practice, the determination is usually made by comparing the EC50 and the K_d. If the EC50 is less than the K_d, spare receptors are said to exist (Figure 2–3). This might result from one of several mechanisms.

Figure 2–2. Quantal dose-response plots from a study of the therapeutic and lethal effects of a new drug in mice. Shaded boxes (and the accompanying curves) indicate the frequency distribution of doses of drug required to produce a specified effect: ie, the percentage of animals that required a particular dose to exhibit the effect. The open boxes (and corresponding curves) indicate the cumulative frequency distribution of responses, which are lognormally distributed. (Reproduced, with permission, from Katzung BG (editor): *Basic & Clinical Pharmacology*, 6th ed. Appleton & Lange, 1995.)

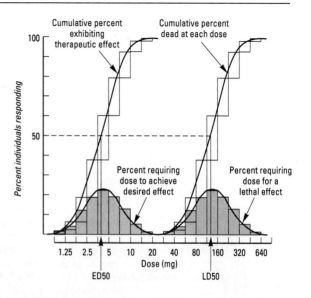

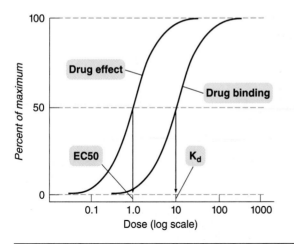

Figure 2–3. In a system with spare receptors, the EC50 is lower than the K_d, indicating that to achieve 50% of maximal effect, fewer than 50% of the receptors must be occupied. Explanations for this phenomenon are discussed in the text.

First, the *effect* of the drug-receptor interaction may persist much longer than the interaction itself (time mechanism). Second, the actual number of *receptors* may exceed the number of *effector* molecules available. The presence of spare receptors increases sensitivity to the agonist.

F. **Inert Binding Sites:** Inert binding sites are components of endogenous molecules that bind a drug without initiating events leading to any of the drug's effects. In some compartments of the body (eg, the plasma), inert binding sites play an important role in buffering the concentration of a drug because bound drug does not contribute directly to the concentration gradient that drives diffusion. The two most important plasma proteins with significant binding capacity are albumin and orosomucoid (α_1-acid glycoprotein).

G. **Agonists and Partial Agonists:** An agonist is a drug capable of fully activating the effector system when it binds to the receptor. A partial agonist produces less than the full effect, even when it has saturated the receptors (Figure 2–4). In the presence of a full agonist, a partial agonist acts like a competitive inhibitor.

H. **Competitive and Irreversible Pharmacologic Antagonists:** Competitive antagonists are drugs that bind to the receptor in a reversible way without activating the effector system for that receptor. In the presence of a competitive antagonist, the log dose-response curve is shifted to higher doses (ie, horizontally to the right on the dose axis) but the same maximum effect is

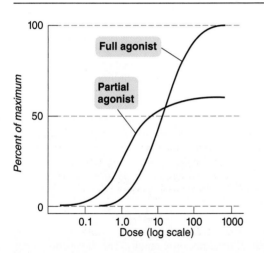

Figure 2–4. Comparison of dose-response curves for a full agonist and a partial agonist. A partial agonist acts on the same receptor system as the full agonist but cannot produce as large an effect, no matter how much the dose is increased. The partial agonist may be more potent (as in the figure), less potent, or equally potent; potency is an independent factor.

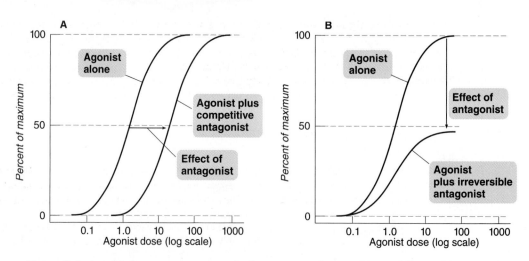

Figure 2–5. Agonist dose-response curves in the presence of competitive and irreversible antagonists. Note the use of a logarithmic scale for drug concentration. **A.** A competitive antagonist has an effect illustrated by the shift of the agonist curve to the right. **B.** A noncompetitive antagonist shifts the agonist curve downward.

reached (Figure 2–5A). In contrast, an irreversible antagonist causes a downward shift of the maximum, with no shift of the curve on the dose axis unless spare receptors are present (Figure 2–5B). The effects of competitive antagonists can be overcome by adding more agonist. Irreversible antagonists cannot be overcome by adding more agonist.

I. Physiologic Antagonists: A physiologic antagonist is a drug that binds to a different receptor, producing an effect opposite to that produced by the drug it is antagonizing. Thus it differs from a pharmacologic antagonist by interacting with a completely different receptor. A common example is the antagonism of the bronchoconstrictor action of histamine (mediated at histamine receptors) by epinephrine's bronchodilator action (mediated at beta adrenoceptors).

J. Chemical Antagonists: A chemical antagonist is a drug that interacts directly with the drug being antagonized to remove it or to prevent it from reaching its target. A chemical antagonist does not depend on interaction with the agonist's receptor (although such interaction may occur). An excellent example of a chemical antagonist is dimercaprol, a chelator of lead and some other toxic metals. Pralidoxime, which combines avidly with the phosphorus in organophosphate cholinesterase inhibitors, is another type of chemical antagonist.

K. Efficacy: Efficacy, often called maximal efficacy, is the maximum effect an agonist can produce if the dose is taken to its maximum. Efficacy is determined mainly by the nature of the receptor and its associated effector system. It can be measured with a graded dose-response curve (Figures 2–1, 2–4) but not with a quantal dose-response curve. By definition, partial agonists have lower maximal efficacy than full agonists.

L. Potency: Potency denotes the amount of a drug needed to produce a given effect. In graded dose-response measurements, the effect usually chosen is 50% of the maximum effect and the dose causing this effect is called the EC50. Potency is determined mainly by the affinity of the receptor for the drug. In quantal dose-response measurements, ED50, TD50, and LD50 are typical potency measurements (effective, toxic, and lethal doses, respectively, in 50% of a population). Thus, potency can be determined from either graded or quantal dose-response curves (eg, Figures 2–1, 2–2), but the numbers obtained are not identical.

M. Therapeutic Index, Therapeutic Window: The therapeutic index is the ratio of the TD50 (or LD50) to the ED50, determined from quantal dose-response curves. The therapeutic index represents an estimate of the safety of a drug, since a very safe drug might be expected to have a very large toxic dose and a small effective dose. For example, in Figure 2–2, the ED50 is approximately 3 mg and the LD50 is approximately 150 mg. The therapeutic index is therefore approximately 50 (150/3). Unfortunately, factors such as the varying slopes of dose-response curves make this estimate a poor safety index. The therapeutic window, a more clinically relevant index of safety, describes the dosage range between the minimum effective therapeutic concentration or dose, and the minimum toxic concentration or dose. For example, if the average minimum therapeutic plasma concentration of theophylline is 8 mg/L and toxic effects are observed at 18 mg/L, the therapeutic window is 8–18 mg/L.

N. Signaling Mechanisms: Once an agonist drug has bound to its receptor, some effector mechanism is activated. For many useful drugs, the effector mechanism resides inside the cell or modifies some intracellular process. Four major types of transmembrane signaling mechanisms for receptor-effector systems have been defined (Figure 2–6):

1. **Receptors that are intracellular:** Some drugs, especially more lipid-soluble or diffusible agents (eg, steroid hormones, nitric oxide) may cross the membrane and combine with an intracellular receptor that affects an intracellular effector molecule.

2. **Receptors located on membrane-spanning enzymes:** Drugs that affect membrane-spanning enzymes combine with a receptor on the extracellular portion of enzymes and modify their intracellular activity. For example, insulin acts on a tyrosine kinase that is located in the membrane. The insulin receptor site faces the extracellular environment and the enzyme catalytic site is on the cytoplasmic side.

3. **Receptors located on membrane ion channels:** Receptors that regulate membrane ion channels may directly cause the opening of an ion channel (eg, acetylcholine at the nicotinic receptor) or modify the ion channel's response to other agents (eg, benzodiazepines at the GABA channel).

4. **Receptors linked to effectors via G proteins:** A very large number of drugs bind to receptors that are linked by coupling proteins to intracellular or membrane effectors. The best defined examples of this group are the sympathomimetic drugs, which activate or inhibit adenylyl cyclase (formerly called adenylate cyclase) by a multistep process: activation of the receptor by the drug results in activation of G proteins that either stimulate or inhibit the cyclase. Many types of G proteins have been identified; some of the most important are listed in Table 2–2.

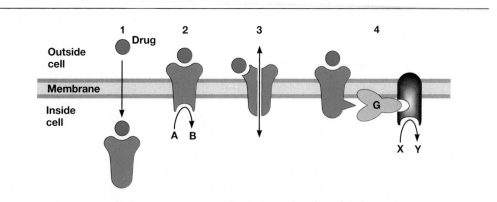

Figure 2–6. Signaling mechanisms for drug effects. Four major signaling mechanisms are recognized: 1) transmembrane diffusion of the drug to bind to an intracellular receptor; 2) transmembrane enzyme receptors, whose outer domain provides the receptor function and inner domain provides the effector mechanism; 3) transmembrane channels that are gated open or closed by the binding of a drug to the receptor site; and 4) G protein-coupled receptors, which utilize a coupling protein to activate a separate effector molecule. (Reproduced, with permission, from Katzung BG (editor): *Basic & Clinical Pharmacology*, 6th ed. Appleton & Lange, 1995.)

Table 2–2. Examples of receptors that are coupled to their effectors by G proteins.

Receptor Types	Coupling Protein	Effector	Effector Substrate	Second Messenger Response	Result
M_1, M_3, α_1	G_q	Phospholipase C	Membrane lipids	↑IP_3 ↑DAG	↑Ca^{2+} ↑Protein kinase activity
β, D_1	G_s	Adenylyl cyclase	ATP	↑cAMP	↑Ca^{2+} influx ↑Enzyme activity
α_2, M_2	G_i	Adenylyl cyclase	ATP	↓cAMP	↓ Ca^{2+} influx and enzyme activity

QUESTIONS

DIRECTIONS: Each of the numbered items or incomplete statements in this section is followed by answers or by completions of the sentence. Select the ONE lettered answer or completion that is BEST in each case.

1. Quantal dose-response curves are
   (A) Used for determining the therapeutic index of a drug
   (B) Used for determining the maximal efficacy of a drug
   (C) Invalid in the presence of inhibitors of the drug being studied
   (D) Obtainable from the study of intact subjects but not from isolated tissue
   (E) Used to determine the statistical variation (standard deviation) of the maximal response to the drug

2. Two drugs, A and B, have the same mechanism of action. Drug A in a dose of 5 mg produces the same magnitude of effect as drug B in a dose of 500 mg.
   (A) Drug B is less efficacious than drug A
   (B) Drug A is about 100 times more potent than drug B
   (C) Toxicity of drug A is less than that of drug B
   (D) Drug A is a better drug if maximal efficacy is needed
   (E) Drug A will have a shorter duration of action than drug B because less of drug A is present

3. The results shown in the graph were obtained in a comparison of positive inotropic agents.
   (A) Drug A is most effective
   (B) Drug B is least potent
   (C) Drug C is most potent
   (D) Drug B is more potent than drug C and more effective than drug A
   (E) Drug A is more potent than drug B and more effective than drug C

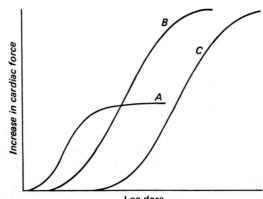

4. In the absence of other drugs, pindolol causes an increase in heart rate by activating beta adrenoceptors. In the presence of highly effective beta stimulants, however, pindolol causes a dose-dependent, reversible decrease in heart rate. Therefore, pindolol is probably
   (A) An irreversible antagonist
   (B) A physiologic antagonist
   (C) A chemical antagonist
   (D) A partial agonist
   (E) A spare receptor agonist

5. All of the following statements about spare receptors are correct EXCEPT
   (A) Spare receptors, in the absence of drug, are identical to nonspare receptors
   (B) Spare receptors do not bind drug when the maximal drug effect first occurs
   (C) Spare receptors influence the sensitivity of the receptor system to the drug
   (D) Spare receptors activate the effector machinery of the cell without the need for a drug
   (E) Spare receptors may be detected by the finding that the EC50 is less than the K_d for the agonist

6. Two drugs, "A" and "B," were studied in a large group of patients; the percentages of the population showing therapeutic and toxic effects were graphed. Based on the graph, it may be concluded that:
   (A) Drug A is safer than drug B
   (B) Drug B is less effective than drug A
   (C) The two drugs act on the same receptors
   (D) The therapeutic index of drug A is 10.
   (E) The therapeutic index of drug B is 10.

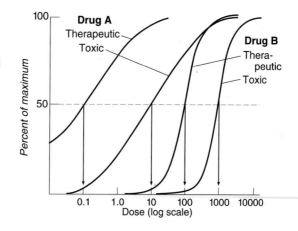

DIRECTIONS: The following section consists of a list of four to twenty-six lettered options followed by several numbered items. For each numbered item, select the ONE option that is most closely associated with it. Each answer may be selected once, more than once, or not at all.

Items 7–9:
   (A) Pharmacologic antagonist
   (B) Partial agonist
   (C) Physiologic antagonist
   (D) Chemical antagonist
   (E) Noncompetitive antagonist

7. This term describes the antagonism of leukotriene's bronchoconstrictor effect (mediated at leukotriene receptors) by terbutaline (acting at adrenoceptors) in a patient with asthma

8. An antagonist that interacts directly with the agonist and not at all, or only incidentally, with the receptor

9. A drug that blocks the action of epinephrine at its receptors by occupying those receptors without activating them

Items 10–12:
    (A) Maximum efficacy
    (B) Therapeutic index
    (C) Drug potency
    (D) Graded dose-response curve
    (E) Quantal dose-response curve
10. Provides information about the standard deviation of sensitivity to the drug in the population studied
11. Provides information about the potency and the maximum efficacy of a drug
12. The largest response a drug can produce, regardless of dose

Items 13–15:
    Each of the curves in the graph may be considered a concentration-effect curve or a concentration-binding curve.
    (A) Curve 1
    (B) Curve 2
    (C) Curve 3
    (D) Curve 4
    (E) Curve 5

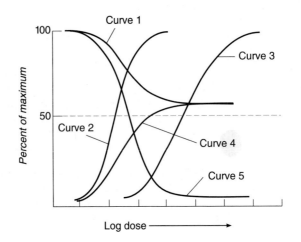

13. Describes the percentage *binding* of a full agonist to its receptors as the concentration of a partial agonist is increased from low to very high levels
14. Describes the percentage *effect* when a full agonist is present throughout the experiment, and the concentration of a partial agonist is increased from low to very high levels
15. Describes the percentage *binding* of the partial agonist whose *effect* is shown by curve 4, if the system has many spare receptors

ANSWERS

1. Graded dose-response curves must be used to determine maximum efficacy (maximal response). Quantal dose-response curves show only the frequency of occurrence of a specified response, which may be therapeutic (ED) or toxic (TD). Dividing the TD50 by the ED50 gives the therapeutic index. The answer is **(A)**.
2. No information is given regarding the magnitude of the maximum response to either drug. Similarly, no information about toxicity is available, since the "response" mentioned is not defined as therapeutic or toxic. The answer is **(B)**.
3. These are straightforward graded dose-response curves. Drug A is the most potent, drug C the least. Drug A is less efficacious than drugs B and C. The answer is **(D)**.
4. **(B)** and **(C)** are clearly incorrect, since pindolol is said to act at beta receptors and to block beta stimulants. The drug effect is reversible, so **(A)** is incorrect. "Spare receptor agonist" is a nonsense distracter. The answer is **(D)**.

5.   There is no difference between "spare" and other receptors. Spare receptors may be defined as those receptors that are not needed for binding drug to achieve the maximal effect. Spare receptors influence the sensitivity of the system to an agonist, since the statistical probability of a drug-receptor interaction increases with the total number of receptors. If they do not have a bound agonist, spare receptors do not activate an effector molecule. EC50 less than K_d is one definition of the presence of spare receptors. The answer is **(D)**.

6.   Note that the therapeutic index of drug A is approximately 100 while that of drug B is approximately 10. Because drug A has a flatter slope, however, patients who require a higher dose of A have a very high risk of toxicity; because drug B has a steeper slope, even patients who require the highest dose of B have a low probability of toxicity. These dose-response curves illustrate the danger in assuming that a drug with a larger therapeutic index must be safer than a drug with a smaller one. The answer is **(E)**.

7.   Because terbutaline interacts with adrenoceptors and leukotriene with leukotriene receptors, terbutaline cannot be a pharmacologic antagonist of leukotriene. Because the results of adrenoceptor activation oppose the effects of leukotriene receptor activation, terbutaline must be a physiologic antagonist. The answer is **(C)**.

8.   A chemical antagonist interacts directly (chemically) with the agonist drug and not with a receptor. The answer is **(D)**.

9.   A pharmacologic antagonist occupies the receptors without activating them. The answer is **(A)**.

10. Quantal dose-response curves provide information about the statistical distribution of sensitivity to a drug. The answer is **(E)**.

11. Only a graded dose-response curve provides information about the maximal efficacy as well as the potency. See question 1. The answer is **(D)**.

12. Maximum efficacy represents the largest response a drug can produce. The answer is **(A)**.

13. The binding of a full agonist will *decrease* as the concentration of a partial agonist is increased to very high levels. As the partial agonist displaces more and more of the full agonist, the percentage of receptors that bind the full agonist will drop to zero, ie, curve 5. The answer is **(E)**.

14. Curve 1 describes the *effect* of combining a large fixed concentration of full agonist and increasing concentrations of partial agonist, since the increasing percentage of receptors binding the partial agonist will finally produce the maximum effect typical of the partial agonist. The answer is **(A)**.

15. Partial agonists, like full agonists, bind 100% of their receptors when present in a high enough concentration. Therefore, the curve will go to 100%. If the effect curve is curve 4 and many spare receptors are present, the binding curve must be displaced to the right of curve 4 (K_d > EC50). Therefore, curve 3 fits the description better than curve 2. The answer is **(C)**.

Pharmacokinetics

3

OBJECTIVES

You should be able to:

- Compute the half-life of a drug based on its clearance and volume of distribution.
- Calculate loading and maintenance dosage regimens for oral or intravenous administration of a drug when given the following information: minimum therapeutic concentration; bioavailability; clearance; and volume of distribution.
- Calculate the dosage adjustment required for a patient with impaired renal function.

Learn the definitions that follow.

Table 3–1. Pharmacokinetic definitions

Term	Definition
Volume of distribution (apparent)	The ratio of the amount of a drug in the body to its concentration in the plasma or blood
Clearance	The ratio of the rate of elimination of a drug to its concentration in plasma or blood
Half-life	The time it takes for the amount or concentration of a drug to fall to 50% of an earlier measurement; this number is a constant, regardless of concentration, for drugs eliminated by first-order kinetics (the great majority of drugs). See Chapter 1. Half-life is not a constant and therefore not particularly useful for drugs eliminated by zero-order kinetics (eg, ethanol)
Bioavailability	The fraction (or percentage) of the administered dose of a drug that reaches the systemic circulation
Area under the curve (AUC)	The graphic area under a plot of drug concentration in plasma versus time, after a single dose of a drug or during a single dosing interval; the AUC is important for calculating the bioavailability of a drug given by any route other than intravenous
Peak & trough concentrations	The maximum and minimum drug concentrations—in plasma or blood—measured during cycles of repeated dosing
Minimum effective concentration (MEC)	The plasma concentration below which a patient's response is too small for therapeutic benefit
First-pass effect	The elimination of drug that occurs after administration but before it reaches the systemic circulation, eg, during passage through the gut wall, portal blood, and liver for an orally administered drug
Extraction	The fraction of drug in the plasma that is removed by an organ as it passes through that organ
Bioequivalence	The equivalence of blood concentrations of two preparations of the same drug measured over time; if the concentration-time plots for the two preparations are nearly superimposable (within certain statistical limits) the preparations are said to be bioequivalent; one preparation may be safely substituted for the other

CONCEPTS

A. Effective Drug Concentration: The effective drug concentration is the concentration of a drug at the receptor site (in contrast to drug concentrations that are more readily measured, eg, in blood). Except for topically active agents, this concentration is often proportionate to the drug's concentration in the plasma. This, in turn, is a function of the rate of input of the drug (by absorption) into the plasma, the rate of distribution to the peripheral tissues (including the target organ), and the rate of elimination, or loss, from the body. These are all functions of time; but if the rate of input is known, the remaining processes are accounted for by two primary properties of the drug: volume of distribution and clearance.

B. Volume of Distribution (Vd): The volume of distribution relates the amount of drug in the body to the plasma concentration (Figure 3–1) according to the following equation:

$$Vd = \frac{\text{Amount of drug in the body}}{\text{Plasma drug concentration}} \quad (1)$$

(Units = volume)

The calculated parameter for the apparent volume of distribution has no direct physical equivalent. If a drug is avidly bound in peripheral tissues, the drug's concentration in plasma may drop to very low values even though the total amount in the body is large. As a result, the volume of distribution may greatly exceed the total volume of the body. For example, 50 thousand liters is the Vd for the drug quinacrine in a person whose physical body volume is 70 liters. On the other hand, a drug that is completely retained in the plasma compartment will have a vol-

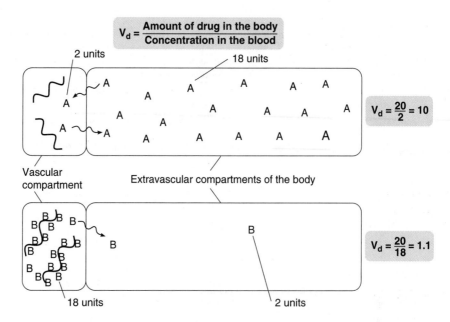

Figure 3–1. Effect of drug binding on volume of distribution. Drug A does not bind to macromolecules (heavy wavy lines) in the vascular or the extravascular compartments of the hypothetical organism in the diagram. Drug A diffuses freely between the two compartments. With 20 units of the drug in the body, the steady-state distribution leaves a blood concentration of 2. Drug B, on the other hand, binds avidly to proteins in the blood. Drug B's diffusion is much more limited. At equilibrium, only 2 units of the total have diffused into the extravascular volume, leaving 18 units still in the blood. In each case the total amount of drug in the body is the same (20 units), but the calculated volumes of distribution are very different.

ume of distribution equal to the plasma volume (about 4% of body weight). The volume of distribution of drugs that are normally bound to plasma proteins such as albumin can be altered by liver disease (through reduced protein synthesis) and kidney disease (through urinary protein loss).

C. Clearance (CL): Clearance relates the rate of elimination to the plasma concentration:

$$CL = \frac{\textbf{Rate of elimination of drug}}{\textbf{Plasma drug concentration}} \qquad (2)$$

(Units = volume per unit time)

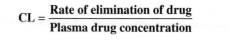

Clearance, CL = $\dfrac{\text{Rate of elimination}}{\text{Plasma concentration (Cp)}}$

Rate of elimination = CL x Cp

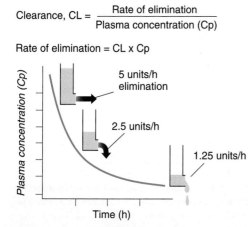

Figure 3–2. The clearance of most drugs is a constant over a broad range of plasma concentrations. Since elimination rate is equal to clearance times plasma concentration, the elimination rate will be rapid at first and slow as the concentration decreases.

For a drug eliminated with first-order kinetics, the clearance is a constant, ie, the ratio of rate of elimination to plasma concentration is the same regardless of plasma concentration (Figure 3–2). The magnitudes of clearance for different drugs range from a small fraction of the blood flow to a maximum of the total blood flow to the organ of elimination. Clearance depends upon the drug and the condition of the organs of elimination in the patient. The clearance of a particular drug by an individual organ is equivalent to the extraction capability of that organ for that drug, times the rate of delivery of drug to the organ. Thus the clearance of a drug that is very effectively extracted by an organ is often flow-limited—ie, the blood is completely cleared of the drug as it passes through the organ. In such a case, the total clearance from the body is a function of blood flow through the eliminating organ, and is limited by the blood flow to the organ. In this situation, other conditions—disease or other drugs that change blood flow—may have more dramatic effects on clearance than disease of the organ of elimination.

D. Half-life: Half-life is a derived parameter, completely determined by volume of distribution and clearance. Half-life can be determined graphically from a plot of the blood level versus time (Figure 1–3), or from the following relationship:

$$t_{1/2} = \frac{0.693 \times Vd}{CL} \tag{3}$$

(Units = time)

One must know both primary variables (Vd and CL) to predict changes in half-life. Disease, age, and other variables usually alter the clearance of a drug much more than its volume of distribution. The half-life of a drug may not change, however, despite a decreased clearance if the volume of distribution decreases at the same time. This occurs, for example, when lidocaine is administered to patients with congestive heart failure. The half-life determines the rate at which blood concentration rises during a constant infusion and falls after administration is stopped (Figure 3–3).

E. Bioavailability: The bioavailability of a drug is the fraction of the administered dose that reaches the systemic circulation. Bioavailability is defined as unity (or 100%) in the case of intravenous administration. After administration by other routes, bioavailability is generally reduced by incomplete absorption, first-pass metabolism, and any distribution into other tissues that occurs before the drug enters the systemic circulation. To account for differing rates of absorption into the blood, the concentration appearing in the plasma must be integrated over time to obtain an integrated total **area under the plasma concentration curve** (AUC, Figure 3–4).

F. Extraction: Removal of a drug by an organ can be specified as the extraction ratio, or the fraction of the drug removed from the perfusing blood during its passage through the organ (Figure 3–5). After steady-state concentration in plasma has been achieved, the extraction ratio

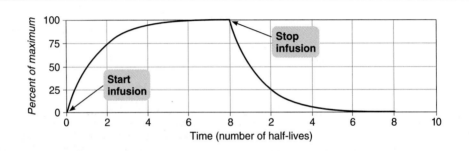

Figure 3–3. Plasma concentration of a drug (plotted as percent of maximum) given by constant IV infusion for 8 half-lives and then stopped. The concentration rises smoothly with time, and always reaches 50% of steady state after one half-life, 75% after two half-lives, 87.5% after three half-lives, and so on. The decline in concentration after stopping drug administration follows the same type of curve: 50% is left after one half-life, 25% after two half-lives, etc.

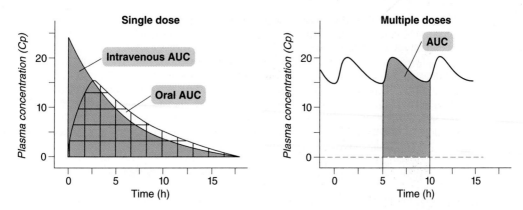

Figure 3–4. The area under the curve is used to calculate the bioavailability of a drug. The AUC can be obtained from either single dose studies (left panel) or multiple dose measurements (right panel). Bioavailability is calculated from $AUC_{(route)}/AUC_{(IV)}$.

is one measure of the elimination of the drug by that organ. Drugs that have a high hepatic extraction ratio have a large first-pass effect; the bioavailability of these drugs after oral administration will be low.

G. Dosage Regimens: A dosage regimen is a plan for drug administration over a period of time. An appropriate dosage regimen results in the achievement of therapeutic levels of the drug in the blood, without exceeding the minimum toxic concentration. To maintain the plasma concentration within a specified range over long periods of therapy, a schedule of **maintenance doses** is used. If it is necessary to achieve the target plasma level rapidly, a **loading dose** is used to "load" the volume of distribution with the drug. Ideally, the dosing plan is based on knowledge of both the minimum therapeutic and minimum toxic concentrations for a given drug, as well as its clearance and volume of distribution.

   1. **Maintenance dose:** Because the maintenance rate of drug administration is equal to the rate of elimination at steady state (this is the definition of steady state), the maintenance dosage is a function of clearance (from equation [2] above).

$$\textbf{Dosing rate} = \textbf{clearance} \times \textbf{desired plasma concentration} \qquad (4)$$

Note that volume of distribution is not directly involved in the above calculation. The dosing rate computed for maintenance dosage is the average dose per unit time. When carrying out such calculations, make certain that the units are in agreement throughout. For example, if clearance is given in mL per minute, the resulting dosing rate is a per-minute rate. For chronic therapy, oral administration is desirable; thus doses should be given only once or a few times per day. The size of the daily dose (dose per minute × 60 min per hour × 24 hours

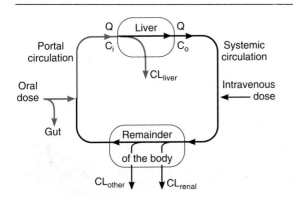

Figure 3–5. The principles of organ extraction and first-pass effect are illustrated. Part of the administered oral dose is lost to metabolism in the gut and the liver before it enters the systemic circulation: this is the first-pass effect. The extraction of drug from the circulation by the liver is equal to blood flow times the difference between entering and leaving drug concentration, ie, Q x (Ci – Co). (Reproduced, with permission, from Katzung BG [editor]: *Basic & Clinical Pharmacology,* 6th ed. Appleton & Lange, 1995.)

per day) is a simple extension of the above information. The number of doses to be given per day is usually determined by the half-life of the drug and the difference between the minimum therapeutic and toxic concentrations (see Therapeutic Window, below).

If it is important to maintain a concentration above the minimum therapeutic level at all times, either a larger dose may be given at long intervals or smaller doses at more frequent intervals. If the difference between the toxic and therapeutic concentrations is small, then smaller, more frequent doses must be administered to avoid toxicity.

2. **Loading dosage:** If the therapeutic concentration must be achieved rapidly and the volume of distribution is large, a large loading dose may be needed at the onset of therapy. This is calculated from the following equation:

$$\textbf{Loading dose = volume of distribution} \times \textbf{desired plasma concentration} \qquad \textbf{(5)}$$

Note that clearance does not enter into this computation. If the loading dose is very large (Vd much larger than blood volume), the dose should be given slowly to avoid excessively high peak plasma levels during the distribution phase.

H. Therapeutic Window: The therapeutic window is the useful "opening" between the minimum therapeutic concentration and the minimum toxic concentration of a drug. The concept is used to determine the range of plasma levels that is acceptable when designing a dosing regimen. Thus the minimum effective concentration will usually determine the desired *trough* levels of a drug given intermittently, while the minimum toxic concentration determines the permissible *peak* plasma concentration. A simple example: the drug theophylline has therapeutic and toxic concentrations which are 7 to 10 and 15 to 20 mg/L, respectively. The therapeutic window for a given patient might thus be fixed in the range from 8 to 17 mg/L (Figure 3–6). Unfortunately, for some drugs the therapeutic and toxic concentrations vary so greatly among patients that it is impossible to predict the therapeutic window in a given patient. Such drugs must be titrated individually in each patient.

I. Adjustment of Dosage When Elimination Is Altered by Disease: Renal disease or reduced cardiac output often reduce the clearance of drugs that depend on renal function. Alteration of clearance by liver disease is less common but may occur. The dosage in renal disease may be corrected by multiplying the dosage estimated for a normal person times the ratio of the patient's altered creatinine clearance to normal creatinine clearance (approximately 100 mL/min or 6 L/h).

$$\textbf{Corrected dose = Average dose} \times \frac{\textbf{Patient's creatinine clearance}}{\textbf{100 mL/min}} \qquad \textbf{(6)}$$

This simplified approach ignores nonrenal routes of clearance that may be significant. If a drug is partly cleared by the kidney and partly by nonrenal clearance, the above equation should be applied to that part of the dose that is eliminated by the kidney. For example, if a

Figure 3–6. The therapeutic window for theophylline in a thirteen year-old patient. The minimum effective concentration in this patient was found to be 8 mg/L; the minimum toxic concentration was found to be 16 mg/L. The therapeutic window is indicated by the gray area. In order to maintain the plasma concentration (Cp) within the window, the drug must be given at least once every half-life (7.5 hours in this patient), since the minimum effective concentration is half the minimum toxic concentration and Cp will decay by 50% in one half-life. (*Note:* This concept applies to drugs given in the ordinary, rapid-release form. Slow-release formulations can often be given at longer intervals.)

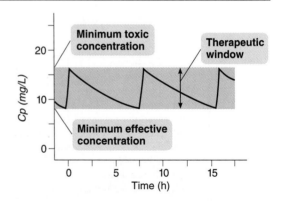

drug is 50% cleared by the kidney and 50% by the liver, and the normal dose is 200 mg/d, the corrected dose in a patient with a creatinine clearance of 20 mL/min will be:

$$\textbf{Dose} = \textbf{100 mg/d} + \textbf{100 mg/d} \times \frac{\textbf{20 mL/min}}{\textbf{100 mL/min}} \tag{7}$$

$$\textbf{Dose} = \textbf{100 mg/d} + \textbf{20 mg/d} = \textbf{120 mg/d}$$

QUESTIONS

DIRECTIONS: Each of the numbered items or incomplete statements in this section is followed by answers or by completions of the sentence. Select the ONE lettered answer or completion that is BEST in each case.

Items 1–2: Mr. Jones is admitted to General Hospital with pneumonia due to gram-negative bacteria. The antibiotic tobramycin is ordered. The CL and Vd of tobramycin in Mr. Jones are 80 mL/min and 40 L respectively.

1. What maintenance dose must be administered intravenously every 6 hours to eventually obtain average steady-state plasma concentrations of 4 mg/L?
   (A) 0.32 mg
   (B) 115 mg
   (C) 160 mg
   (D) 230 mg
   (E) None of the above

2. If you wish to give Mr. Jones a loading dose to achieve the therapeutic plasma concentration of 4 mg/L rapidly, how much should be given?
   (A) 0.1 mg
   (B) 10 mg
   (C) 115.2 mg
   (D) 160 mg
   (E) None of the above

3. Despite your careful adherence to basic pharmacokinetic principles, your patient on digoxin therapy has developed digitalis toxicity. The plasma digoxin level is 4 ng/mL. Renal function is normal, and the plasma $t_{1/2}$ for digoxin in this patient is 1.6 days. How long should you withhold digoxin in order to reach a safer yet probably therapeutic level of 1 ng/mL?
   (A) 1.6 days
   (B) 2.4 days
   (C) 3.2 days
   (D) 4.8 days
   (E) 6.4 days

4. Verapamil and phenytoin are both eliminated from the body by metabolism in the liver. Verapamil has a clearance of 1.5 L/min, approximately equal to liver blood flow, whereas phenytoin has a clearance of 0.1 L/min. When these compounds are administered along with rifampin, a drug that increases hepatic drug-metabolizing enzymes, which of the following is most likely?
   (A) The clearance of both verapamil and phenytoin will be increased
   (B) The clearance of both verapamil and phenytoin will be decreased
   (C) The clearance of verapamil will be unchanged, whereas the clearance of phenytoin will be increased
   (D) The clearance of phenytoin will be unchanged, whereas the clearance of verapamil will be increased

5. Drug X has a narrow therapeutic index: the minimum toxic plasma concentration is 1.5 times the minimum therapeutic plasma concentration. The half-life is 6 hours. It is essential to maintain the plasma concentration above the minimum therapeutic level. Of the following, the most appropriate dosing regimen would be
   (A) Once a day
   (B) Twice a day
   (C) Three times a day

     (D) Four times a day
     (E) Six times a day

6. With regard to design of a dosing regimen,
     (A) When a drug is given at an interval equal to its half-life, the average total amount of drug in the body at steady-state will be 0.693 times the dose
     (B) A drug with a very short half-life will be ineffective unless given at intervals less than the half-life
     (C) The steady-state concentration of a drug in the plasma will be equal to the dose multiplied by 0.693, times the volume of distribution divided by the clearance
     (D) If an immediate therapeutic plasma level is desired, the appropriate loading dose is target plasma concentration times volume of distribution
     (E) The drug should not be given more than 4 times per day

7. The bioavailability of drugs is
     (A) Established by FDA regulation at 100% for preparations for intramuscular injection
     (B) 100% for oral preparations that are not metabolized in the liver
     (C) Equal to the amount of drug in the body at the time of peak concentration relative to the dose administered
     (D) Important in that bioavailability determines what fraction of the administered dose reaches the systemic circulation
     (E) Less than 1 (100%) only for orally administered drugs

8. The pharmacokinetics of theophylline include the following average parameters: Vd 35 L; CL 48 mL/min; half-life 8 hours. If an IV infusion of theophylline is started, how long will it take to reach 93.75% of the final steady state?
     (A) Approximately 6 hours
     (B) Approximately 48 minutes
     (C) Approximately 8 hours
     (D) Approximately 5.8 hours
     (E) Approximately 32 hours

Items 9–10: Your patient with a myocardial infarction has a severe cardiac arrhythmia. You have decided to give lidocaine to correct the arrhythmia.

9. A continuous IV infusion of lidocaine, 1.92 mg/minute, is started at 8 AM. The average pharmacokinetic parameters of lidocaine are: Vd 77 L; CL 640 mL/min; half-life 1.8 hours. The expected steady-state plasma concentration is approximately
     (A) 40 mg/L
     (B) 3.0 mg/L
     (C) 0.025 mg/L
     (D) 7.2 mg/L
     (E) 3.46 mg/L

10. Your patient has been receiving lidocaine for 8 hours and you decide to obtain a plasma concentration measurement. When the results come back, the plasma level is exactly half of what you expected. The most probable explanation is
     (A) The patient's lidocaine volume of distribution is half the average value
     (B) The patient's lidocaine clearance is twice the average
     (C) The patient's lidocaine half-life is half the average
     (D) The patient's infusion rate was accidentally decreased by half
     (E) The laboratory made a mistake in the assay for lidocaine

11. A patient requires an infusion of procainamide. Its half-life is 2 hours. The infusion is begun at 9 AM. At 1 PM the same day a blood sample is taken; the drug concentration is found to be 3 mg/L. What is the probable steady-state drug concentration, eg, after 48 hours of infusion?
     (A) 3 mg/L
     (B) 4 mg/L
     (C) 6 mg/L
     (D) 9.9 mg/L
     (E) 15 mg/L

12. A narcotics addict is brought to the emergency room in a deep coma. His friends state that he took a large dose of morphine 6 hours earlier. A stat (immediate) blood analysis shows a morphine blood level of 0.25 mg/L. Assuming that the pharmacokinetics of morphine in this patient are Vd 200 L and half-life is 3 hours, how much morphine did the patient inject 6 hours earlier?

(A) 25 mg
(B) 50 mg
(C) 100 mg
(D) 200 mg
(E) Too few data to predict

13. A normal volunteer will receive a new drug in a phase I clinical trial. The clearance and volume of distribution in this subject are 1.386 L/h and 80 L respectively. The half-life of the drug in this subject will be approximately
(A) 83 hours
(B) 77 hours
(C) 58 hours
(D) 40 hours
(E) 0.02 hours

14. Gentamicin is often given in intermittent IV bolus doses of 100 mg three times a day to achieve target peak plasma concentrations of about 5 mg/L. Gentamicin's clearance (normally 5.4 L/h/70 kg) is almost entirely by glomerular filtration. Your patient, however, is found to have a creatinine clearance one-third of normal. Your initial dosage regimen for this patient would probably be
(A) 20 mg three times a day
(B) 33 mg three times a day
(C) 72 mg three times a day
(D) 100 mg twice a day
(E) 150 mg twice a day

15. Enalapril, an angiotensin converting enzyme inhibitor, has a half-life of 3 hours but is effective and nontoxic in most patients when given once a day. Assuming IV administration, this indicates that the "therapeutic window" (ratio of minimum toxic to minimum effective concentrations) for enalapril is at least
(A) 2 (ie, the toxic concentration is twice the therapeutic concentration)
(B) 8
(C) 21
(D) 256
(E) The data are insufficient to answer

ANSWERS

1. Maintenance dosage is a function of plasma level and clearance only:

$$\textbf{Rate in = Rate out at steady state}$$
$$\textbf{Dosage = Plasma level}_{(ss)} \times \textbf{clearance}$$
$$= \textbf{4 mg/L} \times \textbf{0.08 L/min}$$
$$= \textbf{0.32 mg/min}$$
$$= \textbf{0.32 mg/min} \times \textbf{60 min/h} \times \textbf{6 h}$$
$$= \textbf{115.2 mg/dose when given at 6 hour intervals}$$

The answer is **(B).**

2. Loading dose is a function of volume of distribution and target plasma concentration:

$$\textbf{Loading dose = 40 L} \times \textbf{4 mg/L = 160 mg}$$

The answer is **(D).**

3. Since the blood level drops by 50% during each half-life, the level will be 2 ng/mL after 1.6 days and 1 ng/mL after 3.2 days. The answer is **(C).**

4. Apparently verapamil is metabolized so rapidly that only the rate of delivery to the liver regulates its disappearance, ie, it is blood flow-limited. Further increases in liver enzymes could not increase its elimination. However, the rate of elimination of phenytoin is apparently limited by its rate of metabolism (clearance is much less than hepatic blood flow). Therefore, the clearance of phenytoin can rise if some agent causes an increase in liver enzymes. The answer is **(C).**

5. If the minimum therapeutic plasma concentration of hypothetical drug X is 100 units, the minimum toxic concentration is 150 units. If a dose is given that brings the plasma concentration to 150 units, it will fall to 75 units in one half-life (6 hours). Since 75 units is less than the minimum therapeutic concentration, this dosing interval is too long. However, in two-thirds as long a dosing interval, the concentration would decrease only about two-thirds as much, ie, by 50 units (based on a linear approximation). Thus, a 4 hour dose interval (with a smaller dose each time) would be appropriate. The answer is **(E)**.

6. It can be shown that at steady state, the average total amount of drug in the body is equal to 1.44 times the dose times the half-life, divided by the dosing interval. Answer **(A)** is incorrect. The efficacy of a particular drug depends on many variables; some drugs are actually more effective when given at long intervals relative to their half-lives. The answer is **(D)**.

7. Bioavailability is calculated from the ratio of the area under the curve after oral administration ($AUC_{(PO)}$) to the AUC after intravenous administration of the same dose ($AUC_{(IV)}$, Figure 3–4). Many drugs given orally are incompletely absorbed or metabolized in the lumen of the gut; they will have a bioavailability less than 1.0 even if they are not metabolized in the liver. Some drugs have a bioavailability of less than 1.0 even when given transdermally or intramuscularly. This parameter is the ratio of the amount found in the circulating blood to the amount administered. The answer is **(D)**.

8. The approach of the drug plasma concentration to steady state concentration during continuous infusion follows a stereotypical curve (Figure 3–3) that rises rapidly at first and gradually levels off. It reaches 50% of steady state at one half-life, 75% at two half-lives, 87.5% at three, 93.75% at four, and progressively halves the difference between its current level and 100% with each half-life. The answer is **(E)**, 32 hours or 4 half-lives.

9. The drug is being administered continuously; the steady-state concentration for a continuously administered drug is given by the equation in question 1. Thus

$$\textbf{Dosage} = \textbf{Plasma level}_{(ss)} \times \textbf{Clearance}$$
$$\textbf{1.92 mg/min} = \textbf{Cp}_{(ss)} \times \textbf{CL}$$

Rearranging:

$$\textbf{Cp}_{(ss)} = \textbf{1.92 mg/min/CL}$$
$$\textbf{Cp}_{(ss)} = \textbf{1.92 mg/min/640 mL/min}$$
$$\textbf{Cp}_{(ss)} = \textbf{0.003 mg/mL or 3 mg/L}$$

The answer is **(B)**.

10. If the half-life is 1.8 hours, the plasma concentration should approach steady state after 8 hours (more than 4 half-lives). As indicated by the equation used in question 9, the steady-state concentration is a function of dosage and clearance, not volume of distribution. If the plasma level is less than predicted, the clearance in this patient must be greater than average. (In a question of this type, do not assume errors of analysis or administration as answers, unless all other possible answers can be positively ruled out.) The answer is **(B)**.

11. According to the curve that relates plasma concentration to infusion time (Figure 3–3), a drug will reach 50% of its final steady-state concentration in one half-life, 75% in two half-lives, etc. From 9 AM to 1 PM is 4 hours or 2 half-lives. Therefore, the measured concentration at 1 PM is 75% of the steady-state value ($0.75 \times Cp_{ss}$). The steady-state concentration will be 3 mg/L divided by 0.75, or 4 mg/L. The answer is **(B)**.

12. According to the curve that relates the decline of plasma concentration to time (in number of half-lives) as the drug is eliminated (Figure 3–3), the plasma concentration was 4 times higher immediately after administration than at the time of the measurement, which occurred 6 hours or two half-lives later. Therefore the initial plasma concentration was 1.0 mg/L. Since the amount in the body is equal to $Vd \times Cp$ (text eqn [1]), the amount injected was 200L × 1 mg/L, or 200 mg. The answer is **(D)**.

13. Half-life can be estimated from

$$t_{1/2} = \textbf{Vd} \times 0.693 / \textbf{CL (text eqn [3])}$$
$$= \textbf{80 L} \times 0.693 / 1.386 \textbf{ L/h}$$
$$= \textbf{80 L} \times 1/2 \textbf{ h/L}$$
$$= \textbf{40 h}$$

The answer is **(D)**.

14. If the drug is cleared almost entirely by the kidney and creatinine clearance is reduced to one third of normal, the total daily dose should also be reduced to one third. The answer is **(B)**.
15. If the drug is given only once a day, it has 24 h/3 h, or 8 half-lives during which it declines in plasma concentration (Figure 3–3). Each half-life results in a decline by half of the preceding level, ie, a power of two (one half-life, to 50%; two half-lives, to 25%; etc). Since the dosing interval is 8 times greater than the half-life of the drug, the peak concentration is roughly 2^8 or 256 times higher than the minimum (trough) concentration. If one assumes that the drug is still effective at its trough concentration, the "opening" of the therapeutic window would be at least 256. The answer is **(D)**.

Drug Metabolism

4

OBJECTIVES

You should be able to:

- List the major phase I and phase II metabolic reactions.
- Describe the mechanism of hepatic enzyme induction and list three drugs that are known to cause it.
- List three drugs that inhibit the metabolism of other drugs.
- List three drugs for which there are well-defined, genetically determined differences in metabolism.
- Discuss the effects of smoking, liver disease, and kidney disease on drug elimination.
- Describe the pathways by which acetaminophen is metabolized (1) to harmless products if taken in normal doses and (2) to hepatotoxic products if taken in overdosage.

Learn the definitions that follow.

Table 4–1. Drug metabolism definitions.

Term	Definition
Phase I reactions	Reactions that convert the parent drug to a more polar (water-soluble) or more reactive product by unmasking or inserting a polar functional group such as –OH, –SH, or –NH$_2$
Phase II reactions	Reactions that increase water solubility by conjugation of the drug molecule with a polar moiety such as glucuronate or sulfate
Enzyme induction	Stimulation of drug-metabolizing capacity; usually manifested in the liver by increased synthesis of smooth endoplasmic reticulum (which contains a high concentration of phase I enzymes)

CONCEPTS

A. Need for Drug Metabolism: All higher organisms require mechanisms for ridding themselves of foreign molecules that are absorbed from the environment, as well as for excreting substances produced within the system. Biotransformation of drugs is one such mechanism. It is an important mechanism by which the body terminates the action of some drugs but also serves in some cases to activate pro-drugs. In most cases, a drug as given is relatively lipid-soluble, to ensure good absorption. The same property would result in very slow removal from

Table 4–2. Examples of phase I drug-metabolizing reactions.

Reaction Type	Typical Drug Substrates
Oxidations, P450-dependent	
Hydroxylations	Barbiturates, amphetamines, phenylbutazone, phenytoin
N-dealkylation	Morphine, caffeine, theophylline
O-dealkylation	Codeine
N-oxidation	Acetaminophen, nicotine, methaqualone
S-oxidation	Thioridazine, cimetidine, chlorpromazine
Deamination	Amphetamine, diazepam
Oxidations, P450-independent	
Amine oxidation	Epinephrine
Dehydrogenation	Ethanol, chloral hydrate
Reductions	Chloramphenicol, clorazepam, dantrolene, naloxone
Hydrolyses	
Esters	Procaine, succinylcholine, aspirin, clofibrate
Amides	Procainamide, lidocaine, indomethacin

the body, because the molecule would also be readily reabsorbed from the urine in the renal tubule. The body hastens excretion by transforming the drug to a less lipid-soluble, less readily reabsorbed, form.

B. Types of Metabolic Reactions:
  1. Phase I reactions: Phase I reactions include oxidation (especially by the cytochrome P450 group of enzymes, mixed-function oxidases), reduction, and hydrolysis. Examples are listed in Table 4–2.
  2. Phase II reactions: Phase II reactions are synthetic reactions that involve addition (conjugation) of subgroups to –OH, –NH$_2$, and –SH functions on the drug molecule. These subgroups include glucuronate (from UDP glucuronic acid), acetate (from acetyl CoA), glutathione, glycine, sulfate, and methyl groups (from S-adenosylmethionine). Note that most of these groups are relatively polar. Examples of phase II reactions are listed in Table 4–3.

C. Sites of Drug Metabolism: The most important organ for drug metabolism is the liver. The kidneys play an important role in the metabolism of some drugs. A few drugs (eg, esters) are metabolized in many tissues (including the blood, intestinal wall, etc) because of the broad distribution of their hydrolyzing enzymes.

D. Determinants of Biotransformation Rate: The rate of biotransformation of a drug may vary markedly among different individuals. This variation is most often due to genetic or drug-induced differences. For a few drugs, age or disease-related differences in drug metabolism are significant. Gender is important for only a few drugs, eg, ethanol. (Women have lower first-pass metabolism of alcohol than do men.) Since the rate of biotransformation is often the primary determinant of clearance, variations in drug metabolism must be considered carefully when designing a dosage regimen. Smoking, a common cause of enzyme induction in the liver, may increase the metabolism of some drugs (eg, theophylline).

Table 4–3. Examples of phase II drug-metabolizing reactions.

Reaction Type	Typical Drug Substrates
Glucuronidation	Acetaminophen, morphine, diazepam, sulfathiazole, digoxin, digitoxin
Acetylation	Sulfonamides, isoniazid, clonazepam, mescaline, dapsone
Glutathione conjugation	Ethacrynic acid, reactive Phase I metabolite of acetaminophen
Glycine conjugation	Salicylic acid, nicotinic acid (niacin), deoxycholic acid
Sulfate conjugation	Acetaminophen, methyldopa, estrone
Methylation	Epinephrine, norepinephrine, dopamine, histamine

Adapted, with permission, from Katzung BG (editor): *Basic & Clinical Pharmacology*, 6th ed. Appleton & Lange, 1995.

Table 4–4. A partial list of drugs that enhance drug metabolism in humans.

Inducer	Drug Whose Metabolism Is Induced
Barbiturates, especially phenobarbital	Barbiturates, warfarin, chloramphenicol, steroids, doxorubicin, phenytoin, chlorpromazine, others
Benzo[a]pyrene (from tobacco smoke)	Theophylline, barbiturates
Chlorcyclizine	Steroid hormones
Griseofulvin	Warfarin
Phenylbutazone	Cortisol, digitoxin
Phenytoin	Cortisol, dexamethasone, digitoxin, theophylline
Rifampin	Warfarin, digitoxin, steroids, methadone, metoprolol, propranolol, quinidine

Adapted, with permission, from Katzung BG (editor): *Basic & Clinical Pharmacology*, 6th ed. Appleton & Lange, 1995.

1. **Genetic factors:** Several drug-metabolizing systems have been shown to differ among families or populations in genetically determined ways.
   a. **Hydrolysis of esters:** Succinylcholine is an ester that is metabolized by plasma cholinesterase ("pseudocholinesterase" or butyrylcholinesterase). In most individuals, this process occurs very rapidly and the drug has a duration of action of about 5 minutes. Approximately one person in 2500 has abnormal variants of this enzyme that result in much slower metabolism of succinylcholine and similar esters. In such individuals, the neuromuscular paralysis produced by succinylcholine may last many hours.
   b. **Acetylation of amines:** Isoniazid and some other amines such as procainamide are inactivated by N-acetylation. Individuals deficient in acetylation capacity, termed slow acetylators, may have prolonged or toxic responses to normal doses of these drugs. Slow acetylators constitute about 50% of white and African-American persons in the USA, and a much smaller fraction of Asian and Inuit (Eskimo) populations. The slow acetylation trait is inherited as an autosomal recessive gene.
   c. **Oxidation:** The rate of oxidation of debrisoquin, sparteine, phenformin, dextromethorphan, metoprolol, and some tricyclic antidepressants by certain P450 isozymes has been shown to be genetically determined.
2. **Other drugs:** Co-administration of certain agents may stimulate or inhibit the metabolism of many drugs. Mechanisms include the following:
   a. **Enzyme induction:** As indicated above, induction usually results from increased synthesis of cytochrome P450-dependent drug-oxidizing enzymes in the liver. Many isozymes of the P450 family exist, and inducers selectively increase subgroups of isozymes. Several days are usually required to reach maximum induction; a similar amount of time is required to regress after withdrawal of the inducer. Common inducers and drugs whose metabolism is increased are indicated in Table 4–4. In addition, some toxic chemicals, such as the carcinogens in cigarette smoke, are hepatic enzyme inducers.

Table 4–5. A partial list of drugs that inhibit drug metabolism in humans.

Inhibitor	Drug Whose Metabolism Is Inhibited
Allopurinol, isoniazid, chloramphenicol	Probenecid, tolbutamide, oral anticoagulants
Cimetidine	Benzodiazepines, warfarin, others
Dicumarol	Phenytoin
Disulfiram	Ethanol, phenytoin, warfarin
Erythromycin	Astemizole, terfenadine
Ethanol	Methanol, ethylene glycol
Ketoconazole	Cyclosporine, terfenadine, astemizole
Phenylbutazone	Phenytoin, tolbutamide
Secobarbital	Secobarbital

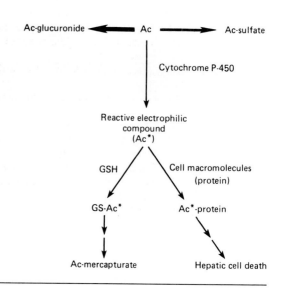

Figure 4–1. Metabolism of acetaminophen to harmless conjugates or to toxic metabolites. Acetaminophen glucuronide, acetaminophen sulfate, and Ac-mercapturate (mercapturate conjugate of acetaminophen) are all nontoxic Phase II conjugates. Ac* is the toxic, reactive Phase I metabolite. Transformation to the reactive metabolite occurs if hepatic stores of sulfate, glucuronide, and glutathione are depleted or overwhelmed. (Reproduced, with permission, from Katzung BG [editor]: *Basic & Clinical Pharmacology*, 6th ed. Appleton & Lange, 1995.)

    b. Metabolism inhibitors: Common inhibitors and the drugs whose metabolism is diminished are indicated in Table 4–5. **Suicide inhibitors** are drugs that are metabolized to products which inhibit the metabolizing enzyme. Such agents include ethinyl estradiol, norethindrone, spironolactone, secobarbital, allobarbital, fluroxene, and propylthiouracil. Metabolism may also be decreased by pharmacodynamic factors such as a reduction in blood flow to the metabolizing organ (eg, propranolol reduces hepatic blood flow).

E. Toxic Metabolism: Drug metabolism is not synonymous with drug inactivation. Some drugs are converted to active products by metabolism. If these products are toxic, severe injury may result under some circumstances. An important example is acetaminophen—when it is taken in a large overdose (Figure 4–1). Acetaminophen is conjugated to harmless glucuronide and sulfate metabolites when it is taken in normal doses. If a large overdose is taken, however, the metabolic pathways are overwhelmed, and a P450-dependent system converts some of the drug to a reactive intermediate. The intermediate is conjugated with glutathione to a third harmless product if glutathione stores are adequate. If glutathione stores are exhausted, however, the reactive intermediate combines with essential hepatic cell proteins, resulting in cell death. Prompt administration of other sulfhydryl donors (eg, acetylcysteine) may be life-saving in such a situation. In severe liver disease, stores of glucuronide, sulfate, and glutathione may be depleted, making the patient more susceptible to hepatic toxicity with near-normal doses of acetaminophen.

QUESTIONS

DIRECTIONS: Each of the numbered items or incomplete statements in this section is followed by answers or by completions of the sentence. Select the ONE lettered answer or completion that is BEST in each case.

    1. Biotransformation (metabolism) usually results in a product that is
        (A) More likely to distribute intracellularly
        (B) Less lipid soluble than the original drug
        (C) More likely to be reabsorbed by kidney tubules
        (D) More lipid soluble than the original drug
        (E) More likely to produce adverse effects
    2. Induction of drug metabolism
        (A) Results in increased smooth endoplasmic reticulum
        (B) Results in increased rough endoplasmic reticulum

    (C) Results in decreased enzymes in the soluble cytoplasmic fraction
    (D) Requires three to four months to reach completion
    (E) Is irreversible

3. A factor that is likely to increase the duration of action of a drug that is partially metabolized in the liver is
    (A) Chronic administration of phenobarbital prior to and during therapy with the drug in question
    (B) Chronic therapy with cimetidine prior to and during therapy with the drug in question
    (C) Displacement from tissue binding sites by another drug
    (D) Increased cardiac output
    (E) Chronic administration of rifampin

4. Which of the following is NOT a phase I drug metabolizing reaction?
    (A) Acetylation
    (B) Deamination
    (C) Hydrolysis
    (D) Oxidation
    (E) Reduction

5. Reports of cardiac arrhythmias caused by unusually high blood levels of two antihistamines, terfenadine and astemizole, are best explained by
    (A) Concomitant treatment with phenobarbital
    (B) Use of these drugs by smokers
    (C) Use of antihistamines by persons of Asian background
    (D) A genetic predisposition to metabolize succinylcholine slowly
    (E) Treatment of these patients with ketoconazole, an antifungal agent

DIRECTIONS: The following section consists of a list of four to twenty-six lettered options followed by several numbered items. For each numbered item, select the ONE option that is most closely associated with it. Each answer may be selected once, more than once, or not at all.
    (A) Succinylcholine
    (B) Debrisoquin
    (C) Procainamide
    (D) Phenobarbital
    (E) Cimetidine

6. Associated with slower metabolism in Caucasians and African-Americans than in most Asians

7. A commonly used drug that may inhibit hepatic microsomal P450 mixed-function oxidizing enzymes

8. An abnormal form of the enzyme that hydrolyzes this agent is found in the plasma of about one out of every 2500 humans

9. Pretreatment with this agent for 5–7 days might increase the toxicity of acetaminophen

ANSWERS

1. Biotransformation usually results in a product that is less lipid soluble. The answer is (B).

2. The smooth endoplasmic reticulum, which contains the mixed-function oxidase drug-metabolizing enzymes, is selectively increased by "inducers." The answer is (A).

3. Phenobarbital induces drug-metabolizing enzymes and thereby *reduces* their duration of action. Displacement of drug from tissue may transiently increase the intensity of the effect, but will decrease the volume of distribution and thereby reduce the half-life. The answer is (B).

4. Acetylation is a phase II reaction. The answer is (A).

5. Treatment with phenobarbital and smoking are associated with increased drug metabolism and lower, not higher, blood levels. Persons of Asian origin have a high probability of metabolizing certain amides (isoniazid, procainamide) *more rapidly;* Asians do not appear to metabolize antihistamines differently from other ethnic groups. Ketoconazole and probably erythromycin slow the metabolism of these "nonsedating" antihistamines. The answer is (E).

6. Procainamide, like hydralazine and isoniazid, is metabolized by N-acetylation, an enzymatic process that is slower than average in about 20% of Asians and about 50% of Caucasians and African-Americans. The answer is (C).

7. Cimetidine is a very commonly used drug and has well-documented ability to inhibit the hepatic metabolism of many drugs. The answer is **(E)**.

8. Succinylcholine is normally hydrolyzed quite rapidly by plasma cholinesterase (pseudocholinesterase). This enzyme is abnormal in about 1/2500 of the human population, resulting in unusually long duration of action of succinylcholine in these patients. The answer is **(A)**.

9. Acetaminophen is normally eliminated by phase II conjugation reactions. The drug's toxicity is dependent on an oxidized reactive metabolite produced by phase I oxidizing P450 enzymes. Drugs that cause induction of P450 enzymes, such as phenobarbital, may increase the production of this toxic metabolite. The answer is **(D)**.

5 Drug Evaluation

OBJECTIVES

Learn the definitions that follow.

Table 5–1. Drug evaluation definitions.

Term	Definition
Single-blind study	A clinical trial in which the investigators, but not the subjects, know which subjects are receiving active drug and which placebo
Double-blind study	A clinical trial in which neither the subjects nor the investigators know which subjects are receiving placebo; the code is held by a third party
IND	Investigational New Drug Exemption; FDA approval to carry out new drug trials in humans; requires animal data
NDA	New Drug Application; FDA approval to market a new drug for ordinary medical use
Placebo	A "dummy" medication made up to resemble the active investigational formulation as much as possible
Phases I, II, and III of clinical trials	Three parts of a clinical trial that must be carried out before submitting an NDA to the FDA
Positive control	A known standard therapy, to be used along with placebo, to fully evaluate the safety and efficacy of a new drug in relation to the others available
Mutagenic	An effect on the inheritable characteristics of a cell or organism; tested in microorganisms with the Ames test
Teratogenic	An effect on the fetal development of an organism resulting in abnormal structure or function; not generally heritable
Carcinogenic	An effect resulting in malignant characteristics
Orphan drug	Drugs developed for diseases in which the expected number of US patients is less than 200,000; bestows certain advantages on companies that develop drugs for unusual diseases

CONCEPTS

A. Safety & Efficacy: Because society expects prescription drugs to be safe and effective, governments have regulated the development and marketing of new drugs. The **Food & Drug Administration (FDA)** is the regulatory body in the USA that proposes and administers these regulations. The FDA requires evidence of relative safety (derived from acute and subacute

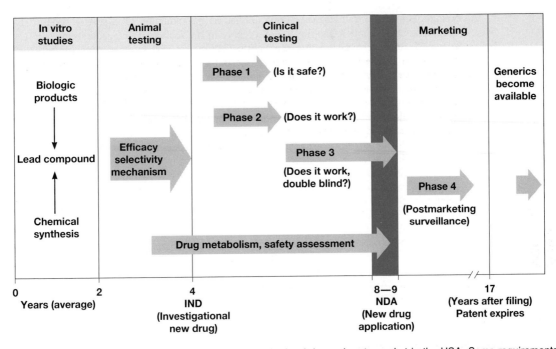

In vitro studies	Animal testing	Clinical testing		Marketing

Phase 1 (Is it safe?)

Generics become available

Biologic products

Phase 2 (Does it work?)

↓

Efficacy selectivity mechanism

Phase 3

Lead compound

(Does it work, double blind?)

↑

Phase 4

(Postmarketing surveillance)

Chemical synthesis

Drug metabolism, safety assessment

0	2	4	8—9	17
Years (average)		IND (Investigational new drug)	NDA (New drug application)	(Years after filing) Patent expires

Figure 5–1. The development and testing process required to bring a drug to market in the USA. Some requirements may be different for drugs used in life-threatening diseases. (Reproduced, with permission, from Katzung BG [editor]: *Basic and Clinical Pharmacology,* 6th ed. Appleton & Lange, 1995.)

toxicity testing in animals) and probable therapeutic action (from the pharmacologic profile in animals) before human testing is permitted. Some information about the pharmacokinetics of a compound is also required before clinical evaluation is begun. Chronic toxicity test results are generally not required before human studies are started. The development of a new drug and its pathway through various levels of testing and regulation are illustrated in Figure 5–1. The cost of development of a new drug, including false starts and discarded molecules, was from $100 million to $300 million dollars in 1994.

B. Animal Testing: The amount of animal testing required before human studies begin is a function of the proposed use and the urgency of the application. Thus, a drug proposed for occasional nonsystemic use requires less extensive testing than one destined for chronic systemic administration. Anticancer drugs and drugs proposed for use in AIDS, because of the urgency of the need for new agents, require less evidence of safety than do drugs used in less threatening diseases, and are often investigated and approved on an accelerated schedule.

    1. Acute toxicity: Acute toxicity studies are required for all drugs. These studies involve single administrations of the agent up to the lethal level in at least two species, eg, one rodent and one nonrodent.

    2. Subacute & chronic toxicity: Subacute and chronic testing are required for most agents, especially those intended for chronic use. Tests are usually carried out for at least the amount of time proposed for human application, ie, 2–4 weeks (subacute) or 6–24 months (chronic), in at least two species.

C. Types of Animal Tests: Tests done with animals often include general screening tests for pharmacologic effects, hepatic and renal function monitoring, blood and urine tests, gross and histopathologic examination of tissues, and tests of teratogenicity, mutagenicity, and carcinogenicity.

    1. Pharmacologic profile: The pharmacologic profile is a description of all the pharmacologic effects of a drug (eg, effects on blood pressure, gastrointestinal activity, respiration, renal function, endocrine function, the central nervous system, etc).

2. **Teratogenesis:** Teratogenesis can be defined as the induction of generally nonheritable developmental defects in the fetus (by exposure of the fetus to a drug, radiation, etc). Teratogenesis is studied by treating pregnant female animals at selected times during early pregnancy when organogenesis is known to take place and later examining the fetuses or neonates for abnormalities. Examples of drugs known to have teratogenic effects include thalidomide, ethanol, glucocorticoids, valproic acid, isotretinoin, warfarin, lithium, and androgens.

3. **Mutagenesis:** Mutagenesis is induction of changes in the genetic material of animals of any age and therefore induction of heritable abnormalities. The **Ames test,** the standard in vitro test for mutagenicity, uses bacteria that naturally depend on specific nutrients in the culture medium. Loss of this dependence during exposure to the test drug signals a mutation. The **dominant lethal test** is an in vivo mutagenicity test carried out in mice. Male animals are exposed to the test substance before mating. Abnormalities in the results of subsequent mating (loss of embryos, deformed fetuses, etc) signal a mutation in the male's germ cells. Many carcinogens (eg, aflatoxin, cancer chemotherapeutic drugs, and other agents that bind to DNA) have mutagenic effects.

4. **Carcinogenesis:** Carcinogenesis is the induction of malignant characteristics in cells. Because carcinogenicity is difficult and expensive to study, the Ames test is often used to screen chemicals, since there is a moderately high degree of correlation between mutagenicity in the Ames test and carcinogenicity in some animal tests. Agents with known carcinogenic effects include coal tar, aflatoxin, dimethylnitrosamine and other nitrosamines, urethane, vinyl chloride, and the polycyclic aromatic hydrocarbons in tobacco smoke, eg, benzo[*a*]pyrene.

D. **Clinical Trials:** Human testing in the USA requires the prior approval of an **Investigational New Drug Exemption** application (IND), which has been submitted by the manufacturer to the FDA (see Figure 5–1). The major testing period is formally divided into three phases before a **New Drug Application** (NDA) can be submitted. The NDA constitutes the request for approval of general marketing of the new agent for prescription use. A fourth phase of study follows NDA approval.

1. **Phase I:** A phase I trial consists of careful evaluation of the dose-response relationship in a small number of normal human volunteers (eg, 20 to 30). An exception is in phase I trials of cancer chemotherapeutic agents; these are carried out by administering the agents to patients with cancer. In phase I studies, the acute effects of the agent are studied over a broad range of dosage, starting with one that produces no detectable effect and progressing to one that produces either a major therapeutic response or a very minor toxic effect.

2. **Phase II:** A phase II trial involves evaluation of a drug in a moderate number of patients (eg, 100 to 300) with the target disease. A placebo or positive control drug is included in a single-blind or double-blind design. The goal is to determine whether the agent has the desired therapeutic effects at doses that are tolerated by sick patients.

3. **Phase III:** A phase III trial consists of a large design involving many patients (eg, 1000 to 5000 or more in many centers) and many clinicians who are using the drug in the manner proposed for its ultimate general use, eg, in outpatients. Such studies usually include placebo and positive controls in a double-blind crossover design. The goal is to explore further the spectrum of beneficial actions of the new drug, to compare it with older therapies, and to discover toxicities, if any, that occur so infrequently as to be undetectable in phase II studies.

4. **Phase IV:** Phase IV represents the post-marketing surveillance phase of evaluation, in which it is hoped that toxicities that occur very infrequently will be detected and reported early enough to prevent major therapeutic disasters. Unlike the first three phases, phase IV is not rigidly regulated by the FDA.

E. **Drug Legislation:** In the USA, many laws regulating drugs have been passed during this century. Refer to Table 5–2 for a partial list of this legislation.

F. **Orphan Drugs:** An orphan drug is a drug for a rare disease (one affecting fewer than 200,000 people). The study of such agents has often been neglected because the sales of an effective agent for an uncommon ailment might not pay the costs of development. In the USA, current legislation provides regulatory incentives encouraging the development of orphan drugs.

Table 5–2. Selected legislation pertaining to drugs in the USA.

Law	Purpose and Effect
Pure Food & Drug Act of 1906	Prohibited mislabeling and adulteration of drugs
Harrison Narcotics Act of 1914	Established regulations for the use of opium, opioids, and cocaine (marijuana added in 1937)
Food, Drug, & Cosmetic Act of 1938	Required that new drugs be safe as well as pure
Kefauver–Harris Amendment (1962)	Required proof of efficacy as well as safety for new drugs
Comprehensive Drug Abuse Prevention & Control Act	Outlined strict controls on the manufacture, distribution, and prescribing of habit-forming drugs; established programs for the treatment and prevention of addiction
Drug Price Competition & Patent Restoration Act of 1984	Abbreviated new drug applications for generic drugs; required bioequivalence data; patent life extended by the amount of time drug was delayed by the review process: cannot exceed 5 years or extend to more than 14 years post-NDA

Modified and reproduced, by permission, from Katzung BG (editor): *Basic & Clinical Pharmacology*, 6th ed, Appleton & Lange, 1995.

QUESTIONS

DIRECTIONS: Each of the numbered items or incomplete statements in this section is followed by answers or by completions of the sentence. Select the ONE lettered answer or completion that is BEST in each case.

1. With regard to clinical trials of new drugs, all of the following are correct EXCEPT
   (A) Phase I involves the study of a small number of normal volunteers by highly trained clinical pharmacologists
   (B) Phase II involves the use of the new drug in a small number of patients (100 to 200) who have the disease to be treated
   (C) Phase III involves the determination of the drug's therapeutic index by the cautious induction of toxicity, conducted by highly trained clinical pharmacologists in a hospital setting
   (D) Phase IV involves the reporting by practitioners of unusual events, especially toxic reactions, after the drug is approved for general prescription use
   (E) Phase II does not require the use of a positive control (a known effective drug) or placebo, but these are often used in this phase

2. Animal testing of potential new therapeutic agents
   (A) Extends over a time period of at least three years in order to discover late toxicities
   (B) Requires the use of at least two primate species, eg, monkey and baboon
   (C) Requires the submission of histopathologic slides and specimens to the FDA for government evaluation
   (D) Has good predictability for drug allergy-type reactions
   (E) May be abbreviated in the case of some very toxic agents used in cancer

3. The "dominant lethal" test involves the treatment of a male adult animal with a chemical before mating; the pregnant female is later examined for fetal death and abnormalities. The dominant lethal test therefore is a test of
   (A) Teratogenicity
   (B) Mutagenicity
   (C) Carcinogenicity
   (D) All of the above
   (E) None of the above

4. An optimal phase III clinical trial of a new analgesic drug would include all of the following EXCEPT
   (A) A negative control (placebo)
   (B) A positive control (current standard therapy)
   (C) Double-blind protocol (neither the patient nor immediate observers of the patient know which agent is active)

    (D)   A group of 200 to 3000 subjects with a clinical condition requiring analgesia

    (E)   Prior submission of an NDA (new drug application) to the FDA

5. In the testing of new compounds (eg, antihypertensives) for potential therapeutic use,

    (A)   Animal tests cannot be used to predict the types of toxicities that may occur because there is no correlation with human toxicity

    (B)   Human studies in normal individuals will be done before the drug is used in diseased individuals

    (C)   Degree of risk must be assessed in at least three species of animals, including one primate species

    (D)   The animal therapeutic index must be known before trial of the agents in humans

ANSWERS

1. The induction of toxicity is not required in any phase of clinical testing, although some toxicity is usually seen. The answer is **(C)**.

2. Drugs proposed for short-term use may not require long-term chronic testing. For some drugs, no primates are used; for other agents, only one species is used. The data from the tests, not the evidence itself, must be submitted to the FDA. Prediction of human drug allergy from animal testing is not very reliable. The answer is **(E)**.

3. The description of the test indicates that a chromosomal change (passed from father to fetus) is the toxicity detected. This is a mutation. The answer is **(B)**.

4. The first four items **(A–D)** are correct. An NDA cannot be acted upon until the first three phases of clinical trials have been completed. The answer is **(E)**.

5. Animal tests in a single species do not always predict human toxicities; but when these tests are carried out in several species, most acute toxicities that occur in humans will also appear in at least one animal species. According to current FDA rules, the "degree of risk" must be determined in at least two species. Use of primates is not always required. The therapeutic index is not required. Except for cancer chemotherapeutic agents, phase I clinical trials are always carried out in normal subjects. The answer is **(B)**.

Part II. Autonomic Drugs

Introduction to Autonomic Pharmacology   6

OBJECTIVES

You should be able to:

- Describe the steps in the synthesis and the termination of action of the major autonomic transmitters.
- Name two cotransmitter substances.
- Describe the organ system effects of stimulation of the parasympathetic and sympathetic systems.
- Name examples of inhibitors of acetylcholine and norepinephrine synthesis, storage, and release. Predict the effects of these inhibitors on the function of the major organ systems.
- List the determinants of blood pressure and describe the baroreceptor reflex response for the following perturbations: (1) blood loss or administration of one of the following: (2) a vasodilator, (3) a vasoconstrictor, (4) a cardiac stimulant, (5) a cardiac depressant.
- Name the major types of receptors found on autonomic effector tissues.
- Describe the differences between the effects of surgical sympathetic ganglionectomy (interruption of ganglionic transmission by surgical removal of the sympathetic ganglia) and those of pharmacologic ganglion block.
- Describe the action of several toxins that affect nerve function: tetrodotoxin, saxitoxin, botulinum toxin, and latrotoxin.

Learn the definitions that follow.

Table 6–1. Autonomic definitions.

Term	Definition
Adrenergic	A nerve ending that releases norepinephrine as the primary transmitter; also a synapse in which norepinephrine is the primary transmitter
Adrenoceptor	A receptor that binds and is activated by one of the catecholamine transmitters (norepinephrine, epinephrine, or dopamine) and related drugs
Autonomic effector cells or tissues	Cells or tissues that have adrenoceptors or cholinoceptors which, when activated, alter the function of those cells or tissues, eg, smooth muscle, heart, glands
Baroreceptor reflex	The neuronal homeostatic mechanism that the body uses in attempting to maintain blood pressure constant; the sensory limb originates in the baroreceptors of the carotid sinus
Cholinergic	A nerve ending that releases acetylcholine as the primary transmitter; also a synapse in which acetylcholine is the primary transmitter
Cholinoceptor	A receptor that binds and is activated by acetylcholine
Dopaminergic	A nerve ending that releases dopamine as the primary transmitter; also a synapse in which dopamine is the primary transmitter
Homeostatic reflex	A neuronal compensatory mechanism for maintaining a body function at a predetermined level, eg, the baroreceptor reflex for blood pressure
Parasympathetic	That part of the autonomic nervous system that originates in the cranial nerves and the sacral part of the spinal cord
Postsynaptic receptor	Receptor located on the distal side of the synapse, eg, on an effector cell; contrast with presynaptic receptors
Presynaptic receptor	Receptor located on the nerve ending in a synapse; modulates the release of transmitter
Sympathetic	That part of the autonomic nervous system that originates in the thoracic and lumbar parts of the spinal cord

CONCEPTS

The autonomic nervous system (ANS) is the major involuntary, unconscious, automatic portion of the nervous system in contrast to the somatic (voluntary) nervous system. The anatomy, neurotransmitter chemistry, receptor characteristics, and functional integration of the ANS are discussed below.

A. Anatomic Aspects of the ANS: The motor (efferent) portion of the ANS is the major pathway for information transmission from the central nervous system (CNS) to the involuntary effector tissues (smooth muscle, vascular endothelium, cardiac muscle, and exocrine glands, Figure 6–1). The **enteric nervous system (ENS)** is a semiautonomous part of the ANS, with specific functions for the control of the gastrointestinal tract. The ENS consists of the myenteric plexus (plexus of Auerbach) and the submucous plexus (plexus of Meissner) and includes many inputs from the parasympathetic and sympathetic nervous systems.

There are many sensory (afferent) fibers in autonomic nerves. These are of considerable importance for the physiologic control of the involuntary organs but are directly influenced by only a few drugs.

1. **Spinal roots of origin:** The parasympathetic preganglionic motor fibers originate in the cranial nerve nuclei (III, VII, IX, X) and the sacral segments (usually S2–S4) of the spinal cord. The sympathetic preganglionic fibers originate in the thoracic (T1–T12) and lumbar (L1–L5) segments of the cord.

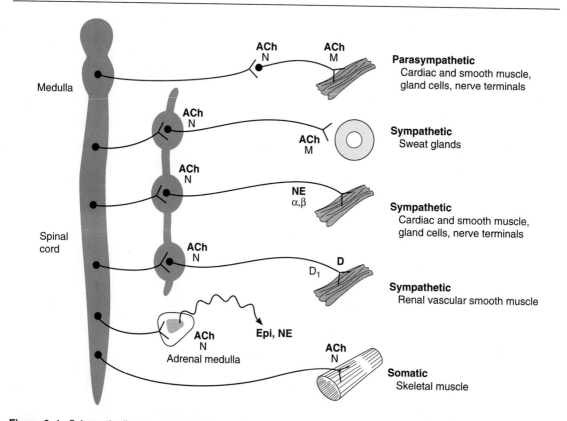

Figure 6–1. Schematic diagram comparing some features of the parasympathetic and sympathetic divisions of the autonomic nervous system with the somatic motor system. Parasympathetic ganglia are not shown as discrete structures because most of them are diffusely distributed in the walls of the organs innervated. ACh, acetylcholine; NE, norepinephrine; D, dopamine. N, nicotinic; M, muscarinic; α, β, alpha and beta adrenoceptors; D₁, dopamine₁ receptors. Reproduced, with permission, from Katzung BG (editor): *Basic & Clinical Pharmacology*, 6th ed. Appleton & Lange, 1995.

2. **Location of ganglia:** Most of the sympathetic ganglia are located in 2 paravertebral chains that lie along the spinal column. A few (the prevertebral ganglia) are located on the anterior aspect of the vertebral column. Most of the parasympathetic ganglia are located in the organs innervated, more distant from the spinal cord.
3. **Length of pre- and postganglionic fibers:** Because of the locations of the ganglia noted above, the preganglionic sympathetic fibers are short and the postganglionic fibers are long. The opposite is true for the parasympathetic system: preganglionic fibers are long and post-ganglionic are short.
4. **Uninnervated receptors:** Some receptors that respond to autonomic transmitters receive no innervation. These include muscarinic receptors on the endothelium of blood vessels, some presynaptic receptors, and in some species, the adrenoceptors on apocrine sweat glands.

B. **Neurotransmitter Aspects of the ANS:** The synthesis, storage, release, and termination of action of the neurotransmitters are important in the action of autonomic drugs (Figure 6–2).
1. **Primary transmitters:** Acetylcholine (ACh) is the primary transmitter in all autonomic ganglia and at the parasympathetic postganglionic neuron-effector cell synapses. Nor-epinephrine (NE) is the primary transmitter at the sympathetic postganglionic neuron-effector cell synapses in most tissues. Important exceptions include sympathetic fibers to thermoregulatory (eccrine) sweat glands and probably vasodilator sympathetic fibers in skeletal muscle, which release ACh. Dopamine (DA) is an important vasodilator transmitter in some splanchnic vessels, especially renal vessels.

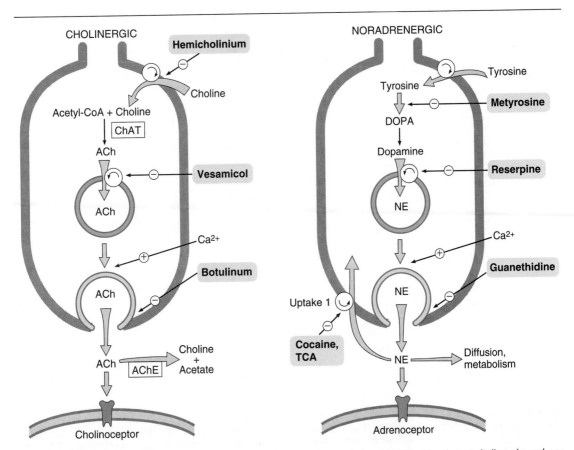

Figure 6–2. Characteristics of transmitter synthesis, storage, release, and termination of action at cholinergic and noradrenergic nerve terminals are shown from the top downward. Circles with rotating arrows represent transporters; ChAT, choline acetyltransferase; ACh, acetylcholine; AChE, acetylcholinesterase; NE, norepinephrine.

2. **Cotransmitters:** Many, perhaps all, autonomic transmitter vesicles contain other cotransmitter molecules in addition to the primary agents described above. In some nerve endings, cotransmitters may be localized in a separate population of vesicles. Substances recognized to date as cotransmitters include ATP, enkephalins, vasoactive intestinal peptide (VIP), neuropeptide Y, substance P, neurotensin, somatostatin, and others. Their role in autonomic function appears to involve modulation of synaptic function. The same substances undoubtedly function as primary transmitters in other synapses.

3. **Synthesis and storage of transmitters:** ACh is synthesized by the enzyme choline acetyltransferase from acetyl-CoA and choline. The rate-limiting step is probably the transport of choline into the nerve terminal. The synthesis of NE is more complex. Tyrosine is hydroxylated (the rate-limiting step) to DOPA (dihydroxyphenylalanine), decarboxylated to dopamine, and hydroxylated to norepinephrine. Both transmitters are actively transported into their vesicles for storage. Drugs that block the synthesis of ACh (eg, hemicholinium), its storage (eg, vesamicol), or its release (eg, botulinum*) are not very useful in therapy because their effects are not sufficiently selective (ie, PANS and SANS ganglia, and somatic neuromuscular junctions, may all be blocked). Drugs that block norepinephrine synthesis (eg, metyrosine) or catecholamine storage (eg, reserpine), or release (eg, guanethidine) are useful in several diseases (eg, hypertension) because their effects are more selective for sympathetic functions.

4. **Termination of action of transmitters:**
   a. **Acetylcholine:** The action of acetylcholine in the synapse is normally terminated by metabolism to acetate and choline by the enzyme acetylcholinesterase. The products are not excreted but are recycled in the body. Inhibition of acetylcholinesterase is an important therapeutic and toxic effect of several drugs.
   b. **Catecholamines:** Metabolism is not responsible for the termination of action of the catecholamine transmitters, norepinephrine and dopamine. Instead, diffusion and reuptake (especially uptake-1, Figure 6–2) reduce their concentration in the synaptic cleft and stop their action. However, these transmitters are also metabolized—by monoamine oxidase (MAO) and catechol-O-methyltransferase (COMT)—and the products of these enzymatic reactions are excreted. Determination of the 24-hour excretion of metanephrine, normetanephrine, 3-methoxy-4-hydroxymandelic acid (VMA), and other metabolites provides a measure of the total body production of catecholamines, a measure useful in diagnosing conditions such as pheochromocytoma. Blockade of MAO increases stores of catecholamines and has both therapeutic and toxicologic potential.

C. **Receptor Characteristics:** The major receptor systems in the ANS include the following:
   1. **Cholinoceptors:** Also referred to as cholinergic receptors, these molecules respond to acetylcholine and its analogues. Cholinoceptors are subdivided as follows (see Table 6–2):
      a. **Muscarinic receptors:** As their name suggests, these receptors respond to muscarine as well as acetylcholine. The effects of activation of these receptors resemble those of postganglionic parasympathetic nerve stimulation. Muscarinic receptors are located primarily on autonomic effector cells (including heart, vascular endothelium, smooth muscle, presynaptic nerve terminals, and exocrine glands). Evidence has been found for five subtypes, of which three are well-defined.
      b. **Nicotinic receptors:** These receptors respond to nicotine, another acetylcholine analogue. The two major subtypes are located in ganglia and in skeletal muscle endplates. The nicotinic receptors are the primary receptors for transmission at these sites.
   2. **Adrenoceptors:** Also referred to as adrenergic receptors, adrenoceptors are divided into several subtypes (Table 6–3).
      a. **Alpha receptors:** Alpha receptors are located on vascular smooth muscle, presynaptic nerve terminals, blood platelets, and fat cells (lipocytes) and in the brain. Alpha receptors are further divided into two major types, α_1 and α_2.
      b. **Beta receptors:** Beta receptors are located on most types of smooth muscle, cardiac muscle, some presynaptic nerve terminals, and lipocytes, as well as in the brain. Beta receptors are divided into three major subtypes, β_1, β_2, and β_3.
   3. **Dopamine receptors:** Dopamine receptors are a subclass of adrenoceptors, but with rather different distribution and function. Dopamine receptors are especially important in the renal and splanchnic vessels and in the brain. Although at least two subtypes exist, the

---

* Botulinum has been used by local injection to achieve a medically useful selective effect.

Table 6–2. Characteristics of the most important cholinoceptors in the ANS.

Receptor	Location	Mechanism	Major Functions
M_1	Nerve endings	G_q-coupled	↑IP_3, DAG cascade
M_2	Heart, some nerve endings	G_i-coupled	↓cAMP, activates K channels
M_3	Effector cells: smooth muscle, glands, endothelium	G_q-coupled	↑IP_3, DAG cascade
N_N	ANS ganglia	Ion channel	Depolarizes, evokes action potential
N_M	Neuromuscular endplate	Ion channel	Depolarizes, evokes action potential

D_1 or DA_1 subtype appears to be the most important peripheral effector-cell dopamine receptor. D_2 (DA_2) receptors are found on presynaptic nerve terminals; both D_1 and D_2 types occur in the CNS.

D. Effects of Activating Autonomic Nerves: Each division of the ANS has specific effects on organ systems. These effects, summarized in Table 6–4, should be memorized.

Dually innervated organs—such as the iris of the eye and the sinoatrial node of the heart—receive both sympathetic and parasympathetic innervation. The pupil has a natural, intrinsic, diameter to which it returns when the influence of both divisions of the ANS is removed. Pharmacologic ganglionic blockade will therefore cause it to move to its intrinsic size. Similarly, the cardiac sinus rate has an intrinsic value in the absence of both ANS inputs. How will these variables change (increase or decrease) if the ganglia are blocked? The answer is predictable if one knows which system is dominant. For example, both the pupil and, in young individuals, the SA node are dominated by the parasympathetic system. The resting pupil diameter and sinus rate are therefore under considerable PANS influence. Therefore, blockade of both systems, with removal of the dominant PANS effect, will result in mydriasis and tachycardia.

E. Sites of Autonomic Drug Action: Because of the number of steps in the transmission of autonomic commands from the CNS to the effector, there are many sites at which autonomic drugs may act. These sites include the CNS centers, the ganglia, the postganglionic nerve terminals, the effector cell receptors, and the mechanisms responsible for termination of transmitter action. The most selective block is achieved by drugs acting at receptors that mediate very selective actions (see Table 6–5). In addition, many natural and synthetic toxins have significant effects on autonomic and somatic nerve function. Some of these toxins are listed in Table 6–5.

F. Nonadrenergic, Noncholinergic Transmission: Some nerve fibers in autonomic effector tissues do not show the histochemical characteristics of either cholinergic or adrenergic fibers. Some of these are motor fibers that cause the release of ATP and possibly other purines related to it. Purine-evoked responses have been identified in the bronchi, gastrointestinal tract, and

Table 6–3. Characteristics of some important adrenoceptors in the ANS.

Receptor	Location	G Protein	Second Messenger	Major Functions
α_1	Effector tissues: smooth muscle, glands	G_q	↑IP_3, DAG	↑Ca^{2+}, cause contraction, secretion
α_2	Nerve endings, some smooth muscle	G_i	↓cAMP	↓Transmitter release, cause contraction
β_1	Cardiac muscle, juxtaglomerular apparatus	G_s	↑cAMP	↑Heart rate, force; ↑ renin release
β_2	Smooth muscle	G_s	↑cAMP	Relax smooth muscle; ↑ glycogenolysis; ↑ heart rate, force
β_3	Adipose cells	G_s	↑cAMP	↑Lipolysis
D_1	Smooth muscle	G_s	↑cAMP	Relax renal vascular smooth muscle

Table 6–4. Direct effects of autonomic nerve activity and autonomic drugs on some organ systems.

Organ	Effect of			
	Sympathetic		Parasympathetic	
	Action[1]	Receptor[2]	Action	Receptor[2]
Eye				
Iris				
Radial muscle	Contracts	α_1	. . .	. . .
Circular muscle	. . .	. . .	Contracts	M_3
Ciliary muscle	[Relaxes]	β	Contracts	M_3
Heart				
Sinoatrial node	Accelerates	β_1	Decelerates	M_2
Ectopic pacemakers	Accelerates	β_1	. . .	. . .
Contractility	Increases	β_1	Decreases (atria)	M_2
Vascular smooth muscle				
Skin, splanchnic vessels	Contracts	α	. . .	. . .
Skeletal muscle vessels	Relaxes	β_2	. . .	. . .
	[Contracts]	α	. . .	. . .
	Relaxes	M^4	. . .	. . .
Endothelium	. . .	. . .	Releases EDRF	$M_3{}^3$
Bronchiolar smooth muscle	Relaxes	β_2	Contracts	M_3
Gastrointestinal tract				
Smooth muscle				
Walls	Relaxes	$\alpha_2{}^5, \beta_2$	Contracts	M_3
Sphincters	Contracts	α_1	Relaxes	M_3
Secretion	. . .	. . .	Increases	M_3
Myenteric plexus	Inhibits	α	Activates	M_1
Genitourinary smooth muscle				
Bladder wall	Relaxes	β_2	Contracts	M_3
Sphincter	Contracts	α_1	Relaxes	M_3
Uterus, pregnant	Relaxes	β_2		
	Contracts	α	Contracts	M_3
Penis, seminal vesicles	Ejaculation	α	Erection	M
Skin				
Pilomotor smooth muscle	Contracts	α	. . .	. . .
Sweat glands				
Thermoregulatory	Increases	M	. . .	. . .
Apocrine (stress)	Increases	α	. . .	. .
Metabolic functions				
Liver	Gluconeogenesis	$\alpha/\beta_2{}^6$	. . .	. . .
Liver	Glycogenolysis	α/β_2	. . .	. . .
Fat cells	Lipolysis	$\beta_3{}^7$	. . .	. . .
Kidney	Renin release	β_1	. . .	. . .
Autonomic nerve endings				
Sympathetic			Decreases NE release	M
Parasympathetic	Decreases ACh release	α		

[1] Less important actions are in brackets.
[2] Specific receptor type: α = alpha, β = beta, M = muscarinic. Muscarinic receptor subtypes are determined mostly in animal tissues.
[3] The endothelium of most blood vessels releases EDRF (endothelium-derived relaxing factor), which causes marked vasodilation, in response to muscarinic stimuli. However, unlike the receptors innervated by sympathetic cholinergic fibers in skeletal muscle blood vessels, these muscarinic receptors are not innervated and respond only to circulating muscarinic agonists.
[4] Vascular smooth muscle in skeletal muscle has sympathetic cholinergic dilator fibers.
[5] Probably through presynaptic inhibition of parasympathetic activity.
[6] Depends on species.
[7] Alpha$_2$ inhibits; β_1 and β_3 stimulate.

urinary tract. Other motor fibers are peptidergic, ie, they release peptides as the primary transmitters (see list above under Cotransmitters).

Other nonadrenergic, noncholinergic fibers have the anatomic characteristics of sensory fibers and contain peptides that are stored in and released from the fiber terminals. These fibers have been termed "sensory-efferent" or "sensory-local effector" fibers because, when activated by a sensory input, they are capable of releasing transmitter peptides from the sensory ending

Table 6–5. Steps in autonomic transmission: Effects of drugs.

Process	Drug Example	Site	Action
Action potential propagation	Local anesthetics, tetrodotoxin[1], saxitoxin[2]	Nerve axons	Block sodium channels; block conduction
Transmitter synthesis	Hemicholinium	Cholinergic nerve terminals: membrane	Blocks uptake of choline and slows synthesis of ACh
	Methyltyrosine (metyrosine)	Adrenergic terminals: cytoplasm	Blocks synthesis of NE
Transmitter storage	Vesamicol	Cholinergic terminals: vesicles	Prevents storage of ACh
	Reserpine	Adrenergic terminals: vesicles	Prevents storage of NE
Transmitter release	Many[3]	Nerve terminal membrane receptors	Modulate release
	ω-Conotoxin GVIA[4]	Nerve terminal calcium channels	Reduces transmitter release
	Botulinus toxin (botulin)	Cholinergic vesicles	Prevents release
	Latrotoxin[5]	Cholinergic and adrenergic vesicles	Causes explosive release
	Tyramine, amphetamine	Adrenergic nerve terminals	Promote release of NE
Transmitter reuptake after release	Cocaine, tricyclic antidepressants	Adrenergic nerve terminals	Inhibit reuptake; increase transmitter effect on post-synaptic receptors
	6-Hydroxydopamine	Adrenergic nerve terminals	Destroys the terminal
Receptor activation/blockade	Norepinephrine	Receptors at adrenergic synapses	Binds and activates α receptors, causes contraction
	Phentolamine	Receptors at adrenergic synapses	Binds and blocks α receptors
	Isoproterenol	Receptors at adrenergic synapses	Binds and activates β receptors
	Propranolol	Receptors at adrenergic synapses	Binds and blocks β receptors
	Nicotine	Receptors at nicotinic synapses	Binds and activates; opens ion channels and depolarizes
	Tubocurarine	Receptors at nicotinic synapses	Binds and blocks nicotinic ion channels
	Bethanechol	Receptors at muscarinic junctions	Binds and activates M receptors
	Atropine	Receptors at muscarinic junctions	Binds and blocks M receptors
Enzymatic inactivation of transmitter	Neostigmine	Cholinergic synapses (cholinesterase)	Inhibits enzyme; prolongs and amplifies transmitter action
	Tranylcypromine	Adrenergic nerve terminals (monoamine oxidase)	Inhibits enzyme; increases stored transmitter

[1] Toxin of the puffer fish, California newt.
[2] Toxin of Gonyaulax (red tide organism).
[3] Norepinephrine, dopamine, acetylcholine, angiotensin II, various prostaglandins.
[4] Toxin of a marine snail.
[5] Black widow spider venom.

itself, from local axon branches, and from collaterals that terminate in the autonomic ganglia. These peptides are potent agonists in many autonomic effector tissues.

G. Integration of Autonomic Function: Functional integration is provided mainly through the mechanism of negative feedback. This process utilizes modulatory pre- and postsynaptic receptors at the local level and homeostatic reflexes at the systemic level.

    1. Local integration: Local feedback control has been found at the level of the nerve endings in many systems. The best documented of these is the negative feedback of norepinephrine upon its own release from the presynaptic adrenergic terminals. This effect is mediated by α_2 receptors located on the presynaptic nerve membrane (Figure 6–3).

Noradrenergic nerve terminal

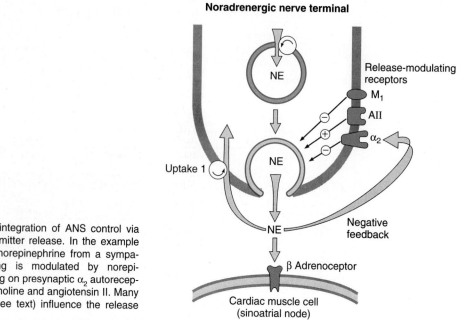

Figure 6–3. Local integration of ANS control via modulation of transmitter release. In the example shown, release of norepinephrine from a sympathetic nerve ending is modulated by norepinephrine itself, acting on presynaptic α_2 autoreceptors, and by acetylcholine and angiotensin II. Many other modulators (see text) influence the release process.

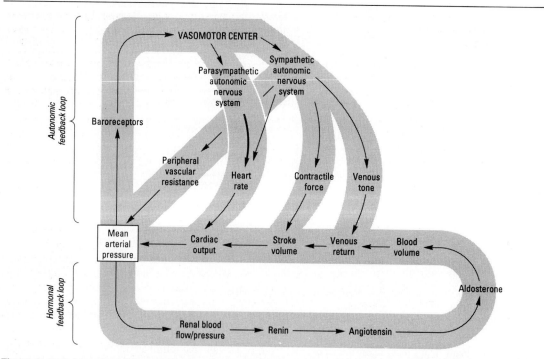

Figure 6–4. Autonomic and hormonal control of cardiovascular function. Note that two feedback loops are present, the autonomic nervous system loop and the hormonal loop. In addition, each major loop has several components. Thus, the sympathetic nervous system directly influences four major variables: peripheral vascular resistance, heart rate, force, and venous tone. The parasympathetic directly influences heart rate. Angiotensin II directly increases peripheral vascular resistance (not shown), and the sympathetic nervous system directly increases renin secretion (not shown). Because these control mechanisms are designed to maintain normal blood pressure, the net feedback effect of each loop is negative; feedback tends to compensate for the change in arterial blood pressure that evoked the response. Thus, decreased blood pressure due to blood loss would be compensated by increased sympathetic outflow and renin release. Conversely, elevated pressure due to the administration of a vasoconstricting drug would cause reduced sympathetic outflow and renin release, and increased parasympathetic (vagal) outflow.

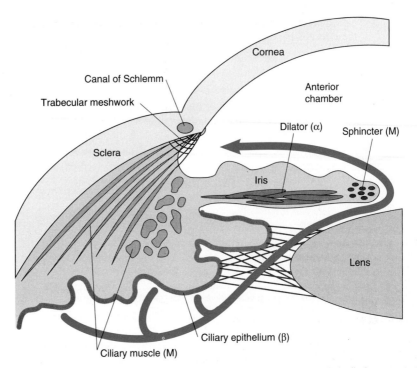

Figure 6–5. Some pharmacologic targets in the eye. The diagram illustrates clinically important structures and their receptors. (M, muscarinic; α, alpha receptor; β, beta receptor.) The heavy arrow (color) indicates the flow of aqueous humor.

Presynaptic receptors that regulate the release of their own transmitter substance are called autoreceptors. Inhibitory control of transmitter release is not limited to inhibition by the transmitter itself. Adrenergic nerve terminals also carry other receptors (heteroreceptors) for acetylcholine (M_1 receptors), histamine, serotonin, prostaglandins, and polypeptides. Presynaptic regulation by a variety of endogenous chemicals probably occurs in all nerve fibers.

Postsynaptic receptors, including two types of muscarinic and at least one type of peptidergic receptor, have been found in ganglionic synapses where nicotinic transmission is primary. These receptors may facilitate or inhibit transmission by evoking slow excitatory or inhibitory postsynaptic potentials (EPSPs or IPSPs).

2. **Systemic reflexes:** Systemic reflexes include mechanisms that regulate blood pressure, especially the baroreceptor neural reflex and the renin-angiotensin-aldosterone hormonal response. (See Figure 6–4.) These homeostatic mechanisms attempt to maintain mean arterial blood pressure at a level determined by the vasomotor center. Any deviation from this blood pressure "set-point" causes a change in ANS activity and renin-angiotensin II-aldosterone levels. These changes are very important in determining the response to conditions or drugs that alter blood pressure. For example, a decrease in blood pressure caused by hemorrhage causes increases in SANS discharge and renin release. Peripheral vascular resistance and venous tone, and heart rate and force are increased by norepinephrine released from sympathetic nerves. Blood volume is replenished by retention of salt and water in the kidney, under the influence of increased levels of aldosterone. These compensatory responses may be large enough to overcome some of the actions of drugs. For example, the treatment of hypertension with a vasodilator such as hydralazine will be unsuccessful if the compensatory tachycardia (via the baroreceptor reflex) and the salt and water retention (via the renin system response) are not prevented through the use of additional drugs. It is therefore essential that the student understand this homeostatic system.

3. **Complex organ control—the eye:** The eye contains multiple tissues with various functions, most of them under autonomic control (Figure 6–5). The pupil, discussed above, is under reciprocal control by the SANS (via alpha receptors) and the PANS (via muscarinic receptors) acting on two different muscles in the iris. The ciliary muscle, which controls accommodation, is under primary control of muscarinic receptors innervated by the PANS, with insignificant contributions from the SANS. The ciliary *epithelium,* on the other hand,

has important beta receptors that appear to facilitate aqueous humor secretion. Each of these receptors is an important target of drugs that are discussed in the following chapters.

DRUG LIST

The following drugs or metabolites are mentioned in this chapter. It is important to know which ones occur in the normal ANS and what their functions are. For those not normally found in the ANS, it is important to know the effects of their administration.

Acetylcholine	3-Methoxy-4-hydroxymandelic acid (VMA)[1]
Amphetamine	Metyrosine (α-methyltyrosine)
Atropine	Neostigmine
Botulinum toxin[1]	Norepinephrine
Cocaine	Propranolol
DOPA	Reserpine
Dopamine	Saxitoxin[1]
Epinephrine	Tetrodotoxin[1]
Guanethidine	Tyramine
Metanephrine[1]	Vesamicol[1]

[1] Not discussed in succeeding chapters; should be learned with this chapter.

QUESTIONS

DIRECTIONS: Each of the numbered items or incomplete statements in this section is followed by answers or by completions of the sentence. Select the ONE lettered answer or completion that is BEST in each case.

1. In the autonomic regulation of blood pressure,
    (A) Cardiac output is maintained constant at the expense of other hemodynamic variables
    (B) Elevation of blood pressure results in elevated aldosterone secretion
    (C) Baroreceptor nerve endings decrease firing rate when arterial pressure increases
    (D) Stroke volume and mean arterial blood pressure are the primary direct determinants of cardiac output
    (E) A condition that reduces the sensitivity of the sensory baroreceptor nerve endings might cause an increase in sympathetic discharge
2. Activation of alpha$_1$ receptors is associated with
    (A) Cardioacceleration
    (B) Vasodepression (vasodilation)
    (C) Pupillary dilation (mydriasis)
    (D) Bronchodilation
    (E) All of the above
3. Probable effects of giving a "pure" arteriolar vasodilator (one that does not act on autonomic receptors) would include
    (A) Tachycardia and increased cardiac contractility
    (B) Tachycardia and decreased cardiac output
    (C) Decreased mean arterial pressure and decreased cardiac contractility
    (D) No change in mean arterial pressure and decreased cardiac contractility
    (E) No change in mean arterial pressure and increased salt and water excretion by the kidney
4. Full activation of the sympathetic nervous system, as in maximal exercise, can produce all of the following responses EXCEPT
    (A) Mydriasis
    (B) Increased renal blood flow
    (C) Decreased intestinal motility
    (D) Bronchial relaxation
    (E) Increased heart rate (tachycardia)

Items 5–7: For the following three questions, use the accompanying diagram. Assume the diagram can represent either the parasympathetic or the sympathetic nervous system.

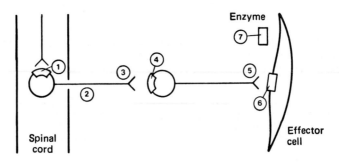

5. Which of the following drugs acts at site 3?
   (A) Tyramine
   (B) Reserpine
   (C) Botulinum toxin
   (D) 6-Hydroxydopamine
   (E) Cocaine

6. Acetylcholine does NOT interact at which one of the following sites in the diagram?
   (A) Site 2
   (B) Site 4
   (C) Site 5
   (D) Site 6
   (E) Site 7

7. Atropine is a useful drug for inducing dilation of the pupil and paralysis of accommodation. These effects of atropine occur at which one of the following sites on the diagram?
   (A) Site 3
   (B) Site 4
   (C) Site 5
   (D) Site 6
   (E) Site 7

8. Mr. Brown has recently had a successful cardiac transplant operation in which his badly damaged and failing heart was replaced by a healthy donor organ. Which of the following drugs would be expected to have the SMALLEST effect on his heart function, as compared to the function of a normal heart?
   (A) Tyramine
   (B) Norepinephrine
   (C) Propranolol
   (D) Bethanechol
   (E) Isoproterenol

9. "Nicotinic" sites include all of the following EXCEPT
   (A) Parasympathetic ganglia
   (B) Sympathetic ganglia
   (C) Skeletal muscle
   (D) Excitatory receptors on Renshaw cells in the spinal cord
   (E) Bronchial smooth muscle

10. The anticholinergic effects of botulinum toxin
    (A) Are caused by acetylcholine receptor blockade
    (B) Occur in preganglionic nerve endings
    (C) Are irreversible
    (D) Are treated with choline infusions
    (E) Are not seen at somatic motor nerve endings at skeletal muscle

DIRECTIONS: The following section consists of a list of four to twenty-six lettered options followed by several numbered items. For each numbered item, select the ONE option that is most closely associated with it. Each answer may be selected once, more than once, or not at all.

(A) Acetylcholine   (F) Metyrosine
(B) Amphetamine   (G) Norepinephrine
(C) Botulinum toxin   (H) Reserpine
(D) Dopamine   (I) Tetrodotoxin
(E) Epinephrine   (J) Vesamicol

11. Agent that is normally released from sympathetic nerve endings innervating thermoregulatory sweat glands

12. Drug that blocks propagation of action potentials in all nerves

13. Drug that inhibits the synthesis of catecholamines such as norepinephrine

14. Indirectly acting drug that releases norepinephrine and dopamine from their nerve endings

15. Drug that prevents the storage of acetylcholine in its vesicles

ANSWERS

1. Baroreceptors increase their firing rate with increased blood pressure. Therefore, a decrease in baroreceptor sensitivity would decrease input to the vasomotor center, which would be interpreted by the vasomotor center as a decrease in blood pressure. This would lead to an increase in sympathetic outflow. The answer is **(E)**. (If you chose a different answer, review the components of the autonomic and hormonal feedback loops for the maintenance of blood pressure, Figure 6–4).

2. Mydriasis can be caused by contraction of the radial fibers of the iris; these smooth muscle cells have alpha-receptors. All the other responses are beta-mediated (Table 6–4). The answer is **(C)**.

3. Because of the baroreceptor reflex, a drug that directly decreases total peripheral resistance will cause a reflex increase in sympathetic outflow, a decrease in parasympathetic outflow, and an increase in renin release. As a result, heart rate and cardiac force will increase. (In addition, salt and water retention will occur.) The answer is **(A)**.

4. Sympathetic autonomic outflow causes constriction of the renal resistance vessels and a fall in renal blood flow. This is the typical response in severe exercise or hypotension. The answer is **(B)**.

5. Each of these agents has a different mechanism of action, yet all but one act on the sympathetic postganglionic nerve terminal (Site 5). Site 3 is a cholinergic nerve ending. The answer is **(C)**.

6. Acetylcholine acts at both the nicotinic ganglionic receptor (Site 4) and at muscarinic receptors on effector cells (Site 6) and presynaptic nerve endings (Site 5). ACh also interacts with acetylcholinesterase (Site 7) but does not influence electrical transmission in axons (Site 2). The answer is **(A)**.

7. In the simplified diagram, the muscarinic receptors blocked by atropine are located only at the smooth muscle effector cells and postganglionic nerve terminals. This type of receptor is also found in ganglia, but higher concentrations of atropine are required to block it. Blocking presynaptic muscarinic receptors would not produce mydriasis and cycloplegia. The answer is **(D)**.

8. Cardiac transplantation requires cutting all postsynaptic sympathetic and presynaptic parasympathetic nerves to the heart. As a result, sympathetic postganglionic nerve endings degenerate and stores of norepinephrine greatly diminish. A drug that acts by releasing stored norepinephrine (ie, an indirectly acting sympathomimetic such as tyramine) will have a greatly reduced effect on a transplanted heart. Directly acting drugs will be unaffected or may produce a greater effect due to receptor up-regulation. The answer is **(A)**.

9. Both types of ganglia and the neuromuscular junction have nicotinic cholinoceptors. Bronchial smooth muscle contains muscarinic cholinoceptors. The Renshaw cell was one of the first central neurons shown to respond to acetylcholine (review physiology of the spinal cord). The answer is **(E)**.

10. Botulinum toxin (botulin) impairs all types of cholinergic transmission, including preganglionic nerve endings and somatic motor nerve endings. The toxin does so by preventing discharge of transmitter vesicles at cholinergic nerve endings. Synthesis of the transmitter is not impaired, so infusion of choline is of no value. The effects of this toxin are very long-lasting but are not irreversible. The answer is **(B)**.

11. Acetylcholine is the transmitter at sympathetic nerve endings innervating thermoregulatory sweat glands. Cholinergic transmission at sympathetic postganglionic nerve endings also occurs to a limited extent in the blood vessels of skeletal muscle. The answer is **(A)**.

12. Tetrodotoxin (and saxitoxin) block propagation of action potentials in all vertebrate nerve axons by blocking voltage-gated sodium channels. The answer is **(I)**.

13. Metyrosine reduces the synthesis of catecholamines such as norepinephrine by inhibiting the rate-limiting enzyme, tyrosine hydroxylase (Figure 6–2). The answer is **(F)**.

14. Amphetamine causes the release of norepinephrine and dopamine from their nerve endings.

Tyramine, a component of certain fermented foods (eg, cheeses, pickled fish, and some wines) has the same effect. The answer is (B).

15. Vesamicol prevents the storage of acetylcholine in its vesicles by inhibiting the carrier molecule that normally transports acetylcholine into the vesicle (Figure 6–2). The answer is (J).

Cholinoceptor-Activating & Cholinesterase-Inhibiting Drugs

7

OBJECTIVES

You should be able to:

- List the locations and types of acetylcholine receptors in the major organ systems (CNS, autonomic ganglia, eye, heart, vessels, bronchi, gut, genitourinary tract, skeletal muscle, exocrine glands).
- Describe the effects of acetylcholine on the major organs.
- Relate the different pharmacokinetic properties of the various choline esters and cholinomimetic alkaloids to their chemical properties.
- List the major clinical uses of cholinomimetic agonists.
- Describe the pharmacodynamic differences between direct- and indirect-acting cholinomimetic agents.
- List the major signs and symptoms of (1) acute nicotine toxicity and (2) organophosphate insecticide poisoning.

Learn the definitions that follow.

Table 7–1. Definitions.

Term	Definition
Choline ester	A cholinomimetic drug consisting of choline (an alcohol) esterified with an acidic substance, eg, acetic or carbamic acid
Cholinergic crisis	The clinical condition of excessive activation of cholinoceptors
Cholinomimetic alkaloid	A drug with weakly basic properties (usually of plant origin) whose effects resemble those of acetylcholine
Cyclospasm	Marked contraction of the ciliary muscle; maximum accommodation
Direct-acting cholinomimetic	A drug that binds and activates cholinoceptors; the effects mimic those of acetylcholine
Endothelium-derived relaxing factor, EDRF	A potent vasodilator substance, largely nitric oxide, released from vascular endothelial cells
Indirect-acting cholinomimetic	A drug that amplifies the effects of endogenous acetylcholine by inhibiting acetylcholinesterase
Muscarinic agonist	A cholinomimetic with primarily muscarine-like actions
Myasthenic crisis	The clinical condition of inadequate activation of nicotinic neuromuscular junction cholinoceptors
Nicotinic agonist	A cholinomimetic with primarily nicotine-like actions
Organophosphate	An ester of phosphoric acid and an organic alcohol that inhibits cholinesterase
Organophosphate aging	A process whereby the organophosphate is chemically modified after binding to cholinesterase and becomes more firmly bound to the enzyme
Parasympathomimetic	A drug whose effects resemble the effects of stimulating the parasympathetic nerves

CONCEPTS

Acetylcholine-like drugs (cholinomimetics) are subdivided in two ways: on the basis of their mode of action (ie, whether they act directly at the acetylcholine receptor [cholinoceptor] or indirectly through inhibition of cholinesterase); and for those that act directly, on the basis of their spectrum of action (ie, whether they act on muscarinic or nicotinic receptors, see Figure 7–1). Acetylcholine may be considered the prototype that acts directly at both muscarinic and nicotinic receptors. Neostigmine is a prototype for the indirect-acting cholinesterase inhibitors (see Appendix I, Keywords).

DIRECT-ACTING CHOLINOMIMETIC AGONISTS

A group of choline esters (acetylcholine, methacholine, carbachol, and bethanechol) and a second group of naturally occurring alkaloids (muscarine, pilocarpine, nicotine, lobeline) comprise this subclass. The members differ in their spectrum of action (amount of muscarinic versus nicotinic stimulation) and in their pharmacokinetics (Table 7–2). Both factors influence their clinical use.

A. Classification: Muscarinic agonists are parasympathomimetic, ie, they mimic the actions of parasympathetic nerve stimulation. Five subgroups of muscarinic receptors have been identified (Table 7–3), but selective agonists for these receptor subtypes are not available for clinical use. Nicotinic agonists are classified on the basis of whether ganglionic or neuromuscular stimulation predominates; agonist selectivity is very limited, however. Nevertheless, relatively selective *antagonists* are available for the two nicotinic receptor types (Chapter 8).

B. Molecular Mechanisms of Action:
  1. Muscarinic mechanism: Several molecular mechanisms of muscarinic action have been defined (Table 7–3). One involves G protein-coupling of muscarinic receptors (especially M_1 and M_3 receptors) to phospholipase C, a membrane-bound enzyme, leading to the release of the second messengers diacylglycerol (DAG) and inositol-1,4,5-trisphosphate (IP_3). DAG modulates the action of protein kinase C, an enzyme important in secretion, while IP_3 evokes the release of calcium from intracellular storage sites, which results in contraction. A second mechanism couples muscarinic receptors (especially M_2 receptors) to adenylyl cyclase through the inhibitory G_i coupling protein. A third mechanism couples the same receptors directly to potassium channels in the heart and elsewhere; muscarinic agonists facilitate opening of these channels.
  2. Nicotinic mechanism: The mechanism of nicotinic action has been clearly defined as a direct coupling of the nicotinic receptor to the opening of ion channels selective for sodium and potassium (ACh channels) on ganglion cells and the neuromuscular endplate. The ACh receptor is located on the channel protein. When the receptor is activated, the channel opens and depolarization of the cell (an excitatory postsynaptic potential, EPSP) results. The EPSP, if large enough, evokes a propagated action potential in the surrounding membrane.

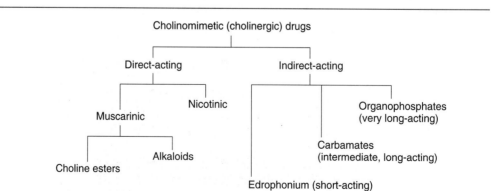

Figure 7–1. Subgroups of cholinomimetic drugs.

Table 7–2. Cholinomimetics: spectrum of action and pharmacokinetics.

Drug	Spectrum of Action[1]	Pharmacokinetic Features
Direct-acting Acetylcholine	B	Rapidly hydrolyzed by cholinesterase (ChE); 5–30 sec duration of action
Bethanechol	M	Resistant to ChE, orally active, poor lipid solubility, 30 min–2 h duration of action
Carbachol	B	Like bethanechol
Pilocarpine	M	Not an ester, good lipid solubility, 30 min–2 h duration of action
Nicotine	N	Like pilocarpine, duration 1–6 h
Indirect-acting Edrophonium	B	Alcohol, quaternary amine, poor lipid solubility, orally inactive, 5–15 min duration of action
Neostigmine	B	Carbamate, quaternary amine, poor lipid solubility, orally active, 30 min–2 h duration
Physostigmine	B	Carbamate, tertiary amine, lipid soluble, 30 min–2 h duration of action
Pyridostigmine, ambenonium	B	Carbamates like neostigmine, duration of action 4–8 h
Echothiophate	B	Organophosphate, moderate lipid solubility, 2–7 day duration
Parathion	B	Organophosphate, high lipid solubility, 7–30 day duration

[1] M, muscarinic; N, nicotinic; B, both.

C. Tissue & Organ Effects: The tissue and organ system effects are summarized in Table 7–4. Note that vasodilation is not parasympathomimetic (ie, it is not evoked by parasympathetic nerve discharge, even though directly acting cholinomimetics cause vasodilation). This action results from the release of endothelium-derived relaxing factor (EDRF: nitric oxide and, possibly, other substances) in the vessels, mediated by uninnervated muscarinic receptors on the endothelial cells. Note also that decreased blood pressure evokes the baroreceptor reflex, resulting in strong compensatory sympathetic discharge to the heart. As a result, injections of small-to-moderate amounts of direct-acting muscarinic cholinomimetics cause tachycardia, not bradycardia.

The tissue and organ level effects of nicotinic ganglionic stimulation depend on the autonomic innervation of the organ involved. The blood vessels are dominated by sympathetic innervation; therefore, nicotinic receptor activation results in vasoconstriction mediated by sympathetic postganglionic nerve discharge. The gut is dominated by parasympathetic control; nicotinic drugs increase motility and secretion because of increased parasympathetic postganglionic neuron discharge. Nicotinic neuromuscular endplate activation by direct-acting drugs results in fasciculations and spasm of the muscles involved. Prolonged activation, which results in paralysis (see Chapter 26), is an important hazard of exposure to nicotine-containing and organophosphate insecticides.

Table 7–3. Identified or cloned cholinoceptors.

Receptor Type	Other Names	Postreceptor Mechanisms
M_1	M_{1a}	↑IP_3, DAG cascade
M_2	M_{2a}, cardiac M_2	↓cAMP production
M_3	M_{2b}, glandular M_2	↑IP_3, DAG cascade
m_4[1]		↓cAMP production
m_5[1]		↑IP_3, DAG cascade
N_M	Endplate receptor	Na,K depolarizing channel
N_N	Ganglion receptor	Na,K depolarizing channel

[1] Cloned; functional receptors have not been identified conclusively.

Table 7–4. Effects of direct-acting cholinoceptor stimulants. Only the direct effects are indicated; homeostatic responses to these direct actions may be important.

Organ	Response
Central nervous system	Complex stimulatory effects; eg, nicotine (elevation of mood), physostigmine (convulsions)
Eye Sphincter muscle of iris	Contraction (miosis)
Ciliary muscle	Contraction for near vision
Heart Sinoatrial node	Decrease in rate (negative chronotropy) but note important reflex response (text)
Atria	Decrease in contractile strength (negative inotropy); decrease in refractory period
Atrioventricular node	Decrease in conduction velocity (negative dromotropy); increase in refractory period
Ventricles	Small decrease in contractile strength
Blood vessels	Dilation (via EDRF)
Bronchi	Contraction (bronchoconstriction)
Gastrointestinal tract Motility	Increase
Sphincters	Relaxation (via enteric nervous system)
Urinary bladder Detrusor	Contraction
Trigone and sphincter	Relaxation
Skeletal muscle	Activation of neuromuscular endplates; contraction of muscle
Glands	Increased secretion: thermoregulatory sweat, lacrimal, salivary, bronchial, gastric, intestinal glands

D. **Clinical Use:** We can predict the major clinical applications of the muscarinic agonists from a consideration of organs and diseases that benefit from an increase in cholinergic activity. They are summarized in Table 7–5. Direct-acting nicotinic agonists have no therapeutic applications except in producing skeletal muscle paralysis (succinylcholine, Chapter 26); indirect-acting agents are superior when increased nicotinic activation is needed (see below).

E. **Toxicity:** The signs and symptoms of overdosage are readily predicted from the general pharmacology of acetylcholine.
1. **Muscarinic toxicity:** These include CNS stimulation (uncommon with direct-acting agonists), miosis, spasm of accommodation, bronchoconstriction, increased gastrointestinal and genitourinary smooth muscle activity, increased secretory activity (sweat glands, airway, gastrointestinal tract), vasodilation, and bradycardia if administered as an intravenous bolus; reflex tachycardia otherwise.
2. **Nicotinic toxicity:** These include CNS stimulation, ganglionic stimulation, and neuromuscular endplate depolarization leading to fasciculations and paralysis. Nicotine is still used in some insecticides.

Table 7–5. Clinical applications of some cholinomimetics.

Drug	Clinical Applications	Action
Direct-acting agonists Bethanechol	Postoperative and neurogenic ileus and urinary retention	Activates bowel and bladder smooth muscle
Carbachol, pilocarpine	Glaucoma	Activates ciliary muscle of eye
Indirect-acting agonists Neostigmine	Postoperative and neurogenic ileus and urinary retention	Amplifies endogenous acetylcholine
Neostigmine, pyridostigmine, edrophonium	Myasthenia gravis, reversal of neuromuscular blockade	Amplifies endogenous acetylcholine; ↑ strength
Physostigmine, echothiophate	Glaucoma	Amplifies effects of ACh

INDIRECT-ACTING AGONISTS

A. Classification & Prototypes: The indirect-acting cholinomimetic drugs fall into two major chemical classes: carbamic acid esters (carbamates; neostigmine is a prototype) and phosphoric acid esters (phosphates, organophosphates; echothiophate is a prototype). Edrophonium is a special case; it is an alcohol (not an ester) with a very short duration of action.

B. Mechanism of Action: Both carbamate and organophosphate inhibitors bind to the enzyme and undergo prompt hydrolysis. The alcohol portion of the molecule is then released. The acidic portion (carbamate or phosphate) is released much more slowly, thus preventing the binding and hydrolysis of acetylcholine.

   1. Carbamates: Carbamates are hydrolyzed and the carbamate residue is released by cholinesterase over a period of 2–8 hours.

   2. Organophosphates: Organophosphates are long-acting drugs; they form an extremely stable phosphate complex with the enzyme and are released over periods of days to weeks.

C. Effects: By inhibiting cholinesterase, the indirect-acting agonists "amplify" the action of endogenous acetylcholine; ie, these agents cause an increase in the concentration and half-life of acetylcholine in synapses where ACh is released physiologically. Therefore, the indirect agents have muscarinic or nicotinic effects, depending on which organ system is under consideration. Cholinesterase inhibitors do not have therapeutic actions at sites where acetylcholine is not normally released.

D. Clinical Use: The major clinical applications of the indirect-acting cholinomimetics include both muscarinic and nicotinic effects. These effects are predictable based on a consideration of the organs and the diseases that benefit from an increase in cholinergic activity. The effects are summarized in Table 7–5. The carbamates, which include neostigmine, physostigmine, ambenonium, and pyridostigmine, are used more commonly in therapeutics than are organophosphates. Some carbamates (eg, carbaryl) are used in agriculture as insecticides. Three organophosphates used in medicine are echothiophate (an antiglaucoma drug), malathion (a scabicide), and metrifonate (an antihelmintic agent). A special use of edrophonium is in the diagnosis of myasthenia and in differentiating myasthenic from cholinergic crisis in patients with this disease. Because cholinergic crisis can result in muscle weakness like that of myasthenic crisis, distinguishing the two conditions may be difficult. Administration of a short-acting cholinomimetic such as edrophonium will improve myasthenic crisis but worsen cholinergic crisis.

E. Toxicity: In addition to their therapeutic uses, some indirect-acting agents have toxicologic importance because of potential accidental exposures to toxic amounts of pesticides. An example of intoxication is described in Case 1 (Appendix II). The most toxic of these drugs, (eg, parathion) are rapidly fatal if exposure is not immediately recognized and treated. Treatment is described in Chapter 8. After first binding to cholinesterase, most organophosphate inhibitors can be removed from the enzyme by the use of "regenerator" compounds such as pralidoxime (see Chapter 8). If the enzyme-inhibitor binding is allowed to persist, however, aging (a further chemical change) occurs and regenerator drugs no longer can remove the inhibitor. Because of their toxicity, organophosphates are used extensively in agriculture as insecticides and antihelmintic agents; examples include malathion and parathion. Some of these agents (eg, malathion, dichlorvos) are relatively safe in humans because they are metabolized rapidly to inactive products in mammals (and birds) but not in insects. Some are pro-drugs (eg, malathion, parathion) and must be metabolized to the active product (malaoxon from malathion, paraoxon from parathion). The signs and symptoms of poisoning are the same as those described for the direct-acting agents, with the following exceptions: vasodilation is a late and uncommon effect; bradycardia is more common than tachycardia; CNS stimulation is common with organophosphate and physostigmine overdosage, and includes convulsions, followed by respiratory and cardiovascular depression. The spectrum of toxicity can be remembered with the aid of the mnemonic "DUMBELS," which stands for diarrhea, urination, miosis, bronchoconstriction, excitation (of skeletal muscle and CNS), lacrimation, and salivation and sweating.

DRUG LIST

The following drugs are important members of the group discussed in this chapter. Prototypes should be learned in detail; the features of major variants should be known well enough to distinguish the variants from prototypes and from each other.

Subclass	Prototypes	Major Variants
Direct-acting drugs Muscarinic agonists	Acetylcholine	Muscarine, carbachol, bethanechol, pilocarpine
Nicotinic agonists	Acetylcholine	Nicotine, carbachol, succinylcholine
Indirect-acting drugs Alcohol	Edrophonium	
Carbamates	Neostigmine	Pyridostigmine, physostigmine, carbaryl
Organophosphates	Echothiophate	Parathion, DFP, malathion, dichlorvos

QUESTIONS

DIRECTIONS: Each of the numbered items or incomplete statements in this section is followed by answers or by completions of the sentence. Select the ONE lettered answer or completion that is BEST in each case.

1. Physostigmine and bethanechol in small doses have similar effects on all of the following EXCEPT
   (A) Neuromuscular junction (skeletal muscle)
   (B) Salivary glands
   (C) Ureteral tone
   (D) Sweat glands
   (E) Gastric secretion

2. Parathion has all of the following characteristics EXCEPT
   (A) It is less persistent in the environment than DDT
   (B) It is more toxic to humans than malathion
   (C) It is inactivated by conversion to paraoxon
   (D) It is very lipid soluble and is well absorbed through skin and lungs
   (E) Its toxicity, if treated early, may be partly reversed by pralidoxime

3. In the treatment of myasthenia gravis, the best agent for distinguishing between myasthenic crisis (insufficient therapy) and cholinergic crisis (excessive therapy) is
   (A) Atropine
   (B) Physostigmine
   (C) Echothiophate
   (D) Pralidoxime
   (E) Edrophonium

4. The cause of death from organophosphate "nerve gas" poisoning would probably be
   (A) Gastrointestinal bleeding
   (B) Hypertension
   (C) Respiratory failure
   (D) Congestive heart failure
   (E) Cardiac arrhythmia

5. Pyridostigmine and neostigmine may cause all of the following EXCEPT
   (A) Reversible inhibition of acetylcholinesterase
   (B) Spasm of accommodation
   (C) Constipation
   (D) Bronchoconstriction
   (E) Some direct nicotinic effects at the neuromuscular endplate

6. Parasympathetic nerve stimulation and a slow infusion of bethanechol will each increase
   (A) Heart rate
   (B) Bladder tone

(C) Both (A) and (B) are correct
(D) Neither (A) nor (B) is correct

7. In the human eye, echothiophate can cause all of the following EXCEPT
   (A) Miosis
   (B) Ciliary spasm
   (C) Reversal of the cycloplegic action of atropine
   (D) Decrease in the incidence of cataracts
   (E) Reduction in intraocular pressure

8. In the comparison of bethanechol and pilocarpine, all of the following are correct EXCEPT
   (A) Both are hydrolyzed by cholinesterase
   (B) Both may cause tachycardia
   (C) Both may increase sweating
   (D) Both activate muscarinic receptors
   (E) Both may increase gastrointestinal motility

9. Typical symptoms of cholinesterase inhibitor toxicity include all of the following EXCEPT
   (A) Nausea, vomiting, diarrhea
   (B) Salivation, sweating
   (C) Miosis
   (D) Paralysis of skeletal muscles
   (E) Paralysis of accommodation

10. Actions of cholinoceptor agonists and their clinical effects include
    (A) Cyclospasm, improved aqueous humor drainage (glaucoma)
    (B) Decreased gastrointestinal motility with resulting postoperative GI stasis (ileus)
    (C) Improved neuromuscular transmission and accelerated recovery (neuromuscular blockade)
    (D) Improved neuromuscular transmission and prevention of cholinergic crisis (myasthenia)
    (E) Both (A) and (C) are correct

DIRECTIONS: The following section consists of a list of four to twenty-six lettered options followed by several numbered items. For each numbered item, select the ONE option that is most closely associated with it. Each answer may be selected once, more than once, or not at all.

(A) Acetylcholine
(B) Pilocarpine
(C) Bethanechol
(D) Neostigmine
(E) Muscarine
(F) Nicotine
(G) Physostigmine
(H) Parathion
(I) Malathion
(J) Echothiophate

11. Direct-acting cholinomimetic that is lipid soluble and is favored in the treatment of glaucoma
12. Indirect-acting cholinomimetic with a duration of many days; used in the treatment of glaucoma
13. Indirect-acting carbamate cholinomimetic; poor lipid solubility; duration of action about 2–4 hours
14. Direct-acting cholinomimetic used for its mood-elevating action and as an insecticide
15. Direct-acting cholinomimetic derived from mushrooms; mainly muscarinic spectrum of action

ANSWERS

1. Because physostigmine acts on the enzyme cholinesterase, which is present at all cholinergic synapses, this drugs increases acetylcholine effects at the nicotinic junctions as well as muscarinic ones. Bethanechol, on the other hand, is a direct-acting agent that is selective for muscarinic junctions. The answer is **(A)**.
2. The "-thion" organophosphates (those containing the P=S bond) are activated, not inactivated, by conversion to "-oxon" (P=O) derivatives. The answer is **(C)**.

3. Since short-acting drugs are usually preferable for diagnostic use, we choose the shortest-acting cholinesterase inhibitor, edrophonium. The answer is **(E)**.

4. Respiratory failure, from neuromuscular paralysis or central nervous system depression, is by far the most important cause of acute deaths in cholinesterase inhibitor toxicity. The answer is **(C)**.

5. Cholinesterase inhibition is typically associated with increased (never decreased) bowel activity. The answer is **(C)**.

6. Choice **(A)** is not correct because the vagus slows the heart. The answer is **(B)**.

7. The long-acting cholinesterase inhibitors are associated with an increased incidence of cataracts in patients receiving them for glaucoma. All the other effects are typical muscarinic actions. The answer is **(D)**.

8. Neither bethanechol nor pilocarpine is hydrolyzed by acetylcholinesterase. The answer is **(A)**.

9. Questions referring to cholinesterase inhibitor toxicity are very common. Skeletal muscle paralysis results from prolonged depolarization of neuromuscular endplates (depolarizing blockade). Cholinomimetics cause cyclospasm, the opposite of paralysis of accommodation (cycloplegia). The answer is **(E)**.

10. Cholinesterase inhibitors may either improve or impair neuromuscular transmission: cholinergic crisis is caused by too much acetylcholine at the endplate. Cholinomimetics never decrease gastrointestinal motility, in fact, they may be used to reverse postoperative ileus. The answer is **(E)**.

11. Pilocarpine is the only direct-acting cholinomimetic on the list that is lipid soluble and also favored in the treatment of glaucoma. Nicotine is also direct acting and lipid soluble, but it is of no value in glaucoma. The answer is **(B)**.

12. Echothiophate is an organophosphate AChE inhibitor with a duration of many days; it is also used in the treatment of glaucoma. The answer is **(J)**.

13. Neostigmine is the prototypical, indirect-acting cholinomimetic; it is a quaternary (charged) substance with poor lipid solubility; its duration of action is about 2 to 4 hours. The answer is **(D)**.

14. Nicotine is a direct-acting cholinomimetic alkaloid with the properties noted. The answer is **(F)**.

15. Muscarine is derived from mushrooms, although the yield from its namesake fungus *Amanita muscaria* is relatively low. Larger amounts are found in other mushrooms, especially those of the *Inocybe* genus. The answer is **(E)**.

8

Cholinoceptor Blockers & Cholinesterase Regenerators

OBJECTIVES

You should be able to:

- Describe the effects of atropine on the major organ systems (CNS, eye, heart, vessels, bronchi, gut, genitourinary tract, exocrine glands, skeletal muscle).
- List the signs, symptoms, and treatment of atropine poisoning.
- List the major clinical indications and contraindications for the use of muscarinic antagonists.
- Describe the autonomic effects of the ganglion-blocking nicotinic antagonists.
- List one antimuscarinic agent promoted for each of the following special uses: mydriasis and cycloplegia; parkinsonism; peptic ulcer; asthma.

Learn the definitions that follow.

Table 8–1. Definitions.

Term	Definition
Atropine fever	Hyperthermia induced by antimuscarinic drugs; caused mainly by inhibition of sweating
Atropine flush	Marked cutaneous vasodilation of the arms and upper torso and head by antimuscarinic drugs; mechanism unknown
Cholinesterase regenerator	A chemical antagonist that binds the phosphorus of organophosphates and displaces acetylcholinesterase
Cycloplegia	Paralysis of accommodation
Depolarizing blockade	Flaccid skeletal muscle paralysis caused by persistent depolarization of the neuro-muscular endplate
Miotic	A drug that constricts the pupil
Mydriatic	A drug that dilates the pupil
Nondepolarizing blockade	Flaccid skeletal muscle paralysis caused by blockade of the nicotinic endplate receptor
Organophosphate aging	A chemical change in the organophosphate molecule that occurs after binding of the organophosphate to cholinesterase for a period of time; aging renders the enzyme-inhibitor complex less susceptible to hydrolysis
Parasympatholytic	A drug that blocks the muscarinic receptors of autonomic effector tissues and reduces the effects of parasympathetic nerve stimulation
Pharmacokinetic selectivity	Selectivity of effect that is achieved by local administration or special distribution, not by receptor selectivity

CONCEPTS

The cholinoceptor antagonists are readily grouped into subclasses on the basis of their spectrum of action (ie, whether the receptors they block are muscarinic or nicotinic, Figure 8–1). These drugs are pharmacologic antagonists. A special subgroup, the cholinesterase regenerators, are not receptor blockers, but rather are chemical antagonists of organophosphate cholinesterase inhibitors.

MUSCARINIC ANTAGONISTS

A. Classification & Pharmacokinetics:

    1. Classification of the muscarinic antagonists: Muscarinic antagonists can be subdivided according to their selectivity for M_1 receptors or the lack thereof. Although the division of muscarinic receptors into subgroups is well documented (Chapters 6, 7), only a few receptor-selective antagonists have reached clinical trials in the USA (eg, pirenzepine, telenzepine). All of the drugs in general use at present are nonselective. These blockers can be further subdivided on the basis of their primary clinical target organs (CNS, eye, bronchi, or gastrointestinal and genitourinary tracts). Drugs used for their effects on the CNS or the eyes must be sufficiently lipid soluble to cross lipid barriers. A major determinant of this

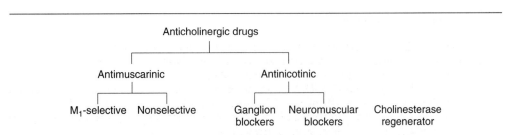

Figure 8–1. Subclasses of anticholinergic drugs and the cholinesterase regenerator discussed in this chapter. (The cholinesterase regenerators are not considered a part of the anticholinergic group.)

property is the presence or absence of a permanently charged (quaternary) amine group in the drug. This is because charged molecules are more polar and therefore less likely to penetrate a lipid barrier like the blood-brain barrier or the cornea of the eye. Atropine is the prototypical nonselective muscarinic blocker.

2. **Pharmacokinetics of atropine:** Atropine is an alkaloid found in *Atropa belladonna* and many other plants. Because it is a tertiary amine, atropine is relatively lipid soluble and readily crosses membrane barriers. The drug is well distributed into the CNS and other organs and is eliminated partially by metabolism in the liver and partially by renal excretion. The elimination half-life is approximately 2 hours, and the duration of action of normal doses is 4–8 hours except in the eye, where effects last for 72 hours or longer.

3. **Pharmacokinetics of other muscarinic blockers:** In ophthalmology, topical activity (the ability to enter the eye after conjunctival administration) and duration of action are important in determining the usefulness of several antimuscarinic drugs (see Clinical Uses). Similar ability to cross lipid barriers is important for the agents used in parkinsonism. In contrast, the drugs used for their antisecretory or antispastic actions in the gut and the bronchi are selected for minimum CNS activity; these drugs often incorporate quaternary amine groups to limit penetration through the blood-brain barrier.

B. **Mechanism of Action:** The muscarinic blocking agents act like competitive (surmountable) pharmacologic antagonists; their blocking effects can be overcome by increased concentrations of muscarinic agonists.

C. **Effects:** The peripheral actions of muscarinic blockers are mostly predictable effects derived from cholinoceptor blockade (Table 8–2). These include the ocular, GI, GU, and secretory effects. The CNS effects are less predictable. Those seen at therapeutic concentrations include sedation, reduction of motion sickness, and, as noted above, reduction of some of the signs of parkinsonism. Cardiovascular effects at therapeutic doses include an initial slowing of heart rate caused by stimulation of the central vagal nucleus, followed by the tachycardia and decreased atrioventricular conduction time that would be predicted from peripheral vagal blockade.

D. **Clinical Uses:** The muscarinic blockers have several useful therapeutic applications in the central nervous system, eye, bronchi, gut, and the urinary bladder. These uses are summarized in Table 8–3.

1. **CNS:** Scopolamine is a standard therapy for motion sickness; this drug is one of the most effective agents available for this condition. A transdermal patch formulation is available.

Table 8–2. Effects of muscarinic blocking drugs.

Organ	Effect	Mechanism
CNS	Sedation, antimotion sickness action, antiparkinson action, amnesia, delirium	Block of muscarinic receptors, unknown subtypes
Eye	Cycloplegia, mydriasis	Block of M_3 receptors
Bronchi	Bronchodilation, especially if constricted	Block of M_3 receptors
GI tract	Relaxation, slowed peristalsis	Block of M_1, M_3 receptors
GU tract	Relaxation of bladder wall, urinary retention	Block of M_3 receptors
Heart	Initial bradycardia, especially at low dose; then tachycardia	Initial bradycardia from stimulation of the vagal nucleus; tachycardia from block of M_2 receptors in the heart
Vessels	Block of muscarinic vasodilation; not manifest unless a muscarinic agonist is present	Block of M_3 receptors on endothelium of vessels
Glands	Marked reduction of salivation; moderate reduction of lacrimation, sweating; less reduction of gastric secretion	Block of M_1, M_3 receptors
Skeletal muscle	No effect	

Table 8–3. Some clinical applications of antimuscarinic drugs.

Organ System	Drugs[1]	Application
CNS	Benztropine, trihexyphenidyl, biperiden	Treat the manifestations of Parkinson's disease
	Scopolamine	Prevent or reduce motion sickness
Eye	Atropine, homatropine, cyclopentolate, tropicamide	Produce mydriasis and cycloplegia
Bronchi	Ipratropium	Bronchodilate in asthma and COPD[2]
GI	Glycopyrrolate, dicyclomine, methscopolamine	Reduce transient hypermotility; adjunct to other anti-ulcer drugs
GU	Oxybutynin, glycopyrrolate, dicyclomine	Treat transient cystitis; postoperative bladder spasms; incontinence (infrequent use)

[1] Only a few of many drugs are listed.
[2] COPD, chronic obstructive pulmonary disease.

Benztropine, biperiden, and trihexyphenidyl are representative of several antimuscarinic agents used in parkinsonism. Although not as effective as L-DOPA (see Chapter 27), these agents may be useful as adjuncts or when patients become unresponsive to L-DOPA. Benztropine is sometimes used parenterally to treat acute dystonias caused by antipsychotic medications.

2. **Eye:** Antimuscarinic drugs are used to dilate the pupil and to paralyze accommodation. They include (in descending order of duration of action) atropine (>72 hours), homatropine (24 hours), cyclopentolate (2–12 hours), and tropicamide (0.5–4 hours). These agents are all well-absorbed from the conjunctival sac into the eye.

3. **Bronchi:** Parenteral atropine has long been used to reduce airway secretions during surgery. Ipratropium is a quaternary antimuscarinic agent used by inhalation to reduce bronchoconstriction in asthma and chronic obstructive pulmonary disease (COPD). Although not as efficacious as beta agonists, ipratropium is less likely to cause cardiac arrhythmias. It has very few antimuscarinic effects outside the lungs because it is poorly absorbed and rapidly metabolized.

4. **Gut:** Atropine, methscopolamine, and propantheline have long been used in acid-peptic disease to reduce acid secretion, but they are not as effective as H_2-blockers such as cimetidine, and they cause more adverse effects. Pirenzepine is an investigational, M_1-selective, muscarinic blocker that may be more useful in peptic ulcer. Muscarinic blockers can also be used to reduce cramping and hypermotility in transient diarrheas, but opioids such as diphenoxylate (Chapter 30) are more effective.

5. **Bladder:** Glycopyrrolate, oxybutynin, methscopolamine, or similar agents may be used to reduce urgency in mild cystitis and to reduce bladder spasms following urologic surgery. Glycopyrrolate and methscopolamine are quaternary molecules that may have fewer CNS effects.

E. **Toxicity:** A traditional mnemonic for atropine toxicity is "Dry as a bone, red as a beet, mad as a hatter." This description reflects both predictable antimuscarinic effects and some unpredictable actions.

1. **Predictable toxicities:** Antimuscarinic actions lead to several important and potentially dangerous effects. In young children, blockade of thermoregulatory sweating may result in hyperthermia or "atropine fever." This is the most dangerous effect of the antimuscarinic drugs and is potentially lethal in infants. In adults, the condition is described by "dry as a bone" because sweating, salivation, and lacrimation are all significantly reduced or stopped. In the elderly, important additional targets include the eye (acute angle-closure glaucoma may occur) and the bladder (urinary retention is possible). Constipation and blurred vision are common adverse effects in all age groups.

2. **Other toxicities:** Toxicities not predictable from peripheral autonomic actions include the following.

   a. **CNS effects:** CNS toxicity includes sedation, amnesia, and delirium or hallucinations ("mad as a hatter"); convulsions may also develop. Central muscarinic receptors are probably involved.

    b. Cardiovascular effects: At toxic doses, intraventricular conduction may be blocked; this action is probably not mediated by muscarinic blockade and is difficult to treat. Dilation of the cutaneous vessels of the arms, head, neck, and trunk also occurs at these doses; the resulting "atropine flush" ("red as a beet") may be diagnostic of overdose with these drugs.

F. Contraindications: The antimuscarinic agents should be used cautiously in infants because of the danger of hyperthermia. The drugs are relatively contraindicated in persons with glaucoma, especially the closed-angle form, and in men with prostatic hypertrophy.

NICOTINIC ANTAGONISTS

A. Classification: Nicotinic receptor antagonists are divided into ganglion-blocking drugs and neuromuscular-blocking drugs.

B. Ganglion-blocking drugs: Blockers of ganglionic nicotinic receptors are now of largely academic interest, though they were important historically for introducing the era of successful therapy of hypertension. Hexamethonium (C6), mecamylamine, and several other ganglion blockers were extensively used for this disease. Unfortunately, the adverse effects of ganglion blockade are so severe (both sympathetic and parasympathetic divisions are blocked) that patients are unable to tolerate them for long periods (Table 8–4). Trimethaphan is the only ganglion blocker still in clinical use. Its action is like that of a competitive pharmacologic antagonist. It is poorly lipid-soluble, inactive orally, and has a short half-life. It is used intravenously to treat severe accelerated hypertension (malignant hypertension) and to produce controlled hypotension. Because ganglion blockers interrupt sympathetic control of venous tone, they cause marked venous pooling; postural hypotension is a major manifestation of this effect.

C. Neuromuscular-blocking drugs: Neuromuscular-blocking drugs are important for producing complete skeletal muscle relaxation in surgery; new ones are frequently introduced. They are discussed in greater detail in Chapter 26.

    1. Nondepolarizing group: Tubocurarine is the prototype. It produces a competitive block at the endplate, causing flaccid paralysis that lasts 30–60 minutes (longer if large doses have been given). Pancuronium, atracurium, vecuronium, and several newer drugs are shorter-acting, nondepolarizing blockers. Gallamine is an older nondepolarizing drug that is used rarely in the USA.

    2. Depolarizing group: Although these drugs are nicotinic agonists, not antagonists, they cause a flaccid paralysis (see Chapter 26). Succinylcholine, the only member of this group used in the USA, produces fasciculations during induction of paralysis; patients may complain of muscle pain after its use. The drug is hydrolyzed by pseudocholinesterase (plasma cholinesterase), and has a half-life of a few minutes in persons with normal plasma cholinesterase. Approximately 1 in 2500 individuals has (genetically determined) abnormal

Table 8–4. Effects of ganglion-blocking drugs.

Organ	Effects
Eye	Moderate mydriasis and cycloplegia
Bronchi	Little effect
GI tract	Markedly reduced motility; constipation may be severe
GU tract	Reduced contractility of the bladder; impairment of erection and ejaculation
Heart	Slight tachycardia; reduction in force of contraction and cardiac output
Vessels	Reduction in arteriolar tone, marked reduction in venous tone; blood pressure decreases and orthostatic hypotension may be severe
Glands	Reductions in salivation, lacrimation, sweating, and gastric secretion
Skeletal muscle	No significant effect

cholinesterase and does not metabolize succinylcholine effectively. The drug's duration of action is grossly prolonged in such individuals.

CHOLINESTERASE REGENERATORS

The cholinesterase regenerators are not receptor antagonists but belong to a class of *chemical* antagonists. These molecules contain an oxime group, which has an extremely high affinity for the phosphorus atom in organophosphate insecticides. Because the affinity of the oxime group for phosphorus exceeds that of the enzyme active site, these agents are able to bind the inhibitor and displace the enzyme—if aging has not occurred. The active enzyme is thus regenerated. Pralidoxime, the oxime currently available in the USA, is often used in the emergency department to treat patients exposed to insecticides such as parathion.

DRUG LIST

The following drugs are important members of the group discussed in this chapter. Prototypes should be learned in detail; features of the major variants should be known well enough to distinguish the variants from prototypes and from each other; the other significant agents should be recognized as belonging to a specific subclass.

Subclass	Prototype	Major Variants	Other Significant Agents
Muscarinic blockers Nonselective	Atropine	Scopolamine, glycopyrrolate, ipratropium, cyclopentolate, benztropine	Homatropine, methscopolamine, tropicamide
M₁-selective	Pirenzepine		Telenzepine
Nicotinic blockers Ganglion blockers	Hexamethonium	Trimethaphan	
Neuromuscular blockers	Tubocurarine		Pancuronium, atracurium
Cholinesterase regenerator	Pralidoxime		

QUESTIONS

DIRECTIONS: Each of the numbered items or incomplete statements in this section is followed by answers or by completions of the sentence. Select the ONE lettered answer or completion that is BEST in each case.

Items 1–2: A 3-year-old child has been admitted to the Emergency Room. Antimuscarinic drug overdose is suspected.

1. Atropine overdosage may cause all of the following EXCEPT
   (A) Blurred vision
   (B) Relaxation of gastrointestinal smooth muscle
   (C) Decrease in gastric secretion
   (D) Pupillary constriction
   (E) Increase in cardiac rate
2. In young children, the most dangerous toxic effect of the belladonna alkaloids is
   (A) Intraventricular heart block
   (B) Dehydration
   (C) Hypertension
   (D) Hyperthermia
   (E) Hallucinations
3. Which of the following pairs of drugs and properties is correct?
   (A) Atropine: Poorly absorbed after oral administration
   (B) Cyclopentolate: Well absorbed from conjunctival sac into the eye
   (C) Scopolamine: Short duration of action when used as antimotion sickness agent

    (**D**) Ipratropium: Well absorbed, long elimination half-life
    (**E**) Benztropine: Quaternary, poor CNS penetration

4. All of the following can be blocked by atropine pretreatment EXCEPT
    (**A**) Vagal bradycardia (slowing of rate caused by vagal stimulation)
    (**B**) Tachycardia induced by infusion of acetylcholine
    (**C**) Sweating induced by injection of pilocarpine
    (**D**) Increased blood pressure induced by nicotine poisoning
    (**E**) Salivation induced by neostigmine

5. In using topical antimuscarinic drugs in ophthalmology,
    (**A**) Atropine is longer acting than cyclopentolate and more efficacious than methscopol-amine
    (**B**) Reversal of excess antimuscarinic effect is more easily achieved with physostigmine than with neostigmine
    (**C**) Both (**A**) and (**B**) are correct
    (**D**) Neither (**A**) nor (**B**) is correct

Items 6 and 7: Two new synthetic drugs (X and Y) are to be studied for their cardiovascular effects. The drugs are given to three anesthetized animals while the blood pressure is recorded. The first animal has received no pretreatment, the second has received an effective dose of a long-acting ganglion blocker, and the third has received an effective dose of a long-acting muscarinic antagonist. The net changes induced by the new drugs (not by the blocking drugs) before and after the onset of action of the blocking drugs are shown in the graph below.

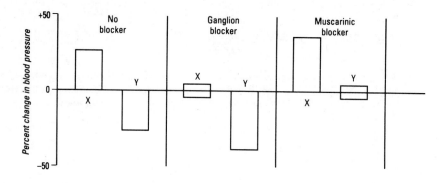

6. Drug X is probably a drug similar to
    (**A**) Acetylcholine
    (**B**) Nicotine
    (**C**) Epinephrine
    (**D**) Atropine
    (**E**) Hexamethonium

7. Drug Y is probably a drug similar to
    (**A**) Acetylcholine
    (**B**) Nicotine
    (**C**) Pralidoxime
    (**D**) Edrophonium
    (**E**) Hexamethonium

8. A 30-year-old man has been treated with several autonomic drugs. He is now showing signs of drug toxicity. Which of the following signs would distinguish between an overdose of a ganglion blocker versus a muscarinic blocker?
    (**A**) Mydriasis
    (**B**) Tachycardia
    (**C**) Postural hypotension
    (**D**) Blurred vision
    (**E**) Dry mouth, constipation

9. All of the following may cause cycloplegia (paralysis of accommodation) when used topically in the eye EXCEPT
   (A) Atropine
   (B) Physostigmine
   (C) Tropicamide
   (D) Atropine
   (E) Scopolamine

10. Atropine therapy in the elderly may be hazardous because
    (A) Atropine can elevate intraocular pressure in patients with glaucoma
    (B) Atropine frequently causes ventricular tachycardia
    (C) Urinary retention may be precipitated in women
    (D) The elderly are particularly prone to develop dangerous hyperthermia
    (E) Atropine often causes excessive vasodilation and hypotension in the elderly

11. When a dose-response study of atropine is carried out in young adults, which of the following effects may be observed?
    (A) Bradycardia
    (B) Tachycardia
    (C) Central nervous system stimulation, eg, hallucinations
    (D) Central nervous system depression, eg, sedation
    (E) All of the above

12. Accepted therapeutic indications for the use of antimuscarinic drugs include all of the following EXCEPT
    (A) Parkinson's disease
    (B) Hypertension
    (C) Traveler's diarrhea
    (D) Motion sickness
    (E) Postoperative bladder spasm

DIRECTIONS: The following section consists of a list of four to twenty-six lettered options followed by several numbered items. For each numbered item, select the ONE option that is most closely associated with it. Each answer may be selected once, more than once, or not at all.
   (A) Atropine
   (B) Benztropine
   (C) Bethanechol
   (D) Botulinum
   (E) Cyclopentolate
   (F) Neostigmine
   (G) Pralidoxime
   (H) Scopolamine
   (I) Trimethaphan
   (J) Tubocurarine

13. This drug is used exclusively in ophthalmology for inducing cycloplegia and mydriasis
14. This drug causes vasodilation that can be blocked by atropine
15. This drug has a very high affinity for the phosphorus atom in parathion and is often used to treat insecticide toxicity

ANSWERS

1. Pupillary dilation, not constriction, is a characteristic atropine effect, as indicated by the origin of the name belladonna ("beautiful lady") from the ancient cosmetic use of extracts of the *Atropa belladonna* plant to dilate the pupils. The answer is **(D)**.

2. Choices **(A)**, **(D)**, and **(E)** are possible effects of the atropine group. In small children, however, the most dangerous effect is hyperthermia. Deaths with body temperatures in excess of 42 °C have occurred after the use of atropine-containing eye drops in children. The answer is **(D)**.

3. Atropine is very well absorbed. Scopolamine has a relatively long duration of action, especially when used as an antimotion sickness transdermal patch. Ipratropium is quaternary and

poorly absorbed from the airways. Benztropine is tertiary, lipid soluble, and penetrates into the CNS well. Only **(B)**is correct.

4. Atropine blocks muscarinic receptors and inhibits parasympathomimetic effects. Nicotine can induce both parasympathomimetic and sympathomimetic effects, by virtue of its ganglion-stimulating action. Hypertension reflects sympathetic discharge and therefore would not be blocked by atropine. The answer is **(D).**

5. Atropine is considerably longer-acting in the eye (about 48–72 hours) than cyclopentolate (about 1 hour) and is also more efficacious, especially in children. Physostigmine (a tertiary amine) penetrates the surface of the eye better than neostigmine (a quaternary amine, Chapter 7). The answer is **(C).**

6. Drug X causes an increase in blood pressure that is blocked by a ganglion-blocker but not by a muscarinic blocker. The pressor response is actually increased by pretreatment with a muscarinic blocker, suggesting that compensatory vagal discharge might have blunted the full response. This description fits a ganglion stimulant like nicotine but not epinephrine, since epinephrine's pressor effects are produced at alpha receptors, not in the ganglia. The answer is **(B).**

7. Drug Y causes a decrease in blood pressure that is blocked by a muscarinic blocker but not by a ganglion-blocker. Therefore, the depressor effect must be evoked at a site distal to the ganglia. In fact, the drop in blood pressure is actually greater in the presence of ganglion blockade, suggesting that compensatory sympathetic discharge might have blunted the full depressor action of drug Y in the untreated animal. The description fits a direct-acting muscarinic stimulant such as acetylcholine (given in high dosage). Indirect-acting cholinomimetics (cholinesterase inhibitors) would not produce this pattern because the vascular muscarinic receptors involved in the depressor response are not innervated. The answer is **(A).**

8. Ganglion blockers and muscarinic blockers can both cause mydriasis, increase resting heart rate, blur vision, and cause dry mouth and constipation, because these are determined largely by parasympathetic tone. Postural hypotension, on the other hand, is a sign of sympathetic blockade, which would occur with ganglion blockers but not muscarinic blockers (Chapter 6). The answer is **(C).**

9. All antimuscarinic agents are, in theory, capable of causing cycloplegia. Physostigmine, on the other hand, is an indirect-acting cholinomimetic. The answer is **(B).**

10. The elderly have a much higher incidence of glaucoma than younger people (and may be unaware of the disease until late in its course). Antimuscarinic agents may increase intraocular pressure in individuals with glaucoma. Elderly men (not women) have a much higher probability of developing urinary retention—because they have a high incidence of prostatic hypertrophy. Cardiac and hyperthermic reactions to atropine are not common in the elderly. The answer is **(A).**

11. All of the effects may be observed. The answer is **(E).**

12. Hypertension is not responsive to antimuscarinic agents. The answer is **(B).**

13. Cyclopentolate is used in ophthalmology to produce mydriasis and cycloplegia. The answer is **(E).**

14. Bethanechol (Chapter 7) causes vasodilation by activating muscarinic receptors on the endothelium of blood vessels. This effect can be blocked by atropine. The answer is **(C).**

15. Pralidoxime has a very high affinity for the phosphorus atom in organophosphate insecticides. The answer is **(G).**

Sympathomimetics 9

OBJECTIVES

You should be able to:

- List tissues that contain significant numbers of alpha receptors of the α_1 or α_2 types.
- List tissues that contain significant numbers of β_1 or β_2 receptors.
- Describe the major organ system effects of a pure alpha agonist, a pure beta agonist, and a mixed alpha and beta agonist. Give examples of each type of drug.
- Describe a clinical situation in which the effects of an indirect sympathomimetic would differ from those of a direct agonist.
- List the major clinical applications of the adrenoceptor agonists.

Learn the definitions that follow.

Table 9–1. Definitions.

Term	Definition
Anorexiant	A drug that causes loss of appetite (anorexia)
Catecholamine	A dihydroxyphenylethylamine derivative, eg, norepinephrine, epinephrine
Decongestant	A drug that reduces nasal, conjunctival, or oropharyngeal mucosal hyperemia and swelling, usually by constricting blood vessels in the submucosal tissue
Direct agonist, indirect agonist	A direct agonist binds and activates the receptor; an indirect one brings about receptor activation by binding to some other molecule, eg, a reuptake carrier
Mydriatic	A drug that causes dilation of the pupil; opposite of miotic
Phenylisopropylamine	A derivative of phenylisopropylamine, eg, amphetamine, ephedrine. Unlike catecholamines, phenylisopropylamines usually have oral activity, a long half-life, some CNS activity, and an indirect mode of action
Selective α-agonist, β-agonist	Drugs that have relatively greater effects on alpha or beta adrenoceptors; none are *absolutely* selective
Sympathomimetic	A drug that mimics stimulation of the sympathetic autonomic nervous system
Reuptake inhibitor	An indirectly acting drug that increases the activity of transmitters in the synapse by inhibiting their reuptake into the presynaptic nerve ending. May act selectively on noradrenergic, serotonergic, or both types of nerve endings

CONCEPTS

A. **Classification:** The adrenoceptor agonists are subdivided in two ways: by mode of action and by spectrum of action (Figure 9–1).
  1. **Mode of action:** The adrenoceptor agonists may directly activate their receptors, or they may act indirectly to increase the concentration of catecholamine transmitter in the synapse. Amphetamine derivatives and tyramine cause the release of stored catecholamines; these sympathomimetics are therefore mainly indirect in their mode of action. Another form of indirect action is seen with cocaine and the tricyclic antidepressants, which inhibit reuptake of catecholamines by nerve terminals and thus also increase the synaptic activity of released transmitter.

  Blockade of metabolism (ie, block of catechol-O-methyltransferase [COMT] and monoamine oxidase [MAO]) has little direct effect on autonomic activity, but MAO inhibition increases the stores of catecholamines in storage vesicles and thus may potentiate the action of indirect-acting sympathomimetics.

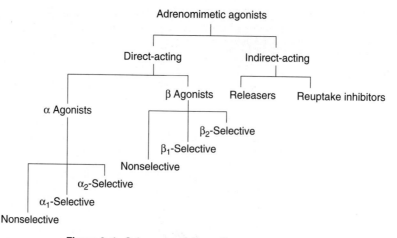

Figure 9–1. Subgroups of drugs discussed in this chapter.

2. **Spectrum of action:** The adrenoceptors are classified as alpha or beta receptors; both groups are further subdivided into 2 (or more) subgroups. The distribution of these receptors is set forth in Table 9–2. Epinephrine may be considered a single prototype with effects at all receptor types (α_1, α_2, β_1, β_2, and β_3). Alternatively, separate prototypes, phenylephrine (alpha) and isoproterenol (beta) may be defined.

B. Chemistry & Pharmacokinetics: The endogenous adrenoceptor agonists (epinephrine, norepinephrine, and dopamine) are catecholamines and are rapidly metabolized by COMT and MAO. As a result, these adrenoceptor agonists are inactive when given by the oral route. After their release from nerve endings, they are again taken up into nerve endings and into perisynaptic cells; these agonists have a short duration of action. When given parenterally, they do not enter the CNS in significant amounts. Isoproterenol, a synthetic catecholamine, is similar to the endogenous transmitters but is not taken up readily into the nerve ending. The phenylisopropylamines such as amphetamine are resistant to MAO; most of them are noncatecholamines and are therefore also resistant to COMT. These agents are orally active; they enter the CNS and their effects last much longer than do those of catecholamines. Tyramine, which is not a phenylisopropylamine, is rapidly metabolized by MAO except in patients who are taking an MAO inhibitor drug.

C. Mechanisms of Action:
1. **Alpha$_1$ receptor effects:** Alpha$_1$ receptor effects are mediated primarily by the coupling protein G_q, which leads to activation of the phosphoinositide cascade and liberates inositol-1,4,5-trisphosphate (IP$_3$) and diacylglycerol (DAG). Calcium is subsequently released in smooth muscle cells and enzymes are activated. Direct gating of calcium channels may also play a role in increasing intracellular calcium concentration.
2. **Alpha$_2$ receptor effects:** Alpha$_2$ receptor activation results in inhibition of adenylyl cyclase (formerly called adenylate cyclase) via the coupling protein G_i.
3. **Beta receptor effects:** Beta receptors (β_1, β_2, and β_3) stimulate adenylyl cyclase via the coupling protein G_s, which leads to an increase in cAMP concentration in the cell.
4. **Dopamine D$_1$ receptor effects:** Dopamine D$_1$ receptors activate adenylyl cyclase in neurons and vascular smooth muscle. Dopamine D$_2$ receptors are most important in the brain but probably also play a significant role as presynaptic receptors on peripheral nerves.

D. Organ System Effects:
1. **CNS:** Catecholamines do not enter the CNS effectively. Sympathomimetics that do enter the CNS (eg, amphetamines) have a spectrum of stimulant effects, beginning with mild alerting or reduction of fatigue, and progressing to anorexia, euphoria, and insomnia. These effects probably represent the release of dopamine in certain dopaminergic tracts. Very high doses lead to marked anxiety or aggressiveness, paranoia, and sometimes, convulsions.

Table 9–2. Types of adrenoceptors, some of the peripheral tissues in which they are found, and the major effects of their activation. Receptor distribution in the CNS is discussed in Chapter 20.

Type	Tissue	Actions
Alpha$_1$	Most vascular smooth muscle	Contracts ($\uparrow$ vascular resistance)
	Pupillary dilator muscle	Contracts (mydriasis)
	Pilomotor smooth muscle	Contracts (erects hair)
	Liver (in some species, eg, rat)	Stimulates glycogenolysis
Alpha$_2$	Adrenergic and cholinergic nerve terminals	Inhibits transmitter release
	Platelets	Stimulates aggregation
	Some vascular smooth muscle	Contracts
	Fat cells	Inhibits lipolysis
	Pancreatic B cells	Inhibits insulin release
Beta$_1$	Heart	Stimulates rate and force
	Juxtaglomerular cells	Stimulates renin release
	Pancreatic B cells	Stimulates insulin release
Beta$_2$	Respiratory, uterine, and vascular smooth muscle	Relaxes
	Liver (human)	Stimulates glycogenolysis
	Somatic motor nerve terminals (voluntary muscle)	Causes tremor
Beta$_3$ (beta$_1$ and beta$_2$ may also contribute)	Fat cells	Stimulates lipolysis
Dopamine$_1$	Renal and other splanchnic blood vessels	Relaxes (reduces resistance)
Dopamine$_2$	Nerve terminals	Inhibits adenylyl cyclase

2. **Eye:** The smooth muscle of the pupillary dilator responds to topical phenylephrine and similar alpha agonists with mydriasis. Accommodation is not affected. Outflow of aqueous humor may be facilitated, with a subsequent reduction of intraocular pressure.

3. **Bronchi:** The smooth muscle of the bronchi relaxes markedly in response to beta$_2$ agonists. These agents are the most efficacious and reliable drugs for reversing bronchospasm.

4. **Gastrointestinal tract:** The gastrointestinal tract is well endowed with both alpha and beta receptors, located on both smooth muscle and on neurons of the enteric nervous system. Activation of either alpha or beta receptors leads to relaxation of the smooth muscle.

5. **Genitourinary tract:** The genitourinary tract contains alpha receptors in the bladder trigone and sphincter area; the receptors mediate contraction of the sphincter. Sympathomimetics are sometimes used to increase sphincter tone. Beta$_2$ agonists may cause significant uterine relaxation in pregnant women near term, but the doses required also cause significant tachycardia.

6. **Vascular system:**
   a. **Alpha$_1$ agonists:** Alpha$_1$ agonists constrict skin and splanchnic blood vessels and increase peripheral vascular resistance and venous pressure. Because these drugs increase blood pressure, they often evoke a compensatory reflex bradycardia.
   b. **Alpha$_2$ agonists:** Alpha$_2$ agonists (eg, clonidine) cause vasoconstriction when administered intravenously or topically (eg, as a nasal spray), but when given orally, they accumulate in the CNS and reduce sympathetic outflow and blood pressure as described in Chapter 11.
   c. **Beta$_2$ agonists:** Beta$_2$ agonists cause significant reduction in arteriolar tone in the skeletal muscle vascular bed and can reduce peripheral vascular resistance and arterial blood pressure.
   d. **Dopamine:** Dopamine causes vasodilation in the splanchnic and renal vascular beds by activating D$_1$ receptors. This effect can be very useful in the treatment of renal failure associated with shock. At higher doses, dopamine activates beta receptors; at still higher doses, alpha receptors are activated.

7. **Heart:** The heart is well supplied with β_1 and β_2 receptors. The β_1 receptors probably predominate in some parts of the heart; both beta receptors, however, mediate increased rate of cardiac pacemakers (normal and abnormal), increased AV node conduction velocity, and increased cardiac force.

8. **Net cardiovascular actions:** Sympathomimetics with both alpha and beta$_1$ effects (eg, norepinephrine) may cause a reflex increase in vagal outflow because they increase blood pressure and evoke the baroreceptor reflex. This reflex bradycardia often dominates any direct beta effects on the heart rate, so that a slow infusion of norepinephrine typically causes increased blood pressure and bradycardia. See Figure 9–2. If the reflex is blocked (eg, by a ganglion blocker), norepinephrine may cause a direct beta$_1$-mediated tachycardia. A pure alpha agonist, eg, phenylephrine, will routinely slow heart rate via the baroreceptor reflex, while a pure beta agonist, eg, isoproterenol, almost always increases the heart rate. The diastolic blood pressure is affected mainly by peripheral vascular resistance and the heart rate. The adrenoceptors with the greatest effects on vascular resistance are alpha and beta$_2$ receptors. The systolic pressure is the sum of the diastolic and the pulse pressures. The pulse pressure is determined mainly by the stroke volume (a function of force of cardiac contraction), which is influenced by beta$_1$ receptors.

9. **Metabolic and hormonal effects:** Beta$_1$ agonists increase renin secretion. Beta$_2$ agonists increase insulin secretion by the pancreas and glycogenolysis in the liver. Hyperglycemia often results, associated initially with hyperkalemia and later with hypokalemia. All beta agonists appear to stimulate lipolysis.

E. Clinical Uses (Table 9–3):

1. **Anaphylaxis:** Epinephrine is the drug of choice in the immediate treatment of anaphylactic shock. The catecholamine is sometimes supplemented with antihistamines and corticosteroids, but these agents are neither as rapid nor as efficacious as epinephrine.

2. **CNS:** The phenylisopropylamines, such as amphetamine, are widely used and abused for their CNS effects. Legitimate applications include narcolepsy, attention deficit disorder, and, with appropriate controls, weight reduction. The anorexiant effect is insufficient to maintain weight loss in patients who do not also receive intensive dietary and psychologic counseling. The drugs are abused or misused for the purpose of deferring sleep and for their mood-elevating, euphoria-producing action.

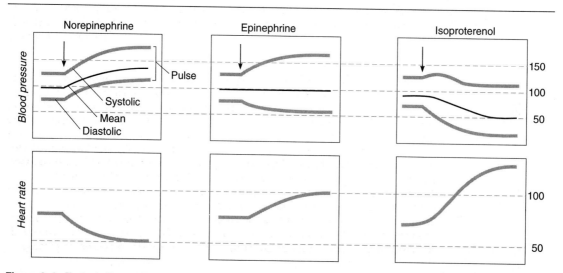

Figure 9–2. Typical effects of principal catecholamines on blood pressure and heart rate. Note that the pulse pressure ("Pulse") is only slightly increased by norepinephrine but is markedly increased by epinephrine and isoproterenol. The reduction in heart rate caused by norepinephrine is the result of baroreceptor reflex activation of vagal outflow to the heart. The blood pressure effects of epinephrine are typically dose-dependent: small doses exhibit more beta effect (isoproterenol-like; large doses exhibit more alpha effect (norepinephrine-like).

Table 9–3. Pharmacokinetics and clinical applications of some sympathomimetics.

Drug	Oral Activity	Duration of Action	Clinical Applications
Catecholamines Epinephrine	No	Minutes	Anaphylaxis, glaucoma, asthma, to cause vasoconstriction
Norepinephrine	No	Minutes	To cause vasoconstriction in hypotension
Isoproterenol	Poor	Minutes	Asthma, atrioventricular block (rare)
Dopamine	No	Minutes	Shock, heart failure
Dobutamine	No	Minutes	Shock, heart failure
Other sympathomimetics Amphetamine, phenmetrazine, others	Yes	Hours	Narcolepsy, obesity, attention deficit disorder
Ephedrine	Yes	Hours	Asthma (obsolete), urinary incontinence, to cause vasoconstriction in hypotension
Phenylephrine	Poor	Hours	To cause mydriasis, vasoconstriction, decongestion
Albuterol, metaproterenol, terbutaline	Yes	Hours	Asthma
Oxymetazoline, xylometazoline	Topical only	Hours	To cause decongestion (long action)
Cocaine	No	Minutes-hours	To cause vasoconstriction and local anesthesia

3. **Eye:** The alpha agonists, especially phenylephrine, are sometimes used topically to produce mydriasis and to reduce the conjunctival itching and congestion caused by irritation or allergy. They do not cause cycloplegia. Epinephrine and a pro-drug, dipivefrin, are sometimes used topically in the treatment of glaucoma. Phenylephrine has also been used for glaucoma, mainly outside the USA.

4. **Bronchi:** The beta agonists, especially the β_2-selective agonists, are drugs of choice in the treatment of acute asthmatic bronchoconstriction.

5. **Cardiovascular applications:**
   a. **Conditions in which an increase in blood flow is desired:** In acute heart failure and some types of shock, an increase in cardiac output and blood flow to the tissues is needed. Beta$_1$ agonists may be useful in this situation because they increase cardiac contractility and reduce afterload (by decreasing the impedance to ventricular ejection through their partial beta$_2$ effect).
   b. **Conditions in which a decrease in blood flow or increase in blood pressure is desired:** Alpha$_1$ agonists are useful in situations in which vasoconstriction is appropriate. These include local hemostasis and decongestant effects as well as spinal shock, in which temporary maintenance of blood pressure may help maintain perfusion of the brain, heart, and kidneys. Shock due to septicemia or myocardial infarction, on the other hand, is usually made worse by vasoconstrictors, since the afterload is increased and tissue perfusion often declines. Alpha agonists are often mixed with local anesthetics to reduce the loss of anesthetic from the area of injection into the circulation.

6. **Genitourinary tract:** Beta$_2$ agonists (ritodrine, terbutaline) have been used in premature labor, but the cardiac stimulant effect may be hazardous to both mother and fetus.

   Long-acting sympathomimetics such as ephedrine are sometimes used to improve urinary continence in children with enuresis and in the elderly. This action is mediated by alpha receptors in the trigone of the bladder and, in men, the smooth muscle of the prostate.

F. **Toxicity:**
1. **Catecholamines:** Because of their limited penetration into the brain, these drugs have little CNS toxicity when given systemically. In the periphery, their adverse effects are extensions of their pharmacologic alpha or beta actions: excessive vasoconstriction, cardiac arrhythmias, myocardial infarction, and pulmonary edema or hemorrhage.

2. **Other sympathomimetics:** The phenylisopropylamines may produce mild to severe CNS toxicity, depending on dosage. In small doses, they induce nervousness, anorexia, and insomnia; in higher doses, they may cause anxiety, aggressiveness, or paranoid behavior. Convulsions may occur. Peripherally acting agents have toxicities that are predictable on the basis of the receptors they activate. Thus, α_1 agonists cause hypertension and β_1 agonists cause sinus tachycardia and serious arrhythmias. Beta$_2$ agonists cause skeletal muscle tremor. It is important to note that none of these drugs is perfectly selective; eg, at high doses, β_1-selective agents have β_2 actions and vice versa. Cocaine is of special importance as a drug of abuse: its major toxicities include cardiac arrhythmias or infarction and convulsions. A fatal outcome is far more common with acute cocaine overdose than with any other sympathomimetic.

DRUG LIST

The following drugs are important members of the group discussed in this chapter. Prototypes should be learned in detail; the features of the major variants should be known well enough to distinguish the variants from prototypes and from each other; the other significant agents should be recognized as belonging to a specific subclass.

Subclass	Prototype	Major Variants	Other Significant Agents
General agonists Direct (α_1, α_2, β_1, β_2)	Epinephrine		
Indirect, releasers	Tyramine	Amphetamine	
Indirect, uptake inhibitors	Cocaine	Tricyclic antidepressants	
Selective agonists α_1, α_2, β_1	Norepinephrine		
$\alpha_1 > \alpha_2$	Phenylephrine		Methoxamine, metaraminol
$\alpha_2 > \alpha_1$	Clonidine	Methylnorepinephrine[1]	
$\beta_1 = \beta_2$	Isoproterenol		
$\beta_1 > \beta_2$	Dobutamine		
$\beta_2 > \beta_1$	Terbutaline		Albuterol, metaproterenol, ritodrine
Dopamine agonist	Dopamine	Bromocriptine, apomorphine	

[1] Active metabolite of methyldopa.

QUESTIONS

DIRECTIONS: Each of the numbered items or incomplete statements in this section is followed by answers or by completions of the sentence. Select the ONE lettered answer or completion that is BEST in each case.

1. Dilation of vessels in muscle, constriction of cutaneous vessels, and positive inotropic and chronotropic effects on the heart are all actions of
   (A) Metaproterenol
   (B) Norepinephrine
   (C) Acetylcholine
   (D) Epinephrine
   (E) Isoproterenol

2. A long-acting indirect sympathomimetic agent sometimes used by the oral route is
   (A) Epinephrine
   (B) Ephedrine
   (C) Dobutamine
   (D) Isoproterenol
   (E) Phenylephrine

3. When pupillary dilation, but not cycloplegia, is desired, a good choice is
   - (A) Homatropine
   - (B) Pilocarpine
   - (C) Isoproterenol
   - (D) Tropicamide
   - (E) Phenylephrine

4. Which of the following act(s) primarily on a receptor located on the membrane of the autonomic effector cell, ie, muscle or glandular tissue?
   - (A) Cocaine
   - (B) Tyramine
   - (C) Clonidine
   - (D) Norepinephrine
   - (E) All of the above

5. When a moderate pressor dose of norepinephrine is given after pretreatment with a large dose of atropine, which of the following is most probable?
   - (A) A decrease in heart rate caused by direct cardiac effect
   - (B) A decrease in heart rate caused by indirect reflex effect
   - (C) An increase in heart rate caused by direct cardiac action
   - (D) An increase in heart rate caused by indirect reflex action
   - (E) No change in heart rate

6. Which of the following may stimulate the central nervous system?
   - (A) Sympathomimetic drugs
   - (B) Antimuscarinic drugs
   - (C) Both (A) and (B) are correct
   - (D) Neither (A) nor (B) is correct

Items 7–8: Mr. Green is to receive a selective β_2 stimulant drug.

7. Beta$_2$-selective stimulants are often effective in
   - (A) Raynaud's syndrome
   - (B) Delayed or insufficiently strong labor
   - (C) Ischemic ulcers of the skin
   - (D) Asthma
   - (E) Coronary insufficiency manifested by angina

8. Beta$_2$ stimulants frequently cause
   - (A) Skeletal muscle tremor
   - (B) Direct stimulation of renin release
   - (C) Vasodilation in the skin
   - (D) Increased cGMP in mast cells
   - (E) All of the above

9. Epinephrine increases the concentration of all of the following EXCEPT
   - (A) Glucose in the blood
   - (B) Free fatty acids in the blood
   - (C) Lactate in the blood
   - (D) cAMP in the heart
   - (E) Triglycerides in the fat cells

10. Phenylephrine
    - (A) Increases skin temperature
    - (B) Causes miosis in the eye
    - (C) Constricts small vessels in the nasal mucosa
    - (D) Increases gastric secretion and motility
    - (E) All of the above

11. A patient was given an IV infusion of a sympathomimetic drug. The blood pressure changed as shown in the diagram on the next page. Which of the following drugs was given?
    - (A) Albuterol
    - (B) Epinephrine
    - (C) Isoproterenol
    - (D) Norepinephrine
    - (E) Phenylephrine

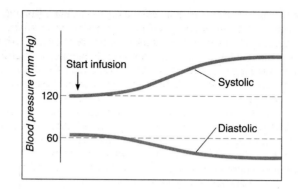

12. A new drug was given by subcutaneous injection to 20 normal subjects in a phase I clinical trial. The cardiovascular effects are summarized in the table below.

Variable	Control	Peak Drug Effect
Systolic BP (mm Hg)	116	144
Diastolic BP (mm Hg)	76	96
Cardiac output (L/min)	5.4	4.7
Heart rate (beats/min)	71.2	54.3

Which of the following drugs does the new experimental agent most resemble?
(A) Bethanechol
(B) Epinephrine
(C) Isoproterenol
(D) Neostigmine
(E) Phenylephrine

DIRECTIONS: The following section consists of a list of four to twenty-six lettered options followed by several numbered items. For each numbered item, select the ONE option that is most closely associated with it. Each answer may be selected once, more than once, or not at all.
(A) Epinephrine
(B) Isoproterenol
(C) Norepinephrine
(D) Phenylephrine
(E) Terbutaline

13. This drug will decrease heart rate in the control situation but if given after a ganglion blocker, will cause no change in heart rate
14. This β_2-selective drug is a drug of choice in acute asthmatic bronchoconstriction
15. This drug is the drug of choice in anaphylaxis

ANSWERS

1. The actions describe the effects of activating alpha, β_1, and β_2 receptors. Of the drugs listed, only epinephrine has all of these actions. The answer is **(D)**.
2. Phenylephrine and ephedrine are the only orally effective agents listed. Phenylephrine has a direct and relatively short action. Although oral ephedrine is almost obsolete, this drug still appears on examinations. The answer is **(B)**.
3. Antimuscarinics (homatropine, tropicamide) are mydriatic and cycloplegic; alpha sympathomimetic agonists are only mydriatic. Pilocarpine causes *miosis*. The answer is **(E)**.
4. The indirect-acting agents (cocaine and tyramine) act on stores of catecholamines in the nerve terminal; clonidine acts primarily on the α_2 receptor of the presynaptic nerve terminal. The answer is **(D)**.

5. Atropine will prevent the normal reflex bradycardia, since that requires integrity of the vagal pathway. The direct action of norepinephrine on the sinus node will be unmasked. The answer is **(C)**.

6. Phenylisopropylamines such as amphetamine are traditional stimulants with a spectrum of effects from mild alerting to paranoid schizophrenia and convulsions; antimuscarinic agents are capable of inducing hallucinations and convulsions. The answer is **(C)**.

7. The absence of β_2 receptors in the cutaneous vascular bed makes beta agonists useless in conditions involving reduced skin blood flow. Furthermore, ischemic ulcers are usually associated with structural occlusion of vessels that is not reversible with vasodilators. Beta agonists increase cardiac rate and force and increase myocardial oxygen demand; they are generally contraindicated in angina. Uterine and bronchiolar smooth muscle are relaxed by beta$_2$ agonists. The answer is **(D)**.

8. Tremor is a common β_2 effect. Blood vessels in the skin have almost exclusively alpha (vasoconstrictor) receptors. Stimulation of renin release is a β_1 effect. The answer is **(A)**.

9. Epinephrine increases free fatty acids by activating lipolysis of triglycerides in fat cells. The answer is **(E)**.

10. Choice **(A)** is incorrect; cutaneous vasoconstriction reduces skin temperature. Choice **(B)** is wrong; phenylephrine is a good mydriatic. Alpha agonists in ordinary dosage have little effect on the gut but may inhibit it. The answer is **(C)**.

11. The drug infusion caused an decrease in diastolic blood pressure and an increase in systolic. Thus there was a significant increase in pulse pressure. The decrease in diastolic pressure with no change in mean pressure suggests that the drug decreased vascular resistance in some beds while increasing it in others, ie, it must have significant alpha *and* beta agonist effects. The fact that it also markedly increased pulse pressure suggests that it strongly increased stroke volume, a beta agonist effect. The drug with this balance of alpha and beta effects is epinephrine (Figure 9–2). The answer is **(B)**.

12. The investigational agent caused a marked increase in diastolic pressure but little increase in pulse pressure (from 40 to 48). These changes suggest a strong alpha effect on vessels but little beta agonist action in the heart. The heart rate decreased markedly, reflecting a baroreceptor reflex compensatory response. Note that the stroke volume increased slightly (cardiac output/heart rate; from 75.8 mL to 86.6 mL). This is to be expected even in the absence of beta effects if venoconstriction causes an increase in venous return to the heart. The drug behaves most like a pure alpha agonist. The answer is **(E)**.

13. A pure alpha agonist will cause a reflex bradycardia in a subject with intact reflexes, but no change in heart rate if the reflexes are blocked. The answer is **(D)**.

14. The drugs of choice in asthmatic bronchoconstriction are the beta$_2$ agonists such as terbutaline, albuterol, and metaproterenol. The answer is **(E)**.

15. The drug of choice in anaphylaxis is epinephrine. The answer is **(A)**.

10   Adrenoceptor Blockers

OBJECTIVES

You should be able to:

- Describe the effects of phentolamine on hemodynamic responses to epinephrine and norepinephrine.
- Compare the effects of propranolol, metoprolol, and pindolol.
- Compare the pharmacokinetics of propranolol, atenolol, esmolol, and nadolol.
- Describe the clinical indications and toxicities of typical alpha- and beta-blockers.

Learn the definitions that follow.

Table 10–1. Definitions.

Term	Definition
Competitive blocker	A surmountable antagonist; one that can be overcome by increasing the dose of agonist
Covalently bound inhibitor	An antagonist that binds irreversibly to its receptor or other binding site
Epinephrine reversal	Conversion of the pressor response (typical of large doses of epinephrine) to a blood pressure-lowering effect; caused by alpha-blockers
Intrinsic sympathomimetic activity (ISA)	Partial agonist action by adrenoceptor blockers; an effect of several beta-blockers, eg, pindolol, acebutolol
Irreversible blocker	An insurmountable inhibitor, usually because of covalent bond formation; eg, phenoxybenzamine
Membrane stabilizing activity (MSA)	Local anesthetic action; typical of several beta-blockers, eg, propranolol
Orthostatic hypotension	Hypotension that is most marked in the upright position; caused by venous pooling or inadequate blood volume; typical of alpha blockade
Partial agonist	A drug (eg, pindolol) that produces a smaller maximal effect than a full agonist and therefore can inhibit the effect of a full agonist
Pheochromocytoma	A tumor that resembles the adrenal medulla; consisting of cells innervated by sympathetic preganglionic neurons and releasing norepinephrine and epinephrine into the circulation
Presynaptic receptor	A receptor located on the presynaptic nerve terminal; the receptor modulates transmitter release from the terminal

CONCEPTS

Alpha- and beta-blocking agents are divided into primary subgroups on the basis of their receptor selectivity (Figure 10–1). Because they differ markedly in their clinical applications, these drugs are considered separately in the following discussion.

ALPHA-BLOCKING DRUGS

A. Classification: Subdivisions of the alpha-blockers are based on selective affinity for α_1 versus α_2 receptors. Other features used to classify the alpha-blocking drugs are their reversibility and duration of action.

    1. Irreversible, long-acting: Phenoxybenzamine is the prototypical long-acting, irreversible alpha-blocker. It is slightly α_1-selective.

    2. Reversible, shorter-acting: Phentolamine (nonselective) and **tolazoline** (slightly α_2-selective) are competitive, reversible blocking agents.

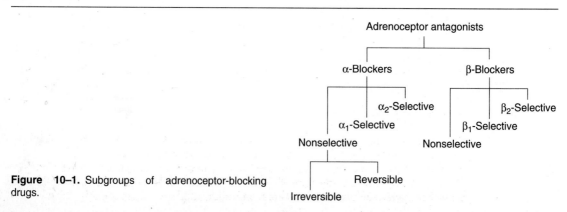

Figure 10–1. Subgroups of adrenoceptor-blocking drugs.

3. **Alpha$_1$-selective:** **Prazosin** is a selective, reversible pharmacologic α_1-blocker. Doxazosin and terazosin are newer drugs with similar properties. The advantage of α_1 selectivity is discussed below.

4. **Alpha$_2$-selective:** **Yohimbine** and **rauwolscine** are alpha$_2$-selective competitive pharmacologic antagonists. They are used primarily in research applications.

B. **Pharmacokinetics:** These drugs are all active by the oral as well as parenteral routes, although phentolamine and tolazoline are rarely given orally. Phenoxybenzamine has a short elimination half-life but a very long duration of action—about 48 hours—because it binds covalently to its receptor. Phentolamine and tolazoline have durations of action of 2–4 hours when used orally and 20–40 minutes when given parenterally. Prazosin acts for 8–10 hours.

C. **Mechanism of Action:** Phenoxybenzamine binds covalently to the alpha receptor, thereby producing an irreversible (insurmountable) blockade. The other agents are competitive pharmacologic antagonists—ie, their effects can be surmounted by increased concentrations of agonist. This difference may be important in the treatment of pheochromocytoma, because massive releases of catecholamines from the tumor may overcome a reversible blockade.

D. **Effects:**
   1. **Nonselective blockers:** These agents cause a predictable blockade of alpha-mediated responses to sympathetic nervous system discharge and exogenous sympathomimetics (ie, the alpha responses listed in Table 9–2). The most important effects of nonselective alpha-blockers are those on the cardiovascular system: a reduction in vascular tone with a reduction of both arterial and venous pressures. There are no significant direct cardiac effects. However, the nonselective alpha-blockers do cause baroreceptor reflex-mediated tachycardia as a result of the drop in mean arterial pressure (Figure 6–4). This tachycardia may be exaggerated because on adrenergic nerve terminals the alpha$_2$ receptors, which normally reduce the net release of norepinephrine, are also blocked (Figure 6–3). **Epinephrine reversal** is a predictable result of the use of this agonist in a patient who has received an alpha-blocker. The term refers to a reversal in the blood pressure effect of moderate-to-large doses of epinephrine, from a pressor response (mediated by alpha-receptors) to a depressor effect (mediated by β_2 receptors) (Figure 10–2). The effect is occasionally seen as an unexpected (but predictable) effect of drugs for which alpha blockade is an adverse effect (eg, some phenothiazine tranquilizers, antihistamines).

   2. **Selective alpha-blockers:** Because prazosin blocks vascular α_1 receptors much more effectively than the α_2-modulatory receptors associated with cardiac sympathetic nerve endings, this drug causes a much less marked tachycardia than the nonselective alpha-blockers when reducing blood pressure.

E. **Clinical Uses:**
   1. **Nonselective alpha-blockers:** Nonselective alpha-blockers have limited clinical applications. The best documented application is in the presurgical management of pheochromocytoma. Such patients may have severe hypertension and reduced blood volume, which should be corrected before subjecting the patient to the stress of surgery. Phenoxybenzamine is usually used during this preparatory phase; phentolamine is sometimes used during surgery. Phenoxybenzamine also has serotonin receptor-blocking effects, which justify its occasional use in carcinoid tumor, and H$_1$ antihistamine effects, leading to its use in mastocytosis.

   Accidental local infiltration of potent alpha agonists such as norepinephrine may lead to tissue ischemia and necrosis if not promptly reversed; infiltration of the ischemic area with phentolamine is sometimes used to prevent tissue damage. Overdose with drugs of abuse such as amphetamine, cocaine, or phenylpropanolamine may lead to severe hypertension because of their indirect sympathomimetic actions. This hypertension will usually respond well to alpha-blockers.

   Raynaud's phenomenon sometimes responds to phenoxybenzamine or phentolamine, but their efficacy is not well documented in this condition. Phentolamine or yohimbine are sometimes used by direct injection to cause penile erection in men with impotence.

   2. **Selective alpha-blockers:** Prazosin and other α_1 blockers are used in hypertension (see Chapter 11). Selective α_1-blockers have also found increasing use in the management of urinary hesitancy and prevention of urinary retention in men with prostatic hypertrophy.

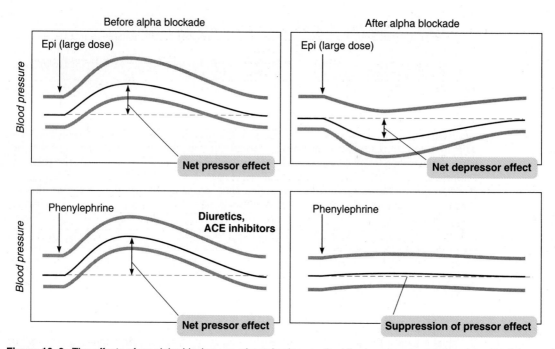

Figure 10–2. The effects of an alpha-blocker, eg, phentolamine, on the blood pressure responses to epinephrine and phenylephrine. The epinephrine response exhibits reversal of the mean blood pressure change, from a net increase (the alpha response) to a net decrease (the beta$_2$ response). The response to phenylephrine is suppressed without reversal, because phenylephrine is a "pure" alpha agonist.

F. Toxicity: The most important toxicities of the alpha-blockers are simple extensions of their alpha-blocking effects. The main manifestations are orthostatic hypotension and for the nonselective agents, reflex tachycardia. In patients with coronary disease, angina may be precipitated by the tachycardia. Oral administration of any of these drugs can cause nausea and vomiting. Prazosin is associated with an exaggerated orthostatic hypotensive response to the first dose in some patients. Therefore, the first dose is usually small and taken just before going to bed.

BETA-BLOCKING DRUGS

A. Classification, Subgroups and Mechanisms: All of the clinically used beta-blockers are competitive pharmacologic antagonists. Propranolol is the prototype. Drugs in this group are usually classified into subgroups on the basis of β_1 versus β_2 selectivity, partial agonist activity, local anesthetic action, and lipid solubility (Table 10–2).

1. **Receptor selectivity:** Beta$_1$ receptor selectivity (β_1 block > β_2 block), is a property of **metoprolol, atenolol, acebutolol,** and other beta-blockers. This property may be an advantage when treating patients with asthma. **Butoxamine,** a β_2-selective drug, is used only in research.

   Labetalol is an unusual agent with combined alpha- and beta-blocking action. This drug has four diastereomers; the alpha-blocking activity resides in the SR enantiomer and the beta-blocking action in the RR enantiomer. The other two enantiomers (RS and SS) are practically inactive.

2. **Partial agonist activity:** Partial agonist activity ("intrinsic sympathomimetic activity") may be an advantage in treating patients with asthma because, even at maximum dosage, these drugs, eg, **pindolol, acebutolol,** will cause some bronchodilation. In contrast, the full antagonists such as propranolol may cause severe asthma in patients with airway disease.

Table 10–2. Properties of several beta-receptor-blocking drugs.[1]

Drug	Selectivity	Partial Agonist Activity	Local Anesthetic Action	Lipid Solubility	Elimination Half-life	Approximate Bioavailability (%)
Acebutolol	β_1	Yes	Yes	Low	3–4 h	50
Atenolol	β_1	No	No	Low	6–9 h	40
Esmolol	β_1	No	No	Low	10 min	...
Labetalol[2]	None	Yes[3]	Yes	Moderate	5 h	30
Metoprolol	β_1	No	Yes	Moderate	3–4 h	50
Nadolol	None	No	No	Low	14–24 h	33
Pindolol	None	Yes[3]	Yes	Moderate	3–4 h	90
Propranolol	None	No	Yes	High	3.5–6 h	30[4]
Timolol	None	No	No	Moderate	4–5 h	50

[1] Modified and reproduced, with permission, from Katzung BG (editor): *Basic & Clinical Pharmacology,* 6th ed. Appleton & Lange, 1995.
[2] Labetalol also causes α_1-selective blockade.
[3] Partial agonist effects at β_2 receptors.
[4] Bioavailability is dose-dependent.

3. **Local anesthetic activity:** Local anesthetic activity ("membrane stabilizing activity" or MSA) is a disadvantage when beta-blockers are used topically in the eye. MSA is absent from **timolol** and several newer beta-blockers.
4. **Pharmacokinetics:** The systemic agents have been developed for chronic oral use, but bioavailability and duration of action vary widely (Table 10–2). Esmolol is a short-acting beta-blocker that is only used parenterally. Nadolol is the longest acting beta-blocker. Acebutolol and atenolol are less lipid soluble than the older beta-blockers and probably enter the CNS to a lesser extent.

B. **Effects and Clinical Uses:** Most of the organ-level effects of beta-blockers (Table 10–3) are predictable from blockade of the beta-receptor-mediated effects of sympathetic discharge. Effects of beta blockade not previously emphasized (and not recognized until beta-blockers became widely used) include reduction of aqueous humor formation in the eye and reduction of skeletal muscle tremor. The cardiovascular and ophthalmic applications are extremely impor-

Table 10–3. Clinical applications of beta-blockers.

Application	Drugs	Effect
Hypertension	Propranolol, metoprolol, timolol, others	Reduced cardiac output, reduced renin secretion
Angina pectoris	Propranolol, nadolol, others	Reduced cardiac rate and force
Arrhythmia prophylaxis after myocardial infarction	Propranolol, metoprolol, timolol	Reduced automaticity of all cardiac pacemakers
Supraventricular tachycardias	Propranolol, esmolol, acebutolol	Slowed AV conduction velocity
Hypertrophic cardiomyopathy	Propranolol	Slowed rate of cardiac contraction
Migraine	Propranolol	Prophylactic, mechanism uncertain
Familial tremor, other types of tremor, "stage fright"	Propranolol	Reduced β_2 alteration of neuromuscular transmission; possible CNS effects
Thyroid storm, thyrotoxicosis	Propranolol	Reduced cardiac rate and arrhythmogenesis; other mechanisms may be involved
Glaucoma[1]	Timolol, others	Reduced secretion of aqueous humor

[1] See Table 10–4 for additional drugs used in glaucoma.

Table 10–4. Drugs used in open angle glaucoma.[1]

Group, Drugs	Mechanism	Methods of Administration
Cholinomimetics Pilocarpine, carbachol, physostigmine, echothiophate	Ciliary muscle contraction, opening of trabecular meshwork; increased outflow	Topical drops or gel; plastic film slow-release insert
Alpha agonists Nonselective Epinephrine, dipivefrin	Increased outflow, probably via the uveoscleral vein	Topical drops
Alpha$_2$-selective Apraclonidine	Decreased aqueous secretion	Topical following ocular laser surgery
Beta-blockers Timolol, betaxolol, carteolol, levobunolol, metipranolol	Decreased aqueous secretion from the ciliary epithelium	Topical drops
Diuretics Acetazolamide	Decreased secretion due to lack of HCO_3^-ion	Oral; topically active carbonic anhydrase inhibitors in clinical trials
Ethacrynic acid (investigational)	Decreased secretion	Intraocular injection at long intervals, eg, annually

[1] Modified and reproduced, with permission, from Katzung BG (editor): *Basic & Clinical Pharmacology,* 6th ed. Appleton & Lange, 1995.

tant. The treatment of open angle glaucoma involves the use of several groups of autonomic drugs and a diuretic. These agents are listed in Table 10–4.

C. Toxicity: Cardiovascular adverse effects, which are extensions of the beta blockade induced by these agents, include bradycardia, atrioventricular blockade, and congestive heart failure. Patients with airway disease may suffer asthmatic attacks. Premonitory symptoms of hypoglycemia from insulin overdosage, eg, tachycardia, tremor, and anxiety, may be masked. CNS adverse effects include sedation, fatigue, and sleep alterations. Atenolol, nadolol, and several other less lipid soluble beta-blockers are claimed to have less marked CNS action because they do not enter the CNS as readily as other members of this group.

DRUG LIST

The following drugs are important members of the group discussed in this chapter. Prototypes should be learned in detail; the features of major variants should be known well enough to distinguish the variants from prototypes and from each other; the other significant agents should be recognized as belonging to a specific subclass.

Subgroup	Prototype	Major Variants	Other Significant Agents
Alpha-blockers Nonselective	Phenoxybenzamine[1]	Phentolamine	
α_1-selective	Prazosin		Terazosin, doxazosin
α_2-selective	Yohimbine		Rauwolscine
Beta-blockers Nonselective	Propranolol	Timolol, nadolol	
β_1-selective	Metoprolol	Atenolol, esmolol	
β_2-selective	Butoxamine		

[1] Compared to prazosin, phenoxybenzamine is only slightly α_1-selective.

QUESTIONS

DIRECTIONS: Each of the numbered items or incomplete statements in this section is followed by answers or by completions of the sentence. Select the ONE lettered answer or completion that is BEST in each case.

1. Which of the following effects of epinephrine would be blocked by phentolamine but not by metoprolol?
   (A) Relaxation of bronchial smooth muscle
   (B) Cardiac stimulation
   (C) Contraction of radial smooth muscle in the iris
   (D) Increase of cAMP in fat
   (E) Relaxation of the uterus
2. Phentolamine and tolazoline
   (A) Are inactive by the oral route
   (B) Induce vasospasm in large doses
   (C) Cause tachycardia
   (D) Cause hypertension
   (E) Block both alpha and beta receptors
3. Propranolol is useful in all of the following EXCEPT
   (A) Hypertension
   (B) Familial tremor
   (C) Idiopathic hypertrophic subaortic cardiomyopathy
   (D) Angina
   (E) Partial atrioventricular heart block
4. Adverse effects that limit the use of adrenoceptor blockers include
   (A) Bronchoconstriction from alpha-blocking agents
   (B) Congestive heart failure from beta-blockers
   (C) Sleep disturbances from alpha-blocking drugs
   (D) Impaired blood sugar response with alpha-blockers
   (E) Increased intraocular pressure with beta-blockers

Items 5–8: Four new synthetic drugs (designated W, X, Y, and Z) are to be studied for their cardiovascular effects. They are given to four anesthetized animals while the heart rate is recorded. The first animal has received no pretreatment, the second has received an effective dose of hexamethonium, the third has received an effective dose of atropine, and the fourth has received an effective dose of phenoxybenzamine. The net changes induced by the new drugs (not by the blocking drugs) are shown in the following graph.

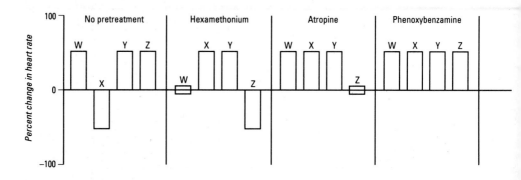

5. Drug W is probably
   (A) A drug similar to acetylcholine
   (B) A vasodilator that does not affect ANS receptors
   (C) A drug similar to norepinephrine
   (D) A drug similar to isoproterenol
   (E) A drug similar to edrophonium

6. Drug X is probably
   (A) A drug similar to acetylcholine
   (B) A vasodilator that does not affect ANS receptors
   (C) A drug similar to norepinephrine
   (D) A drug similar to isoproterenol
   (E) A drug similar to edrophonium

7. Drug Y is probably
   (A) A drug similar to acetylcholine
   (B) A vasodilator that does not affect ANS receptors
   (C) A drug similar to norepinephrine
   (D) A drug similar to isoproterenol
   (E) A drug similar to edrophonium

8. Drug Z is probably
   (A) A drug similar to acetylcholine
   (B) A vasodilator that does not affect ANS receptors
   (C) A drug similar to norepinephrine
   (D) A drug similar to isoproterenol
   (E) A drug similar to edrophonium

9. Phenoxybenzamine is used in the treatment of all of the following EXCEPT
   (A) Pheochromocytoma
   (B) Carcinoid
   (C) Raynaud's phenomenon
   (D) Essential hypertension
   (E) Mastocytosis

10. Pretreatment with phentolamine blocks all of the following EXCEPT
    (A) Vasoconstriction induced by norepinephrine
    (B) Increased cardiac contractile force induced by norepinephrine
    (C) Bradycardia induced by phenylephrine
    (D) Pilomotor erection ("gooseflesh") induced by epinephrine
    (E) Mydriasis induced by phenylephrine

11. Pretreatment with propranolol will block which one of the following?
    (A) Norepinephrine-induced bradycardia
    (B) Methacholine-induced tachycardia
    (C) Nicotine-induced hypertension
    (D) Norepinephrine-induced inhibition of insulin secretion
    (E) All of the above

12. Regarding beta-blocking drugs
    (A) Timolol lacks the local anesthetic potency of propranolol
    (B) Nadolol lacks β_2-blocking action
    (C) Pindolol is a beta antagonist with high membrane-stabilizing (local anesthetic) activity
    (D) Metoprolol blocks β_2 receptors selectively
    (E) All of the above

13. Which of the following bind(s) covalently to the site specified?
    (A) Atenolol—beta receptor
    (B) Labetalol—alpha and beta receptors
    (C) Pindolol—beta receptor
    (D) Phenoxybenzamine—alpha receptor
    (E) None of the above

14. A 60-year-old patient presents with glaucoma. Your therapy might include
    (A) Topical epinephrine
    (B) Topical pilocarpine
    (C) Topical timolol
    (D) Oral acetazolamide
    (E) All of the above

ANSWERS

1. Contraction of the pupillary dilator radial smooth muscle. All the other effects are mediated by beta receptors. The answer is **(C)**.
2. These alpha-blockers cause hypotension and significant reflex tachycardia. The answer is **(C)**.
3. Atrioventricular block is an important *contraindication* to the use of beta-blockers. The answer is **(E)**.
4. Congestive heart failure. Each of the other choices reverses the correct pairing of receptor subtype (alpha versus beta) with effect. The answer is **(B)**.
5. Drug W causes tachycardia that is prevented by ganglion blockade and therefore is probably a compensatory reflex tachycardia. Two of the choices may cause a reflex tachycardia: the nonautonomic vasodilator and acetylcholine. However, the reflex tachycardia evoked by acetylcholine would be blocked by atropine (see answer 8). Thus, drug W must be a nonautonomic vasodilator. The answer is **(B)**.
6. Drug X causes slowing of heart rate, but this is converted into a tachycardia by hexamethonium and atropine—ie, the bradycardia is caused by reflex vagal discharge. Phenoxybenzamine also reverses the bradycardia to a tachycardia, suggesting that alpha receptors are needed to induce the reflex bradycardia and that X has beta agonist actions. The choices that evoke a vagal reflex bradycardia but can also cause a direct tachycardia are limited; the answer is **(C)**.
7. Drug Y causes a direct tachycardia that is not significantly influenced by any of the blockers; the answer is **(D)**.
8. Drug Z causes tachycardia that is converted to a bradycardia by hexamethonium and blocked completely by atropine. This indicates that the tachycardia is a reflex evoked by a direct vascular effect that is blocked by atropine, ie, muscarinic vasodilation. The answer is **(A)**.
9. Phenoxybenzamine is not useful in essential hypertension because it causes tachycardia and marked orthostatic hypotension. The drug is used in Raynaud's phenomenon, but efficacy in this application is controversial. The answer is **(D)**.
10. Phenylephrine induces bradycardia through the baroreceptor reflex. Blockade of this drug's vasoconstrictor effect will prevent the bradycardia. Pilomotor erection is mediated by alpha receptors. The answer is **(B)**.
11. The beta-blocker will not block the vagal slowing induced by norepinephrine hypertension. Nicotine-induced hypertension and norepinephrine-induced inhibition of insulin secretion are mediated by alpha receptors. The answer is **(B)**.
12. Nadolol is a nonselective beta-blocker and metoprolol is a β_1-selective blocker. Timolol is useful in glaucoma because it does not anesthetize the cornea. The answer is **(A)**.
13. The answer is **(D)**, phenoxybenzamine.
14. All of the drugs listed are used in glaucoma. Acetazolamide is discussed in Chapter 15. The answer is **(E)**.

Part III: Cardiovascular Drugs

11   Drugs Used in Hypertension

OBJECTIVES

You should be able to:

- List the four major groups of antihypertensive drugs and give examples of drugs in each group.
- Describe the homeostatic responses to each of the four major types of antihypertensive drugs.
- List the major sites of action of sympathoplegic drugs and give examples of drugs that act at each site.
- List the major antihypertensive vasodilator drugs and describe their actions.
- List the major toxicities of the prototype antihypertensive agents.
- Explain why some combinations of antihypertensive drugs are rational (ie, suited to stepped care) and others are not rational.

Learn the definitions that follow.

Table 11–1. Definitions.

Term	Definition
Baroreceptor reflex	Primary autonomic mechanism for blood pressure homeostasis; involves sensory input from carotid sinus to the vasomotor center and output via the parasympathetic and sympathetic motor nerves
Catecholamine reuptake pump	Nerve terminal transporter responsible for recycling catecholamine transmitters after release into the synapse
Catecholamine vesicle pump	Storage vesicle transporter that pumps amine from cytoplasm into vesicle
End-organ damage	Vascular damage in heart, kidney, retina, or brain; often caused by hypertension
Essential hypertension	Hypertension of unknown etiology; also called "primary" hypertension
False transmitter	Substance stored in vesicles and released into synaptic cleft but lacking the effect of the true transmitter
Malignant hypertension	Accelerated hypertension causing rapid damage to vessels in end organs; a medical emergency
Orthostatic hypotension	Hypotension on assuming upright posture; postural hypotension
Postganglionic neuron blocker	Drug that blocks transmission by an action in the presynaptic postganglionic nerve terminal
Rebound hypertension	Elevated blood pressure resulting from loss of antihypertensive drug effect
Reflex tachycardia	Tachycardia resulting from lowering of blood pressure; mediated by the baroreceptor reflex
Stepped care	Progressive addition of drugs to a regimen, starting with one (usually a diuretic) and adding in stepwise fashion a sympatholytic, a vasodilator, and (sometimes) an ACE inhibitor
Sympatholytic, sympathoplegic	Drug that reduces effects of the sympathetic nervous system

CONCEPTS

Antihypertensive drugs are organized around a clinical indication—the need to treat a disease—rather than a receptor type. As a result, the drugs covered in this unit are much more heterogeneous than those in the preceding chapters on autonomic drugs. The antihypertensive drugs include diuretics, sympathoplegics, vasodilators, and angiotensin antagonists (Figure 11–1).

The strategies for treating high blood pressure are based on the determinants of arterial pressure (see Figure 6–4). These strategies include reduction of blood volume, sympathetic tone, vascular smooth muscle tone, and angiotensin concentration. Because of the baroreceptor reflex, the compensatory homeostatic responses to these drugs may be significant (Table 11–2).

As indicated in Figure 11–2, the compensatory responses can be counteracted with β-blockers or reserpine (for tachycardia) and diuretics or ACE inhibitors (for salt and water retention).

DIURETICS

These drugs are covered in greater detail in Chapter 15 but are mentioned in this chapter because of their importance in hypertension. Diuretics lower blood pressure by reduction of blood volume and by a direct vascular effect that is not yet understood. Those diuretics important for treating hypertension are the **thiazides** (eg, hydrochlorothiazide) and the **loop diuretics** (eg, furosemide). Homeostatic compensatory responses are minimal (Table 11–2). The maximum antihypertensive effect is often achieved with doses of thiazides that are below the maximum diuretic doses.

SYMPATHOPLEGICS

Sympathoplegic agents interfere with sympathetic nerve function in several ways. As predicted from Figure 6–4, the result is a reduction of one or more of the following: venous tone, heart rate, contractile force of the heart, cardiac output, and total peripheral resistance. Compensatory homeostatic responses and adverse effects are significant for some of these agents (Table 11–2). Sympathoplegics are subdivided by anatomic site of action (Figure 11–3).

A. Baroreceptor-Active Agents: The veratrum alkaloids sensitize the carotid sinus baroreceptors. This leads to a reduction in sympathetic outflow, and an increase in parasympathetic outflow. These drugs produce significant adverse gastrointestinal effects and are obsolete.

B. CNS-Active Agents: Alpha$_2$-selective agonists (eg, **clonidine, methyldopa**) cause a decrease in sympathetic outflow by a mechanism that involves activation of α_2 receptors but is not yet completely understood. These drugs accumulate in the CNS when given orally. Methyldopa is a pro-drug; it is converted to alpha-methylnorepinephrine in the brain. Clonidine and methyl-

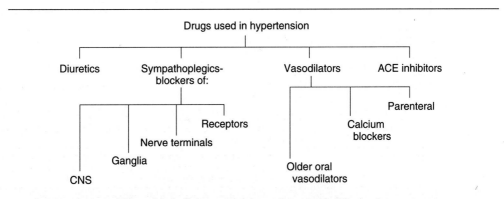

Figure 11–1. Subgroups of drugs discussed in this chapter.

Table 11–2. Compensatory responses to antihypertensive drugs and some of their adverse effects.

Class & Drug	Compensatory Responses	Adverse Effects
Diuretics Hydrochlorothiazide	Minimal	Hypokalemia, slight hyperlipidemia, hyperuricemia, hyperglycemia, lassitude, weakness, impotence
Sympathoplegics		
Veratrum alkaloids	Salt & water retention	Vomiting, diarrhea
Clonidine	Salt & water retention	Dry mouth, severe rebound hypertension if drug is suddenly stopped
Methyldopa	Salt & water retention	Sedation, + Coombs test, hemolytic anemia
Ganglion blockers	Salt & water retention	Orthostatic hypotension, constipation, blurred vision, sexual dysfunction
Reserpine (low dose)	Minimal	Diarrhea, nasal stuffiness, sedation, depression
Guanethidine	Salt & water retention	Orthostatic hypotension, sexual dysfunction
α_1-selective blockers	Salt & water retention, slight tachycardia	Orthostatic hypotension (usually limited to first few doses)
β-blockers	Minimal	Sleep disturbances, sedation, impotence, cardiac disturbances, asthma
Vasodilators Hydralazine	Salt & water retention, marked tachycardia	Lupus-like syndrome (but lacking renal effects)
Minoxidil	Marked salt & water retention, very marked tachycardia	Hirsutism, pericardial effusion
Nifedipine	Minor salt & water retention	Constipation, cardiac disturbances, flushing
Nitroprusside	Salt & water retention	Cyanide toxicity (CN^- released)
ACE inhibitors Captopril	Minimal	Cough, renal damage in pre-existing renal disease and in fetus

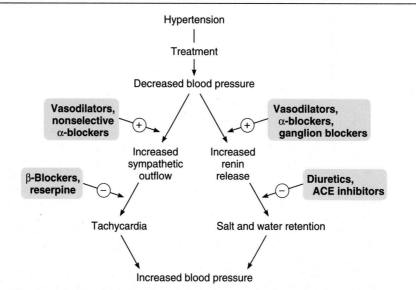

Figure 11–2. Compensatory responses to decreased blood pressure when treating hypertension. Arrows with plus signs indicate drugs that are particularly likely to precipitate the compensatory responses; arrows with minus signs indicate drugs used to minimize the compensatory response.

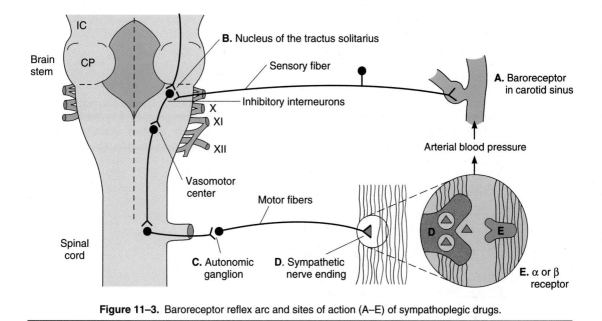

Figure 11–3. Baroreceptor reflex arc and sites of action (A–E) of sympathoplegic drugs.

dopa both reduce blood pressure by reducing cardiac output and vascular resistance to some degree. The major homeostatic response is salt retention. Sudden discontinuation of clonidine causes rebound hypertension, which may be quite severe. This rebound increase in blood pressure can be controlled by reinstitution of clonidine therapy or administration of alpha-blockers such as phentolamine. Methyldopa causes hematologic toxicity, with agglutination of sheep red blood cells (positive Coombs test) initially, and in some patients progressing to hemolytic anemia. Both drugs may cause sedation, methyldopa more so.

C. Ganglion-Blocking Drugs: Nicotinic blockers (eg, trimethaphan) are very efficacious but because of their severe adverse effects are used only in hypertensive emergencies and other acute situations (Table 11–2). Orthostatic hypotension, a prominent feature of the action of ganglion blockers, can be exploited when the patient is asleep by raising the head of the patient's bed. **Trimethaphan** has a short duration of action (minutes) and is given by continuous intravenous infusion. The major homeostatic response is salt retention. Toxicities include parasympathetic blockade (blurred vision, constipation, urinary hesitancy, sexual dysfunction) and sympathetic blockade (sexual dysfunction, orthostatic hypotension).

D. Postganglionic Sympathetic Nerve Terminal Blockers: Drugs that deplete the adrenergic nerve terminal of its norepinephrine stores (eg, **reserpine**), block release of these stores, or both deplete and block release (eg, **guanethidine**) may be useful antihypertensive drugs. The major homeostatic response is salt retention. In high dosages, both reserpine and guanethidine produce a high incidence of adverse effects. Reserpine is still sometimes used in low doses as an adjunct to other agents. Guanethidine is now rarely used. Reserpine readily enters the CNS; guanethidine does not. Both have long durations of action (days to weeks). The most serious toxicity of reserpine is behavioral depression, which may require discontinuation of the drug. The major toxicities of guanethidine are orthostatic hypotension and sexual dysfunction. Guanethidine requires the catecholamine reuptake pump (uptake 1, see Figure 6–2) to reach its intracellular site of action. Therefore, drugs that inhibit this pump (eg, cocaine, tricyclic antidepressants) will interfere with the action of guanethidine.

    MAO inhibitors are of interest in hypertension because they cause the formation of a false transmitter (octopamine) in sympathetic postganglionic neuron terminals. This substance is stored in the vesicles along with smaller amounts of norepinephrine. Normal nerve action potentials release this weak false transmitter with norepinephrine, resulting in diminished vascular and cardiac responses. However, large doses of indirect-acting sympathomimetics (eg, the tyramine in a meal of fermented foods) may cause release of large amounts of stored norepinephrine and result in a hypertensive crisis. Because of this risk (and the availability of better drugs), MAO inhibitors are no longer used in hypertension.

E. Adrenoceptor Blockers: An α_1-selective agent (eg, **prazosin**) or one of many beta-blockers (eg, **propranolol**) is often used. Alpha-blockers reduce vascular resistance. The nonselective alpha-blockers (phentolamine, phenoxybenzamine) are of no value in chronic hypertension because of excessive homeostatic responses, including salt retention and tachycardia. Alpha$_1$-selective adrenoceptor blockers are relatively free of the severe adverse effects of the nonselective alpha-blockers and postganglionic nerve terminal sympathoplegic agents.

Beta-blockers initially reduce cardiac output, but after a few days their action may include a decrease in vascular resistance as a contributing effect. The latter effect may result from reduced angiotensin levels (beta-blockers reduce renin release from the kidney). The beta-blockers are among the most heavily used antihypertensive drugs. Beta-blockers are associated with slightly elevated triglyceride and diminished high-density lipoprotein levels in the blood; other potential adverse effects are listed in Table 11–2.

VASODILATORS

Drugs that dilate blood vessels by acting directly on smooth muscle cells through nonautonomic mechanisms are useful in treating many hypertensive patients. Homeostatic responses may be marked and may include salt retention and tachycardia (Table 11–2, Figure 11–2).

A. Hydralazine & Minoxidil: These older vasodilators have more effect on arterioles than on veins. They are orally active and suitable for chronic therapy. The mechanism of hydralazine is unknown. The toxicity of hydralazine includes compensatory responses (tachycardia, salt and water retention, Figure 11–2, Table 11–2) and a risk of drug-induced lupus erythematosus, which is reversible upon stopping the drug. However, this syndrome is uncommon at dose levels below 200 mg/day.

Minoxidil is extremely efficacious and is thus reserved for severe hypertension. Minoxidil is a pro-drug; its metabolite, minoxidil sulfate, is a potassium channel opener that hyperpolarizes and relaxes vascular smooth muscle. The toxicity of minoxidil consists of severe compensatory responses (Table 11–2, Figure 11–2), hirsutism, and pericardial lesions.

B. Calcium Channel-Blocking Agents: Calcium channel blockers (eg, **nifedipine, verapamil, diltiazem**) are effective vasodilators; because they are orally active, these drugs are suitable for chronic use in hypertension of any severity. They are usually preferred to hydralazine and minoxidil. Their mechanism of action and toxicities are discussed in Chapter 12.

C. Nitroprusside & Diazoxide: These parenteral vasodilators are used in hypertensive emergencies. Nitroprusside is a short-acting agent (duration of action is a few minutes) that must be infused continuously. The drug's mechanism of action is probably similar to that of the nitrates: the release of nitric oxide (NO) stimulates guanylyl cyclase and increases cGMP concentration in smooth muscle. The toxicity of nitroprusside includes excessive hypotension, tachycardia, and if infusion is continued over several days, cumulation of cyanide or thiocyanate ions in the blood.

Diazoxide is given as intravenous boluses and has a duration of action of several hours. Diazoxide opens potassium channels, thus hyperpolarizing and relaxing smooth muscle cells. This drug also reduces insulin release and can be used to treat hypoglycemia caused by an insulin-producing tumor. The toxicity of diazoxide includes hypotension, hyperglycemia, and salt and water retention.

ANGIOTENSIN ANTAGONISTS

The useful members of this group (ACE inhibitors, eg, **captopril**) inhibit the enzyme variously known as angiotensin-converting enzyme, kininase II, and peptidyl dipeptidase. The result is a *re-*

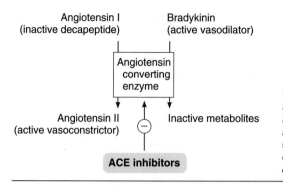

Figure 11–4. Actions of angiotensin-converting enzyme and its inhibitors. The enzyme is responsible for activating angiotensin by conversion of angiotensin I to angiotensin II, and for inactivating bradykinin, a vasodilator normally present in very low concentrations. Block of the enzyme thus decreases the concentration of a vasoconstrictor and increases the concentration of a vasodilator.

duction in blood levels of angiotensin II and aldosterone and probably an *increase* in endogenous vasodilators of the kinin family (bradykinin, Figure 11–4). ACE inhibitors have a low incidence of serious adverse effects when given in normal dosage, and produce minimal homeostatic compensation (Table 11–2). The toxicities of ACE inhibitors include cough (up to 30% of patients), renal damage in occasional patients with pre-existing renal disease, and renal damage in the fetus. These drugs should not be used during pregnancy.

A second type of angiotensin antagonist is represented by **saralasin,** which competitively inhibits angiotensin II at its receptor site (saralasin is a partial agonist). This drug is a polypeptide used only in research. Orally active drugs currently in clinical trials block renin or angiotensin at their receptors.

These drugs reduce aldosterone levels (angiotensin II is a major stimulant of aldosterone release); potassium retention may be noted, especially if the patient is consuming a high potassium diet or taking other drugs that tend to conserve potassium, eg, "potassium sparing" diuretics. Under these circumstances, potassium concentrations may reach toxic levels.

CLINICAL USES

A. Stepped Care: Therapy of hypertension requires attention to the problem of patient compliance, because the disease is symptomless until far advanced and the drugs are expensive and sometimes cause significant toxicities. This requirement gave rise to the concept of using multiple drugs to minimize individual drug toxicities. This approach is still used in patients with severe hypertension. Typically, drugs are added to a patient's regimen in stepwise fashion (stepped care); each additional agent is chosen from a different subgroup until adequate blood pressure control has been achieved. The usual steps include (1) life-style measures such as salt restriction and weight reduction, (2) diuretics, (3) sympathoplegics, (4) vasodilators, and (5) ACE inhibitors. The ability of drugs in steps 2 and 3 to control the homeostatic responses induced by the others should be noted (eg, propranolol reduces the tachycardia induced by hydralazine).

B. Monotherapy: It has been found in large clinical studies that many patients do well on a single drug (eg, an ACE inhibitor, calcium channel blocker, or alpha$_1$-blocker). This approach to the treatment of mild and moderate hypertension has become more popular than stepped care because of its simplicity, better patient compliance, and relatively low incidence of toxicity.

C. Malignant Hypertension: Malignant hypertension is an accelerated phase of severe hypertension with rapidly progressing damage to end organs and rising blood pressure. This condition may be signaled by deterioration of renal function, encephalopathy and retinal hemorrhages, or by angina, stroke, or myocardial infarction. Management of malignant hypertension must be carried out on an emergency basis in the hospital. Powerful vasodilators (nitroprusside or diazoxide) are combined with diuretics (furosemide if necessary) and beta-blockers to lower blood pressure to the 140–160/90–110 range promptly (within a few hours). Further reduction can then be pursued more slowly.

DRUG LIST

The following drugs are important members of the group discussed in this chapter. Prototypes should be learned in detail; features of the major variants should be known well enough to distinguish the variants from prototypes and from each other; the other significant agents should be recognized as belonging to a specific subclass.

Subgroups	Prototypes	Major Variants	Other Significant Agents
Diuretics	Thiazides or loop diuretics, see Chapter 15		
Sympathoplegics Carotid sinus sensitizers	Veratrum alkaloids (obsolete)		
CNS action	Clonidine, methyldopa		
Ganglion blockers	Trimethaphan	Hexamethonium	
Postganglionic neuron blockers	Reserpine, guanethidine		
Receptor blockers	Prazosin, propranolol	See Chapter 10	
Vasodilators	Hydralazine, nifedipine, nitroprusside	Minoxidil, verapamil, diazoxide	
Angiotensin antagonists	Captopril, saralasin		Enalapril, fosinopril

QUESTIONS

DIRECTIONS: Each of the numbered items or incomplete statements in this section is followed by answers or by completions of the sentence. Select the ONE lettered answer or completion that is BEST in each case.

1. A college friend consults you regarding the suitability of the therapy his doctor has prescribed for severe hypertension. He complains of postural and exercise hypotension ("dizziness"), some diarrhea, and problems with ejaculation during sex. Which of the following is most likely to produce the effects that your friend has described?
   (A) Propranolol
   (B) Guanethidine
   (C) Prazosin
   (D) Hydralazine
   (E) Captopril

2. Each of the following can cause bradycardia EXCEPT
   (A) Clonidine
   (B) Propranolol
   (C) Reserpine
   (D) Hydralazine
   (E) Guanethidine

3. In comparing methyldopa and guanethidine, which of the following is correct?
   (A) Guanethidine, but not methyldopa, results in salt and water retention if used without a diuretic
   (B) Guanethidine is less efficacious than methyldopa in severe hypertension
   (C) Guanethidine causes fewer central nervous system adverse effects (such as sedation) than methyldopa
   (D) Methyldopa causes more orthostatic hypotension than guanethidine
   (E) Guanethidine causes more immunologic adverse effects than methyldopa (eg, hemolytic anemia)

4. Captopril and enalapril do all of the following EXCEPT
   (A) Increase renin concentration in the blood
   (B) Inhibit an enzyme

    (C) Competitively block angiotensin II at its receptor

    (D) Decrease angiotensin II concentration in the blood

    (E) Increase sodium and decrease potassium in the urine

  5. After several weeks of treatment, which of the following reduces the release of norepinephrine from the sympathetic nerve terminal in response to vasomotor center discharge?

    (A) Hydralazine

    (B) Prazosin

    (C) Minoxidil

    (D) Guanethidine

    (E) Propranolol

  6. Postural hypotension is a common adverse effect of all of the following types of drugs EXCEPT

    (A) Those that cause venodilation

    (B) Those that cause ganglionic blockade

    (C) Those that cause alpha-receptor blockade

    (D) Those that cause beta-receptor blockade

    (E) Those that cause excessive diuresis and decreased blood volume

  7. Urinary retention in an elderly man is likely to result from

    (A) Trimethaphan

    (B) Reserpine

    (C) Hydralazine

    (D) Guanethidine

    (E) Propranolol

  8. Important (though uncommon) adverse effects of vasodilators include all of the following EXCEPT

    (A) Lupus erythematosus with hydralazine

    (B) Reduced cardiac output or atrioventricular block with verapamil

    (C) Precipitation of gout with prazosin

    (D) Pericardial abnormalities with minoxidil

    (E) Cyanide toxicity with nitroprusside

  9. Comparison of guanethidine and propranolol shows that

    (A) Both increase heart rate

    (B) Both diminish central sympathetic outflow

    (C) Both decrease cardiac output

    (D) Both produce orthostatic hypotension

    (E) None of the above are correct

 10. Reserpine, an alkaloid derived from the root of *Rauwolfia serpentina,*

    (A) Has been used in large doses to control hyperglycemia

    (B) Can cause psychiatric depression

    (C) Can decrease gastrointestinal secretion and motility

    (D) Often causes a reflex increase in heart rate when the drug lowers blood pressure

    (E) Is the safest of the sympathoplegic agents

DIRECTIONS: The following section consists of a list of four to twenty-six lettered options followed by several numbered items. For each numbered item, select the ONE option that is most closely associated with it. Each answer may be selected once, more than once, or not at all.

  (A) Captopril

  (B) Diazoxide

  (C) Guanethidine

  (D) Hydralazine

  (E) Minoxidil

  (F) Prazosin

  (G) Propranolol

  (H) Nifedipine

  (I) Nitroprusside

  (J) Reserpine

  (K) Cocaine

  (L) Vesamicol

11. A drug used in severe hypertensive emergencies; very short acting; must be given by IV infusion
12. A vasodilator that causes hirsutism
13. A postganglionic nerve terminal blocker that has insignificant CNS effects
14. A calcium channel blocker useful in hypertension
15. An angiotensin-converting enzyme inhibitor that may cause renal damage in the fetus
16. A drug that will interfere with the action of guanethidine

ANSWERS

1. Guanethidine is the only one of the three sympathoplegics listed here that is likely to cause the marked adverse effects described. Captopril and hydralazine are not sympathoplegics and are therefore not associated with the adverse effects described. The answer is (**B**).
2. Any sympathoplegic can, in sufficient dosage, cause bradycardia. Conversely, any vasodilator may induce tachycardia and, unless it is also sympathoplegic or a calcium channel blocker, will never slow heart rate. The answer is (**D**).
3. Guanethidine causes many peripheral adverse effects but is poorly distributed into the CNS, so it is relatively free of CNS effects. The answer is (**C**).
4. These converting enzyme inhibitors act on the enzyme, not on the angiotensin receptor. The plasma renin level may increase due to the homeostatic response to reduced angiotensin II. The answer is (**C**).
5. Drugs that act on smooth muscle (hydralazine and minoxidil) and sympathoplegics that act distal to the CNS vasomotor center *increase* sympathetic outflow to a significant degree via the baroreceptor reflex. However, guanethidine blocks release and depletes transmitter stores, despite the increase in central sympathetic outflow. The answer is (**D**).
6. Beta-blocking drugs do not cause orthostatic hypotension. The answer is (**D**).
7. This parasympatholytic effect will occur only with the ganglion blocker. The answer is (**A**).
8. Beta-blockers, not alpha-blockers, are associated with an increase in serum uric acid levels. (Even with beta-blockers, gout is uncommon and usually managed easily.) The answer is (**C**).
9. Neither drug increases heart rate or reduces central sympathetic outflow. Propranolol does not cause orthostatic hypotension. The answer is (**C**).
10. Reserpine is of no value in hyperglycemia. The drug does not induce reflex tachycardia, because it reduces sympathetic neurotransmitter release in the heart as well as the vessels. The answer is (**B**).
11. Diazoxide, nitroprusside, and nifedipine are the drugs in the list that are used in hypertensive emergencies. Diazoxide has a long duration of action and is given by intermittent injection, not by infusion. Nifedipine usually is given orally or sublingually. The answer is (**I**).
12. Minoxidil is the only drug in this list that regularly causes hirsutism. In fact, the drug is also marketed for the treatment of male-pattern baldness. The answer is (**E**).
13. Reserpine and guanethidine are both sympathoplegics that act on the postganglionic sympathetic nerve terminal. Reserpine enters the CNS readily and causes important CNS toxicity. Guanethidine, on the other hand, is too polar to cross the blood brain barrier easily and is almost devoid of central toxicity. The answer is (**C**).
14. Most of the calcium channel blockers are useful in hypertension; nifedipine is one of them. The answer is (**H**).
15. All ACE inhibitors can cause renal damage in patients with pre-existing renal disease and probably cause damage in the developing fetus. Captopril has been shown to have these effects. The answer is (**A**).
16. Cocaine can prevent the uptake of guanethidine into the nerve terminal because the drug blocks uptake 1, the catecholamine reuptake transporter in the nerve terminal membrane. The answer is (**K**).

Vasodilators & the Treatment of Angina   12

OBJECTIVES

You should be able to:

- List the major determinants of cardiac oxygen consumption.
- List the strategies for relief of anginal pain.
- Contrast the therapeutic and adverse effects of nitrates, beta-blockers, and calcium channel blockers when used for angina.
- Explain why a combination of a nitrate with a beta-blocker or a calcium channel blocker may be extremely effective.
- Contrast the effects of medical therapy and surgical therapy of angina.

Learn the definitions that follow.

Table 12–1. Definitions.

Term	Definition
Angina of effort, classic angina, atherosclerotic angina	Angina (crushing, strangling, chest pain) that is precipitated by exertion; increased O_2 demand that cannot be met because of irreversible atherosclerotic obstruction of coronary arteries
Vasospastic angina, variant angina, Prinzmetal's angina	Angina precipitated by reversible spasm of coronary vessels
Coronary vasodilator	Older, incorrect name for drugs useful in angina; drugs that relieve angina of effort do not act primarily through coronary vasodilation; some potent coronary vasodilators are ineffective in angina
Venodilator	Drug that selectively dilates veins, eg, nitrate agent
Monday disease	Industrial disease caused by chronic exposure to vasodilating concentrations of organic nitrates in the workplace; characterized by headache, dizziness, and tachycardia on Mondays
Nitrate tolerance, tachyphylaxis	Loss of effect of a nitrate venodilator when exposure is prolonged
Unstable angina	Rapidly progressing increase in frequency and severity of anginal attacks and pain at rest; probably heralds imminent myocardial infarction
Preload	Filling pressure of the heart; determines end-diastolic fiber length and tension
Afterload	Resistance to ejection of stroke volume; proportionate to arterial blood pressure
Intramyocardial fiber tension	Force exerted by myocardial fibers, especially ventricular fibers at any given time; a primary determinant of O_2 requirement
Double product	The product of heart rate and systolic blood pressure; an estimate of cardiac work
Myocardial revascularization	Mechanical intervention to improve O_2 delivery to the myocardium by angioplasty or bypass grafting

CONCEPTS

PATHOPHYSIOLOGY OF ANGINA

A. **Determinants of Cardiac Oxygen Requirement:** The treatment of coronary insufficiency is based on physiologic factors that control the myocardial oxygen requirement. A major determinant is **myocardial fiber tension,** ie, the higher the tension, the greater the oxygen requirement (Figure 12–1).

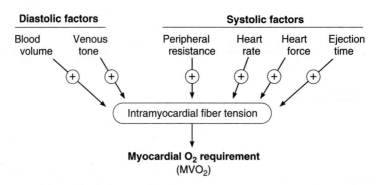

Figure 12–1. Determinants of MVO_2, the minute volume of oxygen required by the heart. Both diastolic and systolic factors contribute to the MVO_2; most of these factors are directly influenced by sympathetic discharge (venous tone, peripheral resistance, heart rate, and heart force).

Several variables contribute to fiber tension:

1. **Preload:** Preload (diastolic filling pressure) is a function of blood volume and venous tone. Because venous tone is mainly controlled by sympathetic outflow, activities that increase sympathetic activity usually increase preload.

2. **Afterload:** Afterload or arterial blood pressure is one of the systolic determinants of oxygen requirement. Arterial blood pressure depends on peripheral vascular resistance, which is determined by sympathetic outflow to the arteriolar vessels.

3. **Heart rate:** Heart rate contributes to time-integrated fiber tension because at fast heart rates, fibers spend more time at systolic tension levels; at faster rates, diastole is abbreviated and diastole constitutes the time available for coronary flow (coronary blood flow is low or nil during systole). Blood pressure and heart rate may be multiplied to yield the **double product,** a measure of cardiac work and therefore oxygen requirement. In patients with atherosclerotic angina, effective drugs reduce the double product.

4. **Cardiac contractility:** Force of cardiac contraction is another systolic factor controlled mainly by sympathetic outflow to the heart. Ejection time for ventricular contraction is inversely related to force of contraction, but is also influenced by impedance to outflow. Increased ejection time increases oxygen requirement.

B. Types of Angina: There are three forms of angina pectoris.

1. **Atherosclerotic angina:** Atherosclerotic angina is also known as angina of effort or classic angina. It is caused by atheromatous occlusion of the coronaries. When cardiac work increases (eg, in exercise), the obstruction of flow results in the accumulation of acidic metabolites and stimulates myocardial pain endings. This form constitutes about 90% of angina cases and may last for years with little change.

2. **Vasospastic angina:** Vasospastic angina is also known as variant angina or Prinzmetal's angina. It involves reversible spasm of coronaries, usually at the site of an atherosclerotic plaque. Spasm may occur at any time, not only during exercise. Vasospastic angina may deteriorate into unstable angina.

3. **Unstable angina:** The third type of angina, unstable or crescendo angina, is caused by diminished coronary flow that results from a combination of a) atherosclerotic plaques, b) platelet aggregation at a fractured plaque, and c) vasospasm. Unstable angina is thought to be the immediate precursor of a myocardial infarction and is treated as a medical emergency.

C. Therapeutic Strategies: The defect that causes anginal pain (coronary oxygen delivery inadequate for the myocardial oxygen requirement) can be corrected in two ways: by increasing oxygen delivery or by reducing oxygen requirement (Figure 12–2). Pharmacologic therapies include the nitrates, the calcium channel blockers, and the beta-blockers. All three groups reduce oxygen requirement in atherosclerotic angina; nitrates and calcium channel blockers (but not beta-blockers) can increase oxygen delivery by reducing vasospasm—only in the vasospastic

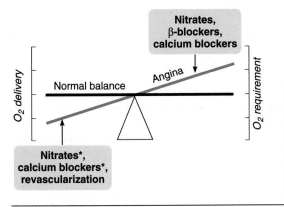

Figure 12–2. Strategies for the treatment of angina pectoris. Angina is characterized by an imbalance in coronary oxygen delivery versus oxygen requirement. In some cases, this can be corrected by increasing oxygen delivery (box on left: revascularization or, in the case of reversible vasospasm, nitrates and calcium channel blockers). More often, drugs are used to reduce oxygen requirement (box on right: nitrates, β-blockers, and calcium channel blockers).

form. Myocardial revascularization surgically corrects coronary obstruction either by bypass grafting or by angioplasty (enlargement of the lumen by means of a special catheter).

NITRATES

A. Classification and Pharmacokinetics: Nitroglycerin (the active ingredient in dynamite) is the most important of the nitrates and is available in forms that provide a range of durations of action from 10–20 minutes (sublingual) to 8–10 hours (transdermal), Table 12–2. Because treatment of acute attacks and prevention of attacks are both important aspects of therapy, the pharmacokinetics of these different dosage forms are clinically significant.

Nitroglycerin (glyceryl trinitrate) is rapidly denitrated in the liver—first to the dinitrate (glyceryl dinitrate), which retains a significant vasodilating effect, and then to the mononitrate, which is much less active. Because of the high enzyme activity in the liver, the first-pass effect for nitroglycerin is large—about 90%. The efficacy of oral (swallowed) nitroglycerin probably results from the high levels of glyceryl dinitrate in the blood. The effects of sublingual nitroglycerin are mainly the result of the unchanged drug.

Other nitrates are similar to nitroglycerin in their pharmacokinetics and pharmacodynamics. After nitroglycerin, isosorbide dinitrate is used most extensively; it is available in sublingual and oral forms. Isosorbide dinitrate is rapidly denitrated in the liver to isosorbide mononitrate, which like glyceryl dinitrate is active. Isosorbide mononitrate is available as a separate drug for oral use. Several other nitrates are available for oral use and, like the oral nitroglycerin preparation, have an intermediate duration of action (4–6 hours). Amyl nitrite is a volatile and rapidly acting vasodilator that was used for angina by the inhalational route but is now rarely prescribed.

B. Mechanism of Action: The nitrates release nitric oxide (NO) in smooth muscle, which stimulates guanylyl cyclase, causes an increase of the second messenger cGMP, and leads to

Table 12–2. Pharmacokinetically distinct forms of nitrate and nitrite drugs used in angina.

Category	Example	Duration of action
Very short	Amyl nitrite inhaled	3–5 minutes
Short	Sublingual nitroglycerin or isosorbide dinitrate	10–30 minutes (isosorbide dinitrate has a somewhat longer half-life than nitroglycerin)
Intermediate	Oral regular or sustained release nitroglycerin or isosorbide dinitrate	4–8 hours (much of the effect is due to active metabolites)
Long	Nitroglycerin (transdermal patch)	8–10 hours (blood levels may persist for 24 hours but tolerance limits the duration of action)

smooth muscle relaxation, probably by dephosphorylation of myosin light chain phosphate. Note that this mechanism is identical to that of nitroprusside (Chapter 11).

C. Organ System Effects:
    1. Cardiovascular: Smooth muscle relaxation leads to peripheral vasodilation, which results in reduced cardiac size and cardiac output through reduced preload. Reduced afterload may contribute to an increase in ejection and a further decrease in cardiac size. Some studies suggest that of the vascular beds, the veins are the most sensitive, arteries less so, and arterioles least sensitive. Venodilation leads to decreased diastolic heart size and fiber tension. Arteriolar dilation leads to reduced peripheral resistance and blood pressure. These changes contribute to an overall reduction in myocardial fiber tension, oxygen consumption, and the double product. Thus, the primary mechanism of therapeutic benefit in atherosclerotic angina is reduction of the oxygen requirement; an increase in coronary flow in ischemic areas is less likely. In vasospastic angina on the other hand, a reversal of spasm and increased flow can be demonstrated. A significant reflex tachycardia is predictable when nitroglycerin reduces the blood pressure.
    2. Other organs: Nitrates relax the smooth muscle of the bronchi, gastrointestinal tract, and genitourinary tract, but these effects are too small to be clinically useful. Intravenous nitroglycerin (sometimes used in unstable angina) reduces platelet aggregation. There are no significant effects on other tissues.

D. Clinical Uses: As previously noted, nitroglycerin is available in several formulations (Table 12–2). The standard form for treatment of acute anginal pain is the sublingual tablet, which has a duration of action of 10–20 minutes. Oral (swallowed) immediate release nitroglycerin has a duration of 4–6 hours. Sustained release oral forms have a somewhat longer duration (Table 12–2). Transdermal formulations (ointment or patch) can maintain blood levels for up to 24 hours. Tolerance develops after about 8 hours, however, with markedly diminishing effectiveness thereafter. It is therefore recommended that nitroglycerin patches be removed after 10–12 hours to allow recovery of sensitivity to the drug.

E. Toxicity of Nitrates & Nitrites: The most common toxic effects of nitrates are the responses evoked by vasodilation. These include tachycardia (from the baroreceptor reflex), orthostatic hypotension (a direct extension of the venodilator effect), and throbbing headache from meningeal artery vasodilation. Nitrites are of greater toxicologic importance because they cause methemoglobinemia at high blood concentrations. This same effect has a potential antidotal action in cyanide poisoning (see below). The nitrates do not cause methemoglobinemia. In the past, the nitrates were responsible for several occupational diseases in munitions plants in which workplace contamination by these volatile chemicals was severe. The most common of these diseases was "Monday disease," or the alternating development of tolerance (during the work week) and loss of tolerance (over the weekend) for the vasodilating action and its associated tachycardia and headache, resulting in headache, tachycardia, and dizziness every Monday.

F. Nitrites in the Treatment of Cyanide Poisoning: Cyanide ion rapidly complexes with the iron in cytochrome oxidase, resulting in a block of oxidative metabolism and cell death. Fortunately, the iron in methemoglobin has a higher affinity for cyanide than does the iron in cytochrome oxidase. Nitrites convert the ferrous iron in hemoglobin to the ferric form, yielding methemoglobin. Cyanide poisoning is therefore treated by (1) immediate exposure to amyl nitrite, followed by (2) IV administration of sodium nitrite, which rapidly increases the methemoglobin level to the degree necessary to remove a significant amount of cyanide from cytochrome oxidase. This is followed by (3) intravenous sodium thiosulfate, which converts cyanomethemoglobin to thiocyanate and methemoglobin. Thiocyanate is much less toxic than cyanide and is excreted by the kidney. (It should be noted that excessive methemoglobinemia is fatal, since methemoglobin is a very poor oxygen carrier.)

CALCIUM CHANNEL-BLOCKING DRUGS

A. Classification and Pharmacokinetics: Several types of calcium channel blockers are approved for use in angina; these drugs are typified by **nifedipine,** a **dihydropyridine,** and several other dihydropyridines; **diltiazem;** and **verapamil.** Although calcium channel blockers differ markedly in structure, all are orally active and most have half-lives of 3 to 6 hours. Newer dihydropyridines possess the same properties of the chemical dihydropyridine family. Nimodipine is another member of the dihydropyridine family with similar properties, but it is approved only for the management of stroke associated with subarachnoid hemorrhage. Bepridil, a new compound that is somewhat similar in structure to verapamil, has a longer duration of action and greater cardiovascular toxicity than the older calcium channel blockers.

B. Mechanism of Action: These drugs block voltage-dependent "L-type" calcium channels, the calcium channels most important in cardiac and smooth muscle. By decreasing calcium influx during action potentials in a frequency- and voltage-dependent manner, these agents reduce intracellular calcium concentration and muscle contractility.

C. Effects: Calcium blockers relax blood vessels, and, to a lesser extent, the uterus, bronchi, and gut. The rate and contractility of the heart are reduced by diltiazem and verapamil. Because they block calcium-dependent conduction in the AV node of the heart, verapamil and diltiazem may be used to treat AV nodal arrhythmias (Chapter 14). Nifedipine and other dihydropyridines evoke greater vasodilation, and the resulting sympathetic reflex prevents bradycardia and may actually increase the heart rate. All the calcium channel blockers reduce blood pressure and reduce the double product in patients with angina.

D. Clinical Use: Calcium blockers are effective as prophylactic therapy in both types of angina; nifedipine can also be used to abort an acute anginal attack. In atherosclerotic angina, these drugs are particularly valuable when combined with nitrates (Table 12–3). In addition to well-established uses in angina, hypertension, and supraventricular tachycardia, these agents are being tried in migraine, preterm labor, stroke, and Raynaud's syndrome. As noted above, nimodipine is approved for use in hemorrhagic stroke.

E. Toxicity: The calcium channel blockers cause constipation, edema, nausea, flushing, and dizziness. More serious adverse effects include congestive heart failure, atrioventricular blockade, and sinus node depression; these are more common with verapamil than with the dihydropyridines. Bepridil may induce *torsade de pointes* arrhythmia.

BETA-BLOCKING DRUGS

A. Classification & Mechanism of Action: These drugs are described in detail in Chapter 10. All beta-blockers are effective in the prophylaxis of atherosclerotic angina attacks.

B. Effects: Actions include both beneficial effects (decreased heart rate, cardiac force, blood pressure) and detrimental effects (increased heart size, longer ejection period, Table 12–3). Like the nitrates and calcium channel blockers, the beta-blockers reduce the double product.

Table 12–3. Effects of nitrates alone and with beta-blockers or calcium channel blockers in angina pectoris.[1]

	Nitrates Alone	β-Blockers or Calcium Blockers	Combined Nitrate and β- or Calcium Blocker
Heart rate	*Reflex increase*	**Decrease**	**Decrease**
Arterial pressure	Decrease	Decrease	**Decrease**
End-diastolic pressure	**Decrease**	*Increase*	**Decrease**
Contractility	*Reflex increase*	**Decrease**	No effect or **decrease**
Ejection time	Reflex decrease	*Increase*	No effect

[1] Undesirable effects (effects that increase myocardial oxygen requirement) are shown in *italics;* major therapeutic effects are shown in **bold.**

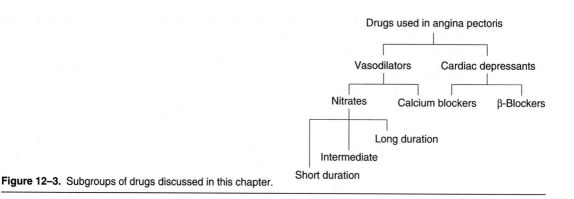

Figure 12–3. Subgroups of drugs discussed in this chapter.

C. Clinical Use: Beta-blockers are used only for prophylactic therapy of angina; they are of no value in an acute attack. They are effective in preventing exercise-induced angina but are ineffective against the vasospastic form. The combination of beta-blockers with nitrates is useful because the adverse reflex effects evoked by the nitrates (tachycardia and increased cardiac force) are prevented or reduced by beta blockade. See Table 12–3.

D. Toxicity: See Chapter 10.

NONPHARMACOLOGIC THERAPY

Myocardial revascularization by coronary artery bypass grafting (CABG) or percutaneous transluminal coronary angioplasty (PTCA) have become important therapies in severe angina. These are the only methods capable of consistently increasing coronary flow in atherosclerotic angina and increasing the double product.

DRUG LIST

The following drugs are important members of the group discussed in this chapter. Prototypes should be learned in detail; features of the major variants should be known well enough to distinguish the variants from prototypes and from each other; the other significant agents should be recognized as belonging to a specific subclass.

Subclass	Prototype	Major Variants	Other Significant Agents
Nitrates	Nitroglycerin	Different dosage forms (sublingual, oral, transdermal)	Isosorbide dinitrate, amyl nitrite
Calcium channel blockers	Nifedipine Verapamil Diltiazem	Nimodipine	Bepridil
Beta-blockers	Propranolol	See Chapter 10	

QUESTIONS

DIRECTIONS: Each of the numbered items or incomplete statements in this section is followed by answers or by completions of the sentence. Select the ONE lettered answer or completion that is BEST in each case.

Items 1–3:   Mr. Green, 60 years old, has severe chest pain when he attempts to carry parcels upstairs to his apartment. The pain rapidly disappears when he rests. A decision is made to treat Mr. Green with nitroglycerin.

1.   Nitroglycerin, either directly or through reflexes, results in all of the following EXCEPT
   (A)   Increased heart rate
   (B)   Decreased cardiac force
   (C)   Increased venous capacitance
   (D)   Decreased intramyocardial fiber tension
   (E)   Decreased afterload

2.   In advising Mr. Green about the adverse effects he may notice, you point out that nitroglycerin in moderate doses often produces certain symptoms. These toxicities result from all of the following EXCEPT
   (A)   Meningeal vasodilation
   (B)   Reflex tachycardia
   (C)   Increased cardiac force
   (D)   Methemoglobinemia
   (E)   Sympathetic discharge

3.   Two years later, Mr. Green returns complaining that his nitroglycerin works well when he takes it for an acute attack, but he is having frequent attacks now and would like something to *prevent* them. Effective drugs for the prophylaxis of angina of effort over 4- to 6-hour periods include all of the following EXCEPT
   (A)   Transdermal nitroglycerin
   (B)   Amyl nitrite
   (C)   Diltiazem
   (D)   Nadolol
   (E)   Oral isosorbide dinitrate

4.   The antianginal effect of propranolol may be attributed to all of the following EXCEPT
   (A)   Block of exercise-induced tachycardia
   (B)   Reduced resting heart rate
   (C)   Decreased cardiac force
   (D)   Increased end-diastolic ventricular volume
   (E)   Decreased systolic fiber tension

5.   The major common determinant of myocardial oxygen consumption is
   (A)   Blood volume
   (B)   Cardiac output
   (C)   Diastolic blood pressure
   (D)   Heart rate
   (E)   Myocardial fiber tension

6.   A new patient presents with severe hypertension and angina. You are considering therapeutic options for her. In considering adverse effects, you note that an adverse effect that nitroglycerin, guanethidine, and trimethaphan have in common is
   (A)   Bradycardia
   (B)   Impaired sexual function
   (C)   Lupus erythematosus syndrome
   (D)   Orthostatic hypotension
   (E)   Throbbing headache

7.   Epidemiologic surveys suggest that, in the past, workers exposed to high levels of organic nitrates in the workplace had
   (A)   A high incidence of methemoglobinemia on the job
   (B)   An increased incidence of angina at work as compared to at home
   (C)   A high incidence of cyanide poisoning in the workplace
   (D)   An increased incidence of headaches on Mondays as compared to other days
   (E)   All of the above

8.   A drug that often causes tachycardia when given in ordinary doses is
   (A)   Isosorbide dinitrate
   (B)   Verapamil
   (C)   Guanethidine
   (D)   Propranolol
   (E)   Diltiazem

9. Drugs that may precipitate angina when used for other indications include all of the following EXCEPT
   (A) Hydralazine
   (B) Terbutaline
   (C) Isoproterenol
   (D) Reserpine
   (E) Cocaine

10. When using nitrates in combination with other drugs for the treatment of angina,
    (A) The actions of beta-blockers and nitrates on end-diastolic cardiac size are additive
    (B) The actions of calcium channel blockers and nitrates on cardiac force are antagonistic
    (C) The actions of calcium channel blockers and nitrates on vascular tone are antagonistic
    (D) The actions of beta-blockers and nitrates on heart rate are additive
    (E) The actions of calcium channel blockers and beta-blockers on cardiac force are antagonistic

DIRECTIONS: The following section consists of a list of four to twenty-six lettered options followed by several numbered items. For each numbered item, select the ONE option that is most closely associated with it. Each answer may be selected once, more than once, or not at all.
   (A) Nitroglycerin (sublingual)
   (B) Nitroglycerin (transdermal)
   (C) Isosorbide mononitrate
   (D) Amyl nitrite
   (E) Verapamil
   (F) Hydralazine
   (G) Nifedipine
   (H) Nimodipine
   (I) Propranolol
   (J) Terbutaline

11. A drug that is approved for the treatment of hemorrhagic stroke
12. A drug used by inhalation; very rapid onset but brief effect
13. A drug capable of maintaining blood levels for 24 hours; but useful therapeutic effects last only about 10 hours.
14. An antihypertensive vasodilator drug that lacks a direct effect on autonomic receptors but may provoke anginal attacks
15. An active metabolite of another drug and an active drug for oral administration in its own right.

ANSWERS

1. Nitroglycerin increases cardiac force because the decrease in blood pressure evokes a reflex increase in sympathetic discharge. The answer is **(B).**
2. Methemoglobinemia never occurs from the doses of nitroglycerin (or other nitrates) used to treat angina. The nitrites cause methemoglobinemia. The answer is **(D).**
3. The calcium channel blockers and the beta-blockers are generally effective in reducing the number of attacks of angina of effort and have durations of 4–8 hours. Oral and transdermal nitrates have similar durations. Amyl nitrite has the shortest duration of action (3–5 minutes) of any drug used in angina and thus is of no value in prophylaxis. The answer is **(B).**
4. Propranolol has all the effects listed, but the increase in end-diastolic volume is not advantageous—it tends to *increase* oxygen consumption. The answer is **(D).**
5. The answer is **(E),** fiber tension. The other variables contribute to this determinant.
6. These drugs all reduce venous return sufficiently to cause some degree of postural hypotension (not very prolonged in the case of nitroglycerin). Throbbing headache is a problem only with the nitrates, bradycardia only with guanethidine, sexual problems only with sympathoplegics (trimethaphan and guanethidine), and lupus with none of them. The answer is **(D).**

7. Nitrites, not nitrates, cause methemoglobinemia in adults. Headache, not angina, increased upon returning to work on Monday. Neither nitrates nor nitrites are related to causation of cyanide poisoning, but nitrites are used as one part of the antidote for cyanide intoxication. The answer is **(D)**.

8. Isosorbide dinitrate (like all the nitrates) causes reflex tachycardia, but all the other drugs listed here slow heart rate. The answer is **(A)**.

9. In general, drugs that induce hypertension or tachycardia—whether directly or by reflex—tend to precipitate angina in individuals with coronary obstruction, unless cardiac work is greatly reduced (as in the case of the nitrates). The answer is **(D)**.

10. The effects of beta-blockers (or calcium channel blockers) and nitrates on heart size are opposite (diastolic size is inversely proportionate to end-diastolic pressure). The answer is **(B)**.

11. Nimodipine, a dihydropyridine calcium channel blocker, is approved only for the treatment of hemorrhagic stroke. The answer is **(H)**.

12. Amyl nitrite, a very volatile liquid, is the only antianginal drug in this list that is usually used by the inhalation route. (Terbutaline is used by aerosol but it *causes* angina in susceptible patients.) The answer is **(D)**.

13. Transdermal formulations of nitroglycerin are capable of maintaining blood concentrations for up to 24 hours. Unfortunately, tolerance develops after about 10 hours of continued exposure, so the effect is limited to about 8–10 hours. The answer is **(B)**.

14. Hydralazine, a direct-acting vasodilator, often precipitates angina in susceptible individuals; the drug should never be used in patients with coronary disease unless heart rate is appropriately controlled. The answer is **(F)**.

15. The organic nitrates are denitrated in the liver after oral administration. Glyceryl dinitrate and isosorbide mononitrate are active metabolites. The latter agent is available as a separate drug. The answer is **(C)**.

13

Cardiac Glycosides & Congestive Heart Failure

OBJECTIVES

You should be able to:

- Describe the strategies and list the major drug groups used in the treatment of congestive heart failure.
- Describe the probable mechanism of action of digitalis.
- Describe the nature and mechanism of digitalis' toxic effects on the heart.
- List some positive inotropic drugs that have been investigated as digitalis substitutes.
- Explain the beneficial effects of vasodilators and ACE inhibitors in congestive heart failure.

Learn the definitions that follow.

Table 13–1. Definitions.

Term	Definition
Bigeminy	An arrhythmia consisting of normal sinus beats coupled with ventricular extrasystoles, ie, "twinned beats"
Cardenolide	The basic chemical structure required for cardiac glycoside action, consisting of a steroid nucleus and a lactone ring at the 17-position
Congestive heart failure	A condition in which the cardiac output is insufficient for the needs of the body. Low output failure is the more common form and is more responsive to positive inotropic drugs than high output failure
End diastolic fiber length	The length of the ventricular fibers at the end of diastole; a determinant of the force of the following contraction
PDE inhibitor	Phosphodiesterase inhibitor; a drug that inhibits one or more enzymes that degrade cAMP (and other cyclic nucleotides). Example: high concentrations of theophylline
Premature ventricular beat	An abnormal beat arising from a cell below the AV node; often from a Purkinje fiber, sometimes from a ventricular fiber
Sodium pump (Na^+/K^+ ATPase)	A transport molecule in the membranes of all vertebrate cells; responsible for the maintenance of normal low intracellular sodium and high intracellular potassium concentrations
Sodium-calcium exchanger	A transport molecule in the membrane of many cells (eg, cardiac cells) that pumps one calcium atom against its concentration gradient (outward) in exchange for 3 sodium ions (moving down their concentration gradient)
Ventricular function curve	The graph that describes the changes in cardiac output, stroke volume, etc, versus increments in filling pressure or end-diastolic fiber length; also known as the Frank-Starling curve
Ventricular tachycardia	An arrhythmia consisting entirely or largely of beats originating below the AV node

CONCEPTS

PATHOPHYSIOLOGY OF CONGESTIVE HEART FAILURE & TREATMENT STRATEGIES

A. Pathophysiology: The fundamental physiologic defect in congestive heart failure is a decrease in cardiac contractility. The result of the defect is that cardiac output is inadequate for the needs of the body. This is best shown by the ventricular function curve (Frank-Starling curve, Figure 13–1). The homeostatic responses of the body to depressed cardiac output are mediated mainly by the sympathetic nervous system and the renin-angiotensin-aldosterone system. While these responses may temporarily improve cardiac output, they also increase the load on the heart; the increased load contributes to a further decline in cardiac function. The ventricular function curve reflects some of these deleterious compensatory responses and may also be used to demonstrate the response to drugs. As ventricular ejection decreases, the end-diastolic fiber length increases as shown by the shift from point A to point B in Figure 13–1. Operation at point B is intrinsically less efficient than operation at shorter fiber lengths because of the increase in myocardial oxygen requirement associated with increased fiber stretch (Figure 11–1).

Other compensatory responses include the following: (1) Tachycardia: an early manifestation of increased sympathetic tone. (2) Increased peripheral vascular resistance: another early response, also mediated by increased sympathetic tone. (3) Retention of salt and water by the kidney: an early compensatory response, mediated by the renin-angiotensin-aldosterone system and by increased sympathetic outflow. Increased blood volume results in edema and pulmonary congestion and contributes to the increased end-diastolic fiber length. (4) Cardiomegaly: enlargement of the heart is a slower compensatory response, mediated at least in part by sympathetic discharge. Angiotensin II may also play a role.

B. Therapeutic Strategies in Congestive Heart Failure: Pharmacologic therapies for congestive heart failure include the removal of retained salt and water with diuretics; direct treat-

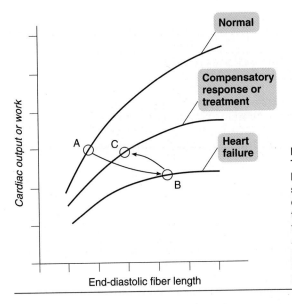

Figure 13–1. Ventricular function (Frank-Starling) curves. The abscissa can be any measure of preload—fiber length, filling pressure, pulmonary capillary wedge pressure, etc. The ordinate is a measure of useful external cardiac work—stroke volume, cardiac output, etc. In congestive heart failure, output is reduced at all fiber lengths and the heart expands because ejection fraction is decreased. As a result, the heart moves from point A to point B. Compensatory sympathetic discharge or effective treatment allows the heart to eject more blood and the heart moves to point C on the middle curve.

ment of the depressed heart with positive inotropic drugs such as digitalis glycosides; reduction of preload or afterload with vasodilators; and reduction of afterload and retained salt and water by angiotensin-converting enzyme inhibitors. In addition, recent evidence suggests that ACE inhibitors also alter the structural changes that often follow myocardial infarction and lead to congestive failure. The use of diuretics is discussed in Chapter 15.

DIGITALIS GLYCOSIDES

A. **Prototypes & Pharmacokinetics:** All cardiac glycosides include a steroid nucleus and a lactone ring; most also have one or more sugar residues. The sugar residues constitute the glycoside portion of the molecule, and the steroid nucleus plus lactone ring comprise the "genin" portion. The cardiac glycosides are often called "digitalis" because several come from the digitalis (foxglove) plant. **Digoxin** is the prototype agent and the one most commonly used in the USA. A very similar molecule, digitoxin, also comes from the foxglove, but is now rarely used. Digitalis-like drugs come from many other plants, and a few come from animals. Ouabain, a shorter-acting glycoside, is derived from a tropical plant. The pharmacokinetics of digoxin, digitoxin, and ouabain are summarized in Table 13–2.

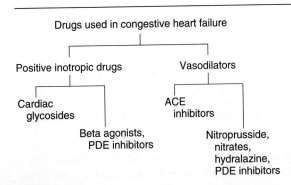

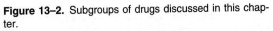

Figure 13–2. Subgroups of drugs discussed in this chapter.

Table 13–2. Pharmacokinetic parameters of typical cardiac glycosides in adults. Digoxin is the cardiac glycoside most commonly used in the USA.

	Digitoxin	Digoxin	Ouabain
Oral bioavailability (%)	90–100	60–85	0
Half-life (hours)	168	36–40	20
Primary organ of elimination	Liver	Kidney	Kidney
Volume of distribution (L/kg)	0.6	6–8	18
Protein bound in plasma (%)	> 90	20–40	0

B. Mechanism of Action: Inhibition of Na^+/K^+ ATPase of the cell membrane by digitalis is well documented and is considered to be the primary biochemical mechanism of action of digitalis (Figure 13–3). The translation of this effect into an increase in cardiac contractility involves the Na^+/Ca^{2+} exchange mechanism. Inhibition of Na^+/K^+ ATPase results in an increase in intracellular sodium. The increased sodium alters the driving force for sodium-calcium exchange so that less calcium is removed from the cell. The increased intracellular calcium is stored in the sarcoplasmic reticulum and upon release, increases contractile force. Other mecha-

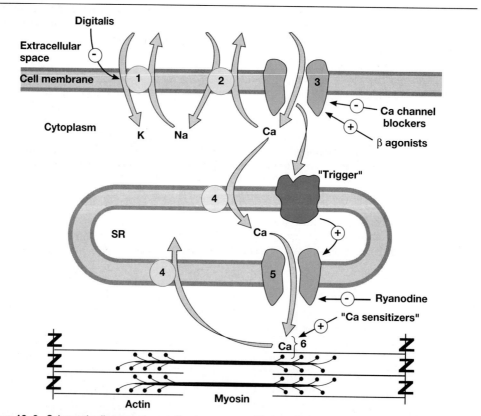

Figure 13–3. Schematic diagram of a cardiac sarcomere with the cellular components involved in contraction. 1, Na^+/K^+ ATPase; 2, Na^+/Ca^{2+} exchanger; 3, voltage-gated calcium channel; 4, calcium pump in the wall of the SR sarcoplasmic reticulum (SR); 5, calcium release channel in the SR; 6, site of calcium interaction with troponin-tropomyosin system. (Reproduced, with permission, from Katzung BG [editor]: *Basic & Clinical Pharmacology*, 6th ed. Appleton & Lange, 1995.)

nisms of action for digitalis have been proposed, but they are probably not as important as the ATPase effect. The consequences of Na^+/K^+ ATPase inhibition are seen in both the mechanical and the electrical function of the heart. Digitalis also modifies autonomic outflow, and this action has effects on the electrical properties of the heart.

C. Cardiac Effects:

1. **Mechanical effects:** The increase in contractility evoked by digitalis results in increased ventricular ejection, decreased end-systolic and end-diastolic size, increased cardiac output, and increased renal perfusion. These beneficial effects permit a decrease in the compensatory sympathetic and renal responses previously described. The decrease in sympathetic tone is especially beneficial: reduced heart rate, preload, and afterload permit the heart to function more efficiently (point C in Figure 13–1).

2. **Electrical effects:** Electrical effects include early cardiac parasympathomimetic responses and later arrhythmogenic responses. They are summarized in Table 13–3.

   a. **Early responses:** Increased PR interval, caused by the decrease in atrioventricular conduction velocity, and flattening of the T wave are often seen. The effects on the atria and AV node are largely parasympathetic in origin and can be partially blocked by atropine. The increase in the atrioventricular nodal refractory period is particularly important when atrial flutter or fibrillation is present because the refractoriness of the AV node determines the ventricular rate in these arrhythmias. The effect of digitalis is to slow ventricular rate. Inversion of the T wave and ST depression may occur later.

   b. **Toxic responses:** Increased automaticity, caused by intracellular calcium overload, is the most important manifestation of toxicity. It results from delayed afterdepolarizations, which may evoke extrasystoles, tachycardia, or fibrillation in any part of the heart. In the ventricles, the extrasystoles are recognized as premature ventricular beats (PVBs). When PVBs are coupled to normal beats in a 1:1 fashion, the rhythm is called bigeminy (Figure 13–4).

D. Clinical Uses:

1. **Congestive heart failure:** Digitalis is the traditional positive inotropic agent used in the treatment of congestive heart failure. However, other agents (diuretics, ACE inhibitors, vasodilators) may be equally effective and less toxic in some patients. Because the half-lives of both digoxin and digitoxin are long, the drugs accumulate significantly in the body and dosing regimens must be carefully designed and monitored.

2. **Atrial fibrillation:** In atrial flutter and fibrillation, it is desirable to reduce the conduction velocity or increase the refractory period of the atrioventricular node so that ventricular rate is decreased. The parasympathomimetic action of digitalis effectively accomplishes this therapeutic objective.

Table 13–3. Major actions of cardiac glycosides on cardiac electrical functions. (PANS, parasympathomimetic actions, direct membrane actions.)

	Tissue		
Variable	**Atrial Muscle**	**AV Node**	**Purkinje System, Ventricles**
Effective refractory period	↓ (PANS)	↑ (PANS)	↓ (Direct)
Conduction velocity	↑ (PANS)	↓ (PANS)	Negligible
Automaticity	↑ (Direct)	↑ (Direct)	↑ (Direct)
Electrocardiogram Before arrhythmias	Negligible	↑ PR interval	↓ QT interval; T wave inversion; ST segment depression
Arrhythmias	Atrial tachycardia, fibrillation	AV nodal tachycardia; AV blockade	Premature ventricular contractions (beats), ventricular tachycardia, ventricular fibrillation

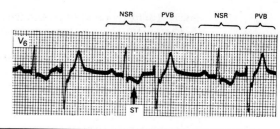

Figure 13–4. ECG record showing digitalis-induced bigeminy. The complexes marked NSR are normal sinus rhythm beats; an inverted T wave and depressed ST segment are present. The complexes marked PVB are premature ventricular beats.

E. Interactions: Quinidine causes a well-documented reduction in digoxin clearance and often increases the serum digoxin level if digoxin dosage is not adjusted. Several other drugs have been shown to have the same effect (amiodarone, verapamil, others) but the interactions with these drugs are not clinically significant. Digitalis effects are inhibited by extracellular potassium and magnesium and facilitated by extracellular calcium. Loop diuretics and thiazides, often used in treating heart failure, may significantly reduce serum potassium and thus precipitate digitalis toxicity. Digitalis-induced vomiting may deplete serum magnesium and similarly facilitate toxicity. These ionic interactions are important in treating digitalis toxicity (see below).

F. Digitalis Toxicity: The major signs of digitalis toxicity are arrhythmias, nausea, vomiting, and diarrhea. Rarely, confusion or hallucinations and visual aberrations may occur. The treatment of digitalis arrhythmias is important because this manifestation of digitalis toxicity is common and dangerous. Chronic intoxication is an extension of the therapeutic effect of the drug, and is caused by excessive calcium accumulation in cardiac cells (calcium overload). This overload triggers abnormal automaticity and the arrhythmias noted in Table 13–3. Digitalis arrhythmia is more likely if serum potassium or magnesium is lower than normal or if serum calcium is higher than normal.

Severe, acute, intoxication is caused by suicidal or accidental extreme overdose and results in cardiac depression leading to cardiac arrest rather than tachycardia or fibrillation. A case of severe intoxication is described in Case 2 (Appendix IV).

Treatment of digitalis toxicity includes the following:

1. Potassium or magnesium alterations: Correction of potassium deficiency is useful in chronic digitalis intoxication. Mild toxicity may often be managed by omitting one or two doses of digitalis and giving oral or parenteral K+ supplements. Similarly, if hypomagnesemia is present, it should be treated by normalizing serum magnesium. Severe acute intoxication (as in suicidal overdoses) usually causes marked hyperkalemia and should not be treated with supplemental potassium.

2. Antiarrhythmic drugs: Antiarrhythmic drugs may be useful if increased automaticity is prominent and does not respond to normalization of serum potassium. Agents that do not severely impair cardiac contractility (eg, lidocaine) are favored. Severe acute digitalis overdose usually causes suppression of all pacemaker cells. Antiarrhythmic drugs would be dangerous in such patients.

3. Digoxin antibodies: Digoxin antibodies (FAB fragments, Digibind) are extremely effective and should always be used if other therapies appear to be failing. They are effective for both digoxin and digitoxin overdose and may save severely poisoned patients who would otherwise die.

OTHER DRUGS USED IN CONGESTIVE HEART FAILURE

The major agents used with or as alternatives to digitalis in heart failure include diuretics, ACE inhibitors, β_1-selective sympathomimetics, phosphodiesterase inhibitors, and vasodilators.

A. Diuretics: Furosemide is a very useful agent for immediate reduction of the pulmonary congestion and severe edema associated with acute congestive heart failure. Thiazides such as hydrochlorothiazide are often used in the management of chronic failure even before digitalis is considered. The pharmacologic characteristics of the diuretics are discussed in Chapter 15.

B. Angiotensin-Converting Enzyme Inhibitors: These agents have been shown to be as effective as digitalis—or more so—in the management of chronic heart failure. Although they have no direct positive inotropic action, ACE inhibitors reduce aldosterone secretion, salt and water retention, and vascular resistance. They reduce symptoms and appear to prolong life in patients with heart failure. They are now considered among the first line drugs for chronic heart failure, along with diuretics and digitalis.

C. Beta$_1$-Selective Adrenoceptor Agonists: Dobutamine and dopamine are useful in some cases of acute failure. However, they are not appropriate for chronic failure because of tolerance, lack of oral efficacy, and significant arrhythmogenic effects.

D. Phosphodiesterase Inhibitors: Amrinone and milrinone are the major representatives of this infrequently used group, although theophylline (in the form of its salt, aminophylline) was commonly used in the past. These drugs increase cAMP by inhibiting its breakdown by phosphodiesterase and cause an increase in cardiac intracellular calcium similar to that produced by beta adrenoceptor agonists. Phosphodiesterase inhibitors also cause vasodilation, which may be responsible for a major part of their beneficial effect. At sufficiently high concentrations, these agents may increase the sensitivity of the contractile protein system to calcium (site 6 in Figure 13–3).

E. Vasodilators: Vasodilator therapy with nitroprusside or nitroglycerin is often used for acute severe congestive failure. The use of these vasodilator drugs is based on the reduction in cardiac size and improved efficiency that can be realized with proper adjustment of venous return and reduction of resistance to ventricular ejection. Vasodilator therapy can be dramatically effective, especially in cases in which increased afterload is a major factor in causing the failure (eg, hypertension in an individual who has just had an infarct). Chronic congestive heart failure sometimes responds favorably to oral vasodilators such as hydralazine or isosorbide dinitrate.

DRUG LIST

The following drugs are important members of the group discussed in this chapter. Prototypes should be learned in detail; features of the major variants should be known well enough to distinguish the variants from the prototypes and from each other; the other significant agents should be recognized as belonging to a specific subclass.

Subclass	Prototype	Major Variants	Other Significant Agents
Cardiac glycosides	Digoxin	Digitoxin	Ouabain
Positive inotropic digitalis substitutes	Dobutamine, amrinone		Milrinone, theophylline
ACE inhibitors	Captopril		Enalapril, lisinopril
Diuretics	Furosemide, hydrochlorothiazide		
Vasodilators	Nitroprusside	Nitroglycerin, hydralazine	Isosorbide, theophylline

QUESTIONS

DIRECTIONS: Each of the numbered items or incomplete statements in this section is followed by answers or by completions of the sentence. Select the ONE lettered answer or completion that is BEST in each case.

1. Drugs that have been found to be useful in one or more types of heart failure include all of the following EXCEPT
   (A) Na⁺/K⁺ ATPase inhibitors
   (B) Alpha adrenoceptor agonists
   (C) Beta adrenoceptor agonists
   (D) Thiazide diuretics
   (E) ACE inhibitors

2. The biochemical mechanism of action of digitalis is associated with
   (A) A shortening of the action potential duration
   (B) An increase in ATP synthesis
   (C) A modification of the actin molecule
   (D) An increase in systolic intracellular calcium levels
   (E) A block of sodium/calcium exchange

3. A common effect of digoxin (at therapeutic blood levels) that can be almost entirely blocked by atropine is
   (A) Tachycardia
   (B) Decreased appetite
   (C) Increased atrial contractility
   (D) Increased PR interval on the ECG
   (E) Headaches

4. A 65-year-old woman has been admitted to the coronary care unit with a myocardial infarction. If this patient develops acute severe congestive failure, all of the following might be useful EXCEPT
   (A) Nitroprusside
   (B) Digoxin
   (C) Furosemide
   (D) Propranolol
   (E) Dobutamine

5. Important effects of digitalis on the heart include
   (A) Increased force of contraction
   (B) Decreased atrioventricular conduction velocity
   (C) Increased ectopic automaticity
   (D) Decreased ejection time
   (E) All of the above

6. Which of the following situations constitutes an added risk of drug toxicity?
   (A) Digoxin therapy in a patient with hypocalcemia
   (B) Digoxin therapy in a patient with hyperkalemia
   (C) Digoxin therapy in a patient with hypermagnesemia
   (D) Digoxin therapy in a patient taking captopril
   (E) Digoxin therapy in a patient taking quinidine

7. Which row in the following table correctly shows the major pharmacokinetic characteristics of the cardiac glycosides?

Row	Variable	Digoxin	Digitoxin	Ouabain
(A)	Oral bioavailability	28%	75%	98%
(B)	Half-life	36 hours	168 hours	20 hours
(C)	Volume of distribution	0.6 L/kg	6.3 L/kg	18 L/kg
(D)	Percent protein bound in plasma	> 90%	50–60%	0%
(E)	Organ of excretion	Liver	Kidney	Liver

8. Effects of digitalis on electrical functions of the heart include all of the following EXCEPT
   (A) Prolonged atrioventricular refractory period
   (B) Slowed sinoatrial nodal rate
   (C) Increased atrial rate in atrial flutter

    (D) Decreased ventricular rate in atrial fibrillation

    (E) Decreased ectopic automaticity

9. Drugs associated with clinically useful or physiologically important positive inotropic effects include all of the following EXCEPT

    (A) Amrinone

    (B) Captopril

    (C) Digoxin

    (D) Dobutamine

    (E) Norepinephrine

10. The effects of digoxin include all of the following EXCEPT

    (A) Increased cardiac intracellular potassium

    (B) Increased cardiac intracellular sodium

    (C) Increased cardiac intracellular calcium

    (D) Increased force of cardiac contraction

    (E) Reduced sympathetic outflow to the heart

DIRECTIONS: The following section consists of a list of four to twenty-six lettered options followed by several numbered items. For each numbered item, select the ONE option that is most closely associated with it. Each answer may be selected once, more than once, or not at all.

    (A) Enalapril

    (B) Furosemide

    (C) Potassium

    (D) Dobutamine

    (E) Digoxin

    (F) Digitoxin

    (G) Magnesium

    (H) Digibind antibodies

    (I) Quinidine

    (J) Lidocaine

11. Administration of this monovalent cation would tend to decrease or reverse a mild-to-moderate digitalis-induced arrhythmia

12. Shown to prolong life in patients with chronic congestive failure but has no direct positive inotropic action

13. A β_1-selective agent sometimes used in acute congestive failure

14. Drug of choice in treating suicidal overdose of digoxin

15. Antiarrhythmic drug that is used to suppress digoxin-induced arrhythmias in some patients

ANSWERS

1. All the drugs listed are commonly used in heart failure except alpha agonists. These agents increase vascular resistance and would decrease the stroke volume of the weakened heart even more. The answer is **(B)**.

2. Digitalis does shorten the action potential in some parts of the heart and at some doses but this action is another *result,* not the *mechanism,* of digitalis biochemical action. Sodium/calcium exchange is not blocked, it is merely altered. The most accurate description of digitalis' mechanism in this list is that it increases intracellular calcium. The answer is **(D)**.

3. The parasympathomimetic effects of digitalis can be blocked by muscarinic blockers such as atropine. The only parasympathomimetic effect in the list provided is increased PR interval, representing slowing of AV conduction. The answer is **(D)**.

4. Acute severe congestive failure often requires vasodilators to reduce intravascular pressures in the lungs and the periphery. Both nitroprusside and furosemide have such vasodilating actions in the context of acute failure. Positive inotropic agents such as digoxin and dobutamine are traditional agents for heart failure. Beta antagonists such as propranolol, on the other hand, are usually contraindicated in heart failure; they are used only if the failure is due to certain cardiomyopathies. The answer is **(D)**.

5. The effects of digitalis include all the effects listed. The answer is **(E)**.

6. Digitalis toxicity is facilitated by hypercalcemia, hypokalemia, or hypomagnesemia. It is also

more likely if a patient begins taking quinidine after being stabilized on a dose of digitalis, because quinidine reduces the clearance of digoxin. The answer is **(E)**.

7. Review the pharmacokinetics of the cardiac glycosides. Note that the order of the drugs in this table (digoxin, digitoxin, ouabain) is not the same as the order in Table 13–2 (digitoxin, digoxin, ouabain). The answer is **(B)**.

8. The major cause of digitalis arrhythmias is *increased* automaticity. All the other effects listed are seen frequently. The answer is **(E)**.

9. Although they are extremely useful in congestive heart failure, captopril and the other ACE inhibitors have no positive inotropic effect on the heart. The answer is **(B)**.

10. Digoxin increases intracellular sodium and calcium and reduces sympathetic outflow to the heart (because the drug replaces the need for constant stimulation of contractility). However, digoxin does not increase intracellular potassium; blockade of Na^+/K^+ ATPase increases intracellular sodium and calcium, and very slightly reduces intracellular potassium. The answer is **(A)**.

11. Potassium is the only monovalent cation in the list that is used for reversing mild to moderate digitalis toxicity. The answer is **(C)**.

12. The ACE inhibitors have been shown to prolong life in heart failure patients even though these drugs have no direct positive inotropic action on the heart. The answer is **(A)**.

13. Dobutamine is a β_1-selective agonist often used in acute heart failure. The answer is **(D)**.

14. The drug of choice in severe, massive, digitalis overdose is digitalis antibody, Digibind. The answer is **(H)**.

15. Although quinidine may have this beneficial effect, it is also much more likely than lidocaine to precipitate digitalis toxicity. The answer is **(J)**.

14 Antiarrhythmic Drugs

OBJECTIVES

You should be able to:

- Describe the distinguishing features of the four major groups of antiarrhythmic drugs and adenosine.
- List two or three of the most important drugs in each of the four groups.
- List the major toxicities of those drugs.
- Describe the mechanism of selective depression by local anesthetic antiarrhythmic agents.
- Explain how hyperkalemia, hypokalemia, or an antiarrhythmic drug can cause an arrhythmia.

Learn the definitions that follow.

Table 14–1. Definitions.

Term	Definition
Abnormal automaticity	Pacemaker activity that originates anywhere other than in the sinoatrial node
Abnormal conduction	Conduction of an impulse that does not follow the path defined in Figure 14–1 or reenters tissue previously excited
Atrial, ventricular fibrillation	Arrhythmias involving rapid reentry and chaotic movement of impulses through the tissue of the atria or ventricles; ventricular, but not atrial, fibrillation is fatal within a few minutes if not terminated
Group I, II, III, and IV drugs	A method for classifying antiarrhythmic drugs, sometimes called the Vaughan Williams classification; based loosely on the channel or receptor affected
Reentrant arrhythmia	Arrhythmias of abnormal conduction; they involve the repetitive movement of an impulse through tissue previously excited by the same impulse
Effective refractory period	The period that must pass after the upstroke of a conducted impulse in a part of the heart before a new action potential can be propagated in that cell or tissue
Selective depression	The ability of certain drugs to selectively depress areas of excitable membrane that are most susceptible, leaving other areas relatively unaffected
Supraventricular tachycardia	A reentrant arrhythmia that travels through the AV node; it may also be conducted through atrial and ventricular tissue as part of the reentrant circuit
Ventricular tachycardia	A very common arrhythmia, associated often with myocardial infarction; ventricular tachycardia (a) may involve abnormal automaticity or abnormal conduction, (b) usually impairs cardiac output, and (c) may deteriorate into ventricular fibrillation; requires prompt management

CONCEPTS

Cardiac arrhythmias are the most common cause of death in patients who have had a myocardial infarction. They are also the most serious manifestation of digitalis toxicity.

PATHOPHYSIOLOGY

A. What Is an Arrhythmia? Normal cardiac function is dependent on generation of an impulse in the normal pacemaker (the sinoatrial [SA] node), and its conduction through the atrial muscle, through the atrioventricular (AV) node, through the Purkinje conduction system, to the ventricular muscle (Figure 14–1). Normal pacemaking and conduction require normal action potentials (dependent on sodium, calcium, and potassium channel activity), under appropriate autonomic control. Arrhythmias are therefore defined by exclusion—ie, any rhythm that is not a normal sinus rhythm (NSR) is an arrhythmia.

B. Arrhythmogenic Mechanisms: Abnormal automaticity and abnormal (reentry) conduction are the two major mechanisms for arrhythmias. A few of the clinically important arrhythmias are: atrial flutter, atrial fibrillation (AF), atrioventricular nodal reentry (a common type of supraventricular tachycardia [SVT]), premature ventricular beats (PVBs), ventricular tachycardia (VT), and ventricular fibrillation (VF). Examples of ECG recordings of normal sinus rhythm and some of these common arrhythmias are shown in Figure 14–2.

C. Normal Electrical Activity in the Cardiac Cell: The cellular action potentials shown in Figure 14–1 are the result of ion fluxes through voltage-gated channels and carrier mechanisms. These processes are diagrammed in Figure 14–3. In most parts of the heart, sodium current (I_{Na}) dominates the upstroke of the action potential and is the most important determinant of conduction of that action potential. In the AV node, calcium current (I_{Ca}) dominates the upstroke. The carrier processes (sodium pump and sodium/calcium exchanger) contribute little to the shape of the action potential. Antiarrhythmic drugs act on one or more of the three major currents (I_{Na}, I_{Ca}, I_K) or on the second messenger systems that modulate these currents.

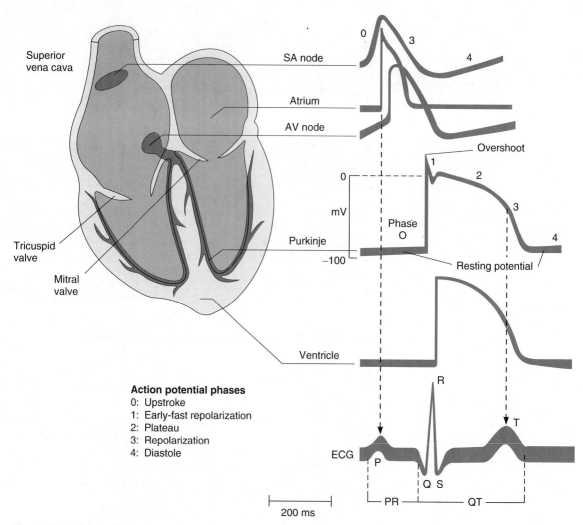

Figure 14–1. Schematic representation of the heart and normal cardiac electrical activity (intracellular recordings from areas indicated and ECG). The ECG is the body surface manifestation of the depolarization and repolarization waves of the heart. The P wave is generated by atrial depolarization, the QRS by ventricular muscle depolarization, and the T wave by ventricular repolarization. Thus the PR interval is a measure of conduction time from atrium to ventricle, and the QRS duration indicates the time required for all of the ventricular cells to be activated (ie, the intraventricular conduction time). The QT interval reflects the duration of the ventricular action potential.

D. Drug Group Classification: The antiarrhythmic agents are often classified using a system loosely based on the channel or receptor involved (Figure 14–4). This system specifies four groups, usually denoted by Roman numerals I through IV:

    I. Sodium channel blockers
    II. Beta adrenoceptor blockers
    III. Potassium channel blockers
    IV. Calcium channel blockers

A miscellaneous group includes adenosine, digitalis, potassium ion, and magnesium ion.

GROUP I (LOCAL ANESTHETICS)

A. Prototypes: The group I drugs are further characterized on the basis of their effects on action potential duration. Group IA agents (prototype, quinidine) prolong the action potential.

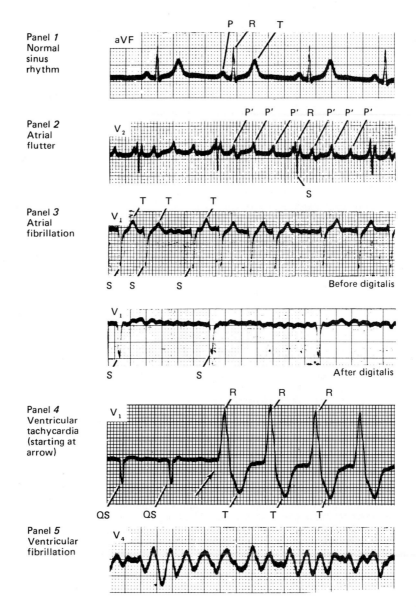

Figure 14–2. Typical electrocardiograms of normal sinus rhythm and some common arrhythmias. Major waves (P, Q, R, S, and T) are labeled in each electrocardiogram record except in panel 5, in which electrical activity is completely disorganized and none of these deflections are recognizable. (Modified and reproduced, with permission, from Goldman MJ: *Principles of Clinical Electrocardiography,* 11th ed. Lange, 1982.)

Group IB drugs shorten the action potential in some cardiac tissues (prototype, lidocaine). Group IC drugs have no effect on action potential duration (prototype, flecainide).

B. Mechanism of Action: As local anesthetics, all group I drugs slow or block conduction (especially in depolarized cells) and slow or abolish abnormal pacemakers wherever these processes depend on sodium channels. Useful sodium (and calcium) channel-blocking drugs bind to their receptors much more readily when the channel is open or inactivated than when it is fully repolarized and recovered from its previous activity. Ion channels in arrhythmic tissue spend more time in the open or inactivated states than do channels in normal tissue. Therefore, these antiarrhythmic drugs block channels in abnormal tissue more effectively than channels in

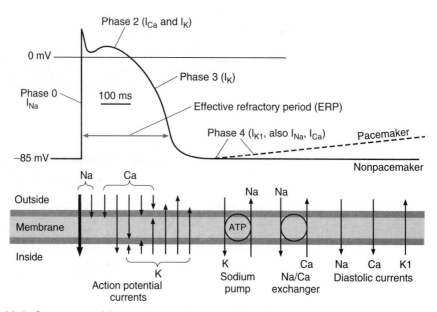

Figure 14–3. Components of the membrane action potential (AP) in a typical Purkinje or ventricular cardiac cell. The deflections of the AP, designated as phases 0 through 3, are generated by different ionic currents. The actions of the sodium pump and sodium/calcium exchanger are mainly involved in maintaining ionic steady state during repetitive activity. These actions are omitted from the following diagrams. Note that small but significant currents occur during diastole (phase 4) in addition to the pump and exchanger activity. In nonpacemaker cells, the outward potassium current is sufficient to maintain a stable negative resting potential, as shown by the solid line at the right end of the tracing. In pacemaker cells, however, the potassium current is smaller and the depolarizing currents (sodium, calcium, or both) are large enough to gradually depolarize the cell during diastole (shown by the dashed line).

normal tissue. As a result, antiarrhythmic sodium (and calcium) channel blockers are state-dependent in their action, ie, selectively depressant on tissue that is frequently depolarizing (eg, during a fast tachycardia) or is relatively depolarized during rest (eg, by hypoxia). The effects of the major antiarrhythmic group I drugs are summarized in Table 14–2 and Figure 14–5.

1. **Drugs with group IA action:** Quinidine is the Group IA prototype. Other drugs with IA actions include amiodarone, procainamide, and disopyramide. They affect both atrial and ventricular arrhythmias. These drugs increase action potential (AP) duration and the effective refractory period (ERP). The increase in action potential duration generates an increase in QT interval (Table 14–2). Amiodarone has similar effects on sodium current and has the greatest AP-prolonging effect. It is often considered a group III drug even though it also blocks sodium channels, a group I action.

2. **Drugs with group IB actions:** Lidocaine is the prototype IB drug. Mexiletine and tocainide are other IB agents. Lidocaine affects ischemic or depolarized Purkinje and ventric-

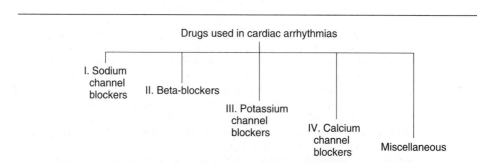

Figure 14–4. Subgroups of drugs discussed in this chapter.

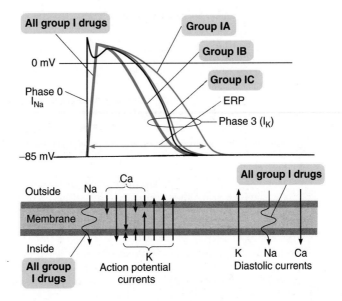

Figure 14–5. Schematic diagram of the effects of Group I agents. Note that all group I drugs reduce both phase 0 and phase 4 sodium currents in susceptible cells (shown as wavy lines). Group IA drugs also reduce potassium current (I_K) and prolong the AP duration. This results in significant prolongation of the effective refractory period. Group IB and IC drugs have different (or no) effects on potassium current and thus shorten or have no effect on the action potential.

ular tissue and has little effect on atrial tissue; the drug reduces action potential duration, but because it slows recovery of sodium channels from inactivation, it does not shorten (or may even prolong) the effective refractory period. Mexiletine and tocainide have similar effects. Because these agents have little effect on normal cardiac cells, they have little effect on the ECG (Table 14–2).

3. **Drugs with group IC action:** Flecainide is the prototype drug with group IC actions. Encainide (recently withdrawn), moricizine, and propafenone are also members of this group. These drugs have no effect on ventricular action potential duration or the QT interval. They are powerful depressants of sodium current, however, and can markedly slow conduction velocity in atrial and ventricular cells.

C. **Pharmacokinetics:**   See Table 14–2.

D. **Clinical Uses & Toxicities:**
1. **Group IA drugs:**   Quinidine is used in all types of arrhythmias, especially chronic ones requiring outpatient treatment. Both atrial and ventricular arrhythmias may be responsive. Procainamide and disopyramide have similar uses.

   Quinidine causes cinchonism (headache, tinnitus); cardiac depression; gastrointestinal upset; and allergic reactions (eg, thrombocytopenic purpura). As noted in Chapter 13, quinidine reduces the clearance of digoxin and may increase the serum concentration of the glycoside to dangerous levels. Procainamide causes a reversible syndrome similar to lupus erythematosus. Disopyramide has marked antimuscarinic effects and may precipitate congestive heart failure. All the group IA drugs may precipitate new arrhythmias. One arrhythmia, called *torsade de pointes,* is particularly associated with quinidine and other drugs that prolong AP duration (except amiodarone). Hyperkalemia usually exacerbates the cardiac toxicity of group I drugs. Treatment of overdose with these agents is usually carried out with sodium lactate (to reverse drug-induced arrhythmias) and pressor sympathomimetics (to reverse drug-induced hypotension).

2. **Group IB drugs:**   Lidocaine is useful in acute ventricular arrhythmias, especially those involving ischemia, eg, following myocardial infarction. Atrial arrhythmias are not respon-

sive unless caused by digitalis. Lidocaine is usually given intravenously, but IM administration is also possible. Mexiletine and tocainide have similar actions but can be given orally.

Lidocaine, mexiletine, and tocainide cause typical local anesthetic toxicity (ie, CNS stimulation, including convulsions); cardiovascular depression (usually minor); allergy (usually rashes but may extend to anaphylaxis). Tocainide may cause agranulocytosis. These drugs may also precipitate arrhythmias, but this is less common than with group IA drugs. Hyperkalemia, however, increases cardiac toxicity.

3. **Group IC drugs:** Flecainide is effective in both atrial and ventricular arrhythmias, but is approved only for (a) refractory ventricular tachycardias that tend to progress to VF at unpredictable times, resulting in "sudden death," and (b) certain intractable supraventricular arrhythmias.

Flecainide and its congeners are more likely than other antiarrhythmic drugs to exacerbate or precipitate arrhythmias (proarrhythmic effect). For this reason, the group IC drugs are limited to last resort applications in refractory tachycardias. These drugs also cause local anesthetic-like CNS toxicity. Hyperkalemia increases the cardiac toxicity of these agents.

4. **Amiodarone, a special case:** Amiodarone is effective in most types of arrhythmias, and may be considered the most efficacious antiarrhythmic drug. This may be because it has a broad spectrum: it blocks sodium, calcium, and potassium channels and beta adrenoceptors. Because of its toxicities, however, amiodarone must be reserved for use in arrhythmias that are resistant to other drugs.

Amiodarone causes thyroid dysfunction (hyper- or hypothyroidism), paresthesias, tremor, microcrystalline deposits in the cornea and skin, and pulmonary fibrosis. Amiodarone rarely causes new arrhythmias.

GROUP II (BETA-BLOCKERS)

A. **Prototypes, Mechanisms, & Effects:** Propranolol and esmolol are the prototype antiarrhythmic beta-blockers. Their mechanism in arrhythmias is primarily cardiac beta blockade and reduction in cAMP, which results in the reduction of both sodium and calcium currents and the suppression of abnormal pacemakers. The AV node is particularly sensitive to beta-blockers; the PR interval is frequently prolonged by group II drugs (Table 14–2). Under some conditions, they may have some direct local anesthetic (membrane stabilizing) effect in the heart, but this is probably rare at the concentrations achieved clinically.

B. **Clinical Uses & Toxicities:** Esmolol, a very short-acting beta-blocker for intravenous administration, is used almost exclusively in acute surgical arrhythmias. Propranolol, metoprolol, and timolol are commonly used as prophylactic drugs in patients who have had a myocardial infarction. These drugs provide a protective effect for two years or more after the infarct.

The toxicities of beta-blockers are the same when used as antiarrhythmics or in any other application. However, patients with arrhythmias are often more prone to β-blocker-induced depression of cardiac output than are patients with normal hearts.

GROUP III (POTASSIUM CHANNEL BLOCKERS)

A. **Prototypes:** Sotalol and bretylium. Amiodarone is often classified as a group III drug because it markedly prolongs AP duration as well as blocking sodium channels. Sotalol is a chiral compound, ie, it has two optical isomers. One isomer is an effective beta-blocker, the other provides most of the antiarrhythmic action. The clinical preparation contains both isomers. Bretylium is an older drug that combines sympathoplegic actions and a potassium channel-blocking effect.

B. **Mechanism & Effects:** The hallmark of group III drugs is prolongation of the action potential duration. This AP prolongation is caused by blockade of potassium channels that are responsible for the repolarization of the action potential (Figure 14–6). Sotalol and amiodarone (and quinidine, see above) produce this effect on most cardiac cells; the action of these drugs is

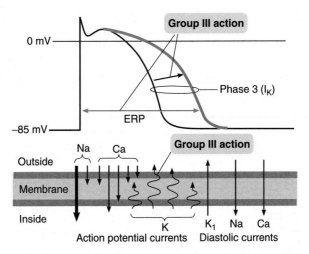

Figure 14–6. Schematic diagram of the effects of Group III agents. All group III drugs prolong the AP duration in susceptible cardiac cells by reducing the outward phase 3 potassium current (I_K, wavy lines). The main effect is to prolong the effective refractory period. Note that the phase 4 diastolic potassium current (I_{K1}) is not affected by these drugs.

therefore apparent in the ECG. N-acetylprocainamide (NAPA), a metabolite of procainamide, also significantly prolongs the action potential and the QT interval. Bretylium, on the other hand, produces AP prolongation mainly in ischemic cells, and causes little change in the ECG. AP prolongation results in an increase in effective refractory period and reduces the ability of the heart to respond to rapid tachycardias.

C. Clinical Uses & Toxicities: Bretylium is used only in the treatment of refractory post-myocardial infarction arrhythmias, eg, recurrent ventricular fibrillation. The drug is rarely used. It may precipitate new arrhythmias or marked hypotension. Sotalol is more generally useful and is available by the oral route (Table 14–2). Sotalol may precipitate *torsade de pointes* arrhythmia, as well as signs of excessive beta blockade such as sinus bradycardia or asthma. The toxicities of amiodarone and other group IA drugs (which share the potassium channel-blocking action of group III agents) are discussed with the group IA drugs.

GROUP IV (CALCIUM CHANNEL BLOCKERS)

A. Prototype: Verapamil is the prototype. Diltiazem is also an effective antiarrhythmic drug although it is not approved for this purpose. Nifedipine and the other dihydropyridines are not useful as antiarrhythmics, probably because they decrease arterial pressure sufficiently to evoke a compensatory sympathetic discharge to the heart. The latter effect would facilitate rather than suppress arrhythmias.

B. Mechanism & Effects: Verapamil and diltiazem are effective in arrhythmias that must traverse calcium-dependent cardiac tissue (eg, the atrioventricular node). These agents cause a state-dependent selective depression of calcium current in tissues that require the participation of L-type calcium channels (Figure 14–7). Conduction velocity is decreased and effective refractory period is increased by these drugs. PR interval is consistently increased (Table 14–2).

C. Clinical Use & Toxicities: Calcium channel blockers were drugs of choice in atrioventricular nodal reentry (also known as nodal tachycardia and supraventricular tachycardia) until adenosine became available; they are highly effective in this type of arrhythmia. Their major use now is in the prevention of these nodal arrhythmias. These drugs are orally active; verapamil is also available for parenteral use (Table 14–2). The most important toxicity of verapamil as an antiarrhythmic relates to excessive pharmacologic effect, since cardiac contractility

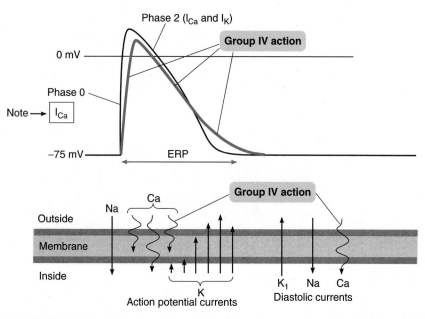

Figure 14–7. Schematic diagram of the effects of group IV drugs in a calcium-dependent cardiac cell in the AV node (note that the AP upstroke is due mainly to calcium current). Group IV drugs reduce inward calcium current during the action potential and during phase 4 (wavy lines). As a result, conduction velocity is slowed in the AV node and refractoriness is prolonged. Pacemaker depolarization during phase 4 is slowed as well, if caused by the calcium current.

can be significantly depressed. See Chapter 12 for additional discussion of toxicity. Amiodarone has moderate calcium channel-blocking activity.

MISCELLANEOUS ANTIARRHYTHMIC DRUGS

A. Adenosine: Adenosine is a normal component of the body, but when given in high dosage (6–12 mg) as an intravenous bolus, the drug markedly slows conduction in the atrioventricular node (Table 14–2). Adenosine is extremely effective in abolishing AV nodal arrhythmias and, because of its very low toxicity, has become the drug of choice for this arrhythmia. Adenosine has an extremely short duration of action (about 15 seconds). Toxicity includes flushing and hypotension, but because of the short duration of action these effects do not limit the use of the drug.

B. Digitalis: The actions of digitalis were discussed in Chapter 13. The cardiac parasympathomimetic action of digoxin is sometimes exploited in the treatment of rapid atrial or AV nodal arrhythmias. In atrial flutter or fibrillation, digitalis slows AV conduction sufficiently to protect the ventricles from excessively high rates. In AV nodal reentrant arrhythmias, digitalis may exert enough depressant effect to abolish the arrhythmia. The latter application of digitalis has become less common since the development of calcium channel blockers and adenosine as antiarrhythmic drugs.

C. Potassium Ion: Potassium depresses ectopic pacemakers, including those caused by digitalis toxicity. Hypokalemia is associated with increased incidence of arrhythmias, especially in patients receiving digitalis. Conversely, excessive potassium levels depress conduction and can cause reentry arrhythmias. Therefore, when treating arrhythmias, serum potassium should be measured and, if abnormal, normalized.

D. Magnesium Ion: Magnesium has not been as well studied as potassium but appears to have similar depressant effects on digitalis-induced arrhythmias. Magnesium also appears to be effective in some cases of *torsade de pointes* arrhythmia.

DRUG LIST: See Table 14–2.

Table 14–2. Properties of the prototype antiarrhythmic drugs.

	Group	Half-life	Route	PR Interval	QRS Duration	QT interval
Adenosine	Misc	3 sec	IV	↑	–	–
Amiodarone	IA, III	1–10 weeks	Oral, parenteral	↑	↑↑	↑↑↑↑
Bretylium	III	4 h	IV	–	–	–[1]
Disopyramide	IA	6–8 h	Oral	↓ or ↑[2]	↑	↑
Esmolol	II	10 min	IV	↑↑	–	–
Flecainide	IC	20 h	Oral	↑(slight)	↑↑	–
Lidocaine	IB	1–2 h	IV	–	–[3]	–
Mexiletine, tocainide	IB	12 h	Oral	–	–[3]	–
Procainamide	IA	3–4 h	Oral, IV	↓ or ↑[2]	↑	↑↑
Propranolol	II	8 h	Oral, IV	↑↑	–	–
Quinidine	IA	6 h	Oral, IV	↓ or ↑[2]	↑	↑↑↑
Sotalol	III	7 h	Oral	↑[4]	–	↑↑↑
Verapamil	IV	7 h	Oral, IV	↑↑	–	–

[1] Bretylium increases action potential duration in ischemic cells.
[2] PR may decrease through antimuscarinic action or increase through channel-blocking action.
[3] Lidocaine, mexiletine, and tocainide slow conduction velocity in ischemic, depolarized ventricular cells but not in normal tissue.
[4] Sotalol in its racemic formulation has beta-blocking effects that increase PR interval.

QUESTIONS

DIRECTIONS: Each of the numbered items or incomplete statements in this section is followed by answers or by completions of the sentence. Select the ONE lettered answer or completion that is BEST in each case.

Items 1–3: An elderly patient with rheumatoid arthritis and chronic heart disease is being considered for treatment with quinidine. She is already receiving digoxin, hydrochlorothiazide, and potassium supplements for her cardiac condition.

1. In making your decision to treat with quinidine, all of the following statements would be important EXCEPT
   (A) Quinidine may worsen or precipitate arrhythmias
   (B) Quinidine is not effective for atrial arrhythmias
   (C) Quinidine prolongs the effective refractory period in atrial and ventricular cells
   (D) Quinidine may induce thrombocytopenia
   (E) Quinidine may induce nausea, headache, and tinnitus

2. In deciding on a treatment regimen with quinidine for this patient, which of the following statements is MOST correct?
   (A) Quinidine is not active by the oral route
   (B) Quinidine has a duration of action of 20–30 hours
   (C) The serum potassium level should be as high as possible to reduce the likelihood of quinidine toxicity
   (D) A possible drug interaction with digoxin suggests that digoxin blood levels should be obtained before and after starting quinidine
   (E) Because of its beta-blocking effect, quinidine cannot be used if the patient has asthma

3. If this patient should manifest severe quinidine toxicity, rational therapy would entail the immediate administration of
   (A) KCl
   (B) Digitalis
   (C) A calcium chelator such as EDTA
   (D) Nitroprusside
   (E) Sodium lactate

4. When used as an antiarrhythmic drug, lidocaine typically
   - (A) Reduces abnormal automaticity
   - (B) Reduces resting potential
   - (C) Increases action potential duration
   - (D) Increases PR interval
   - (E) Increases contractility

5. All of the following can be used for chronic oral therapy of arrhythmias EXCEPT
   - (A) Esmolol
   - (B) Disopyramide
   - (C) Amiodarone
   - (D) Verapamil
   - (E) Procainamide

6. The antiarrhythmic of choice in most cases of acute supraventricular tachycardia (nodal tachycardia) is
   - (A) Propranolol
   - (B) Quinidine
   - (C) Flecainide
   - (D) Amiodarone
   - (E) Adenosine

7. Antiarrhythmic substances and their ECG effects include all of the following EXCEPT
   - (A) Quinidine: increased QRS and QT intervals
   - (B) Flecainide: increased PR, QRS, and QT intervals
   - (C) Verapamil: increased PR interval
   - (D) Lidocaine: no consistent ECG effect
   - (E) Metoprolol: increased PR interval

8. Drugs that consistently reduce potassium (I_K) current and thereby prolong the action potential duration include all of the following EXCEPT
   - (A) Quinidine
   - (B) Procainamide
   - (C) Amiodarone
   - (D) Sotalol
   - (E) Lidocaine

9. Recognized adverse effects of quinidine include all of the following EXCEPT
   - (A) Cinchonism
   - (B) Constipation
   - (C) Thrombocytopenic purpura
   - (D) Reduction of digoxin clearance with possible digoxin toxicity
   - (E) Precipitation of *torsade de pointes* arrhythmia

10. A drug that consistently hyperpolarizes the AV node and prevents conduction of impulses is
   - (A) Digoxin
   - (B) Quinidine
   - (C) Lidocaine
   - (D) Adenosine
   - (E) Verapamil

DIRECTIONS: The following section consists of a list of four to twenty-six lettered options followed by several numbered items. For each numbered item, select the ONE option that is most closely associated with it. Each answer may be selected once, more than once, or not at all.
   - (A) Adenosine
   - (B) Amiodarone
   - (C) Disopyramide
   - (D) Esmolol
   - (E) Flecainide
   - (F) Lidocaine
   - (G) Mexiletine
   - (H) Procainamide
   - (I) Quinidine
   - (J) Verapamil

11. Orally active drug that blocks sodium channels and decreases action potential duration
12. Slows conduction through the atrioventricular node; primary action is directly on calcium channels
13. Longest half-life of all antiarrhythmic drugs
14. Blocks sodium channels and prolongs action potential duration; duration of action is 6–8 hours
15. Very useful in supraventricular tachycardia; duration of action is 10–15 seconds
16. Causes thyroid abnormalities; may induce either hypo- or hyper-thyroidism
17. Orally active drug that may cause purpuric rash
18. Derived from the bark of the cinchona tree; may cause tinnitus and diarrhea
19. Causes reversible lupus erythematosus
20. Sodium channel blocker with little effect on AP duration; high incidence of arrhythmia induction

ANSWERS

1. Quinidine is effective for both atrial and ventricular arrhythmias. All of the other statements are true. The answer is **(B)**.
2. Quinidine is active by the oral route and has a duration of action of 6–8 hours. Hyperkalemia facilitates quinidine toxicity. Quinidine does have a well-documented interaction with digoxin: the clearance of the latter is reduced. Quinidine has little or no beta-blocking action. The answer is **(D)**.
3. The most effective therapy for quinidine toxicity appears to be concentrated sodium lactate. This drug may (a) increase sodium current by increasing the ionic gradient and (b) reduce drug-receptor binding by alkalinizing the tissue. The answer is **(E)**.
4. Lidocaine reduces automaticity in the ventricles; the drug does not alter resting potential or AP duration and does not increase contractility. The answer is **(A)**.
5. Esmolol is an ester that is rapidly metabolized even when given intravenously; it is inactive by the oral route. Therefore, esmolol would not be suitable for chronic therapy. The answer is **(A)**.
6. Calcium channel blockers are effective in supraventricular tachycardias. However, adenosine is just as effective in most supraventricular tachycardias and is less toxic because of its extremely short duration of action. The answer is **(E)**.
7. All the associations listed are correct except flecainide. This IC drug has little effect on QT interval. The answer is **(B)**.
8. All of the IA drugs and group III agents reduce potassium current during phase 3 and prolong the action potential. Lidocaine, the prototype IB drug, actually shortens the duration under some circumstances. The answer is **(E)**.
9. Quinidine has a wide spectrum of adverse effects but causes increased, not decreased, GI motility and often results in diarrhea. The answer is **(B)**.
10. The only antiarrhythmic agent that consistently alters the resting potential is adenosine. It apparently activates potassium channels in the AV node, thus forcing the membrane potential closer to the Nernst potassium potential; ie, adenosine significantly hyperpolarizes this tissue, preventing the conduction of action potentials. The answer is **(D)**.
11. Group IB drugs such as lidocaine and mexiletine typically block sodium channels and decrease the action potential duration. Mexiletine, but not lidocaine, is orally active. The answer is **(G)**.
12. Verapamil is the calcium channel blocker in this list. (Adenosine and beta-blockers also slow AV conduction but do not act directly on calcium channels.) The answer is **(J)**.
13. Amiodarone has the longest half-life of all the antiarrhythmics (Table 14–2). The answer is **(B)**.
14. Quinidine, procainamide, and amiodarone all block sodium channels and prolong the action potential. The duration of amiodarone action, however, is very long (question 12); that of procainamide is shorter than 6–8 hours (Table 14–2). The answer is **(I)**.
15. The only drug in the list with a half-life of seconds is adenosine. The answer is **(A)**.
16. Amiodarone is the only antiarrhythmic drug that is associated with thyroid toxicity. The answer is **(B)**.
17. Quinidine may cause thrombocytopenia; this can lead to punctate hemorrhages under the skin (purpura). The answer is **(I)**.
18. Quinidine is derived, along with quinine, from cinchona bark. The answer is **(I)**.

19. Procainamide frequently results in a positive antinuclear antibody (ANA) test after a prolonged therapy; this may progress to typical signs of drug-induced lupus (joint, skin, and systemic but not renal changes). The answer is **(H)**.
20. The IC antiarrhythmic drugs have little effect on AP duration; they have been associated with a high incidence of drug-induced arrhythmias. The answer is **(E)**.

15

Diuretic Agents

OBJECTIVES

You should be able to:

- List five major types of diuretics and relate them to their sites of action.
- Describe two drugs that reduce potassium loss during a sodium diuresis.
- Describe a therapy that will reduce calcium excretion in patients who have recurrent urinary stones.
- Describe a treatment for severe hypercalcemia in a patient with advanced carcinoma.
- Describe a method for reducing urine volume in nephrogenic diabetes insipidus.
- List the major applications and the toxicities of thiazides, loop diuretics, and potassium-sparing diuretics.

Learn the definitions that follow.

Table 15-1. Definitions.

Term	Definition
Bicarbonate diuretic	A diuretic that selectively increases sodium bicarbonate excretion. Example: a carbonic anhydrase inhibitor
Diluting segment	A segment of the nephron that removes solute without water; the thick ascending limb and the distal convoluted tubule are active salt-absorbing segments that are not permeant to water
Hyperchloremic metabolic acidosis	A shift in body electrolyte and pH balance involving elevated chloride, diminished bicarbonate concentration, and a decrease in pH in the blood. Typical result of bicarbonate diuresis
Hypokalemic metabolic alkalosis	A shift in body electrolyte balance and pH involving a decrease in serum potassium and an increase in blood pH. Typical result of loop and thiazide diuretics
Nephrogenic diabetes insipidus	Loss of urine-concentrating ability in the kidney caused by lack of responsiveness to antidiuretic hormone (ADH is present)
Pituitary diabetes insipidus	Loss of urine-concentrating ability in the kidney caused by lack of antidiuretic hormone (ADH is absent)
Potassium-sparing diuretic	A diuretic that reduces the exchange of potassium for sodium in the collecting tubule; a drug that increases sodium and reduces potassium excretion. Example: aldosterone antagonists
Uricosuric diuretic	A diuretic that increases uric acid excretion, usually by inhibiting uric acid reabsorption in the proximal tubule. Example: ethacrynic acid

CONCEPTS

RENAL TRANSPORT & DIURETIC DRUG GROUPS

A. Renal Transport Mechanisms: Each segment (proximal convoluted tubule, PCT; thick ascending limb of the loop of Henle, TAL; distal convoluted tubule, DCT; and cortical collecting tubule, CCT) has a different mechanism for reabsorbing sodium and other ions. The subgroups of the diuretics are based upon these sites in the nephron (Figure 15–1). The effects of the diuretic agents are predictable from a knowledge of the function of the segment of the nephron in which they act (Figure 15–2).

1. **Proximal convoluted tubule (PCT):** This segment carries out isosmotic reabsorption of amino acids, glucose, and cations. This is also the major site for bicarbonate reabsorption. The mechanism for bicarbonate reabsorption is shown in Figure 15–3. Although bicarbonate itself is not reabsorbed through the luminal membrane, conversion of bicarbonate to carbon dioxide permits rapid reabsorption; sodium is reabsorbed in exchange for hydrogen ions. Bicarbonate can then be regenerated within the tubular cell and reabsorbed back into the blood. Carbonic anhydrase, the enzyme required for this bicarbonate reabsorption process, is the target of carbonic anhydrase inhibitor diuretic drugs. The proximal tubule is responsible for 40–50% of the total reabsorption of sodium. Active secretion and reabsorption of weak acids and bases also occurs in the PCT. Uric acid transport is especially important and is targeted by some of the drugs used in treating gout (Chapter 35).

2. **Thick portion of the ascending limb of the loop of Henle (TAL):** This segment pumps sodium, potassium, and chloride out of the lumen into the interstitium of the kidney. It is also a major site of calcium and magnesium reabsorption, as shown in Figure 15–4. Reabsorption of sodium, potassium, and chloride are all carried out by a single carrier, which is the target of the loop diuretics. This cotransporter provides the concentration gradient for the countercurrent-concentrating mechanism in the kidney and is responsible for the reabsorption of 30–40% of the sodium filtered at the glomerulus. Because potassium is pumped into the cell from both the luminal and basal sides, an escape route must be provided; this occurs into the lumen via a channel. Since the potassium diffusing back is not accompanied by an anion, a net positive charge is set up in the lumen. This positive potential drives the reabsorption of calcium and magnesium.

3. **Distal convoluted tubule (DCT):** This segment actively pumps sodium and chloride out of the lumen of the nephron via the carrier shown in Figure 15–5. This cotransporter is the target of the thiazide diuretics. The distal convoluted tubule is responsible for approximately 10% of sodium reabsorption. Calcium is also reabsorbed in this segment, under the control of parathyroid hormone (PTH). Removal of the reabsorbed calcium back into the blood requires the sodium/calcium exchange process, discussed in Chapter 13.

4. **Collecting tubule (CCT):** The final segment of the nephron is the last tubular site of sodium reabsorption and is controlled by aldosterone (Figure 15–6). The aldosterone recep-

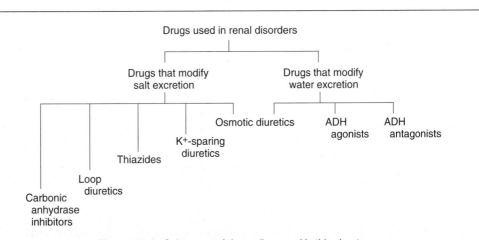

Figure 15–1. Subgroups of drugs discussed in this chapter.

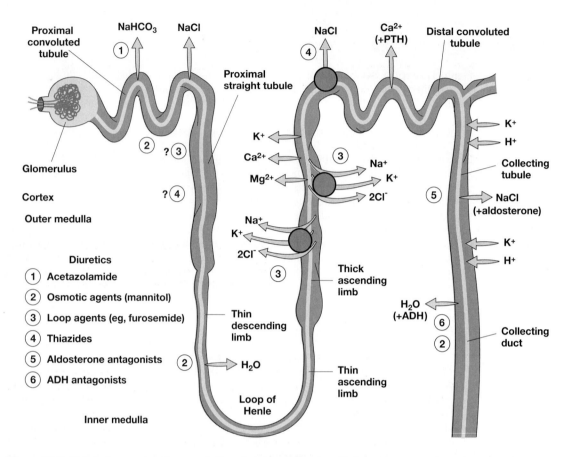

Figure 15–2. Tubule transport systems and sites of action of diuretics. Circles with arrows denote known ion cotransporters that are targets of the diuretics indicated by the numerals. Question marks denote preliminary or incompletely documented suggestions for the location of certain drug effects. (Reproduced, with permission, from Katzung BG [editor]: *Basic & Clinical Pharmacology,* 6th ed. Appleton & Lange, 1995.

tor and the sodium channels are sites of potassium-sparing diuretic action. This segment is responsible for reabsorbing 2–4% of the total filtered sodium. This reabsorption of sodium occurs via channels and is accompanied by an equivalent loss of potassium or hydrogen ions. The CCT is thus the primary site of acidification of the urine. Reabsorption of water occurs here and in the medullary collecting tubule under the control of antidiuretic hormone (ADH).

B. Diuretic Drug Groups: Because the mechanisms for reabsorption of salt and water differ in each of the four segments discussed above, the diuretics acting in these segments each have differing mechanisms of action. Most diuretics act from the luminal side of the membrane and must be present in the urine. They are filtered at the glomerulus and some are also secreted by the weak acid secretory carrier in the proximal tubule. An exception is the aldosterone receptor antagonist spironolactone, which enters from the basolateral side and binds to the cytoplasmic aldosterone receptor.

CARBONIC ANHYDRASE INHIBITORS

A. Prototypes and Mechanism of Action: Acetazolamide is the prototype agent. These diuretics are sulfonamide derivatives. The mechanism of action is inhibition of carbonic anhydrase in the brush border and intracellular carbonic anhydrase in the PCT cells (Figure 15–3). Inhibition of carbonic anhydrase by acetazolamide occurs in other tissues of the body as well as in the kidney.

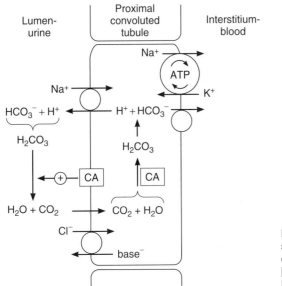

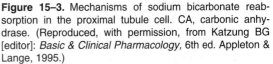

Figure 15–3. Mechanisms of sodium bicarbonate reabsorption in the proximal tubule cell. CA, carbonic anhydrase. (Reproduced, with permission, from Katzung BG [editor]: *Basic & Clinical Pharmacology,* 6th ed. Appleton & Lange, 1995.)

B. Effects: The major renal effect is a bicarbonate diuresis (ie, sodium bicarbonate is excreted); body bicarbonate is depleted, and a metabolic acidosis results. As increased sodium is presented to the cortical collecting tubule, some of the excess sodium is reabsorbed and potassium is secreted, resulting in significant potassium "wasting" (Table 15–2). As a result of bicarbonate depletion, sodium bicarbonate excretion slows—even with continued diuretic administration—and the diuresis is self-limiting within 2–3 days. The inhibitory effect of acetazolamide occurs throughout the body; secretion of bicarbonate into aqueous humor by the ciliary epithelium in the eye and into the cerebrospinal fluid by the choroid plexus is reduced. In the eye, a useful reduction in intraocular pressure can be achieved. This effect is not self-limiting. In the CNS, acidosis of the CSF results in hyperventilation, which can protect against high altitude sickness.

C. Clinical Uses: The major application of carbonic anhydrase inhibitors is in the treatment of glaucoma. These drugs must be used orally, but topical analogues are becoming available (eg, dorzolamide). Carbonic anhydrase inhibitors are also used to prevent development of acute

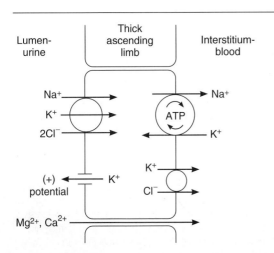

Figure 15–4. Mechanisms of sodium, potassium, and chloride reabsorption in the thick ascending limb of the loop of Henle. Note that pumping of potassium into the cell from both the lumen and the interstitium would result in unphysiologically high intracellular K^+ concentration. This is avoided by movement of K^+ down its concentration gradient back into the lumen, carrying with it excess positive charge. This positive charge drives the reabsorption of calcium and magnesium. (Reproduced, with permission, from Katzung BG [editor]: *Basic & Clinical Pharmacology,* 6th ed. Appleton & Lange, 1995.)

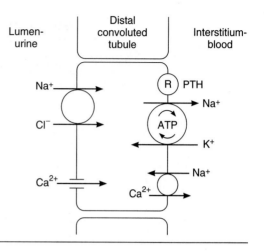

Figure 15–5. Mechanism of sodium and chloride reabsorption in the distal convoluted tubule. A separate reabsorptive mechanism, modulated by parathyroid hormone, is present for movement of calcium into the cell from the urine. This calcium must be transported via the sodium/calcium carrier back into the blood. (Reproduced, with permission, from Katzung BG [editor]: *Basic & Clinical Pharmacology,* 6th ed. Appleton & Lange, 1995.)

mountain (high altitude) sickness. These agents are used for their diuretic effect only if edema is accompanied by significant metabolic alkalosis.

D. Toxicity: Drowsiness and paresthesias are commonly reported. Cross allergenicity occurs between these and all other sulfonamide derivatives. Alkalinization of the urine by these drugs may cause precipitation of calcium salts and formation of renal stones. Renal potassium wasting may be marked. Patients with hepatic impairment may develop hepatic encephalopathy because of increased ammonia reabsorption.

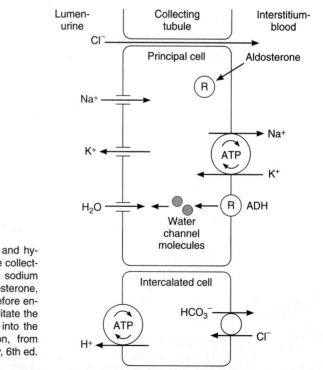

Figure 15–6. Mechanisms of sodium, potassium, and hydrogen ion movement and water reabsorption in the collecting tubule cells. Synthesis of Na^+/K^+ ATPase and sodium and potassium channels is under the control of aldosterone, which combines with an intracellular receptor, *R,* before entering the nucleus. ADH acts on its receptor to facilitate the insertion of water channels from storage vesicles into the luminal membrane. (Reproduced, with permission, from Katzung BG [editor]: *Basic & Clinical Pharmacology,* 6th ed. Appleton & Lange, 1995.)

Table 15–2. Electrolyte changes produced by diuretic drugs.

Drug Group	Urine			Body	
	NaCl	NaHCO$_3$	K$^+$	Cl$^-$	pH
Carbonic anhydrase inhibitors	↑	↑↑↑	↑	↑	Acidosis
Loop diuretics	↑↑↑↑	–	↑	↓	Alkalosis
Thiazides	↑↑	↑, –	↑	↓	Alkalosis
K$^+$-sparing diuretics	↑	–	↓	–, ↓	Acidosis

LOOP DIURETICS

A. Prototypes & Mechanism of Action: Furosemide is the prototype loop agent. Furosemide, bumetanide, and torsemide are sulfonamide derivatives. Ethacrynic acid is a phenoxyacetic acid derivative; it is not a sulfonamide but acts by the same mechanism. Loop diuretics inhibit the cotransporter of sodium, potassium, and chloride (Figure 15–4). The loop diuretics are relatively short-acting (diuresis usually occurs over the 4 hours following a dose).

B. Effects: The loop of Henle is responsible for a large proportion of total renal sodium chloride reabsorption; therefore, a full dose of a loop diuretic produces a massive sodium chloride diuresis. If tissue perfusion is adequate, edema fluid is rapidly excreted and blood volume may be significantly reduced. The diluting ability of the nephron is reduced because the loop of Henle is the site of significant dilution of urine. Inhibition of the transporter also results in loss of the lumen-positive potential, which reduces reabsorption of divalent cations as well. As a result, calcium excretion is significantly increased. Ethacrynic acid is a moderately effective uricosuric drug if blood volume is maintained. The presentation of large amounts of sodium to the cortical collecting tubule may result in significant potassium wasting and excretion of protons; hypokalemic alkalosis may result (Table 15–2). The loop diuretics also have potent pulmonary vasodilating effects; the mechanism is not understood.

C. Clinical Use: The major application of loop diuretics is in the treatment of edematous states (eg, congestive heart failure and ascites). They are particularly valuable in acute pulmonary edema, in which the pulmonary vasodilating action often plays a useful role. They are sometimes used in hypertension, if response to thiazides is inadequate; but the short duration of action of loop diuretics is a disadvantage in this condition. A less common but important application is in the treatment of severe hypercalcemia (eg, that induced by malignancy). This life-threatening condition can often be managed with large doses of furosemide coupled with parenteral volume and electrolyte (sodium and potassium chloride) supplementation. It should be noted that diuresis *without* volume replacement will result in hemoconcentration; serum calcium concentration then will not diminish and may even increase further.

D. Toxicity: Loop diuretics usually induce a hypokalemic metabolic alkalosis. Because large amounts of sodium are presented to the collecting tubules, wasting of potassium (which is excreted by the kidney in an effort to conserve sodium) may be severe. Because they are so efficacious, the loop diuretics can cause hypovolemia and cardiovascular complications. Ototoxicity is an important toxic effect of the loop agents. The sulfonamides in this group may cause typical sulfonamide allergy.

THIAZIDE DIURETICS

A. Prototypes & Mechanism of Action: Hydrochlorothiazide, the prototype agent, is a sulfonamide derivative. A few sulfonamide derivatives that lack the typical thiazide ring in their structure nevertheless have effects identical to those of thiazides and are therefore considered thiazide-like. Indapamide is a relatively new thiazide-like agent with a significant vasodilating effect. Thiazides are active by the oral route and have a duration of action of 6–12 hours, considerably longer than the loop diuretics. The major action of thiazides is to inhibit sodium chloride transport in the early segment of the distal convoluted tubule (Figure 15–5).

B. Effects: In full doses, thiazides produce a moderate but sustained sodium and chloride diuresis. A hypokalemic metabolic alkalosis may occur. Reduction in the transport of sodium into the tubular cell reduces intracellular sodium and promotes sodium/calcium exchange. As a result, reabsorption of calcium from the urine is increased and urine calcium content is decreased—the *opposite* of the effect of loop diuretics.

Thiazides reduce the blood pressure (Chapter 11). Initially, the reduction reflects the reduction of blood volume, but with continued use, these agents appear to reduce vascular resistance as well. The vascular effect is modest but significant and is maximal at doses lower than the maximal diuretic dosage. Compared to older thiazides and thiazide-like agents, indapamide may have a greater ratio of vasodilating effect relative to its sodium diuretic effect.

When a thiazide is used with a loop diuretic, a synergistic effect occurs with marked diuresis.

C. Clinical Use: The major application of thiazides is in hypertension, for which their long duration and moderate intensity of action are particularly useful. Chronic therapy of edematous conditions such as congestive heart failure is another common application. Chronic renal calcium stone formation can sometimes be controlled with thiazides because of their ability to reduce urine calcium concentration.

D. Toxicity: A massive sodium diuresis with hyponatremia is an uncommon but dangerous early effect of thiazides. Chronic therapy is often associated with potassium wasting, since an increased sodium load is presented to the collecting tubules. Diabetic patients may have significant hyperglycemia. Serum uric acid and lipid levels are also increased in some individuals. Thiazides are sulfonamides and share sulfonamide allergenicity.

POTASSIUM-SPARING DIURETICS

A. Prototypes & Mechanism of Action: Spironolactone, a steroid derivative, is a pharmacologic antagonist of aldosterone in the collecting tubules. By combining with the intracellular aldosterone receptor, spironolactone reduces the expression of the genes controlling synthesis of sodium ion channels and Na^+/K^+ ATPase. Amiloride and triamterene act by blocking the sodium channels in the same portion of the nephron (Figure 15–6). Spironolactone has a slow onset and offset of action (24–72 hours). Amiloride and triamterene have durations of action of 12–24 hours.

B. Effects: All three drugs in this class cause an increase in sodium clearance and a decrease in potassium and hydrogen ion excretion, and therefore qualify as "potassium-sparing" diuretics. These drugs may cause hyperchloremic metabolic acidosis.

C. Clinical Use: Aldosteronism (eg, the elevated serum aldosterone levels that occur in cirrhosis) is an important indication for spironolactone. Potassium wasting caused by chronic therapy with loop or thiazide diuretics, if not controlled by dietary potassium supplements, will usually respond to these drugs. The most common use is in the form of products that combine a thiazide with a potassium-sparing agent in a single pill.

D. Toxicity: The most important toxic effect is hyperkalemia. These drugs should never be given with potassium supplements. Other aldosterone antagonists (such as ACE inhibitors), if used at all, should be used with great caution. Spironolactone may cause endocrine abnormalities, including gynecomastia and anti-androgenic effects.

OSMOTIC DIURETICS

A. Prototypes & Mechanism of Action: Mannitol, the prototype osmotic diuretic, is given intravenously. Other drugs often classified with mannitol (but rarely used) include glycerin, isosorbide, and urea. Because it is filtered at the glomerulus but poorly reabsorbed from the tubule, mannitol "holds" water in the lumen by virtue of its osmotic effect. The major location for this action is the proximal convoluted tubule, where the bulk of isosmotic reabsorption normally takes place. Reabsorption of water is also reduced in the descending limb of the loop of Henle and the collecting tubule.

B. Effects: The volume of urine is increased. Most filtered solutes will be excreted in larger amounts unless they are actively reabsorbed. Sodium excretion is usually increased because the rate of urine flow through the tubule is greatly accelerated and sodium transporters cannot handle the volume rapidly enough. Mannitol can also reduce brain volume and intracranial pressure by osmotically extracting water from the tissue into the blood. A similar effect occurs in the eye.

C. Clinical Use: These drugs are used to maintain high urine flow (eg, when renal blood flow is reduced and in conditions of solute overload from severe hemolysis or rhabdomyolysis). Mannitol (and several other osmotic agents) are useful in reducing intraocular pressure in acute glaucoma and intracranial pressure in neurologic conditions.

D. Toxicity: Removal of water from the intracellular compartment may cause hyponatremia and pulmonary edema. Headache, nausea, and vomiting are common.

ANTIDIURETIC HORMONE AGONISTS & ANTAGONISTS

A. Prototypes & Mechanism of Action: Antidiuretic hormone (ADH) and desmopressin are prototype antidiuretic hormone agonists. They are peptides and must be given parenterally. Demeclocycline and lithium ion are ADH antagonists that can be used orally.

ADH facilitates water reabsorption from the collecting tubule by activation of adenylyl cyclase. The increased cAMP causes the insertion of additional water channels into the luminal membrane in this part of the tubule (Figure 15–6). Demeclocycline and lithium inhibit the action of ADH at some point distal to the generation of cAMP and presumably interfere with the insertion of water channels into the membrane.

B. Effects & Clinical Uses: ADH and desmopressin reduce urine volume and increase its concentration. ADH and desmopressin are useful in pituitary diabetes insipidus. They are of no value in the nephrogenic form of the disease, but salt restriction, thiazides, and loop diuretics may be used.

ADH antagonists oppose the actions of ADH and other naturally occurring peptides that act on the same V_2 receptor. Such peptides are produced by certain tumors (eg, small cell carcinoma of the lung) and can cause significant water retention and dangerous hyponatremia. This syndrome of inappropriate ADH secretion (SIADH) can be treated with demeclocycline.

C. Toxicity: In the presence of ADH and desmopressin, a large water load may cause dangerous hyponatremia. Large doses of either peptide may cause hypertension in some individuals.

In children under 8 years of age, demeclocycline (like other tetracyclines) causes bone and teeth abnormalities. Lithium causes nephrogenic diabetes insipidus as a toxic effect; the drug is never used to treat SIADH because of its other toxicities.

DRUG LIST

The following drugs are important members of the group discussed in this chapter. Prototypes should be learned in detail; the features of major variants should be known well enough to distinguish the variants from prototypes and from each other; the other significant agents should be recognized as belonging to a specific subclass.

Subclass	Prototype	Major Variants	Other Significant Agents
Carbonic anhydrase inhibitors	Acetazolamide		
Loop diuretics	Furosemide	Ethacrynic acid	
Thiazides and thiazide-like drugs	Hydrochlorothiazide	Indapamide	Metolazone
Potassium-sparing diuretics	Spironolactone Amiloride		Triamterene
Osmotic diuretics	Mannitol		
ADH agonists	Vasopressin (ADH)	Desmopressin	
ADH antagonists	Demeclocycline	Lithium	

QUESTIONS

DIRECTIONS: Each of the numbered items or incomplete statements in this section is followed by answers or by completions of the sentence. Select the ONE lettered answer or completion that is BEST in each case.

1. Which of the following drugs has a rapid diuretic effect plus smooth muscle effects that prove useful in the treatment of acute pulmonary edema?
   (A) Furosemide
   (B) Thiazide diuretic
   (C) Spironolactone
   (D) Triamterene
   (E) Acetazolamide

2. The most useful agent in the treatment of recurrent calcium stones is
   (A) Mannitol
   (B) Furosemide
   (C) Spironolactone
   (D) Hydrochlorothiazide
   (E) Acetazolamide

3. When used chronically to treat hypertension, thiazide diuretics have all of the following properties or effects EXCEPT
   (A) Reduce blood volume or vascular resistance or both
   (B) Have maximal effects on blood pressure at doses below the maximal diuretic dose
   (C) May cause an elevation of plasma uric acid and triglyceride levels
   (D) Decrease the urinary excretion of calcium
   (E) Cause ototoxicity

4. Which of the following drugs is correctly associated with its site of action and maximal diuretic efficacy?
   (A) Thiazides—distal convoluted tubule—10% of filtered Na^+
   (B) Spironolactone—distal convoluted tubule—10%
   (C) Bumetanide—thick ascending limb—15%
   (D) Metolazone—collecting tubule—2%
   (E) All of the above

5. Which of the following agents would be least harmful in a patient with severe hyperkalemia?
   (A) Amiloride
   (B) Captopril
   (C) Hydrochlorothiazide
   (D) Spironolactone
   (E) Triamterene

6. Which of the following would be most useful in a patient with cerebral edema?
   (A) Acetazolamide
   (B) Amiloride
   (C) Ethacrynic acid
   (D) Furosemide
   (E) Mannitol

7. Which of the following is NOT a complication of therapy with thiazide diuretics?
   (A) Hypercalciuria
   (B) Hyponatremia
   (C) Hypokalemia
   (D) Hyperuricemia
   (E) Metabolic alkalosis

8. Which of the following therapies would be most useful in the management of severe hypercalcemia?
   (A) Amiloride plus saline infusion
   (B) Furosemide plus saline infusion
   (C) Hydrochlorothiazide plus saline infusion
   (D) Mannitol plus saline infusion
   (E) Spironolactone plus saline infusion

9. A 70-year-old woman is admitted to the Emergency Room because of a "fainting spell" at home. She appears to have suffered no trauma from her fall, but her blood pressure is 110/60 when lying down and 60/40 when she sits up. Neurologic exam and an ECG are within normal limits when she is lying down. Questioning reveals that she has been on "water pills" (diuretics) for a heart condition. All of the following statements about this case are reasonable EXCEPT
   (A) The fainting spell could have resulted from postural hypotension caused by an inadvertent overdose with furosemide
   (B) The fainting spell could have resulted from a transient arrhythmia caused by furosemide-induced hypokalemia
   (C) The fainting spell could be unrelated to her diuretic therapy
   (D) The fainting spell could have resulted from furosemide-induced hyperuricemia
   (E) Management should include careful evaluation of her apparent blood volume

10. A patient complains of paresthesias and occasional nausea associated with one of her drugs. She is found to have a hyperchloremic metabolic acidosis. She is probably taking
    (A) Acetazolamide for glaucoma
    (B) Amiloride for edema associated with aldosteronism
    (C) Furosemide for severe hypertension and congestive failure
    (D) Hydrochlorothiazide for hypertension
    (E) Mannitol for cerebral edema

DIRECTIONS: The following section consists of a list of four to twenty-six lettered options followed by several numbered items. For each numbered item, select the ONE option that is most closely associated with it. Each answer may be selected once, more than once, or not at all.
    (A) Acetazolamide
    (B) Amiloride
    (C) Demeclocycline
    (D) Desmopressin
    (E) Ethacrynic acid
    (F) Furosemide
    (G) Metolazone
    (H) Mannitol
    (I) Spironolactone
    (J) Triamterene

11. Causes a self-limiting diuresis and a hyperchloremic metabolic acidosis
12. Not a thiazide but has its major effect in the distal convoluted tubule
13. Increases the formation of dilute urine in water-loaded subjects; used to treat SIADH
14. Useful in glaucoma and high altitude sickness
15. Acts in the loop of Henle thick ascending limb; no cross allergenicity with thiazides
16. Can reduce the binding of aldosterone to its receptor

ANSWERS

1. Furosemide has a rapid onset of action, is very efficacious, and appears to have significant direct smooth muscle-relaxing effects, especially in the pulmonary vessels. The answer is **(A).**

2. The thiazides are useful in the prevention of calcium stones because these drugs inhibit the renal excretion of calcium. In contrast, the loop agents facilitate calcium excretion. The answer is **(D)**.

3. Thiazides do not cause ototoxicity, loop diuretics do. The answer is **(E)**.

4. Spironolactone acts in the collecting tubule, not the distal convoluted tubule. This drug is not capable of causing a 10% sodium diuresis. Bumetanide, a loop diuretic, can produce a 30–40% increase in sodium excretion. Metolazone, a thiazide-like drug, acts in the distal convoluted tubule, not in the collecting tubule. The answer is **(A)**.

5. Hyperkalemia should not be treated with drugs that interfere with aldosterone production (eg, captopril) or collecting tubule potassium excretion (eg, amiloride, spironolactone, triamterene). These agents are all capable of increasing serum potassium. Hydrochlorothiazide would not reduce serum potassium rapidly, but it would not increase it. The answer is **(C)**.

6. An osmotic agent is needed to remove water from the cells of the edematous brain and reduce intracranial pressure. The answer is **(E)**.

7. Thiazides produce all of the effects listed except hypercalciuria. They *reduce* urine calcium and for this reason are useful in chronic stone formers. The answer is **(A)**.

8. Diuretic therapy of hypercalcemia requires a reduction in calcium reabsorption in the thick ascending limb. However, a loop diuretic alone would reduce blood volume around the remaining calcium so that serum calcium would not decrease appropriately. Therefore, saline infusion should accompany the loop diuretic. The answer is **(B)**.

9. The clinical vignette and the choice of answers suggests that the patient is taking a diuretic. Complications of diuretics that could result in syncope (fainting) include both postural hypotension (which this patient exhibits) due to excessive reduction of blood volume and arrhythmias due to excessive potassium loss. On the other hand, we have not ruled out other possible causes; the syncope may be unrelated to her diuretic therapy. Management would certainly include evaluation of her hemodynamic status, especially the level of hydration and blood volume. Both loop and thiazide diuretics may cause hyperuricemia. However, diuretic-induced hyperuricemia is not a cause of syncope but may cause acute gout in patients with gout as a pre-existing condition. The answer is **(D)**.

10. Paresthesias and gastrointestinal distress are common adverse effects of acetazolamide, especially when it is taken chronically, as in glaucoma. The observation that the patient has metabolic acidosis confirms the use of acetazolamide. The answer is **(A)**.

11. The carbonic anhydrase inhibitors, as suggested in question 10, cause metabolic acidosis; the diuresis is self-limiting because of bicarbonate depletion associated with this acidosis. The answer is **(A)**.

12. Metolazone, though not a thiazide, is a sulfonamide that is often used as a thiazide substitute. Metolazone's actions and toxicities (including sulfonamide allergy) are indistinguishable from the thiazides. The answer is **(G)**.

13. Inability to form dilute urine in the fully hydrated condition is characteristic of SIADH. Antagonists of ADH are needed to treat this condition. The answer is **(C)**.

14. Carbonic anhydrase inhibitors are useful in glaucoma and altitude sickness. The answer is **(A)**.

15. A loop agent that does not demonstrate cross allergenicity with thiazides is not a sulfonamide derivative. The answer is **(E)**.

16. Spironolactone is a pharmacologic antagonist of aldosterone, ie, it binds to the same receptor as the salt-retaining hormone. The answer is **(I)**.

Part IV. Drugs With Important Actions on Smooth Muscle

Histamine, Serotonin, & the Ergot Alkaloids

16

OBJECTIVES

You should be able to:

- List the major organ system effects of histamine and serotonin.
- List two or three different antihistamines of the H_1 and H_2 types.
- List two antiserotonin drugs and their major applications; describe the action and indication for sumatriptan.
- List the major organ system effects of the ergot alkaloids.
- Describe the major clinical applications of the ergot drugs.

Learn the definitions that follow.

Table 16–1. Definitions.

Term	Definition
Acid-peptic disease	Disease of the upper digestive tract caused by acid and pepsin; includes erosions and ulcers
Autacoids	Endogenous substances with complex physiologic and pathophysiologic functions; commonly taken to include histamine, serotonin, prostaglandins, and peptides
Carcinoid	A neoplasm of the bronchi or gastrointestinal tract that may secrete serotonin and a variety of peptides
Ergotism ("St. Anthony's Fire")	Disease caused by excess ergot alkaloid; classically an epidemic caused by consumption of grain (in bread, etc) that is contaminated by the ergot fungus
Gastrinoma	A tumor that produces large amounts of gastrin; associated with hypersecretion of gastric acid and pepsin leading to ulceration
IgE-mediated immediate reaction	An allergic response caused by interaction of an antigen with IgE antibodies on a mast cell; results in the release of histamine and other mediators of allergy
Oxytocic	A substance that causes contraction of the uterus
Prolactinoma	A tumor of the anterior pituitary that produces large amounts of prolactin and leads to amenorrhea/galactorrhea
Zollinger-Ellison syndrome	Hypersecretory syndrome, often caused by gastrinoma; associated with severe acid-peptic ulceration and diarrhea

CONCEPTS

Autacoids have obvious effects when studied as drugs, but these endogenous substances have poorly defined physiologic roles. Histamine and serotonin (5-hydroxytryptamine, 5-HT) are two of the most important autacoids. Both are synthesized in the body from amino acid precursors and then eliminated by pathways very similar to those used for catecholamine synthesis and metabolism. The ergot alkaloids are a heterogeneous group of drugs that interact with serotonin receptors, dopamine receptors, and adrenoceptors. They are included in this chapter because of their effects on serotonin receptors and on smooth muscle.

HISTAMINE

Histamine is formed from the amino acid histidine and is stored in high concentrations in mast cells. Histamine is metabolized by amine oxidase enzymes. Excess production of histamine in the body can be detected by measurement of imidazoleacetic acid, its major metabolite, in the urine. Because it is released from mast cells in response to IgE-mediated (immediate) allergic reactions, this autacoid plays an important pathophysiologic role in seasonal rhinitis (hay fever), urticaria, and angioneurotic edema. Histamine may also play a physiologic role in the control of acid secretion in the stomach.

A. Receptors & Effects: Two receptors for histamine, H_1 and H_2, mediate most of the well-defined actions; a third (H_3) has been identified (Table 16–2).

    1. H_1 receptor: This receptor is important in smooth muscle effects, especially those caused by IgE-mediated responses. IP_3 and DAG are released. Bronchoconstriction and vasodilation, the latter by release of endothelium-derived relaxing factor (EDRF), are typical responses of smooth muscle. Capillary endothelium, in addition to releasing EDRF, also contracts, opening gaps in the permeability barrier and resulting in the formation of local edema. These effects are manifest in allergic reactions and in mastocytosis, a rare neoplasm of mast cells.

    2. H_2 receptor: This receptor mediates gastric acid secretion by parietal cells in the stomach. It also has a cardiac stimulant effect. A third action is to reduce histamine release from mast cells—a negative feedback effect. These actions are mediated by activation of adenylyl cyclase, which increases intracellular cAMP.

    3. H_3 receptor: This receptor appears to be involved mainly in presynaptic modulation of histaminergic neurotransmission in the central nervous system. In the periphery, it appears to be a presynaptic heteroreceptor with modulatory effects on the release of other transmitters.

B. Clinical Use: Histamine has no therapeutic applications, but drugs that block histamine's effects are very important in clinical medicine.

HISTAMINE H_1 ANTAGONISTS

A. Classification & Prototypes: A wide variety of antihistaminic H_1 blockers are available from several different chemical families. Diphenhydramine and chlorpheniramine may be considered prototypes. Because they have been developed for use in chronic conditions, H_1 block-

Table 16–2. Histamine and serotonin receptor subtypes.[1]

Receptor Subtype	Distribution	Postreceptor Mechanism	Prototype Antagonist
H_1	Smooth muscle	↑ IP_3, DAG	Diphenhydramine
H_2	Stomach, heart, mast cells	↑ cAMP	Cimetidine
H_3	Nerve endings, CNS	G protein-coupled	Impromidine
$5-HT_{1d}$	Brain	↓ cAMP	–
$5-HT_2$	Smooth muscle, platelets	↑ IP_3, DAG	Ketanserin
$5-HT_3$	Area postrema (CNS), sensory and enteric nerves	Gated cation channel	Ondansetron

[1] Many other serotonin receptors are recognized in the CNS. They are discussed in Chapter 20.

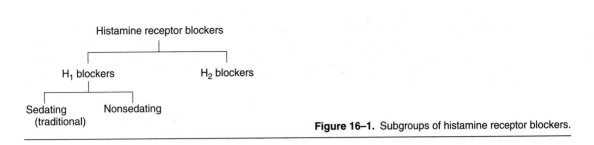

Figure 16–1. Subgroups of histamine receptor blockers.

ers are all active by the oral route. Most are metabolized extensively in the liver. Half-lives of the older H_1 blockers vary from 4 to 12 hours. Several newer agents (eg, terfenadine, astemizole) have half-lives of 12 to 24 hours and decreased CNS penetration.

B. Mechanism & Effects: H_1 blockers are competitive pharmacologic antagonists at the H_1 receptor; these drugs have no effect on histamine release from storage sites. Because their structure closely resembles that of muscarinic blockers and alpha adrenoceptor blockers, many of these agents are pharmacologic antagonists at these autonomic receptors. A few also block serotonin receptors. However, they have negligible effects at H_2 receptors.

H_1-blocking drugs have sedative and antimotion sickness effects in the CNS. In the periphery, they competitively inhibit the effects of histamine (especially if given before histamine release occurs). In addition, they may block muscarinic, alpha adrenoceptor-mediated, and serotonin-mediated effects. Many H_1 blockers are potent local anesthetics.

C. Clinical Use: H_1 blockers have major applications in allergies of the immediate type (ie, those caused by antigens acting on IgE antibody-sensitized mast cells). These conditions include hay fever and urticaria. The drugs have a broad spectrum of adverse effects that limit their usefulness but can sometimes be used to good effect (eg, the sedative effect is used in over-the-counter sleep aids). Dozens of H_1-blocking compounds are available.

D. Toxicity & Interactions: Sedation is common, especially with diphenhydramine and promethazine. It is much less common with newer agents that do not enter the CNS readily (eg, terfenadine, astemizole). Antimuscarinic effects such as dry mouth and blurred vision occur with some drugs in some patients. Alpha-blocking actions may cause orthostatic hypotension.

Interactions occur between older antihistamines and other drugs with sedative effects, eg, benzodiazepines and alcohol. Drugs that inhibit hepatic metabolism may result in dangerously high levels of nonsedating antihistaminic drugs that are taken concurrently. For example, ketoconazole inhibits metabolism of astemizole and terfenadine. In the presence of this antifungal drug, the plasma concentration of either antihistamine may increase and precipitate lethal arrhythmias.

HISTAMINE H_2 ANTAGONISTS

A. Classification & Prototypes: Four H_2 blockers are available; cimetidine is the prototype. These drugs do not resemble H_1 blockers structurally. They are orally active, with half-lives of 1–3 hours. Because they are relatively nontoxic, they can be given in large doses, so that the duration of action of a single dose may be 12–24 hours.

B. Mechanism & Effects: These drugs produce a surmountable pharmacologic blockade of histamine H_2 receptors. They are relatively selective and have no significant blocking action at H_1 or autonomic receptors.

The only therapeutic effect of clinical importance is the reduction of gastric acid secretion, but this is a very useful action. Blockade of cardiovascular H_2 receptor-mediated effects can be demonstrated, but has no clinical significance.

C. Clinical Use: In acid-peptic disease, especially duodenal ulcer, these drugs reduce symptoms, accelerate healing, and prevent recurrences. Acute ulcer is usually treated with two or more doses per day, while recurrence of the ulcer can often be prevented with a single bedtime dose. H_2 blockers are also effective in accelerating healing and preventing recurrences of gastric peptic ulcers. In Zollinger-Ellison syndrome, these drugs are very helpful (though large doses are required and they are not as effective as omeprazole) in controlling symptoms (acid hypersecretion, severe recurrent peptic ulceration, gastrointestinal bleeding, and diarrhea). Similarly, the H_2 blockers have been used in gastroesophageal reflux disease (GERD), but they are not as effective as omeprazole.

D. Toxicity: Cimetidine is a potent inhibitor of hepatic drug-metabolizing enzymes and may reduce hepatic blood flow. Cimetidine also has significant antiandrogen effects in many patients. Ranitidine has a weaker inhibitory effect on hepatic drug metabolism; neither it nor the newer H_2 blockers appear to have endocrine effects.

SEROTONIN (5-HYDROXYTRYPTAMINE, 5-HT) & RELATED AGONISTS

Serotonin is produced from tryptophan and stored in the enterochromaffin cells of the gut and in the CNS. Excess production in the body can be detected by measuring its major metabolite, 5-hydroxyindoleacetic acid, in the urine. Serotonin appears to play a physiologic role as a neurotransmitter in both the CNS and the enteric nervous system, and possibly as a local hormone that modulates gastrointestinal activity. Serotonin is also stored (but synthesized to only a minimal extent) in platelets. Only one drug is in use for its serotonin agonist effects; several are in use or under investigation as serotonin antagonists (Figure 16–2).

A. Receptors & Effects:

1. **5-HT$_1$ receptors:** 5-HT$_1$ receptors are most important in the brain and mediate synaptic inhibition via increased potassium conductance (Table 16–2). Peripheral 5-HT$_1$ receptors mediate both excitatory and inhibitory effects in various smooth muscle tissues.

2. **5-HT$_2$ receptors:** 5-HT$_2$ receptors are important in both brain and peripheral tissues. These receptors mediate synaptic excitation in the CNS and smooth muscle contraction (gut, bronchi, uterus, vessels) or dilation (vessels). The mechanism involves (in different tissues) decreased potassium conductance, decreased cAMP, and increased IP$_3$. In carcinoid tumor, this receptor probably mediates some of the vasodilation, diarrhea, and bronchoconstriction characteristic of the disease.

3. **5-HT$_3$ receptors:** 5-HT$_3$ receptors are found in the CNS, especially in the chemoreceptive area and vomiting center, and in peripheral sensory and enteric nerves. These receptors mediate excitation via a 5-HT-gated cation channel (ie, the mechanism of serotonin at the 5-HT$_3$ receptor resembles that of ACh at nicotinic cholinergic cation channels). Antagonists acting at this receptor have proved to be useful antiemetic drugs.

B. Clinical Use: Serotonin has no clinical applications.

C. Other Serotonin Agonists: **Sumatriptan,** a substituted indole compound, is a 5-HT$_{1d}$ agonist. It is effective in the treatment of acute migraine and cluster headache attacks, an observation that strengthens the association of serotonin abnormalities with these headache syndromes. At present it is available only for parenteral injection, unlike the ergot antimigraine medications, which are available for oral and rectal (suppository) use.

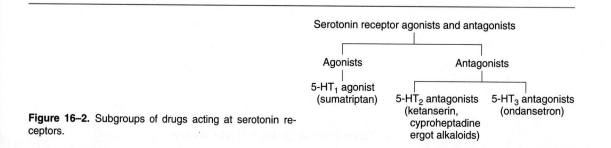

Figure 16–2. Subgroups of drugs acting at serotonin receptors.

A number of important antidepressant drugs act at serotonergic synapses by inhibiting the re-uptake carrier for 5-HT. These drugs are discussed in Chapter 29.

SEROTONIN ANTAGONISTS

A. Classification & Prototypes: **Ketanserin** is a 5-HT$_2$ and alpha adrenoceptor blocker. **Phenoxybenzamine** (an alpha adrenoceptor blocker) and **cyproheptadine** (an H$_1$ blocker) are also good 5-HT$_2$ blockers. **Ondansetron** is a 5-HT$_3$ blocker. The **ergot alkaloids** are partial agonists at 5-HT (and other) receptors (see below).

B. Mechanisms & Effects: Ketanserin and cyproheptadine are competitive pharmacologic antagonists. Phenoxybenzamine is an irreversible blocker.

Ketanserin, cyproheptadine, and phenoxybenzamine are weakly selective agents. In addition to inhibition of serotonin effects, they also have alpha-blocking effects (ketanserin, phenoxybenzamine) or H$_1$ blocking effects (cyproheptadine). Ondansetron, which is more selective for 5-HT$_3$ receptors, has a very significant central antiemetic action.

C. Clinical Uses: Ketanserin is under investigation as an antihypertension drug. Ketanserin, cyproheptadine, and phenoxybenzamine may be of value (separately or in combination) in the treatment of carcinoid tumor, a neoplasm that secretes large amounts of serotonin (and peptides) and causes diarrhea, bronchoconstriction, and flushing. Ondansetron is used to control postoperative vomiting and vomiting associated with cancer chemotherapy.

D. Toxicity: Adverse effects of ketanserin are those of alpha blockade and H$_1$ blockade. The toxicities of ondansetron include diarrhea and headache.

ERGOT ALKALOIDS

These complex molecules are produced by a fungus found in wet or spoiled grain. They are responsible for the epidemics of "St. Anthony's Fire" (ergotism) described during the Middle Ages. There are at least twenty naturally occurring members of the family, but only a few of these and a handful of semisynthetic derivatives are used as therapeutic agents. The ergot alkaloids are partial agonists at alpha adrenoceptors and 5-HT receptors. The balance of agonist versus antagonist effect varies from compound to compound. Some are also agonists at the dopamine receptor.

A. Classification & Prototypes: The ergot alkaloids may be subdivided into three major groups on the basis of the organ or tissue in which they have their primary effects (Figure 16–3). This division is not absolute, since most of the alkaloids have some effects on several tissues.

The brain is a target organ for several natural ergot alkaloids that cause the hallucinations and chemical psychoses associated with epidemics of ergotism. The most important derivatives acting in the CNS, however, are the semisynthetic drugs, **LSD** and **bromocriptine.** The uterus is very sensitive to ergot alkaloids as term pregnancy nears but is less sensitive at other times. **Ergonovine** is a prototype oxytocic ergot alkaloid. Blood vessels are sensitive to another group of ergot drugs, of which **ergotamine** is the prototype.

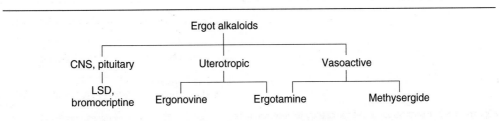

Figure 16–3. Subgroups of ergot alkaloids.

B. Effects: The receptor effects of the ergot alkaloids are summarized in Table 16–3 and include the following:

1. **Vessels:** Ergot alkaloids can produce marked and prolonged alpha receptor-mediated vasoconstriction. An overdose can cause ischemia and gangrene of the limbs.

2. **Uterus:** A powerful contraction occurs in this tissue near term. This is sufficient to cause abortion or miscarriage. Earlier in pregnancy (and in the nonpregnant uterus) much higher doses of ergot alkaloids are needed to produce this effect. After delivery of the placenta, ergonovine or ergotamine can produce a useful contraction of the uterus that reduces blood loss.

3. **Brain:** Hallucinations may be prominent with the naturally occurring ergots and with LSD, but are less common with therapeutic ergots. Although LSD is a potent 5-HT$_2$ blocker in peripheral tissues, its actions in the CNS are believed to be due to actions at dopamine receptors. In the pituitary, some ergot alkaloids are potent dopamine-like inhibitors of prolactin secretion. Bromocriptine is one of the most potent of the semisynthetic derivatives at these dopamine D$_2$ receptors and at similar receptors in the basal ganglia.

C. Clinical Uses:

1. **Migraine:** Ergotamine is a mainstay of treatment of acute attacks. Methysergide and ergonovine are used prophylactically.

2. **Obstetric bleeding:** Ergonovine and ergotamine are effective agents for the reduction of postpartum bleeding.

3. **Hyperprolactinemia and parkinsonism:** Bromocriptine is used to reduce prolactin secretion (dopamine is the physiologic prolactin release inhibitor). Bromocriptine also appears to reduce the size of pituitary tumors of the prolactin-secreting cells. This drug is also useful in the treatment of Parkinson's disease (Chapter 27).

4. **Other uses:** Methysergide has been used in carcinoid tumor.

D. Toxicity: The toxic effects of ergot alkaloids are quite important, both from a public health standpoint (epidemics of ergotism from spoiled grain) and from the toxicity of overdose or abuse by individuals.

1. **Vascular effects:** Severe prolonged vasoconstriction can result in ischemia and gangrene. The only consistently effective antagonist is nitroprusside. When used for long periods, methysergide produces an unusual hyperplasia of connective tissue, which may be a response to chronic ischemia in this tissue. This fibroplasia may be retroperitoneal, retropleural, or subendocardial and can cause hydronephrosis or cardiac valvular and conduction system malfunction. Similar lesions are found in some patients with carcinoid, indicating that this action is probably mediated by agonist effects at serotonin receptors.

2. **Gastrointestinal effects:** Most ergot alkaloids cause gastrointestinal upset (nausea, vomiting, diarrhea) in many individuals.

3. **Uterine effects:** Marked uterine contractions may be produced. The uterus becomes progressively more sensitive to ergot alkaloids during pregnancy. Although abortion due to use for migraine is rare, most obstetricians recommend avoidance or very conservative use of these drugs as pregnancy progresses.

Table 16–3. Effects of ergot alkaloids at several receptors.[1,2]

Ergot Alkaloid	Alpha Adrenoceptor	Dopamine Receptor (D$_2$)	Serotonin Receptor (5-HT$_2$)	Uterine Smooth Muscle Stimulation
Bromocriptine	–	+++	–	0
Ergonovine	+	+	– (PA)	+++
Ergotamine	– – (PA)	0	+ (PA)	+++
Lysergic acid diethylamide (LSD)	0	+++	– – –	++
Methysergide	0/+	+/0	– – – (PA)	0

[1] Reproduced, with permission, from Katzung BG (editor): *Basic & Clinical Pharmacology*, 6th ed. Appleton & Lange, 1995.
[2] Agonist effects are indicated by +, antagonist by –, no effect by 0. Relative affinity for the receptor is indicated by the number of + or – signs. PA means partial agonist..

4. **CNS effects:** Hallucinations resembling psychosis are common with LSD but less common with the other ergot alkaloids. Methysergide has occasionally been used as an LSD substitute by users of "recreational drugs."

DRUG LIST

The following drugs are important members of the group discussed in this chapter. Prototypes should be learned in detail; features of the major variants should be known well enough to distinguish them from the prototypes and from each other; the other significant agents should be recognized as belonging to a specific subclass.

Subclass	Prototype	Major Variants	Other Significant Agents
Histamine agonists	Histamine		
H₁ blockers	Diphenhydramine Terfenadine		Chlorpheniramine, cyproheptadine, promethazine, astemizole
H₂ blockers	Cimetidine		Ranitidine, famotidine, nizatidine
5-HT agonists	Serotonin, sumatriptan		
5-HT antagonists	Ketanserin, ondansetron		Cyproheptadine, ergot alkaloids
Ergot alkaloids	Bromocriptine Ergonovine Ergotamine	LSD, methysergide	

QUESTIONS

DIRECTIONS: Each of the numbered items or incomplete statements in this section is followed by answers or by completions of the sentence. Select the ONE lettered answer or completion that is BEST in each case.

Questions 1–2 refer to the following clinical case. Your patient has been diagnosed with a rare metastatic carcinoid tumor. This neoplasm is releasing serotonin, bradykinin, and several unknown peptides.

1. The effects of serotonin in this patient may include all of the following EXCEPT
   (A) Episodes of bronchospasm
   (B) Diarrhea
   (C) Hypersecretion of gastric acid
   (D) Instability of blood pressure
   (E) Retroperitoneal fibroplasia

2. In recommending treatment for your carcinoid patient, you will consider all of the following EXCEPT
   (A) Cyproheptadine
   (B) Methysergide
   (C) Phenoxybenzamine
   (D) Sumatriptan
   (E) Ketanserin

3. Drugs that can reverse one or more smooth muscle effects of circulating histamine in humans include all of the following EXCEPT
   (A) Epinephrine
   (B) Cyproheptadine
   (C) Ketanserin
   (D) Chlorpheniramine
   (E) Phenylephrine

4. Many antihistamines (H₁ blockers) have additional effects; these are likely to include all of the following EXCEPT
   (A) Antimuscarinic reduction in bladder tone
   (B) Local anesthetic effects if the drug is injected

      (**C**) Antimotion sickness effect

      (**D**) Increase in total peripheral resistance

      (**E**) Sedation

5. All of the following are H_2-blocking drugs EXCEPT

      (**A**) Cimetidine

      (**B**) Famotidine

      (**C**) Nizatidine

      (**D**) Ranitidine

      (**E**) Terfenadine

6. Toxicities of H_1 antihistamines include all of the following EXCEPT

      (**A**) Blurred vision

      (**B**) Diarrhea

      (**C**) Orthostatic hypotension

      (**D**) Sleepiness

7. All of the following statements about possible pharmacologic causes of 16th and 17th century accounts of witchcraft are reasonable EXCEPT

      (**A**) Ingestion of bread made with flour from spoiled grain could cause painful burning sensations in the limbs, leading naive individuals to suspect supernatural evil forces

      (**B**) Similar ingestion could cause "epidemics" of abortions, with similar interpretations

      (**C**) Similar ingestion by elderly women might cause them to have hallucinations and exhibit behaviors interpretable by others as "casting spells"

      (**D**) The major substance now known to occur in spoiled grain is methysergide, a substance similar to PCP

8. A patient undergoing cancer chemotherapy is vomiting frequently. A drug that might help in this situation is

      (**A**) Bromocriptine

      (**B**) Cimetidine

      (**C**) Ketanserin

      (**D**) Ondansetron

      (**E**) Terfenadine

9. Characteristics of H_2 histamine blockers include all of the following EXCEPT

      (**A**) All have short half-lives of 2–4 hours

      (**B**) All available H_2 blockers have approximately equal efficacy but widely varying potency

      (**C**) Cimetidine is associated with more drug interactions than other H_2 blockers, due to inhibition of hepatic P450 systems

      (**D**) Cimetidine is associated with antiandrogenic effects in some patients

      (**E**) H_2 blockers must be given 4 to 5 times per day for therapeutic effect

10. Correct applications of drugs include the following clinical indications EXCEPT

      (**A**) Astemizole: for hay fever

      (**B**) Ergonovine: for postpartum bleeding

      (**C**) Methysergide: for recurrent migraine headache

      (**D**) Ondansetron: for acute migraine headache

      (**E**) Ranitidine: for prophylaxis of duodenal ulcer

DIRECTIONS: The following section consists of a list of four to twenty-six lettered options followed by several numbered items. For each numbered item, select the ONE option that is most closely associated with it. Each answer may be selected once, more than once, or not at all.

      (**A**) Bromocriptine

      (**B**) Cimetidine

      (**C**) Ergotamine

      (**D**) Ketanserin

      (**E**) LSD

      (**F**) Methysergide

      (**G**) Nitroprusside

      (**H**) Ondansetron

      (**I**) Phenoxybenzamine

      (**J**) Sumatriptan

11. Useful in the treatment of hyperprolactinemia

12. Effective in the treatment of peptic ulcer disease
13. Serotonin agonist useful for aborting an acute migraine headache; parenteral only
14. Used in management of severe ergot-induced vasospasm
15. Causes inhibition of hepatic metabolism of many drugs; some antiandrogenic effects
16. Useful irreversible antagonist for treatment of some carcinoid tumors

ANSWERS

1. The effects of serotonin include all of those listed except gastric acid hypersecretion; serotonin actually decreases acid secretion. The answer is **(C)**.
2. All of the drugs listed have significant blocking effects on 5-HT receptors except sumatriptan, which is an agonist at 5-HT$_{1d}$ receptors. The answer is **(D)**.
3. Each of the drugs listed is a pharmacologic antagonist (chlorpheniramine, cyproheptadine) or physiologic antagonist (epinephrine, phenylephrine) of histamine except ketanserin, a pharmacologic antagonist of 5-HT at 5-HT$_2$ receptors. The answer is **(C)**.
4. H$_1$ blockers do not activate receptors that mediate vasoconstriction; some of these drugs actually block alpha adrenoceptors, causing significant vasodilation. The answer is **(D)**.
5. Terfenadine is a nonsedating H$_1$ blocker. The answer is **(E)**.
6. None of the H$_1$ blockers cause diarrhea as a prominent adverse effect, and many have antimuscarinic actions that result in constipation (see also question 4). The answer is **(B)**.
7. It has been proposed by historians that many of the behaviors described for accused "witches" during the Salem witch trials period of American history resemble the signs of ergotism. Ergotism is caused by a mixture of naturally occurring ergot alkaloids, not methysergide, a semisynthetic ergot derivative. Methysergide is not similar to PCP (phencyclidine). The answer is **(D)**.
8. Ondansetron has significant antiemetic effects. The answer is **(D)**.
9. H$_2$ blockers have short half-lives but can be given in very large doses that provide adequate blood levels for 12 to 24 hours. The answer is **(E)**.
10. Ondansetron has no value in migraine headache; the drug is used only as an antiemetic during chemotherapy and for postoperative vomiting. The answer is **(D)**.
11. Bromocriptine is an effective dopamine agonist in the CNS with the advantage of oral activity. The drug inhibits prolactin secretion by activating pituitary dopamine receptors. The answer is **(A)**.
12. An H$_2$ blocker is appropriate for peptic ulcer; cimetidine is such a drug. The answer is **(B)**.
13. Sumatriptan, an agonist at 5-HT$_{1d}$ receptors, is indicated for parenteral treatment of migraine. Ergotamine is also effective for acute migraine but it is given orally or rectally. The answer is **(J)**.
14. A very powerful vasodilator is necessary to reverse ergot-induced vasospasm; nitroprusside is such a drug. The answer is **(G)**.
15. Cimetidine is well known for causing drug interactions because of its ability to inhibit hepatic P450 isozymes. The drug also has weak antiandrogenic effects. The answer is **(B)**.
16. Phenoxybenzamine is the only irreversible blocker in this list. The drug has significant affinity for histamine and 5-HT$_2$ receptors as well as for alpha receptors, and has been found useful in some patients with carcinoid, presumably because of this agent's ability to block 5-HT$_2$ receptors. The answer is **(I)**.

17

Vasoactive Peptides

OBJECTIVES

You should be able to:

- Name a partial agonist inhibitor of angiotensin and at least two drugs that reduce the formation of angiotensin II.
- Outline the major effects of bradykinin and atrial natriuretic peptide (ANP).
- Describe the functions of converting enzyme (peptidyl dipeptidase, kininase II).
- Describe the effects of vasoactive intestinal peptide (VIP), substance P, and neuropeptide Y.

CONCEPTS

A. Classification & Prototypes: Vasoactive peptides comprise a large class of endogenous substances that function as neurotransmitters and as local and systemic hormones. Many are still poorly understood, in terms of the physiologic or pathophysiologic roles they play and their possible clinical potential. They include angiotensin, bradykinin, atrial natriuretic peptide, vasoactive intestinal peptide, substance P, calcitonin gene-related peptide, vasopressin, glucagon, and opioid peptides. Vasopressin is discussed in Chapters 15 and 36. Glucagon is discussed in Chapter 40, and the opioids in Chapter 30. The peptides discussed in this chapter and their effects are summarized in Table 17–1.

B. Mechanisms: These agents probably all act on cell surface receptors. As indicated in Table 17-1, most act via G protein-coupled receptors and cause the production of second messengers; a few may open ion channels.

ANGIOTENSIN & ITS ANTAGONISTS

A. Source & Disposition: Angiotensin I is produced from angiotensinogen by renin, an enzyme released from the juxtaglomerular apparatus of the kidney. An inactive decapeptide, angiotensin I is converted into angiotensin II (AII), an octapeptide, by angiotensin-converting enzyme (ACE), also known as peptidyl dipeptidase or kininase II (Fig 11–3). Angiotensin II, the active form of the peptide, is rapidly degraded by peptidases (angiotensinases).

Table 17–1. Some vasoactive peptides and their properties.

Peptide	Properties
Angiotensin II (AII)	↑ IP_3, DAG. Constricts arterioles, increases aldosterone secretion
Atrial natriuretic peptide (ANP)	↑ cGMP. Dilates vessels, inhibits aldosterone secretion and effects, increases glomerular filtration
Bradykinin	↑ IP_3, DAG; ↑ cAMP, ↑ NO. Dilates arterioles, increases capillary permeability, stimulates sensory pain endings
Calcitonin gene-related peptide (CGRP)	Causes hypotension and tachycardia by unknown mechanisms
Endothelin	↑ IP_3, DAG. Constricts most vessels and contracts other smooth muscle
Neuropeptide Y (NPY)	Causes vasoconstriction and stimulates heart; mediated in part by IP_3
Substance P	Dilates arterioles, contracts veins and intestinal and bronchial smooth muscle, causes diuresis; transmitter in sensory pain neurons
Vasoactive intestinal peptide (VIP)	Dilates vessels, relaxes bronchi and intestinal smooth muscle

B. **Effects:** Angiotensin II is a potent arteriolar vasoconstrictor and stimulant of aldosterone release. AII directly increases peripheral vascular resistance and, through aldosterone, causes renal sodium retention. AII also facilitates the release of norepinephrine from adrenergic nerve endings via presynaptic heteroreceptor action.

C. **Clinical Role:** Angiotensin II was used in the past by intra-arterial infusion to control bleeding in difficult-to-access sites. The peptide is no longer used for this indication. Its major clinical significance is as a pathophysiologic mediator in some cases of hypertension (high renin hypertension) and in congestive heart failure. Thus, AII antagonists are of considerable clinical interest.

D. **Antagonists:** As noted in Chapter 11, two types of antagonists are available. **Saralasin** is a partial agonist inhibitor at the angiotensin II receptor. **Angiotensin-converting enzyme inhibitors** (eg, captopril, enalapril, etc) are important agents for the treatment of hypertension. Block by either of these inhibitors is often accompanied by a compensatory increase in renin and angiotensin I. Several orally active renin and AII *receptor* inhibitors are in clinical trials. **Losartan** is one of the more promising: it blocks AII receptors and has been shown to be effective in some patients with hypertension.

BRADYKININ

A. **Source & Disposition:** Bradykinin is one of several vasodilator kinins produced from kininogen by a family of enzymes, the kallikreins. Bradykinin is rapidly degraded by various peptidases, including angiotensin-converting enzyme.

B. **Effects:** Bradykinin is one of the most potent vasodilators known. The peptide is thought to be involved in inflammation (causing edema and pain when released or injected into tissue). Bradykinin can be released into saliva, but the peptide's function there is unknown. Bradykinin may play a role in stimulating the secretion of saliva.

C. **Clinical Role:** Although it has no therapeutic application, bradykinin may play a role in the antihypertensive action of angiotensin-converting enzyme inhibitors, as previously noted (Chapter 11, Fig 11–4). There are no clinically important bradykinin antagonists.

ATRIAL NATRIURETIC PEPTIDE

A. **Source & Disposition:** Atrial natriuretic peptide (ANP) is synthesized and stored in the cardiac atria of mammals. ANP is released from the atria in response to distension of the chambers.

B. **Effects:** Atrial natriuretic peptide activates guanylyl cyclase in many tissues. ANP is a vasodilator as well as a natriuretic (sodium excretion-enhancing) agent. Its renal action includes increased glomerular filtration, decreased proximal tubular sodium reabsorption, and inhibitory effects on renin secretion. The peptide also inhibits the actions of angiotensin II and aldosterone. Although it lacks positive inotropic action, ANP may play an important compensatory role in congestive heart failure by limiting sodium retention.

C. **Clinical Role:** ANP has been studied for possible use in the treatment of congestive heart failure, but results have not been encouraging. There are no clinically important products that act as agonists or antagonists at ANP receptors.

ENDOTHELIN

Endothelin is a peptide formed in and released by endothelial cells in blood vessels. Endothelin is believed to function as an autocrine and paracrine hormone in the vasculature. Three different endothelin peptides (ET-1, ET-2, and ET-3) with minor variations in amino acid sequence have been identified in man. Two receptors have been identified, both of which are G protein-coupled.

Endothelin is much more potent than norepinephrine as a vasoconstrictor and has a relatively long-lasting effect. The peptide also stimulates the heart, increases ANP release, and activates smooth muscle proliferation. The peptide may be involved in some forms of hypertension and other types of cardiovascular pathology. Antagonists have recently become available for research use.

VASOACTIVE INTESTINAL PEPTIDE, SUBSTANCE P, CALCITONIN GENE-RELATED PEPTIDE, & NEUROPEPTIDE Y

Vasoactive intestinal polypeptide (VIP) is an extremely potent vasodilator but probably is physiologically more important as a neurotransmitter. It is found in the central and peripheral nervous systems and in the gastrointestinal tract. No clinical role has been found for this peptide thus far.

Substance P is another neurotransmitter polypeptide with potent vasodilator action. Relaxant effects, however, are restricted to arterioles; substance P is a potent *stimulant* of veins and of intestinal and airway smooth muscle. The peptide may also function as a local hormone in the gastrointestinal tract. Highest concentrations of substance P are found in those parts of the nervous system that contain neurons subserving pain. At the present time, there are no clinical applications for substance P or its antagonists. However, **capsaicin,** the "hot" component of chili peppers, releases substance P from its stores in nerve endings and depletes the peptide. Capsaicin has been approved for topical use on arthritic joints.

Calcitonin gene-related peptide (CGRP) is found (along with calcitonin) in high concentrations in the thyroid, but is also present in most smooth muscle tissues. The presence of CGRP in smooth muscle suggests a function as a cotransmitter in autonomic nerve endings. CGRP is the most potent hypotensive agent discovered to date and causes reflex tachycardia. There is no clinical application for this peptide.

Unlike the three preceding peptides in this section, neuropeptide Y (NPY) is a potent *vasoconstrictor* that stimulates the heart. NPY is found in both the CNS and the peripheral nerves. In the periphery, NPY is most commonly localized as a cotransmitter in adrenergic nerve endings. Several receptor subtypes have been identified.

DRUG LIST: See Table 17–1.

QUESTIONS

DIRECTIONS: Each of the numbered items or incomplete statements in this section is followed by answers or by completions of the sentence. Select the ONE lettered answer or completion that is BEST in each case.

1. Regarding polypeptides,
    (A) Angiotensin I (a decapeptide) is the most potent of the series that includes angiotensinogen and angiotensin II (an octapeptide)
    (B) Bradykinin is a potent vasodilator with pain-inducing and edema-inducing effects
    (C) Atrial natriuretic peptide (ANP) increases cardiac contractility in congestive heart failure
    (D) Because they cannot cross the blood-brain barrier, polypeptides are not found in the brain
    (E) Bradykinin is inactivated by the enzyme kallikrein
2. Which of the following, if given intravenously, will cause increased gastrointestinal motility or diarrhea?
    (A) Bethanechol
    (B) Bradykinin
    (C) Angiotensin
    (D) Renin
    (E) All of the above
3. A polypeptide that causes increased capillary permeability and edema is
    (A) Captopril
    (B) Histamine
    (C) Bradykinin
    (D) Saralasin
    (E) Angiotensin II

4. Agents that produce arterial vasoconstriction include all of the following EXCEPT
   (A) Angiotensin II
   (B) Epinephrine
   (C) Methysergide
   (D) Serotonin
   (E) Substance P
5. A vasodilator that can be inactivated by proteolytic enzymes is
   (A) Neuropeptide Y
   (B) Vasoactive intestinal peptide
   (C) Histamine
   (D) Angiotensin I
   (E) Isoproterenol

DIRECTIONS: The following section consists of a list of four to twenty-six lettered options followed by several numbered items. For each numbered item, select the ONE option that is most closely associated with it. Each answer may be selected once, more than once, or not at all.
   (A) Angiotensin I
   (B) Angiotensin II
   (C) Atrial natriuretic peptide
   (D) Calcitonin gene-related peptide
   (E) Vasoactive intestinal peptide
   (F) Endothelin
   (G) Substance P
   (H) Neuropeptide Y
   (I) Bradykinin
   (J) Renin

6. Produced in traumatized tissue; causes pain and edema
7. Decapeptide precursor of a vasoconstrictor substance
8. Arterial vasodilator found in peripheral and CNS nerves; causes contraction of veins and airway smooth muscle; associated with sensory pain fibers
9. Octapeptide vasoconstrictor that increases in the blood of hypertensive patients treated with large doses of diuretics
10. Vasodilator that increases in the blood or tissues of patients treated with captopril
11. Most potent vasodilator discovered to date; found in high concentrations in the thyroid
12. Peptide cotransmitter in many autonomic nerve endings; directly relaxes vascular, airway, and GI smooth muscle

ANSWERS

1. Angiotensin I is an inactive precursor. Atrial natriuretic peptide has no effect on cardiac contractility. Polypeptides are found in high concentrations in parts of the brain because they are synthesized there. The answer is **(B)**.
2. The polypeptides listed here are not associated with marked increases in gastrointestinal motility. Bethanechol, a muscarinic cholinoceptor stimulant, is an effective stimulant of the gut. The answer is **(A)**.
3. Histamine and bradykinin both cause marked increase in permeability that is often associated with edema, but histamine is not a peptide. The answer is **(C)**.
4. Substance P is a potent arterial vasodilator. The answer is **(E)**.
5. A peptide, but not an amine, would be altered by proteolytic enzymes. Vasoactive intestinal peptide is the only polypeptide in the list that is a vasodilator. The answer is **(B)**.
6. Bradykinin is a mediator in damaged tissue. The answer is **(I)**.
7. Angiotensin I is a decapeptide. The answer is **(A)**.
8. Substance P is a vasodilator that is also a pain-mediating neurotransmitter. The answer is **(G)**.
9. Angiotensin II, an octapeptide, increases because the compensatory cardiovascular response causes an increase in renin secretion. The answer is **(B)**.
10. Bradykinin increases because the enzyme inhibited by captopril, converting enzyme, normally degrades kinins as well as synthesizing angiotensin II (see Fig 11–4). The answer is **(I)**.

11. The most potent vasodilator discovered to date is calcitonin gene-related peptide. The answer is **(D)**.

12. Vasoactive intestinal peptide is a general smooth muscle relaxant that is also an important co-transmitter in ANS nerves. The answer is **(E)**.

18 Prostaglandins & Other Eicosanoids

OBJECTIVES

You should be able to:

- List the major effects of PGE_2, PGF_2, LTB_4, LTC_4, and LTD_4.
- List important sites of synthesis and the effects of thromboxane and prostacyclin in the vascular system.
- Explain the differing effects of aspirin on prostaglandin synthesis and on leukotriene synthesis.

Learn the definitions that follow.

Table 18–1. Definitions.

Term	Definition
Abortifacient	A drug used to cause an abortion. Example: Prostaglandin $F_{2\alpha}$
Cyclooxygenase	Enzyme that converts arachidonic acid to PGG and PGH, the precursors of the prostaglandins
Dysmenorrhea	Painful uterine cramping activated by prostaglandins released during menstruation
Endoperoxide	General term for prostaglandin precursors, eg, PGG, PGH
Great vessel transposition	Congenital anomaly in which the pulmonary artery exits from the left ventricle and the aorta from the right ventricle. Incompatible with life unless a large patent ductus or ventricular septal defect is present
Lipoxygenase	Enzyme that converts arachidonic acid to leukotriene precursors (HPETEs)
NSAID	Nonsteroidal anti-inflammatory drug, eg, aspirin, ibuprofen. Inhibitor of cyclooxygenase
Patent ductus arteriosus	Persistence after birth of the fetal connection between the pulmonary artery and aorta
Phospholipase A_2	Enzyme in the cell membrane that generates arachidonic acid from membrane lipid constituents
Slow-reacting substance of anaphylaxis (SRS-A)	Material originally identified by bioassay from tissues of animals undergoing anaphylactic shock; now recognized as a mixture of leukotrienes, especially LTB_4, LTC_4, and LTD_4

CONCEPTS

The eicosanoids are an important group of fatty-acid derivatives that are produced from arachidonic acid derived from cell membrane lipids.

EICOSANOID AGONISTS

A. Classification: The principal eicosanoids are the prostaglandins, prostacyclin, thromboxanes, and leukotrienes. Prostacyclin and thromboxane are often considered members of the prostaglandins since they are also cyclized derivatives. The leukotrienes retain the straight chain configuration of arachidonic acid. There are several series for most of the principal subgroups; these series are based on different substituents (indicated by A, B, C, etc) and different numbers of double bonds (indicated by the subscript 2, 3, 4, etc) in the molecule.

B. Synthesis: See Figure 18–1. Active eicosanoids are synthesized in response to various stimuli, eg, tissue injury. These stimuli activate phospholipases in the cell membrane, and arachidonic acid is produced from membrane lipid. Arachidonic acid can be metabolized to straight chain products by **lipoxygenase,** finally producing leukotrienes. Alternatively, cyclization by the enzyme **cyclooxygenase** may occur, resulting in the production of prostacyclin, prostaglandins, or thromboxane. Cyclooxygenase (Cox) exists in at least two forms. **Cox I** is found in many tissues; the prostaglandins produced in these tissues by Cox I appear to be important for a variety of normal physiologic processes. In contrast, **Cox II** is found primarily in inflammatory cells; the products of its actions play a major role in tissue injury, eg, inflammation. Thromboxane is preferentially synthesized in platelets, whereas prostacyclin is synthesized in the endothelial cells of vessels. Naturally occurring eicosanoids have very short half-lives (seconds to minutes) and are inactive by the oral route.

C. Mechanism of Action: Most eicosanoid effects appear to be brought about by activation of cell surface receptors that are coupled by G proteins to adenylyl cyclase (producing cAMP) or the phosphatidylinositol cascade (producing IP_3 and DAG) second messengers.

D. Effects: A vast array of effects are produced on smooth muscle, platelets, the CNS, and other tissues. Some of the most important effects are summarized in Table 18–2. Eicosanoids most directly involved in pathologic processes include $PGF_{2\alpha}$, thromboxane (TXA_2), and the leukotrienes LTC_4 and LTD_4. LTC_4 and LTD_4 comprise the important mediator of bronchoconstriction, "slow-reacting substance of anaphylaxis" (SRS-A). Leukotriene LTB_4 is a chemotactic factor important in inflammation. PGE_2 and prostacyclin may play important roles as naturally occurring vasodilators. PGE derivatives have significant protective effects on the gastric mucosa. The mechanism may involve increased secretion of bicarbonate and mucous, de-

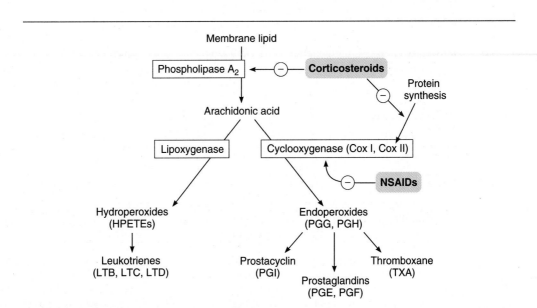

Figure 18–1. Synthesis of eicosanoids and sites of inhibitory effects of corticosteroids and nonsteroidal anti-inflammatory drugs (NSAIDs).

Table 18–2. Effects of some important eicosanoids.[1]

Effect	PGE$_2$	PGF$_{2\alpha}$	PGI$_2$	TXA$_2$	LTB$_4$	LTC$_4$	LTD$_4$
Vascular tone	↓	↑ or ↓	↓↓	↑↑↑	?	↑,↓	↑,↓
Bronchial tone	↓↓	↑	↓	↑↑↑	?	↑↑↑↑	↑↑↑↑
Uterine tone	↑↑	↑↑↑	↓		?	?	?
Platelet aggregation	↑ or ↓	?	↓↓↓	↑↑↑	?	?	?
Leukocyte chemotaxis	?	?	?	?	↑↑↑↑	?	?

[1] ?, unknown effect.

creased acid secretion, or both. PGE$_2$ and PGF$_{2\alpha}$ are released in large amounts from the endometrium during menstruation and may play a physiologic role in labor. Dysmenorrhea is associated with uterine contractions induced by prostaglandins, especially PGF$_{2\alpha}$. Platelet clotting is strongly activated by thromboxane. Therapeutic effects of prostaglandins are described under Clinical Uses.

E. Clinical Uses:

1. **Obstetrics:** PGE$_2$ and PGF$_{2\alpha}$ produce a strong contraction of the uterus. They are useful as abortifacients in the second trimester of pregnancy. Although effective in inducing labor at term, they produce more adverse effects (nausea, vomiting, diarrhea) than do other oxytocics used for this application. In Europe, the PGE$_1$ analogue **misoprostol** has been used with mifepristone (RU486) as an extremely effective and safe abortifacient combination.

2. **Pediatrics:** PGE$_1$ is given as an infusion to maintain patency of the ductus arteriosus in infants with transposition of the great vessels until surgical correction can be undertaken.

3. **Dialysis:** Prostacyclin (PGI$_2$) is occasionally used to prevent platelet aggregation in dialysis machines.

4. **Peptic ulcer associated with NSAID use:** Misoprostol is approved in the USA for the prevention of peptic ulcers in patients who must take high doses of nonsteroidal anti-inflammatory drugs for arthritis and have a history of ulcer associated with this use.

EICOSANOID ANTAGONISTS

Phospholipase A$_2$ and cyclooxygenase can be inhibited by drugs; these inhibitors are mainstays in the treatment of inflammation (Figure 18–1; Chapter 35). No selective inhibitors of lipoxygenase are currently available; some cyclooxygenase inhibitors, however, exert a mild inhibitory effect on leukotriene synthesis. Inhibitors of the receptors for the prostaglandins and the leukotrienes are being actively sought, but none are currently available.

A. Corticosteroids: As indicated in Figure 18–1, corticosteroids inhibit the production of arachidonic acid by phospholipases in the membrane. This effect is mediated by intracellular steroid receptors that, when activated by an appropriate steroid, increase expression of specific proteins that are capable of inhibiting phospholipase. It has also been reported that steroids inhibit the synthesis of Cox II. These actions are thought to be the major mechanisms of the important anti-inflammatory action of corticosteroids.

B. NSAIDs: Aspirin and other nonsteroidal (ie, noncorticosteroid) anti-inflammatory drugs inhibit cyclooxygenase and the production of the thromboxane, prostaglandin, and prostacyclin branch of the synthetic path (Figure 18–1). Unfortunately, none of the currently available NSAIDs selectively inhibit Cox II, the isoform of the enzyme thought to be responsible for the production of inflammatory prostaglandins. In fact, most inhibit Cox I more effectively than Cox II.

Inhibition of cyclooxygenase by aspirin, unlike that of other NSAIDs, is irreversible. It is thought that some cases of aspirin allergy result from diversion of arachidonic acid to the leukotriene pathway when the cyclooxygenase-catalyzed prostaglandin pathway is blocked. The antiplatelet action of aspirin results from the fact that inhibition of thromboxane synthesis is essentially permanent in platelets; they lack the machinery for new protein synthesis. In contrast, inhibition of prostacyclin synthesis in the vascular endothelium is temporary because these cells can synthesize new enzyme. Inhibition of prostaglandin synthesis also results in important anti-inflammatory effects. Inhibition of synthesis of fever-inducing prostaglandins in the brain produces the antipyretic action of NSAIDs. Closure of a patent ductus arteriosus in an otherwise normal infant can be accelerated with a potent NSAID such as indomethacin.

DRUG LIST

The following drugs are important members of the group discussed in this chapter. Prototypes should be learned in detail; features of the major variants should be known well enough to distinguish the variants from prototypes and from each other; the other significant agents should be recognized as belonging to a specific subclass.

Subclass	Prototype	Major Variants	Other Significant Agents
Prostaglandins	PGE_2, $PGF_{2\alpha}$		PGE_1
Prostacyclin	PGI_2		
Thromboxane	TXA_2		
Leukotrienes	LTC_4	LTB_4	LTD_4
Phospholipase inhibitors	Prednisone, hydrocortisone	(See Chapter 38)	
Cyclooxygenase inhibitors	Aspirin	Ibuprofen, etc (see Chapter 35)	

QUESTIONS

DIRECTIONS: Each of the numbered items or incomplete statements in this section is followed by answers or by completions of the sentence. Select the ONE lettered answer or completion that is BEST in each case.

1. Which of the following is (are) frequently associated with increased gastrointestinal motility and diarrhea?
    (A) Timolol
    (B) Prostaglandin E_1
    (C) Corticosteroids
    (D) Leukotriene LTB_4
    (E) All of the above
2. Which of the following drugs inhibits cyclooxygenase irreversibly?
    (A) Acetylsalicylic acid
    (B) Histamine
    (C) Hydrocortisone
    (D) Ibuprofen
    (E) Nitroprusside
3. Agents that often cause vasoconstriction include all of the following EXCEPT
    (A) Angiotensin II
    (B) Prostacyclin
    (C) Methysergide
    (D) $PGF_{2\alpha}$
    (E) Thromboxane
4. A uterine stimulant derived from membrane lipid is
    (A) Serotonin (5-HT)
    (B) Histamine
    (C) Prostacyclin (PGI_2)
    (D) Prostaglandin E_2
    (E) Angiotensin (AII)
5. Inflammatory prostaglandins are produced from arachidonic acid by
    (A) Phospholipase A_2
    (B) Lipoxygenase

    (C) Cyclooxygenase I
    (D) Cyclooxygenase II
    (E) Glutathione-S-transferase

6. Recognized clinical indications for eicosanoids or their inhibitors include all of the following EXCEPT
    (A) Patent ductus arteriosus
    (B) Primary dysmenorrhea
    (C) Abortion
    (D) Hypertension
    (E) Transposition of the great arteries

7. All of the following have direct or indirect bronchoconstrictor action EXCEPT
    (A) Leukotriene LTD_4
    (B) Prostaglandin E_2
    (C) Prostaglandin $F_{2\alpha}$
    (D) Thromboxane A_2
    (E) Slow-reacting substance of anaphylaxis (SRS-A)

DIRECTIONS: The following section consists of a list of four to twenty-six lettered options followed by several numbered items. For each numbered item, select the ONE option that is most closely associated with it. Each answer may be selected once, more than once, or not at all.
    (A) Prednisone
    (B) Ibuprofen
    (C) LTC_4
    (D) Acetylsalicylic acid
    (E) Prostacyclin

8. Reversible inhibitor of platelet cyclooxygenase
9. Component of SRS-A (slow-reacting substance of anaphylaxis)
10. Reduces the activity of phospholipase A_2
11. Increased levels may be responsible, in part, for some cases of aspirin hypersensitivity
12. Extremely potent vasodilator

ANSWERS

1. Neither beta-blockers (eg, timolol) nor corticosteroids increase gastrointestinal activity. LTB_4 is a chemotactic factor. The answer is **(B)**.
2. Hydrocortisone and other corticosteroids inhibit phospholipase, and histamine and nitroprusside have no recognized effect on the enzymes involved in eicosanoid synthesis. Ibuprofen inhibits cyclooxygenase reversibly. The answer is **(A)**, acetylsalicylic acid (aspirin).
3. Prostacyclin PGI_2 is a very potent vasodilator. The answer is **(B)**.
4. While serotonin and, in some species, histamine may cause uterine stimulation, these substances are not derived from membrane lipid. Prostacyclin relaxes the uterus (Table 18–2). The answer is **(D)**.
5. Phospholipase A_2 converts membrane phospholipid to arachidonic acid. Cyclooxygenases convert arachidonic acid to prostaglandins. Cox II is the enzyme believed to be responsible for this reaction in inflammatory cells. The answer is **(D)**.
6. None of the vasodilator eicosanoids have a long enough duration of action or sufficient bioavailability to be useful in hypertension. The answer is **(D)**.
7. PGE_2 is a very potent bronchodilator. Unfortunately, it is an irritant and causes coughing when inhaled. The answer is **(B)**.
8. NSAIDs other than aspirin are reversible inhibitors of cyclooxygenase. The answer is **(B)**.
9. The leukotriene C and D series are major components of SRS-A. The answer is **(C)**.
10. Corticosteroids cause inhibition of phospholipase A2, the enzyme that produces arachidonic acid. The answer is **(A)**.
11. It is thought that the leukotrienes may be produced in increased amounts when cyclooxygenase is blocked; in patients with aspirin hypersensitivity, this might precipitate the bronchoconstriction often observed in this condition. The answer is **(C)**.
12. Prostacyclin is the only potent vasodilator in the list. The answer is **(E)**.

Bronchodilators & Other Agents Used in Asthma

19

OBJECTIVES

You should be able to:

- List the major classes of drugs used in asthma.
- Describe the mechanisms of action of these drug groups.
- List the major adverse effects of the most important asthma drugs.
- Explain why both bronchodilators and anti-inflammatory drugs are important in asthma.

Learn the definitions that follow.

Table 19–1. Definitions.

Term	Definition
Bronchial hyperreactivity	Pathologic increase in the bronchoconstrictor response to antigens and irritants; caused by bronchial inflammation
IgE-mediated disease	Disease caused by excessive or misdirected immune response mediated by IgE antibodies. Example: asthma
Mast cell degranulation	Exocytosis of granule contents from mast cells with release of mediators of inflammation and bronchoconstriction
Phosphodiesterase, PDE	Enzyme that degrades cAMP (active) to AMP (inactive)
Tachyphylaxis	Rapid loss of responsiveness to a stimulus, eg, a drug. Rapid tolerance

CONCEPTS

A. Pathophysiology of Asthma: Asthma is a disease characterized by airway inflammation and episodic, reversible bronchospasm. The immediate cause of the bronchial smooth muscle contraction is the release of several mediators from sensitized mast cells and other cells involved in immunologic responses (Figure 19–1). These mediators include the leukotrienes, LTC_4 and LTD_4. In addition, chemoattractant mediators such as LTB_4 attract inflammatory cells to the airways. Chronic inflammation leads to marked bronchial hyperreactivity to various provocative inhaled substances including antigens, histamine, muscarinic agonists, and irritants such as SO_2 and cold air. This reactivity is partially mediated by vagal reflexes.

B. Subgroups of Antiasthmatic Drugs: Drugs useful in asthma include bronchodilators (smooth muscle relaxants) and anti-inflammatory drugs (Figure 19–2).

Bronchodilators include sympathomimetics, especially β_2-selective agonists, muscarinic antagonists, and methylxanthines.

The most important anti-inflammatory drugs in the treatment of asthma are the corticosteroids and drugs that inhibit release of mediators from mast cells and other inflammatory cells.

BETA ADRENOCEPTOR AGONISTS

A. Prototypes & Pharmacokinetics: The most important sympathomimetics used in asthma are the β_2-selective agonists, although epinephrine and isoproterenol are still used occasionally. Of the selective agents, terbutaline, albuterol, and metaproterenol are the most important in the USA. Salmeterol and formoterol are new, long-acting prophylactic β_2 agonists. Beta agonists

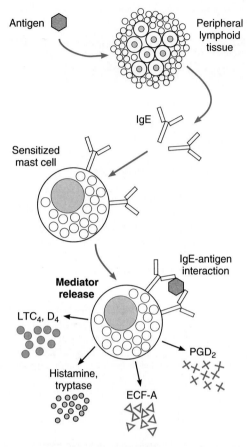

Figure 19–1. Immunologic model for the pathogenesis of asthma. Exposure to antigen causes synthesis of IgE, which binds to and sensitizes mast cells and other inflammatory cells. When such sensitized cells are challenged with antigen, a variety of mediators are released that can account for most of the signs of the early bronchoconstrictor response in asthma. LTC_4, D_4, leukotrienes; PGD_2, prostaglandin; ECF, eosinophil chemotactic factor. (Modified and reproduced, with permission, from Gold WW: Cholinergic pharmacology in asthma. In: *Asthma Physiology, Immunopharmacology, and Treatment.* Austen KF, Lichtenstein LM [editors]. Academic Press, 1974.)

are given almost exclusively by inhalation, usually from pressurized aerosol canisters but occasionally by nebulizer. The inhalational route decreases the systemic dose (and adverse effects) while delivering a locally effective dose to the airway smooth muscle. The older drugs have durations of 6 hours or less; salmeterol and formoterol have durations of action of 12 hours or more.

B. Mechanism & Effects: These agents act by stimulating adenylyl cyclase and increasing cAMP in smooth muscle cells, as described in Chapter 9. The increase in cAMP results in a powerful bronchodilator response (Figure 19–3).

C. Clinical Use: Sympathomimetics are used very extensively in asthma. In almost all patients, the beta agonists are the most effective bronchodilators available.

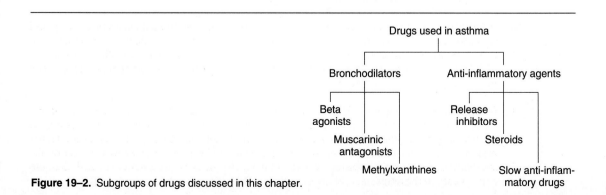

Figure 19–2. Subgroups of drugs discussed in this chapter.

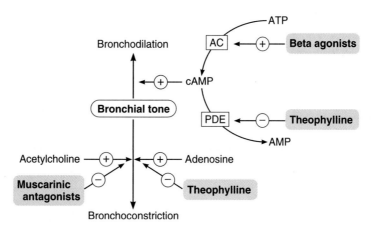

Bronchodilation

Bronchial tone

Acetylcholine

Muscarinic antagonists

Adenosine

Theophylline

Bronchoconstriction

ATP

AC — (+) — Beta agonists

cAMP

PDE — (−) — Theophylline

AMP

Figure 19–3. Possible mechanisms of beta agonists, muscarinic antagonists, and theophylline in altering bronchial tone in asthma. AC, adenylyl cyclase; PDE, phosphodiesterase.

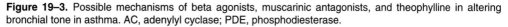

D. Toxicity: Skeletal muscle tremor is a common adverse β_2 effect. Beta$_2$-selectivity is relative. At high clinical dosage, these agents have significant β_1 effects. Even when they are given by inhalation, some cardiac effect (tachycardia) is common. Other adverse effects are rare. When the agents are used excessively, arrhythmias may occur. Loss of responsiveness (tolerance or tachyphylaxis) is another unwanted effect.

METHYLXANTHINES

A. Prototypes & Pharmacokinetics: The methylxanthines are purine derivatives. Three major groups of methylxanthines are found in plants and provide the stimulant effects of three common beverages: caffeine (in coffee), theophylline (tea), and theobromine (cocoa). Theophylline is the only methylxanthine important in the treatment of asthma. The drug is orally active and available as the salt and the base, and in rapid and slow release forms. Theophylline is eliminated by metabolism in the liver. Clearance varies with age (highest in young adolescents), smoking status (higher in smokers), and concurrent use of other drugs that inhibit or induce hepatic enzymes.

B. Mechanism of Action: The methylxanthines inhibit phosphodiesterase (PDE), the enzyme that degrades cAMP to AMP (Figure 19–3), and thus increase cAMP. This anti-PDE effect, however, requires high concentrations of the drug. Methylxanthines also block adenosine receptors in the CNS and elsewhere, but a relationship between this action and the bronchodilating effect has not been clearly established. It is possible that bronchodilation is caused by a third, as yet unrecognized, action.

C. Effects: In asthma, bronchodilation is the most important therapeutic action. Increased strength of skeletal muscle (diaphragm) contraction has been demonstrated in some patients. Other effects include CNS stimulation, cardiac stimulation, vasodilation, a slight increase in blood pressure (probably caused by the release of norepinephrine from adrenergic nerves), and increased gastrointestinal motility.

D. Clinical Use: The major clinical indication for the use of any methylxanthine is for asthma; theophylline is the most important methylxanthine in clinical use. A newer methylxanthine derivative, pentoxifylline, is promoted as a remedy for intermittent claudication; this effect is said to result from decreased viscosity of the blood. Of course, the nonmedical use of the methylxanthines in coffee, tea, and cocoa is far greater, in total quantities consumed, than the clinical uses of the drugs.

E. Toxicity: The common adverse effects include gastrointestinal distress, tremor, and insomnia. Severe nausea and vomiting, cardiac arrhythmias, and convulsions may result from overdosage. Very marked overdose is potentially lethal because of the arrhythmias and convulsions. Beta-blockers are useful antidotes in such severe overdose.

MUSCARINIC ANTAGONISTS

A. Prototypes & Pharmacokinetics: Atropine and other naturally occurring belladonna alkaloids were used for many years in the treatment of asthma, with only modest success. A quaternary antimuscarinic agent designed for aerosol use, **ipratropium,** has achieved much greater success. This drug is delivered by pressurized aerosol and has little systemic action. When absorbed, ipratropium is rapidly metabolized.

B. Mechanism of Action: When given as an aerosol, ipratropium competitively blocks muscarinic receptors in the airways and effectively prevents bronchoconstriction mediated by vagal discharge. Given systemically, the drug is indistinguishable from other short-acting muscarinic blockers.

C. Effects: Ipratropium reverses bronchoconstriction in some asthma patients (especially children) and in many patients with chronic obstructive pulmonary disease (COPD).

D. Clinical Use: Asthma. Muscarinic blockers are not useful in as large a fraction of the asthmatic population as are the β_2 agonists. In chronic obstructive pulmonary disease, however, the antimuscarinics may be more effective (or less toxic) than β agonists.

E. Toxicity: Because ipratropium is delivered directly to the airway and is minimally absorbed, systemic effects are small. When given in excessive dosage, minor atropine-like toxic effects may occur (Chapter 8). In contrast to the β_2 agonists, ipratropium does not cause tremor or arrhythmias.

CROMOLYN & NEDOCROMIL

A. Prototypes & Pharmacokinetics: Cromolyn (disodium cromoglycate) and nedocromil are unusual chemicals: they are extremely insoluble, so that even massive doses result in minimal systemic blood levels. They are given by aerosol for asthma. Cromolyn is the older compound and is the prototype of this group.

B. Mechanism of Action: Cromolyn's mechanism is still poorly understood but appears to involve a decrease in the release of mediators (such as the leukotrienes and histamine) from mast cells. The drug has no bronchodilator action but can prevent bronchoconstriction caused by a challenge with antigen to which the patient is allergic. Cromolyn is capable of preventing both early and late responses (Figure 19–4).

C. Effects: Because they are not absorbed from the airway, cromolyn and nedocromil have only local effects. When administered orally, cromolyn has some efficacy in preventing food allergy. Similar actions have been demonstrated after local application in the conjunctiva of the eye and the nasopharyngeal tract.

D. Clinical Uses: Asthma (especially in children) is by far the most important use for cromolyn and nedocromil. Nasal inhaler and eyedrop formulations of cromolyn are available for hay fever, and an oral formulation is used for food allergy.

E. Toxicity: These drugs may cause cough and irritation of the airway. Rare instances of drug allergy have been reported.

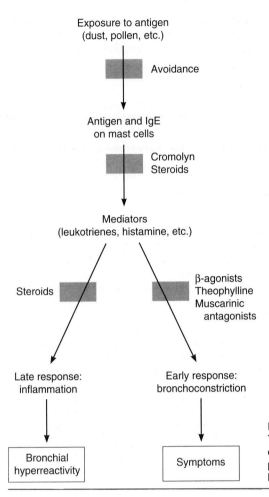

Figure 19–4. Summary of treatment strategies in asthma. Therapeutic interventions are shown as shaded bars. (Redrawn from Cockcroft DW: The bronchial late response in the pathogenesis of asthma and its modulation by therapy. Ann Allergy 1985;55:857.)

CORTICOSTEROIDS

A. Prototypes & Pharmacokinetics: All of the corticosteroids, eg, cortisol and prednisone, are potentially beneficial in severe asthma (see Chapter 38). However, because of their toxicity, systemic (oral) corticosteroids are used only as a last resort. In contrast, local aerosol administration of surface-active corticosteroids (eg, **beclomethasone, budesonide**) is relatively safe; inhaled corticosteroids are becoming more common as first or second line therapy for individuals with moderate to severe asthma.

B. Mechanism of Action: The mechanism of action may be to block the synthesis of arachidonic acid by phospholipase A_2 (see Chapter 18, Figure 18–1). It has also been suggested that corticosteroids increase the responsiveness of beta adrenoceptors in the airway.

C. Effects: See Chapter 38. Glucocorticoids react with intracellular receptors and, in bound form, activate glucocorticoid response elements (GREs) in the nucleus, resulting in synthesis of substances that prevent the full expression of inflammation and allergy. Reduced activity of phospholipase A_2 is thought to be particularly important in asthma because the leukotrienes that result from eicosanoid synthesis are extremely potent bronchoconstrictors and may also participate in the late inflammatory response (Figure 19–4).

D. Clinical Use: Inhaled glucocorticoids are now considered appropriate in most cases of moderate asthma that are not fully responsive to aerosol beta agonists (even in children). It is believed that such early use may prevent the severe, progressive inflammatory changes characteristic of long-standing asthma. This is a shift from earlier beliefs that steroids should be used only in severe, refractory asthma. In such cases of severe asthma, patients are usually hospitalized and stabilized on daily systemic prednisone and then switched to inhaled or alternate-day oral therapy before discharge. (See Chapter 38 for other uses.)

E. Toxicity: See Chapter 38. Local aerosol administration can result in adrenal suppression, but this is rarely significant. More commonly, changes in oropharyngeal flora result in candidiasis. If oral therapy is required, adrenal suppression can be reduced by using alternate day therapy—ie, by giving the drug in slightly higher dosage every other day, rather than smaller doses every day. The major systemic toxicities of the glucocorticoids described in Chapter 38 are much more likely if systemic treatment for more than a few weeks is required, as in severe, refractory asthma.

DRUG LIST:

The following drugs are important members of the group discussed in this chapter. Prototypes should be learned in detail; features of the major variants should be known well enough to distinguish the variants from prototypes and from each other; the other significant agents should be recognized as belonging to a specific subclass.

Subclass	Prototype	Major Variants	Other Significant Agents
Beta agonists	Terbutaline	Salmeterol	Metaproterenol, albuterol, formoterol
Methylxanthines	Theophylline	Aminophylline (a theophylline salt)	Caffeine, theobromine
Muscarinic antagonist	Ipratropium		
Release inhibitors	Cromolyn		Nedocromil
Glucocorticoids	Beclomethasone	Prednisone	

QUESTIONS

DIRECTIONS: Each of the numbered items or incomplete statements in this section is followed by answers or by completions of the sentence. Select the ONE lettered answer or completion that is BEST in each case.

1. One effect that theophylline, nitroglycerin, isoproterenol, and histamine have in common is
   (A) Direct stimulation of cardiac contractile force
   (B) Tachycardia
   (C) Increased gastric acid secretion
   (D) Postural hypotension
   (E) Throbbing headache

2. Which of the following is NOT a recognized action of terbutaline?
   (A) Diuretic effect
   (B) Positive inotropic effect
   (C) Skeletal muscle tremor
   (D) Smooth muscle relaxation
   (E) Tachycardia

3. Of the following, the most likely to have adverse effects when used over long periods for severe asthma in a 10-year-old child is
   (A) Daily administration of albuterol by aerosol
   (B) Daily administration of prednisone by mouth
   (C) Daily administration of beclomethasone by aerosol
   (D) Daily administration of cromolyn by inhaler
   (E) Daily administration of theophylline in long-acting oral form

4. Cromolyn has as its major action
   (A) Smooth muscle relaxation in the bronchi
   (B) Stimulation of cortisol release by the adrenals
   (C) Block of calcium channels in lymphocytes
   (D) Block of mediator release from mast cells
   (E) Block of phosphodiesterase in mast cells and basophils

5. Drugs that can reverse existing bronchospasm during an acute asthmatic attack include all of the following EXCEPT
   (A) Epinephrine
   (B) Terbutaline
   (C) Nedocromil
   (D) Theophylline
   (E) Ipratropium

6. Successful strategies currently in use for asthma include all of the following EXCEPT
   (A) Blockade of leukotriene receptors
   (B) Avoidance of antigen exposure
   (C) Inhibition of release of mediators from mast cells and leukocytes
   (D) Activation of beta receptors
   (E) Inhibition of phospholipase A_2

DIRECTIONS: The following section consists of a list of four to twenty-six lettered options followed by several numbered items. For each numbered item, select the ONE option that is most closely associated with it. Each answer may be selected once, more than once, or not at all.
   (A) Aminophylline
   (B) Ipratropium
   (C) Prednisone
   (D) Epinephrine
   (E) Cromolyn

7. Bronchodilator; useful in chronic obstructive pulmonary disease; least likely to cause cardiac arrhythmia

8. Nonselective but very potent and efficacious bronchodilator; not active by the oral route

9. Prophylactic agent that appears to stabilize mast cells

10. Direct bronchodilator useful in asthma by the oral route

11. Parenteral form is life-saving in severe status asthmaticus; inhibits phospholipase A_2

12. Overdose toxicity includes insomnia, arrhythmias, convulsions

ANSWERS

1. Aminophylline does not cause headache. Nitroglycerin does not increase gastric acid secretion. Isoproterenol does not cause either. Histamine may cause all of the effects listed. The answer is **(B)**.

2. Terbutaline is a "selective" β_2-receptor agonist, but in moderate to high doses it induces β_1 cardiac effects as well as β_2-mediated smooth and skeletal muscle effects. The answer is **(A)**.

3. If oral corticosteroids must be used, alternate-day therapy is preferred because it interferes less with normal growth in children. The answer is **(B)**.

4. The answer is **(D)**, inhibition of mediator release from mast cells. The mechanism for this effect is not known.

5. Neither nedocromil nor cromolyn are capable of reversing bronchospasm; they are limited to preventing it. The answer is **(C)**.

6. See Figure 19–4. Leukotriene receptor blockers are not yet available although there is considerable research activity directed at finding such compounds. The answer is **(A)**.

7. Ipratropium is the bronchodilator that is most likely to be useful in COPD without causing arrhythmias. The answer is **(B)**.

8. Epinephrine is still one of the most potent and efficacious agents available for asthma. However, because it is nonselective, β2-selective agents are preferred. The answer is **(D)**.

9. Cromolyn is only useful for prophylaxis. The drug stabilizes mast cells, ie, prevents mediator release. The answer is **(E)**.

10. Aminophylline, a salt of theophylline, is a bronchodilator that is active by the oral route. The answer is **(A)**.

11. Parenteral corticosteroids such as prednisone are life-saving in status asthmaticus. They probably act by reducing production of leukotrienes (see Chapter 18). The answer is **(C)**.

12. Aminophylline is a salt of theophylline. Like the base theophylline, aminophylline can cause severe and potentially lethal overdose toxicity. The answer is **(A)**.

Part V. Drugs That Act in the Central Nervous System

Introduction to CNS Pharmacology   20

OBJECTIVES

You should be able to:

- List the criteria for accepting a chemical as a neurotransmitter.
- Describe the mechanisms by which drugs cause presynaptic and postsynaptic modulation of synaptic transmission.
- List the major excitatory central neurotransmitters.
- List the major inhibitory central neurotransmitters.
- Identify the major receptor subtypes of CNS neurotransmitters.

Learn the definitions that follow.

Table 20–1. Definitions.

Term	Definition
Voltage-gated ion channels	Transmembrane ion channels regulated by changes in membrane potential; also called electrically gated channel
Receptor-operated ion channels	Transmembrane ion channels that are regulated by interactions between neurotransmitters and their receptors; also called chemically gated channel
EPSP	Excitatory postsynaptic potential; a depolarizing potential change
IPSP	Inhibitory postsynaptic potential; a hyperpolarizing potential change
CNS neurotransmitter	A chemical that interacts with synaptic membrane receptors in the central nervous system to cause excitatory or inhibitory neuronal responses
Synaptic mimicry	Ability of an administered drug to mimic the actions of the natural synaptic transmitter; a criterion for identification of a putative neurotransmitter

CONCEPTS

A. Targets of CNS Drug Action: Most drugs that act on the CNS appear to do so by changing ion flow through transmembrane channels.

    1. Types of receptor-channel coupling: Coupling may be (1) through a receptor that acts directly on the channel protein, (2) through a receptor that is coupled to the ion channel through second messengers, or (3) through a perturbation of the channel that results from changes in the lipid environment caused by the solubility of the drug in the lipid. (It is not clear whether the third mechanism is specific for certain ion channels or involves a non-selective interaction with lipids and other membrane molecules.)

    2. Types of ion channels: Transmembrane ion channels can be divided into voltage-sensitive (electrically gated) and transmitter-sensitive (chemically gated or receptor-operated) groups. Some electrically gated channels (eg, calcium channels) are closely regulated by chemical transmitters. Electrically gated channels are usually concentrated on the axons of nerve cells, whereas chemically gated ones are found on cell bodies and on both sides of synapses.

3. **Role of the ion current carried by the channel:** In general, excitatory postsynaptic potentials (EPSPs) are generated by opening channels that conduct sodium or calcium. In some instances these depolarizing potentials result from *closing* potassium channels. Inhibitory postsynaptic potentials (IPSPs) are generated by opening potassium or chloride channels.

B. **Sites & Mechanisms of Drug Action:** Most therapeutically important CNS drugs act on chemically gated channels. Their sites of action are therefore in synapses. Possible mechanisms are indicated in Figure 20–1. Drugs may act presynaptically by altering the production, storage, release, reuptake, or metabolism of transmitter chemicals. Other agents activate or block postsynaptic receptors for specific transmitters. A few toxic substances damage or kill the nerve cell (eg, kainic acid; 6-hydroxydopamine; 1-methyl-4-phenyl-1,2,3,6-tetrahydropyridine [MPTP]).

C. **Role of CNS Organization:** The CNS contains two types of neuronal systems, hierarchic and nonspecific (or diffuse).

1. **Hierarchic systems:** These systems are clearly delimited in their anatomic distribution and generally contain large, myelinated, rapidly conducting fibers. Hierarchic systems control major sensory and motor functions. The excitatory transmitters include aspartate and glutamate. These systems also include numerous small inhibitory interneurons, which utilize gamma-aminobutyric acid (GABA) or glycine as transmitters. Drugs that affect these systems tend to have well-defined effects.

2. **Diffuse systems:** Diffuse systems are broadly distributed, with single cells frequently sending processes to many different areas. The axons are fine and branch repeatedly to form synapses with many cells. Axons commonly have periodic enlargements (varicosities) that contain vesicles. The transmitters are often amines (norepinephrine, dopamine, sero-

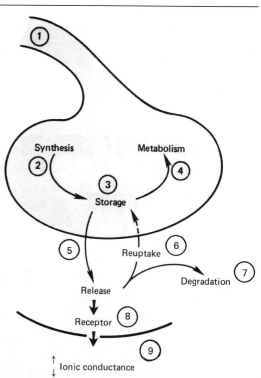

Figure 20–1. Sites of drug action. Drugs may alter the (1) action potential in the presynaptic fiber; (2) synthesis of transmitter; (3) storage of transmitter; (4) metabolism of transmitter within the nerve ending; (5) release of transmitter; (6) reuptake or (7) extracellular disposition of transmitter; (8) postsynaptic receptor; or (9) postsynaptic effect of the receptor. (Reproduced, with permission, from Katzung BG [editor]: *Basic & Clinical Pharmacology,* 6th ed. Appleton & Lange, 1995.)

Table 20–2. Nonpeptide neurotransmitter pharmacology in the central nervous system.[1]

Transmitter	Anatomical Distribution	Receptor Subtypes	Receptor Mechanisms
Acetylcholine	Cell bodies at all levels, short and long axons	Muscarinic, M_1; blocked by pirenzepine and atropine	Excitatory; decrease in K^+ conductance
		Muscarinic, M_2; blocked by atropine	Inhibitory; increase in K^+ conductance
	Motoneuron-Renshaw cell synapse	Nicotinic, N	Excitatory; increase in cation conductance
Dopamine	Cell bodies at all levels, short, medium, and long axons	D_1; blocked by phenothiazines	Inhibitory; increases cyclic AMP
		D_2; blocked by phenothiazines and haloperidol	Inhibitory, increase in K^+ conductance
Norepinephrine	Cell bodies in pons and brain stem project to all levels	$Alpha_1$; blocked by prazosin	Excitatory; decrease in K^+ conductance
		$Alpha_2$; activated by clonidine	Inhibitory; increase in K^+ conductance
		$Beta_1$; blocked by propranolol	Excitatory; cAMP-mediated decrease in K^+ conductance
		$Beta_2$; blocked by propranolol	Inhibitory; ? increase in electrogenic sodium pump
Serotonin (5-hydroxytryptamine)	Cell bodies in midbrain and pons project to all levels	$5\text{-}HT_{1A}$; buspirone is a partial agonist	Inhibitory; increase in K^+ conductance
		$5\text{-}HT_{2A}$; blocked by ketanserin, clozapine, and risperidone	Excitatory; decrease in K^+ conductance
		$5\text{-}HT_3$; blocked by ondansetron	Excitatory; increase in K^+ conductance
		$5\text{-}HT_4$	Excitatory; cAMP-mediated decrease in K^+ conductance
GABA	Supraspinal interneurons; spinal interneurons involved in presynaptic inhibition	$GABA_A$; facilitated by benzodiazepines	Inhibitory; increase in Cl^- conductance
		$GABA_B$; activated by baclofen	Inhibitory; decrease in Ca^{2+} conductance (presynaptic), increase in K^+ conductance (postsynaptic)
Glutamate, aspartate	Relay neurons at all levels	Three subtypes; NMDA subtype blocked by phencyclidine	Excitatory; increase in Ca^{2+} or cation conductance; decrease in K^+ conductance
Glycine	Interneurons in spinal cord and brain stem	Single subtype; blocked by strychnine	Inhibitory; increase in Cl^- conductance

[1] Adapted, with permission, from Katzung BG (editor): *Basic & Clinical Pharmacology,* 6th ed, Appleton & Lange, 1995.

tonin) or peptides. Drugs that affect these systems will often have very general effects (eg, on sleep or mood).

D. Transmitters at Central Synapses:

1. Criteria for transmitter status: To be accepted as a neurotransmitter, a candidate chemical must be present in higher concentration in the synaptic area than in other areas (ie, must be localized in appropriate areas), must be released by electrical or chemical stimulation, and must produce the same sort of postsynaptic response that is seen with physiologic activation of the synapse (ie, must exhibit synaptic mimicry).

2. **Recognized nonpeptide transmitters:** A list of these is given in Table 20–2.
   a. **Acetylcholine:** Most CNS responses to ACh are mediated by a large family of G protein-coupled muscarinic M_1 receptors which, on activation, lead to slow excitation.
   b. **Dopamine:** This amine exerts inhibitory actions at synapses in diffuse neuronal systems. In addition to the two receptors listed in Table 20–2, several other dopamine receptor subtypes have been identified (D_3, D_4, and D_5). The dopamine D_4 receptor has a high affinity for the atypical antipsychotic drug, clozapine.
   c. **Norepinephrine:** Noradrenergic neuron cell bodies are mainly located in the locus ceruleus and the lateral tegmental area of the pons. These neurons fan out broadly to provide most regions of the CNS with diffuse noradrenergic input. Excitatory effects are produced by activation of $alpha_1$ and $beta_1$ receptors. Inhibitory effects are caused by activation of $alpha_2$ and $beta_2$ receptors.
   d. **Serotonin:** Most serotonergic pathways originate from cell bodies in the Raphe or midline regions of the pons and upper brain stem; these pathways innervate most regions of the CNS. Serotonin is inhibitory at most CNS sites but can cause excitation of some neurons, depending on the receptor subtype activated. Both excitatory and inhibitory actions can occur on the same neuron if appropriate receptors are present.
   e. **Excitatory amino acids:** Most neurons in the brain are excited by glutamic and aspartic acid. *Ionotropic* receptors directly gate cation-selective channels. Subtypes include the NMDA (N-methyl-D-aspartate) receptor, which is blocked by phencyclidine (PCP). Activation of *metabotropic* glutamate receptors modulates G-protein-coupled second messenger systems.
   f. **GABA and glycine:** GABA is the primary neurotransmitter mediating IPSPs in neurons in the brain. GABA is also important in the spinal cord. Fast IPSPs are blocked by $GABA_A$ receptor antagonists and slow IPSPs are blocked by $GABA_B$ receptor antagonists. Glycine receptors, which are important in the cord, are blocked by strychnine, a "spinal convulsant."
3. **Peptide transmitters:** Many peptides have been identified in the CNS and meet most or all of the criteria for acceptance as neurotransmitters. The best defined of this group are the opioid peptides (beta-endorphin, met- and leu-enkephalin, and dynorphin). Peptide transmitters differ from nonpeptide transmitters in that: (1) the peptides are synthesized in the cell body and transported to the nerve ending via axonal transport and (2) no reuptake or specific enzyme mechanisms have been identified for terminating the action of these peptides.

QUESTIONS

DIRECTIONS: Each of the numbered items or incomplete statements in this section is followed by answers or by completions of the sentence. Select the ONE lettered answer or completion that is BEST in each case.

1. Each of the following is recognized as a central neurotransmitter EXCEPT
   (A) Glutamic acid
   (B) Norepinephrine
   (C) GABA
   (D) Cyclic AMP
   (E) Glycine
2. Most drugs with CNS effects influence synaptic transmission. Valid **presynaptic** mechanisms of action include all of the following EXCEPT
   (A) Inhibition of reuptake of peptide neurotransmitters into the nerve terminal
   (B) Increase in neurotransmitter synthesis
   (C) Increased release of transmitter from the nerve terminal
   (D) Inhibition of neurotransmitter metabolism
   (E) Depletion of neurotransmitter storage in synaptic vesicles
3. Neurotransmitters may
   (A) Increase chloride conductance, resulting in an IPSP
   (B) Increase potassium conductance, resulting in an EPSP

(C) Increase sodium conductance, resulting in an IPSP
(D) Increase calcium conductance, resulting in an IPSP
(E) All of the above

4. All of the following compounds have been shown to **decrease** K$^+$ ion conductance EXCEPT
   (A) Acetylcholine
   (B) Dopamine
   (C) Glutamic acid
   (D) Serotonin
   (E) Norepinephrine

DIRECTIONS: The following section consists of a list of four to twenty-six lettered options followed by several numbered items. For each numbered item, select the ONE option that is most closely associated with it. Each answer may be selected once, more than once, or not at all.

   (A) Norepinephrine
   (B) GABA
   (C) Acetylcholine
   (D) Glutamic acid
   (E) Dopamine
   (F) Beta-endorphin
   (G) Substance P
   (H) Serotonin

5. Acts on supraspinal receptors to increase chloride ion conductance
6. A peptide that excites spinal cord neurons activated by painful stimuli
7. Ondansetron acts as an antagonist at a receptor activated by this neurotransmitter
8. It is estimated that over 50% of CNS neurons are responsive to this exclusively excitatory neurotransmitter
9. The extrapyramidal effects of haloperidol result from antagonism at receptors for this neurotransmitter
10. This neurotransmitter is found at high concentrations in cell bodies in the locus ceruleus; at some sites release of transmitter is autoregulated via presynaptic inhibition

ANSWERS

1. Cyclic AMP is undoubtedly important as a second messenger in the CNS, but there is no evidence that cAMP acts as a neurotransmitter. The answer is **(D)**.
2. No uptake mechanism for peptides has been demonstrated. All of the other mechanisms listed have been identified. Examples include: (B), levodopa increases dopamine synthesis; (C), amphetamine releases norepinephrine and dopamine; (D), MAO inhibitors decrease the metabolism of catecholamines and serotonin; and (E), reserpine depletes catecholamines and serotonin. The answer is **(A)**.
3. Chloride and potassium currents result in IPSPs. Sodium and calcium currents cause EPSPs. The answer is **(A)**.
4. A decrease in K$^+$ conductance is associated with neuronal excitation. All of the neurotransmitters listed are able to cause excitation by this mechanism at certain neurons in the CNS except dopamine. The answer is **(B)**.
5. The interaction of both GABA and glycine with their receptors can cause membrane hyperpolarization via increased chloride ion conductance. Glycine is thought to elicit IPSPs in the spinal cord, but not in neurons of higher brain structures. The GABA-mediated increase in chloride ion conductance is facilitated by benzodiazepines and barbiturates. The answer is **(B)**.
6. Though not mentioned in the text, substance P is a neuroactive peptide present in certain small unmyelinated neurons of the spinal cord and brain stem. It is postulated that substance P is an excitatory neurotransmitter involved in the activation of primary sensory fibers by nociceptive stimuli. Note that opioid peptides are generally inhibitory at CNS neurons. The answer is **(G)**.

7. Ondansetron, an effective antiemetic drug, blocks 5-HT$_3$ receptors. The precise neuroanatomical site of action of the drug is uncertain, but may involve the brain stem, where the vomiting center is located. The answer is **(H).**

8. Virtually all neurons in the brain are strongly excited by glutamic acid. Depending on the glutamate receptor subtype activated, the mechanism of excitation may involve direct or indirect (second messenger-mediated) effects on ion conductance. The answer is **(D).**

9. Conventional antipsychotic drugs, including phenothiazines and haloperidol, block the dopamine D$_2$ receptor on striatal neurons innervated by the nigrostriatal tract. This results in adverse effects resembling parkinsonism when such drugs are used in the treatment of schizophrenia. The answer is **(E).**

10. Cell bodies of many noradrenergic neurons are located in the locus ceruleus. Agents that activate alpha$_2$ receptors, located presynaptically on such neurons, decrease their activity. Norepinephrine is thought to function in autoregulation via its actions on presynaptic alpha$_2$ receptors (Figure 6–3). The answer is **(A).**

21

Sedative-Hypnotic Drugs

OBJECTIVES

You should be able to:

- Identify the major chemical classes of sedative-hypnotics.
- Describe the sequence of CNS effects of a typical sedative-hypnotic over the entire dose range.
- Describe the pharmacodynamics of benzodiazepines, including interactions with neuronal membrane receptors.
- Compare the pharmacokinetics of commonly used benzodiazepines and barbiturates and discuss how differences among them affect clinical use.
- Describe the clinical uses of sedative-hypnotics.

Learn the definitions that follow.

Table 21–1. Definitions.

Term	Definition
Sedation	Reduction of anxiety
Hypnosis	Induction of sleep
REM sleep	Phase of sleep associated with rapid eye movements; most dreaming takes place during REM sleep
Tolerance	Reduction in drug effect requiring an increase in dosage to maintain the same response
Physical dependence	The state of response to a drug whereby removal of the drug evokes unpleasant symptoms, usually the opposite of the drug's effects
Anxiolytic	A drug that reduces anxiety, a sedative
Anesthesia	Loss of consciousness associated with absence of response to pain
Coma	Extremely deep anesthesia or depression of brain activity; precursor to respiratory and circulatory failure
Psychologic dependence	The state of response to a drug whereby the drug taker feels compelled to use the drug and suffers anxiety when separated from the drug

CONCEPTS

A. Classification & Pharmacokinetics:

1. **Subgroups:** The sedative-hypnotics belong to a chemically heterogeneous class of drugs that produces dose-dependent CNS depressant effects (Figure 21–1). The most important subgroup is the **benzodiazepines,** but representatives of other subgroups, including **barbiturates,** and miscellaneous agents (**carbamates, alcohols,** and **cyclic ethers**) are still used. The steepness of the dose-response curve varies among drug groups; those with flatter curves, such as benzodiazepines, are safer for clinical use.

2. **Absorption and distribution:** Most of these drugs are lipid-soluble and are absorbed well from the gastrointestinal tract, with good distribution to the brain. Drugs with the highest lipid solubility (eg, **thiopental**) enter the CNS rapidly and can be used as induction agents in anesthesia. The CNS effects of thiopental are terminated by rapid **redistribution** of the drug from brain to other tissues.

3. **Metabolism and excretion:** Sedative-hypnotics are metabolized prior to elimination from the body, mainly by hepatic enzymes. Metabolic rates and pathways vary among different drugs. Many benzodiazepines are converted initially to **active metabolites** with long half-lives. After several days of therapy with such drugs (eg, diazepam, flurazepam), accumulation of active metabolites can lead to excessive sedation. Lorazepam and oxazepam do not form active metabolites. With the exception of phenobarbital, which is excreted partly unchanged in the urine, the barbiturates are extensively metabolized via oxidation at the C5 position. Chloral hydrate is oxidized to trichloroethanol, an active metabolite. The duration of CNS actions of sedative-hypnotic drugs ranges from a few hours (eg, chloral hydrate, pentobarbital, triazolam) to more than 30 hours (eg, chlordiazepoxide, clorazepate, diazepam, phenobarbital).

B. Mechanism of Action: No single mechanism of action for sedative-hypnotics has been identified, and the different chemical subgroups may have different actions. Certain drugs (eg, benzodiazepines) facilitate neuronal membrane inhibition by actions at specific receptors.

1. **Benzodiazepines:** Receptors for benzodiazepines are present in many brain regions, including the thalamus, limbic structures, and the cerebral cortex. These receptors form part of a GABA$_A$ receptor-chloride ion channel macromolecular complex. Binding of benzodiazepines to these receptors appears to facilitate the inhibitory actions of GABA, which are exerted through increased chloride ion conductance (Figure 21–2). Benzodiazepines increase the *frequency* of GABA-mediated chloride ion channel opening. Flumazenil, an antagonist at benzodiazepine receptors, reverses the central nervous system effects of benzodiazepines. Certain beta-carbolines have high affinity for benzodiazepine receptors and can elicit anxiogenic and convulsant effects. These drugs are classified as **inverse agonists.**

2. **Barbiturates:** Barbiturates depress neuronal activity in the midbrain reticular formation, facilitating and prolonging the inhibitory effects of GABA and glycine. They do not bind to benzodiazepine or GABA receptors, but appear to interact with other sites on the chloride channel. Barbiturates increase the *duration* of GABA-mediated chloride ion channel opening. They may also block the excitatory transmitter, glutamic acid, and at high concentration, sodium channels.

3. **Other sedative-hypnotics:** The newer anxiolytic drug **buspirone** interacts with the 5-HT$_{1A}$ subclass of brain serotonin receptors as a partial agonist, but the precise mechanism of its

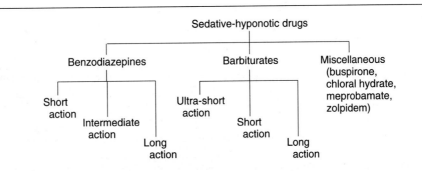

Figure 21–1. Subgroups of drugs discussed in this chapter.

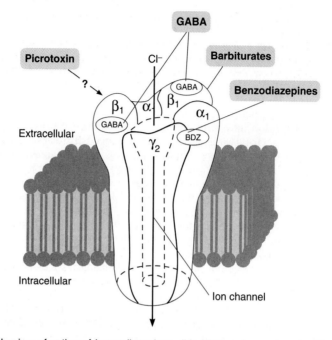

Figure 21–2. Mechanism of action of benzodiazepines. (Modified and reproduced, with permission, from Zorumski CF, Isenberg KE: Insights into the structure and function of GABA-benzodiazepine receptors: Ion channels and psychiatry. Am J Psychiat 1991;148:162.

anxiolytic effect is unknown. The hypnotic drug **zolpidem,** though not a benzodiazepine, appears to exert its CNS effects via interaction with benzodiazepine receptors.

C. Effects: The CNS effects of the sedative-hypnotics depend on dose, as shown in Figure 21–3. These effects range from sedation and relief of anxiety (anxiolysis), through hypnosis (facilitation of sleep), to anesthesia and coma. Depressant effects are additive when two or more drugs are given together.

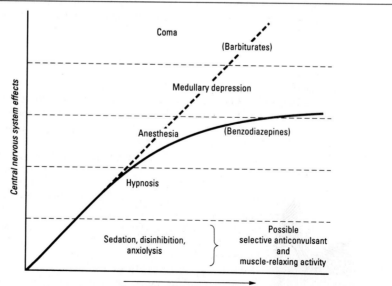

Figure 21–3. Relationships between sedative-hypnotic dose and the CNS effects for the benzodiazepines and the barbiturates.

1. **Sedation:** Sedative actions, with relief of anxiety, occur with all drugs in this class. Behavioral disinhibition may also occur. In animals, punishment-suppressed behavior is released.

2. **Hypnosis:** Sedative-hypnotics promote sleep onset and increase the duration of the sleep state. Rapid eye movement (REM) sleep stages are usually decreased at high dose; upon withdrawal from chronic drug use, a rebound increase in REM sleep may occur.

3. **Anesthesia:** At high doses, loss of consciousness occurs, with amnesia and suppression of reflexes. Anesthesia can be produced by most barbiturates (eg, thiopental) and certain benzodiazepines (eg, midazolam).

4. **Anticonvulsant actions:** Suppression of seizure activity occurs with high doses of most of the barbiturates and some of the benzodiazepines, but this is at the cost of marked sedation. A selective anticonvulsant action (ie, suppression of convulsions at doses that do not cause severe sedation) occurs only with a few drugs (eg, phenobarbital, diazepam) that reduce the spread of epileptiform activity without excessive CNS depression. High doses of intravenous diazepam, lorazepam, or phenobarbital are used in status epilepticus. In this condition, marked sedation is desirable.

5. **Muscle relaxation:** Relaxation of skeletal muscle occurs at high dosage for most sedative-hypnotics, but diazepam is effective at sedative dose levels for specific spasticity states, including cerebral palsy.

6. **Medullary depression:** High doses can cause depression of medullary neurons leading to respiratory arrest, hypotension, and cardiovascular collapse. These effects are the cause of death in suicidal overdose.

7. **Tolerance and dependence:** Tolerance, a decrease in responsiveness, occurs when sedative-hypnotics are used continuously or in high dosage. Cross-tolerance may occur among different chemical subgroups. Psychologic dependence occurs frequently with most sedative-hypnotics and involves the compulsive use of these drugs to reduce anxiety. Physical dependence constitutes an altered state that leads to an abstinence syndrome (withdrawal state) when the drug is discontinued. Withdrawal signs, which may include anxiety, tremors, hyperreflexia and seizures, occur more commonly with shorter-acting drugs such as pentobarbital and secobarbital. Buspirone is not schedule-controlled because dependence is unlikely to occur with this drug.

D. **Clinical Use:** Most of these uses can be predicted from the pharmacodynamic effects outlined above. Drugs with intermediate or long durations of action are usually favored in the treatment of anxiety states, while those with short durations of action are used for the management of sleep disorders. Special uses include the management of grand mal seizures (diazepam, phenobarbital), status epilepticus (diazepam), muscle spasticity (diazepam), phobic anxiety states (alprazolam), induction of anesthesia (thiopental), and general anesthesia (midazolam). Longer-acting sedative-hypnotics are also used in the detoxification of physically dependent patients. The anxiolytic effects of buspirone occur without marked sedation, but take several days to develop.

E. **Toxicity:**
   1. **Excess CNS depression:** This includes decreased psychomotor functioning and unwanted daytime sedation following use as hypnotics. These adverse effects occur most often with benzodiazepines that have active metabolites with long half-lives (eg, flurazepam). The dosage of a sedative-hypnotic should be reduced in the elderly patient to avoid excessive daytime sedation, which has been shown to increase the risk of falls and fractures.
      a. **Interactions:** Additive CNS depression occurs when sedative-hypnotics are used with other drugs in the class, as well as with antihistamines, antipsychotic drugs, and ethanol. This is the most common type of drug interaction involving sedative-hypnotics. Ethanol is less likely to cause additive CNS depression with buspirone than with other sedative-hypnotics.
      b. **Overdosage:** Overdosage causes severe respiratory and cardiovascular depression and is more likely to occur with alcohols, barbiturates, and carbamates than with benzodiazepines. Management of intoxication requires maintenance of a patent airway and ventilatory support. Flumazenil may reverse CNS depressant effects of benzodiazepines, but has no beneficial actions in overdosage with other sedative-hypnotics.
   2. **Other effects:** Short-acting hypnotics, especially triazolam, may cause daytime anxiety

and amnesia. Anterograde amnesia may also occur with other benzodiazepines when used at high dosage. Barbiturates and carbamates (but not benzodiazepines) induce the formation of the liver microsomal enzymes that metabolize drugs. This enzyme induction may lead to multiple drug interactions. Barbiturates may also precipitate acute intermittent porphyria in susceptible patients. Chloral hydrate may displace coumarins from plasma protein binding sites and increase anticoagulant effects.

DRUG LIST

The following drugs are important members of the group discussed in this chapter. Prototypes should be learned in detail; features of the major variants should be known well enough to distinguish the variants from prototypes and from each other; the other significant agents should be recognized as belonging to a specific subclass.

Subclass	Prototype	Major Variants	Other Significant Agents
Benzodiazepines	Chlordiazepoxide, diazepam, temazepam	Alprazolam	Flurazepam, lorazepam, nitrazepam, oxazepam, triazolam
Barbiturates	Phenobarbital, pentobarbital, thiopental		Secobarbital, methohexital
Carbamates	Meprobamate		
Alcohols	Ethanol	Chloral hydrate	
Others	Buspirone, zolpidem		

QUESTIONS

DIRECTIONS: Each of the numbered items or incomplete statements in this section is followed by answers or by completions of the sentence. Select the ONE lettered answer or completion that is BEST in each case.

1. All of the following may be caused by treatment with moderate to large doses of a benzodiazepine EXCEPT
   (A) Decreased performance on tests of psychomotor function
   (B) Anterograde amnesia with continued use as hypnotic agents
   (C) Hyperreflexia and seizures with abrupt discontinuance after chronic use
   (D) Increase in the activity of ALA synthetase with continued use
   (E) Additive depression of the central nervous system with alcoholic beverages

2. All of the following statements concerning the barbiturates are accurate EXCEPT
   (A) With physical dependence, the symptoms of the abstinence syndrome are most severe during withdrawal from use of shorter-acting barbiturates
   (B) Renal elimination of phenobarbital is increased by urinary alkalinization
   (C) Barbiturates are contraindicated in patients with acute intermittent porphyria
   (D) In terms of CNS depressant effects, barbiturates exhibit a steeper dose-response relationship than benzodiazepines
   (E) Flumazenil is an appropriate antidote in barbiturate overdosage

3. Concerning the clinical uses of sedative-hypnotics, all of the following are recognized indications EXCEPT
   (A) Diazepam is used for muscle spasticity in patients with cerebral palsy
   (B) Symptoms of the alcohol withdrawal state may be alleviated by treatment with chlordiazepoxide
   (C) Alprazolam has selective anxiolytic effects in patients who suffer from panic attacks and phobic disorders
   (D) Phenobarbital is effective in the long-term management of patients with psychotic disorders
   (E) Intravenous diazepam is used in status epilepticus

4.   Characteristic properties of sedative-hypnotic drugs include all of the following EXCEPT
   (A) A patient who regularly uses alcoholic beverages is likely to be tolerant to the CNS actions of sedative-hypnotics
   (B) Administration to a pregnant patient during the immediate predelivery period will result in depression of neonatal vital functions
   (C) High doses lead to increases in the time spent in REM sleep
   (D) Sedative-hypnotics may cause respiratory depression in patients with chronic obstructive pulmonary disease
   (E) Toxic levels depress myocardial contractility and reduce vascular tone

5.   Which ONE of the following best describes the mechanism of action of benzodiazepines?
   (A) They act as GABA receptor agonists in the CNS
   (B) They inhibit GABA transaminase leading to increased levels of GABA
   (C) They block glutamate receptors in the CNS
   (D) They facilitate GABA-mediated increases in chloride ion conductance
   (E) They inhibit brain monoamine oxidase

Items 6–7:   An 82-year-old woman, otherwise healthy for her age, has difficulty sleeping. Triazolam is prescribed for her at one-half of the conventional adult dose.

6.   All of the following statements about the use of triazolam in this 82-year-old patient are accurate EXCEPT
   (A) The drug may cause ambulatory difficulties in the elderly patient
   (B) She may experience rebound insomnia when she stops taking the drug
   (C) Additive CNS depressant effects are likely if she takes over-the-counter cold medications
   (D) Hypertension is a common problem with flurazepam in patients over 75 years of age
   (E) She may experience amnesia, especially if she also drinks alcoholic beverages

7.   The most likely explanation for the increased sensitivity of elderly patients to a single dose of triazolam and other sedative-hypnotic drugs is
   (A) Changes in brain function that accompany the aging process
   (B) Decreased renal function
   (C) Increased cerebral blood flow
   (D) Decreased hepatic metabolism of lipid-soluble drugs
   (E) Changes in plasma protein binding

DIRECTIONS: The following section consists of a list of four to twenty-six lettered options followed by several numbered items. For each numbered item, select the ONE option that is most closely associated with it. Each answer may be selected once, more than once, or not at all.
   (A) Buspirone
   (B) Triazolam
   (C) Clorazepate
   (D) Lorazepam
   (E) Zolpidem
   (F) Alprazolam
   (G) Secobarbital
   (H) Phenobarbital
   (I) Chloral hydrate
   (J) Flurazepam

8.   This drug has the most rapid onset of action, and the shortest half-life of the benzodiazepines listed; widely used as a hypnotic, the drug may cause daytime anxiety and amnestic effects

9.   This pro-drug is biotransformed to an active metabolite; it may increase anticoagulant effects by displacement of warfarin from plasma protein binding sites

10.   Commonly used as a sleeping pill, this drug has caused a high incidence of unwanted daytime sedation in elderly patients; it has a long duration of action due to the formation of several active metabolites with half-lives greater than 24 hours

11.   Of the drugs listed, this drug is least likely to alleviate withdrawal symptoms in a patient who has abruptly discontinued use of high doses of a barbiturate

12.   This drug is useful in the management of anxiety states and for grand mal; chronic use may lead to an increase in the rates of metabolism of warfarin, phenytoin and digitalis compounds

ANSWERS

1. In contrast to the barbiturates and carbamates, chronic therapy with benzodiazepines does not lead to increased activity of liver drug-metabolizing enzymes or of enzymes involved in porphyrin synthesis. However, the benzodiazepines are CNS depressants that exert additive effects with ethanol. With chronic use, tolerance and both psychologic and physical dependence occur. The answer is **(D)**.

2. Flumazenil is an antagonist at BDZ receptors and is used in emergency and operating rooms to reverse CNS depressant effects of benzodiazepines. In severe overdosage the efficacy of flumazenil is questionable; use of the drug does not obviate the need for ventilatory support. Flumazenil does *not* reverse the CNS depressant actions of alcohols, barbiturates, or carbamates. Note that, as a weak acid (pK_a=7), phenobarbital will exist mainly in the ionized (nonprotonated) form in the urine at alkaline pH, and will not be reabsorbed in the renal tubule. The answer is **(E)**.

3. Sedative-hypnotic drugs have no long-term benefit in the management of psychotic disorders, though they are sometimes used in the short-term control of violent behavior in schizophrenia or drug-induced psychoses. The answer is **(D)**.

4. A decrease in the time spent in REM sleep is a characteristic effect of sedative-hypnotics, especially when they are used as hypnotics. Increases in REM sleep (rebound) may occur during withdrawal from use of sedative-hypnotics. Note that all drugs in this class cross the placental barrier and may depress APGAR score in the neonate. The answer is **(C)**.

5. Benzodiazepines are thought to exert most of their CNS effects through the mediation of the inhibitory neurotransmitter GABA, which causes membrane hyperpolarization through an increase in chloride ion conductance. Benzodiazepines interact with specific receptors (BDZ receptors) that are components of the $GABA_A$ receptor-chloride ion channel macromolecular complex. Benzodiazepines are not GABA receptor *agonists,* because they do not interact directly with this component of the complex. The answer is **(D)**.

6. In elderly patients taking benzodiazepines, hypotension is far more likely to occur than elevation of blood pressure. All of the other statements are accurate. The answer is **(D)**.

7. Decreased blood flow to vital organs, including the liver and kidney, occurs during the aging process. These changes may contribute to cumulative effects of sedative-hypnotic drugs. However, this does not explain the enhanced sensitivity of the elderly patient to a *single* dose of a central depressant, which appears to be due to changes in brain function that accompany aging. The answer is **(A)**.

8. Triazolam is widely prescribed as a hypnotic drug. Oversedation occurs infrequently with triazolam, presumably due to its short plasma half-life. However, side effects of triazolam include disinhibition, hyperexcitability, daytime anxiety, and effects on memory. A rebound increase in REM sleep has occurred on discontinuance of triazolam after only a few days of administration. The answer is **(B)**.

9. Chloral hydrate is a pro-drug that is metabolized to trichloroethanol, the active moiety. It displaces certain drugs from plasma protein binding sites and may cause bleeding when administered to patients given warfarin. The chronic use of chloral hydrate has been associated with an increased incidence of neoplastic disease. Clorazepate is also a pro-drug hydrolyzed to form nordiazepam, the active metabolite. The benzodiazepines do not displace other drugs from plasma protein binding sites. The answer is **(I)**.

10. The formation of long-acting metabolites can lead to cumulative CNS depressant effects when flurazepam is used daily in the treatment of sleep disorders. The incidence of unwanted sedative actions is highest in the elderly patient. For such patients, it seems preferable to use a benzodiazepine that does not form active metabolites, such as oxazepam. The answer is **(J)**.

11. Buspirone is a novel anxiolytic drug that appears to interact with a subclass of brain serotonin receptors. The effects of the drug develop slowly; while it is less likely than conventional sedative-hypnotics to exert additive CNS depressant effects with ethanol, caution is advised. Buspirone does not exhibit cross-tolerance with conventional sedative-hypnotics and does *not* reduce the severity of withdrawal symptoms in patients who have become physically dependent on such drugs. The answer is **(A)**.

12. With chronic administration, barbiturates increase the activity of hepatic drug-metabolizing enzymes, including cytochromes P450. This may lead to increases in the rate of metabolism of many drugs administered concomitantly, with decreases in the intensity and duration of their effects. Secobarbital is used for hypnosis and has no selective actions in seizure disorders. The answer is **(H)**.

Alcohols

22

OBJECTIVES

You should be able to:

- Describe the pharmacodynamics and pharmacokinetics of acute ethanol ingestion.
- List the toxic effects of chronic ethanol ingestion.
- Outline the treatment of (a) ethanol overdosage and (b) the alcohol withdrawal syndrome.
- Describe the toxicity and treatment of acute poisoning with (a) methanol and (b) ethylene glycol.

Learn the definitions that follow.

Table 22–1. Definitions.

Term	Definition
Alcoholism	Compulsive use of ethanol
Psychologic and physical dependence	States wherein deprivation of the drug results in severe anxiety (psychologic dependence) and physical symptoms (physical dependence)
Tolerance, cross-tolerance	State of adaptation to a drug that results in reduced effects at a given dosage; cross-tolerance is tolerance to a second drug developed as a result of exposure to a first drug
Wernicke-Korsakoff syndrome	Destruction of brain neurons that results from acute thiamine deficiency; most commonly occurs in alcoholics (see text)
Acute ethanol intoxication	The signs and symptoms of acute ingestion of a large quantity of ethanol (see text)
Alcohol withdrawal syndrome	The syndrome engendered by deprivation in an individual who has become physically dependent
Fetal alcohol syndrome	The syndrome of teratogenic effects of alcohol consumed by a pregnant woman (see text)

CONCEPTS

Ethanol, a sedative-hypnotic drug, is the most important alcohol of pharmacologic interest. It has few medical applications, but its abuse as a recreational drug is responsible for major medical and socio-economic problems. Other alcohols of toxicologic importance are methanol and ethylene glycol.

ETHANOL

A. Pharmacokinetics: After ingestion, ethanol is rapidly and completely absorbed; the drug is then distributed to all body tissues, and its volume of distribution is equivalent to that of total body water. Two enzyme systems metabolize ethanol to acetaldehyde.

1. Alcohol dehydrogenase: This cytosolic, NAD-dependent enzyme, found mainly in the liver and gut, accounts for the metabolism of low to moderate doses of ethanol. Because of the limited supply of the coenzyme NAD, the reaction has zero-order kinetics that result in a fixed capacity for ethanol metabolism of about 7-10 g/h. In chronic ethanol use, the use of NAD for its metabolism leads to a deficiency of the coenzyme for its normal metabolic functions. Gut metabolism of ethanol is lower in women than in men.

2. Microsomal ethanol-oxidizing system (MEOS): This liver microsomal mixed-function oxidase system increases in activity with chronic exposure to ethanol or inducing agents such as barbiturates. This increase may be partially responsible for the tolerance to ethanol that develops with chronic use.

Acetaldehyde formed from the oxidation of ethanol is rapidly metabolized to acetate by aldehyde dehydrogenase, a mitochondrial enzyme found in the liver and many other tissues. Aldehyde dehydrogenase is inhibited by **disulfiram,** and by other drugs including **metronidazole, oral hypoglycemics,** and certain **cephalosporin antibiotics.**

B. Acute Effects: The mechanisms underlying the CNS actions are not fully understood but are believed to involve effects of ethanol on neuronal membrane fluidity and synaptic transmission. The major acute effects of ethanol on the CNS include sedation, loss of inhibition, impaired judgment, slurred speech, and ataxia. Impairment of driving ability is thought to occur at ethanol blood levels between 60 and 80 mg/dL. Blood levels of 120 to 160 mg/dL are associated with gross drunkenness. Still higher levels (> 300 mg/dL) lead to loss of consciousness, anesthesia, and coma with fatal respiratory and cardiovascular depression. Lethal blood levels are usually >400 mg/dL. Chronic alcoholics function almost normally at much higher blood levels than occasional drinkers. Additive CNS depression occurs with concomitant administration of sedative-hypnotics, phenothiazines, and tricyclic antidepressants. Ethanol, even at relatively low concentrations in the blood, significantly depresses the heart. Vascular smooth muscle is relaxed, which leads to vasodilation, sometimes with marked hypothermia. Ethanol relaxes uterine smooth muscle. The drug also enhances the hypoglycemic effects of sulfonylureas and the antiplatelet actions of aspirin.

C. Chronic Effects:
1. **Tolerance and dependence:**   Tolerance occurs mainly as a result of CNS adaptation but may be partly caused by an increased rate of ethanol metabolism. There is cross-tolerance to other sedative-hypnotic drugs. Both psychologic and physical dependence are marked, the latter demonstrated by an abstinence syndrome upon abrupt discontinuance of ethanol intake by the chronic user.
2. **Liver:**   Gluconeogenesis is reduced and hypoglycemia and fat accumulation may occur as a result of NAD depletion; nutritional deficiencies may contribute to this process. Progressive loss of liver function occurs with hepatitis and cirrhosis. Hepatic dysfunction is often more severe in females, perhaps because higher concentrations of alcohol reach the liver in women. Ethanol may induce an increase in the activity of hepatic microsomal drug-metabolizing enzymes.
3. **Gastrointestinal system:**   Irritation, inflammation, bleeding, and scarring of the gut wall occur after chronic heavy use of ethanol and may cause absorption defects and exacerbate nutritional deficiencies.
4. **CNS:**   Peripheral neuropathies are the most common neurologic abnormalities in chronic alcoholics. More rarely, thiamine deficiency with ethanol use leads to the **Wernicke-Korsakoff** syndrome, which is characterized by ataxia, confusion, and paralysis of the extraocular muscles. Prompt treatment with parenteral thiamine is essential to prevent permanent brain damage.
5. **Endocrine system:**   Gynecomastia, testicular atrophy, and salt retention occur, partly because of altered steroid metabolism in the cirrhotic liver.
6. **Cardiovascular system:**   Chronic ethanol use is associated with an increased incidence of hypertension, anemia, and myocardial infarction.
7. **Fetal alcohol syndrome:**   Ethanol use in pregnancy is associated with teratogenic effects that include mental retardation, growth deficiencies, microencephaly, and characteristic malformations of the face and head.
8. **Neoplasia:**   Ethanol is not a primary carcinogen, but its chronic use is associated with an increased incidence of neoplastic diseases including breast carcinoma.

D. Treatment of Acute & Chronic Alcoholism:
1. **Excessive CNS depression:**   Intoxication due to acute ingestion of ethanol is managed by maintenance of vital signs and prevention of aspiration after vomiting. The administration of dextrose and the adjustment of electrolyte imbalance may also be required.
2. **Alcohol withdrawal syndrome:**   In the chronic user of ethanol, discontinuance can lead to a withdrawal syndrome characterized by insomnia, tremor, anxiety, and, in severe cases, delirium tremens (DTs) and life-threatening convulsions. Peripheral effects include nausea, vomiting, diarrhea, and arrhythmias. The abstinence syndrome is usually managed by treat-

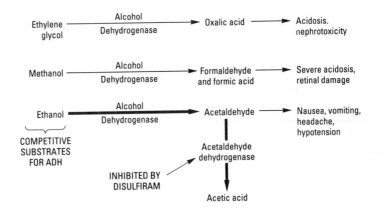

Figure 22–1. Toxic metabolites of alcohols. The oxidation of alcohols by alcohol dehydrogenase (ADH) results in the formation of metabolites that cause serious toxicities. Ethanol, a preferred substrate for ADH, is used in methanol or ethylene glycol poisoning to slow the rate of formation of the toxic metabolites of these alcohols. Acetaldehyde formed from ethanol is oxidized rapidly by aldehyde dehydrogenase except in the presence of disulfiram.

ment with a long-acting sedative-hypnotic (eg, diazepam), but the intensity of the syndrome may also be reduced by clonidine or propranolol.

3. **Treatment of alcoholism:** This is a complex sociomedical problem, and the disease of alcoholism is characterized by a high relapse rate. The aldehyde dehydrogenase inhibitor disulfiram is used adjunctively in some treatment programs. If ethanol is consumed by a patient who has taken disulfiram, acetaldehyde accumulation leads to nausea, headache, flushing, and hypotension (Figure 22–1).

OTHER ALCOHOLS

A. **Methanol:** Methanol is sometimes used by alcoholics when they are unable to obtain ethanol. Intoxication from methanol alone may include visual dysfunction, gastrointestinal distress, shortness of breath, loss of consciousness, and coma. Methanol is metabolized to formaldehyde, which can cause severe acidosis, retinal damage, and blindness. The formation of this toxic metabolite is retarded by prompt intravenous administration of ethanol, which acts as a preferred substrate for alcohol dehydrogenase and competitively inhibits the oxidation of methanol (Figure 22-1).

B. **Ethylene Glycol:** Industrial exposure to ethylene glycol (by inhalation or skin absorption) or self-administration (eg, by drinking antifreeze products) leads to severe acidosis and renal damage from the metabolism of ethylene glycol to oxalic acid. Prompt treatment with ethanol may slow or prevent formation of this toxic metabolite via competition for oxidation by alcohol dehydrogenase. Alcohol dehydrogenase is also inhibited by **fomepizole (4-methylpyrazole),** an orphan drug that is used on an experimental basis as an antidote in methanol and ethylene glycol toxicity.

QUESTIONS

DIRECTIONS: Each of the numbered items or incomplete statements in this section is followed by answers or by completions of the sentence. Select the ONE lettered answer or completion that is BEST in each case.

1. All of the following may occur after acute ingestion of ethanol EXCEPT
   (A) Hypertension
   (B) Additive CNS depression with over-the-counter antihistaminic drugs

    (C) Relaxation of uterine smooth muscle
    (D) Inhibition of liver microsomal drug-metabolizing enzymes
    (E) Myocardial depression

2. All of the following are signs or symptoms of regular ethanol use EXCEPT
    (A) Distal bilateral paresthesias
    (B) Gynecomastia and testicular atrophy
    (C) Fatty liver and hepatitis
    (D) Gastric irritation and bleeding
    (E) Increased coronary heart disease

3. All of the following statements about the biodisposition of ethanol are accurate EXCEPT
    (A) Ethanol is absorbed at all levels of the gastrointestinal tract
    (B) Acetaldehyde is the initial product of ethanol metabolism
    (C) After an intravenous dose, plasma levels of ethanol are higher in women than in men
    (D) The metabolism of ethanol follows zero-order kinetics
    (E) Methanol is a less effective substrate for alcohol dehydrogenase than ethanol

4. All of the following statements about ethanol are correct EXCEPT
    (A) Primary objectives in the management of ethanol intoxication include the support of respiration and the prevention of aspiration of vomitus
    (B) Flushing, headache, nausea, and vomiting are likely effects of drinking alcoholic beverages in patients who have consumed disulfiram
    (C) The Wernicke-Korsakoff syndrome occurs following withdrawal from chronic use of ethanol
    (D) The main objective of drug therapy in ethanol withdrawal is to prevent seizures, delirium, and arrhythmias
    (E) Long-acting benzodiazepines are used in ethanol detoxification

Items 5–6: A homeless middle-aged male patient presents in the emergency room in a state of intoxication. You note that he is behaviorally disinhibited and rowdy. He tells you that he has recently consumed about a pint of a red-colored liquid that his friends were using to "get high." He complains that his vision is blurred and that it is "like being in a snowstorm." His breath smells a bit like formaldehyde.

5. The most likely cause of his intoxicated state is the ingestion of
    (A) Ethylene glycol
    (B) Ethanol
    (C) Isopropanol
    (D) Methanol
    (E) Hexane

6. Your management of this patient may include all of the following EXCEPT
    (A) Airway and respiratory support if needed
    (B) Administration of activated charcoal
    (C) Administration of bicarbonate to counteract metabolic acidosis
    (D) Administration of ethanol before laboratory diagnosis is confirmed
    (E) Initiation of dialysis procedures, since it is likely to be an important step in the management of this patient

DIRECTIONS: The following section consists of a list of four to twenty-six lettered options followed by several numbered items. For each numbered item, select the ONE option that is most closely associated with it. Each answer may be selected once, more than once, or not at all.
    (A) Aldehyde dehydrogenase
    (B) NADH dehydrogenase
    (C) Alcohol dehydrogenase
    (D) Monoamine oxidase
    (E) Microsomal ethanol oxidizing system

7. A cytoplasmic zinc-containing enzyme that is primarily responsible for the oxidation of low to moderate doses of ethanol

8. The clinical use of disulfiram depends on its ability to inhibit this enzyme

9. This enzyme utilizes NADPH as a coenzyme; its activity may be increased with chronic ingestion of ethanol

10. Fomepizole (4-methylpyrazole) is a potent inhibitor of this enzyme

ANSWERS

1. The emphasis in this question is on the word *acute*. An acute dose of ethanol relaxes both vascular and uterine smooth muscle. Vasodilation occurs and at high doses may lead to hypothermia. Blood pressure is not raised acutely, though chronic use of alcohol is a risk factor for hypertension. The effect of ethanol on the uterus is to prolong labor. Note that most non-prescription antihistaminic drugs act as sedatives and will cause additive CNS depression if ethanol is consumed. The answer is **(A)**.

2. Compared to those who abstain, individuals who regularly ingest modest quantities of ethanol (1–2 drinks daily) are reported to have a *decreased* risk of coronary heart disease. All of the other items are signs and symptoms of chronic ethanol use. The answer is **(E)**.

3. There are no differences between men and women in plasma levels of ethanol following its intravenous administration. The higher plasma levels of ethanol in women after its *oral* ingestion may be due to the fact that they have lower activity of gastric alcohol dehydrogenase than men. A characteristic feature of ethanol biodisposition is that its elimination via metabolism follows zero-order kinetics. This results from limited availability of NAD, the cofactor in alcohol dehydrogenase-mediated ethanol oxidation. The answer is **(C)**.

4. The Wernicke-Korsakoff syndrome occurs with ethanol use, not withdrawal, but it may be difficult to distinguish from the acute confusional state that often accompanies alcohol withdrawal. The syndrome is characterized by paralysis of the external eye muscles, ataxia, and altered mentation. The syndrome is associated with thiamine deficiency but is rarely seen in the absence of alcoholism. The answer is **(C)**.

5. Behavioral disinhibition is a feature of early intoxication due to ethanol and most other alcohols, but not ingestion of the solvent, hexane. Ocular dysfunction, including horizontal nystagmus and diplopia, is also a common finding in poisoning with alcohols, but the complaint of "flickering white spots before the eyes" or "being in a snowstorm" is pathognomonic for methanol intoxication. In some cases, the odor of formaldehyde may be present on the breath. In this patient, blood methanol levels should be determined as soon as possible. The answer is **(D)**.

6. In all poisoning situations, it is important to establish adequate respiration. Bicarbonate may be needed to counteract metabolic acidosis. In patients with suspected methanol intoxication, ethanol (10%) is often given intravenously before laboratory diagnosis is confirmed, to block the formation of toxic products of ADH-catalyzed metabolism of methanol. Blood levels of methanol in excess of 50 mg/dL are an absolute indication for hemodialysis. Activated charcoal does not bind alcohols. The answer is **(B)**.

7. Alcohol dehydrogenase, a cytosolic enzyme that contains zinc, is the main enzyme involved in the oxidation of low to moderate doses of ethanol. NAD is required as a cofactor, and its concentration is rate-limiting. The enzyme also oxidizes methanol to formaldehyde, and ethylene glycol to oxalic acid (Figure 22-1). Ethanol—as a preferred substrate for ADH—competitively decreases the metabolism of the other alcohols and is used clinically in the management of methanol and ethylene glycol toxicity. The answer is **(C)**.

8. Disulfiram is an inhibitor of aldehyde dehydrogenase, the enzyme that converts acetaldehyde (formed from ethanol) to acetate. Disulfiram is sometimes used adjunctively in alcoholic rehabilitation programs, since ethanol ingestion leads to toxic accumulation of acetaldehyde in the presence of the drug. Disulfiram does not inhibit alcohol dehydrogenase (ADH) and thus does not block the metabolism of methanol or ethylene glycol to their aldehydes. The answer is **(A)**.

9. MEOS is a mixed function oxidase enzyme that requires NADPH as a cofactor. It plays a significant role in ethanol oxidation to acetaldehyde only when blood alcohol levels are high. With chronic exposure to ethanol, the activity of MEOS may increase via enzyme induction, and this may play a role in "metabolic tolerance." The answer is **(E)**.

10. A potent inhibitor of alcohol dehydrogenase (ADH), 4-methylpyrazole blocks the conversion of methanol and ethylene glycol to their toxic metabolites. The answer is **(C)**.

23

Antiepileptic Drugs

OBJECTIVES

You should be able to:

- List the major drugs used for partial seizures, generalized tonic-clonic seizures, absence and myoclonic seizures, and status epilepticus.
- Describe the main biodispositional features and the major adverse effects of each drug.
- Describe the pharmacokinetic factors that must be considered in designing a dosage regimen for antiepileptic drugs.

CONCEPTS

A. Classification: Epilepsy comprises a group of chronic syndromes that involve the recurrence of seizures, ie, limited periods of abnormal discharge of cerebral neurons. Subgroups of antiepileptic drugs are selective in their therapeutic effects for specific types of seizures (see Figure 23–1). Several chemical subgroups of antiepileptic drugs are structurally related; these include **hydantoins** (eg, phenytoin), **barbiturates** (eg, phenobarbital) and **succinimides** (eg, ethosuximide). There are also several unrelated subgroups including **carbamazepine** and **oxcarbazepine,** tricyclic compounds; **valproic acid,** a carboxylic acid; **benzodiazepines** (eg, diazepam, clonazepam); **felbamate,** a carbamate; **GABA derivatives** (eg, vigabatrin); and **lamotrigine,** a phenyltriazine.

B. Pharmacokinetics: Antiepileptic drugs are commonly used for long periods of time and can cause adverse effects. Consideration of their pharmacokinetic properties is important for avoiding toxicity and drug interactions. For some of these drugs (eg, phenytoin), determination of plasma levels and clearance rates in individual patients may be necessary for optimum therapy. In general, antiepileptic drugs are well absorbed orally and have good bioavailability. They are usually metabolized by hepatic enzymes, and in some cases (eg, primidone, trimethadione) active metabolites are formed.

Pharmacokinetic drug interactions are common in this drug group. In the presence of drugs that inhibit antiepileptic drug metabolism or displace anticonvulsants from plasma protein binding sites, plasma concentrations of the antiepileptic agents may reach toxic levels. On the other hand, drugs that induce hepatic drug-metabolizing enzymes (eg, rifampin) may result in plasma levels of the antiepileptic agents that are inadequate for seizure control.

1. Phenytoin: The oral bioavailability of phenytoin is variable due to variations in first-pass metabolism. Phenytoin metabolism is nonlinear; elimination kinetics shift from first-order to zero-order at moderate to high dose levels. The drug binds extensively to plasma proteins (97–98%) and free (unbound) phenytoin levels in plasma are increased by drugs that compete for binding (eg, sulfonamides, valproic acid). The metabolism of phenytoin is enhanced in the presence of inducers of liver metabolism (eg, phenobarbital, rifampin), and inhibited by other drugs (eg, cimetidine, isoniazid).

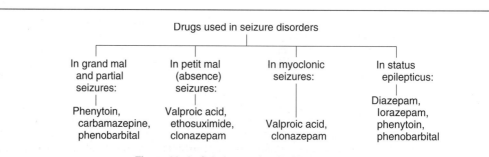

Figure 23–1. Subgroups of antiepileptic drugs.

2. **Carbamazepine:** The drug induces formation of liver drug-metabolizing enzymes that increase metabolism of the drug itself and may increase the clearance rates of many other anticonvulsant drugs. Carbamazepine metabolism can be inhibited by other drugs (eg, propoxyphene, valproic acid).

3. **Valproic acid:** In addition to competing for phenytoin plasma protein binding sites, valproic acid inhibits the metabolism of phenytoin and of phenobarbital. In some patients, the hepatic biotransformation of valproic acid leads to formation of a toxic metabolite that has been implicated in the hepatotoxicity of the drug.

C. **Mechanisms of Action:** The general effect of antiepileptic drugs is to suppress repetitive action potentials in epileptic foci in the brain. The mechanisms by which this occurs are not identical for all antiepileptic drugs. In the case of some anticonvulsants, multiple mechanisms may contribute to their antiseizure activities. Some of the recognized mechanisms are listed below.

1. **Sodium channel blockade:** At therapeutic concentrations, phenytoin and carbamazepine appear to block sodium channels in neuronal membranes. This action is use-dependent (ie, dependent on the frequency of neuronal discharge) and results in prolongation of the inactivated state of the Na^+ channel and the refractory period of the neuron. Phenobarbital and valproic acid may exert similar effects at high doses, and a new drug, lamotrigine, also appears to prolong inactivation of neuronal Na^+ channels.

2. **GABA-related targets:** As described in Chapter 21, benzodiazepines interact with specific receptors on the $GABA_A$ receptor-chloride ion channel macromolecular complex; these drugs facilitate the inhibitory effects of GABA. In the presence of benzodiazepines, the *frequency* of chloride ion channel opening is increased. Phenobarbital and other barbiturates also enhance the inhibitory actions of GABA, but interact with a different receptor site on chloride ion channels that results in an increased *duration* of chloride ion channel opening.

   GABA transaminase is an important enzyme in the termination of action of GABA. The enzyme is inhibited by valproic acid at very high concentrations, and is irreversibly inactivated by the new drug, vigabatrin, at therapeutic levels. This action may lead to enhanced inhibitory effects of GABA at synaptic sites.

3. **Calcium channel blockade:** Ethosuximide inhibits low-threshold (T-type) Ca^{2+} currents, especially in thalamic neurons that act as pacemakers to generate rhythmic cortical discharge.

4. **Other mechanisms:** Valproic acid causes neuronal membrane hyperpolarization, possibly through an action on K^+ channels to enhance potassium ion permeability. In addition to its actions on sodium channels and GABA-chloride channels, phenobarbital also blocks the quisqualate receptor subclass of the excitatory neurotransmitter glutamic acid.

D. **Clinical Use:** Diagnosis of a specific seizure type is important for prescribing the most appropriate antiseizure drug (or combination of drugs). Drug choice is usually made on the basis of established efficacy in the specific seizure state that has been diagnosed, the prior responsiveness of the patient, and the anticipated toxicity of the drug.

1. **Generalized tonic-clonic (grand mal) and partial seizures:** Carbamazepine, phenytoin, and phenobarbital (for children) continue to be the mainstay of treatment of grand mal epilepsy in the United States. Of these three agents, carbamazepine is usually the preferred drug for partial seizures. Primidone, a barbiturate with active metabolites (phenobarbital and phenylethylmalonamide), is sometimes used. Valproic acid is also effective in some patients with generalized tonic-clonic seizures. In addition, the newer drugs, felbamate, gabapentin, lamotrigine, and vigabatrin, all appear to be effective in partial seizures.

2. **Absence (petit mal) seizures:** Ethosuximide and valproic acid are the preferred drugs, since they cause minimal sedation. Ethosuximide is the drug of choice for uncomplicated absence seizures, but valproic acid may be more useful in patients who have concomitant tonic-clonic seizures. Clonazepam is effective, but has the disadvantages of causing sedation and the development of tolerance. Lamotrigine may be useful in children with petit mal.

3. **Myoclonic syndromes:** Myoclonic seizure syndromes are usually treated with valproic acid. Clonazepam can be effective, but the high doses required cause sedation and drowsiness. Lamotrigine is also reported to be effective in myoclonic syndromes in children.

4. **Status epilepticus:** Intravenous diazepam and lorazepam are effective in terminating attacks. For prolonged therapy, intravenous phenytoin is usually employed, since it is highly

Table 23–1. Possible adverse effects and complications of the use of antiepileptic drugs.

Antiepileptic Drug	Adverse Effects and Complications
Benzodiazepines	Sedation, tolerance, dependence
Carbamazepine	Diplopia, ataxia, enzyme induction, blood dyscrasias
Ethosuximide	Gastrointestinal distress, lethargy, headache
Phenobarbital	Sedation, enzyme induction, tolerance, dependence
Phenytoin	Nystagmus, diplopia, ataxia, sedation, gingival hyperplasia, hirsutism, anemias, enzyme induction
Valproic acid	Gastrointestinal distress, hepatotoxicity (rare but possibly fatal), inhibition of drug metabolism

effective and less sedating than benzodiazepines or barbiturates. Phenobarbital has also been used in status epilepticus, especially in children. In very severe status epilepticus that does not respond to these measures, general anesthesia may be employed.

5. **Infantile spasms:** Corticotropin and corticosteroids are commonly used, but cause characteristic cushingoid side effects. Benzodiazepines and other anticonvulsants may also be used, but their efficacy is limited.

E. **Toxicity:** Chronic therapy with antiepileptic drugs is associated with specific toxic effects, some of which are listed in Table 23-1.

1. **Teratogenicity:** Children born of mothers taking antiepileptic drugs have an increased risk of congenital malformations. Neural tube defects (spina bifida) are associated with the use of valproic acid, and a fetal hydantoin syndrome has been described following phenytoin use by pregnant women. Trimethadione should not be used in pregnancy because of its high risk of teratogenicity.

2. **Overdosage toxicity:** Respiratory depression, the major problem of overdosage, should be treated supportively (airway management and artificial ventilation).

3. **Withdrawal:** Withdrawal from antiepileptic drugs should be accomplished gradually to prevent increased seizure frequency and severity. In general, withdrawal from anti-absence drugs is more easily accomplished than from drugs used in partial or generalized tonic-clonic seizure states.

DRUG LIST

The following drugs are important members of the group discussed in this chapter. Prototypes should be learned in detail; features of the major variants should be known well enough to distinguish the variants from prototypes and from each other; the other significant agents should be recognized as belonging to a specific subclass.

Subclass	Prototype	Major Variant	Other Significant Agents
Barbiturates	Phenobarbital	Primidone	Mepharbital
Benzodiazepines	Diazepam	Lorazepam, clorazepate	Clonazepam, nitrazepam
Carboxylic acids	Valproic acid	Sodium valproate	
Hydantoins	Phenytoin		Mephenytoin
Succinimides	Ethosuximide	Phensuximide	
Tricyclics	Carbamazepine	Oxcarbazepine	
Newer agents	Felbamate, Gabapentin, Lamotrigine, Vigabatrin		

QUESTIONS

DIRECTIONS: Each of the numbered items or incomplete statements in this section is followed by answers or by completions of the sentence. Select the ONE lettered answer or completion that is BEST in each case.

1. Drugs useful in the treatment of partial seizures include all of the following EXCEPT
   (A) Lamotrigine
   (B) Phenytoin
   (C) Ethosuximide
   (D) Carbamazepine
   (E) Primidone

2. This drug is effective in absence seizure states, but has the disadvantages of dose-related sedation and the development of tolerance.
   (A) Valproic acid
   (B) Phenobarbital
   (C) Ethosuximide
   (D) Clonazepam
   (E) Diazepam

3. All of the following statements concerning proposed mechanisms of action of antiepileptic drugs are correct EXCEPT
   (A) Phenytoin prolongs the inactivated state of the Na^+ ion channel
   (B) Ethosuximide selectively blocks K^+ ion channels in thalamic neurons
   (C) Diazepam facilitates GABA-mediated inhibitory actions
   (D) Phenobarbital has multiple actions including enhancement of the effects of GABA, antagonism of glutamate receptors, and blockade of Na^+ ion channels
   (E) Vigabatrin elevates brain GABA by irreversible inhibition of GABA-transaminase

4. Which of the following antiseizure drugs is most likely to elevate the plasma levels of other drugs administered concomitantly?
   (A) Carbamazepine
   (B) Diazepam
   (C) Phenobarbital
   (D) Phenytoin
   (E) Valproic acid

Items 5–6: A young female patient employed as a computer programmer suffers from myoclonic jerking with no overt signs of neurologic deficit. There is no history of generalized tonic-clonic seizures. You are considering drug therapy for this patient.

5. If the seizures are to be effectively controlled without excessive sedation, the most appropriate drug is
   (A) Acetazolamide
   (B) Carbamazepine
   (C) Clonazepam
   (D) Phenytoin
   (E) Valproic acid

6. In the drug management of this case, all of the following are important considerations EXCEPT
   (A) Liver enzymes should be monitored
   (B) The patient should be examined periodically for deep tendon reflex activity
   (C) Abdominal pain and "heartburn" are likely side effects
   (D) The patient should not take barbiturates
   (E) She should contact her physician immediately if she becomes pregnant

7. All of the following statements concerning the pharmacokinetics of antiseizure drugs are correct EXCEPT
   (A) At high doses, phenytoin elimination follows zero-order kinetics
   (B) Phenobarbital may increase the activity of hepatic ALA synthase
   (C) The administration of phenytoin to patients in methadone maintenance programs has led to symptoms of opioid overdose, including respiratory depression

    (D) Although ethosuximide has a half-life of approximately 40 hours, the drug is usually taken twice a day

    (E) Treatment with carbamazepine may reduce the effectiveness of oral contraceptives

DIRECTIONS: The following section consists of a list of four to twenty-six lettered options followed by several numbered items. For each numbered item, select the ONE option that is most closely associated with it. Each answer may be selected once, more than once, or not at all.

    (A) Lorazepam
    (B) Phenytoin
    (C) Ethosuximide
    (D) Felbamate
    (E) Primidone
    (F) Carbamazepine
    (G) Valproic acid
    (H) Phenobarbital
    (I) Clonazepam
    (J) Vigabatrin

8. This drug is used for both partial and generalized tonic-clonic seizures. It should be used cautiously in pregnancy because of possible teratogenicity. Hirsutism and gingival hyperplasia are relatively common side effects

9. In addition to its uses in seizure states, this drug is effective in the management of trigeminal neuralgia and can be used in bipolar affective disorders in patients intolerant to lithium

10. The risk of hepatotoxicity due to this drug is greatest in children under 2 years of age; most fatalities have occurred within 4 months after initiation of therapy

11. This drug can be used by the intravenous route in status epilepticus; it interacts with specific receptors that are components of the $GABA_A$ receptor-chloride ion channel macromolecular complex

12. Concerns about its hematotoxicity have restricted the use of this drug in the management of partial seizures; the agent is structurally related to meprobamate, but has minimal sedative effect

ANSWERS

1. Phenytoin, carbamazepine, and barbiturates are used for both generalized tonic-clonic and partial seizures. Valproic acid and several newer drugs, including lamotrigine, are also useful in partial seizures. Succinimides (ethosuximide, phensuximide) are not effective in grand mal or in partial seizures. The answer is **(C)**.

2. Three drugs are effective in absence seizures (petit mal). Ethosuximide and valproic acid are not sedating and tolerance does not develop to their antiseizure activity. Clonazepam is effective but exerts troublesome CNS depressant effects, and tolerance develops with chronic use. At high doses, the drug has a dependence liability like most benzodiazepines. The answer is **(D)**.

3. Though not completely understood, the mechanism of action of ethosuximide is thought to involve blockade of T-type Ca^{2+} ion channels in thalamic neurons. The drug does not block K^+ ion channels, which in any case would be likely to result in an increase (rather than a decrease) in neuronal excitability. The answer is **(B)**.

4. With chronic use, the anticonvulsant barbiturates, carbamazepine, and phenytoin all induce the formation of hepatic drug-metabolizing enzymes. This action may lead to a *decrease* in the plasma levels of other drugs used concomitantly. Valproic acid, an inhibitor of drug metabolism, can increase the plasma levels of many drugs including carbamazepine, phenobarbital, and phenytoin. Benzodiazepines have no major effects on the metabolism of other drugs. The answer is **(E)**.

5. Valproic acid is highly effective in specific myoclonic syndromes and is usually considered to be the drug of choice since it is nonsedating. Clonazepam is a back-up drug, since the high doses required cause excessive drowsiness. None of the other drugs listed are effective. Acetazolamide is rarely used in seizure states because tolerance develops rapidly; this drug may be useful in women who experience seizures at the time of menses. The answer is **(E)**.

6. Valproic acid often causes gastrointestinal distress and is potentially hepatotoxic. The use of this drug in pregnancy has been associated with teratogenicity (neural tube defects). Valproic acid inhibits the metabolism of barbiturates; marked CNS depression may result if such drugs are given concomitantly. Peripheral neuropathy, in the form of diminished deep tendon reflexes in the lower extremities, is associated with chronic use of phenytoin. The answer is **(B)**.

7. Monitoring of plasma levels of phenytoin may be critical in establishing an effective dosage, since the drug exhibits non-linear elimination kinetics. Due to possible induction of liver enzymes, barbiturates are contraindicated in patients with porphyrias; similarly, carbamazepine may enhance estrogen metabolism. The enzyme-inducing activity of phenytoin has led to symptoms of opioid *withdrawal,* presumably due to an increase in the rate of metabolism of methadone. Twice-a-day dosage of ethosuximide is common, since it reduces the severity of adverse gastrointestinal effects. The answer is **(C)**.

8. The use of antiseizure drugs in pregnancy is associated with an increased incidence of congenital abnormalities. Of the drugs listed, carbamazepine, phenytoin, and valproic acid are the most frequently implicated teratogens. The most frequent adverse effects of phenytoin are nystagmus, diplopia, and ataxia; gingival hyperplasia and hirsutism occur to some degree in most patients. The answer is **(B)**.

9. Carbamazepine is usually the drug of choice in partial seizures and it is also effective in the management of grand mal. Though clonazepam has been used in manic-depressive disorders, it has minimal efficacy in trigeminal neuralgia. The answer is **(F)**.

10. The idiosyncratic hepatotoxicity of valproic acid may be related to the formation of a reactive metabolite, via a minor pathway of hepatic biotransformation of the drug. Careful monitoring of liver function is recommended; hepatotoxicity may be reversible if the drug is withdrawn immediately. The answer is **(G)**.

11. Diazepam (not listed) is the drug most commonly administered intravenously for initial treatment of status epilepticus. Of the drugs listed, lorazepam, phenobarbital, and phenytoin may also be used. Phenytoin is the primary drug used for longer-term management. The actions of lorazepam result from binding to benzodiazepine receptors, leading to the facilitation of the inhibitory effects of GABA. The answer is **(A)**.

12. Idiosyncratic blood dyscrasias have occurred with carbamazepine, mostly in elderly patients treated for trigeminal neuralgia. However, their infrequent occurrence when the drug is used in seizure states has not limited its clinical use. The new drug, felbamate, is highly effective in partial seizures and does not cause drowsiness. Recent reports of agranulocytosis have severely restricted the use of felbamate in the United States. The answer is **(D)**.

General Anesthetics

24

OBJECTIVES

You should be able to:

- Identify the main inhalational and intravenous anesthetic agents and describe their pharmacodynamic properties.
- Describe the relationship between the blood:gas partition coefficient of an inhalation anesthetic and the speed of onset (and offset) of anesthesia.
- Describe how changes in pulmonary ventilation and blood flow can influence the speed of onset (and offset) of inhalation anesthesia.
- Describe the pharmacokinetics of the commonly used intravenous anesthetics.

Learn the definitions that follow.

Term	Definition
Balanced anesthesia	Anesthesia produced by a mixture of drugs, often including both inhaled and intravenous agents
Inhalation anesthesia	Anesthesia induced by inhalation of drug
Minimal alveolar anesthetic concentration (MAC)	The alveolar concentration required to eliminate the response to a standardized painful stimulus in 50% of patients
Analgesia	A stage of decreased awareness of pain, sometimes with amnesia
General anesthesia	A state of unconsciousness, analgesia, and amnesia, with skeletal muscle relaxation and loss of reflexes

Table 24–1. Definitions.

CONCEPTS

A. General Anesthesia: General anesthesia is characterized by a state of unconsciousness, analgesia, and amnesia, with skeletal muscle relaxation and loss of reflexes. General anesthetics are CNS depressants with actions that can be induced and terminated more rapidly than those of sedative-hypnotics. Modern general anesthetics act very rapidly and achieve deep anesthesia quickly. With older, slowly acting anesthetics, the progressively greater depth of central depression associated with increasing dose or time of exposure is reflected by the traditional **stages of anesthesia:**

1. **Analgesia:** Stage 1 is a stage of decreased awareness of pain, sometimes with amnesia. Consciousness may be impaired, but not lost.
2. **Disinhibition:** In stage 2, the patient appears to be delirious and excited. Amnestic effects are prominent, reflexes are enhanced, and respiration is typically irregular; retching and incontinence may occur.
3. **Surgical anesthesia:** In stage 3, the patient is unconscious and has no pain reflexes; respiration is very regular and blood pressure is maintained.
4. **Medullary depression:** In stage 4, the patient experiences severe respiratory and cardiovascular depression that requires mechanical and pharmacologic support.

B. Anesthesia Protocols: For minor procedures, **conscious sedation** is often used, combining intravenous agents with local anesthetics. For more extensive procedures, **balanced anesthesia** may be used. This consists of short-acting intravenous anesthetics, plus nitrous oxide and opioids. For major surgery, anesthesia protocols commonly include the use of intravenous drugs to induce the anesthetic state, inhaled anesthetics to maintain anesthesia, and neuromuscular blocking agents to effect muscle relaxation.

C. Mechanisms of Action: The mechanisms of action of general anesthetics are unclear, but these drugs usually increase the threshold for firing of CNS neurons. The potency of most in-

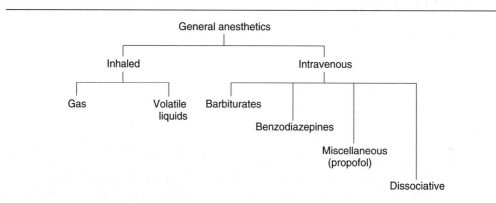

Figure 24–1. Subgroups of drugs discussed in this chapter.

haled anesthetics correlates positively with their lipid solubility. Possible mechanisms of action include block of ion channels by interactions with membrane lipids or proteins, as well as effects on central neurotransmitter mechanisms. CNS neurons in different regions of the brain have different sensitivities to general anesthetics; inhibition of neurons involved in pain pathways occurs before inhibition of neurons in the midbrain reticular formation.

INHALED ANESTHETICS

A. Classification & Pharmacokinetics of Onset of Action: The agents currently used in inhalation anesthesia are nitrous oxide (a gas) and several easily vaporized liquid halogenated hydrocarbons, including halothane, desflurane, enflurane, isoflurane, and methoxyflurane. They are administered as gases; the partial pressure, or "tension," of a particular anesthetic is a measure of its concentration in the body. The speed of induction of anesthetic effects depends on several factors:

1. **Inspired gas concentration:** A high partial pressure of the gas in the lungs results in more rapid achievement of anesthetic levels in the blood. Advantage is taken of this effect by the initial administration of gas concentrations higher than those required for maintenance of anesthesia.

2. **Blood:gas partition coefficient:** The more rapidly a drug equilibrates with the blood, the more quickly the drug passes into the brain to produce anesthetic effects. Drugs with low blood solubility (eg, nitrous oxide) equilibrate more rapidly than do drugs with a higher partition coefficient (eg, halothane), as illustrated in Figure 24–2. Partition coefficients for inhalational anesthetics are shown in Table 24–2.

3. **Ventilation rate:** The greater the ventilation, the more rapid the rise in alveolar and blood concentration of the agent and the more rapid the onset of anesthesia (Figure 24–3). Advantage is taken of this effect in the induction of the anesthetic state.

4. **Pulmonary blood flow:** At high pulmonary blood flows, the gas partial pressure rises at a slower rate; thus, the speed of onset of anesthesia is reduced. At low flow rates, onset is

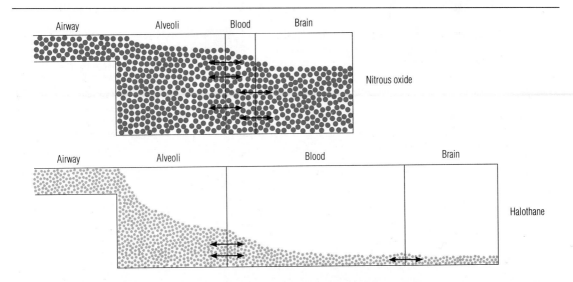

Figure 24–2. Why induction of anesthesia is slower with more soluble anesthetic gases and faster with less soluble ones. In this schematic diagram, solubility is represented by the size of the blood compartment (the more soluble, the larger the compartment). For a given concentration or partial pressure of the two anesthetic gases in the inspired air, it will take much longer with halothane than with nitrous oxide for the blood partial pressure to rise to the same partial pressure as in the alveoli. Since the concentration in the brain can rise no faster than the concentration in the blood, the onset of anesthesia will be much slower with halothane than with nitrous oxide. (Reproduced, with permission, from Katzung BG [editor]: *Basic & Clinical Pharmacology,* 6th ed. Appleton & Lange, 1995.)

Table 24–2. Properties of inhalational anesthetics.[1]

Anesthetic	Blood:Gas Partition Coefficient	Blood:Brain Partition Coefficient	Minimum Alveolar Concentration[2] (percent)
Nitrous oxide	0.47	1.1	>100
Desflurane	0.42	1.3	6–7
Isoflurane	1.40	2.6	1.40
Enflurane	1.80	1.4	1.68
Halothane	2.30	2.9	0.75
Methoxyflurane	12.00	2.0	0.16

[1] Modified and reproduced, with permission, from Katzung BG [editor]: *Basic & Clinical Pharmacology,* 6th ed. Appleton & Lange, 1995.
[2] Minimum alveolar concentration (MAC) is the anesthetic concentration that eliminates the response in 50% of patients exposed to a standardized painful stimulus.

faster. In circulatory shock, this effect may accelerate the rate of onset of anesthesia with agents of high blood solubility.

5. **Arteriovenous concentration gradient:** Uptake of soluble anesthetics into highly perfused tissues may decrease gas tension in mixed venous blood. This can influence the rate of onset of anesthesia, since achievement of equilibrium is dependent on the difference in anesthetic tension between arterial and venous blood.

B. Elimination: Anesthesia is terminated by redistribution of the drug from the brain to the blood and elimination of the drug through the lungs. The rate of recovery from anesthesia using agents with high blood:gas partition coefficients is slower than that of anesthetics with low blood solubility. Halothane and methoxyflurane are metabolized by liver enzymes to a significant extent; however, the rate of their metabolism does not influence speed of recovery from anesthesia.

C. Minimum Alveolar Anesthetic Concentration (MAC): The potency of inhaled anesthetics is best measured by the minimum alveolar anesthetic concentration (MAC). This is defined as the alveolar concentration required to eliminate the response to a standardized painful stimu-

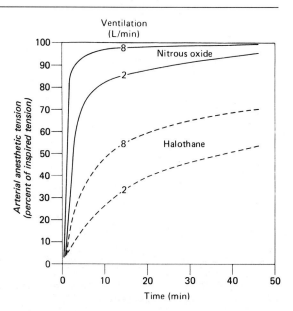

Figure 24–3. Ventilation rate and arterial anesthetic tensions. (Reproduced, with permission, from Katzung BG [editor]: *Basic & Clinical Pharmacology,* 6th ed. Appleton & Lange, 1995.)

lus in 50% of patients (see Table 24–2). Each anesthetic has a defined MAC, but this value may vary among different patients depending on age, cardiovascular status, use of adjuvant drugs, etc. MACs for elderly patients are lower than those for young adults. When several anesthetic agents are used simultaneously, their MAC values are additive.

D. Effects of Inhaled Anesthetics:
   1. **CNS effects:** Inhaled anesthetics reduce brain metabolic rate but reduce vascular resistance and thus increase cerebral blood flow. This may lead to an increase in intracranial pressure. High concentrations of enflurane may cause spike-and-wave activity and muscle twitching. Though nitrous oxide has low anesthetic potency (ie, a high MAC), it exerts marked analgesic and amnestic actions.
   2. **Cardiovascular effects:** Most inhaled anesthetics decrease arterial blood pressure moderately. Enflurane and halothane are myocardial depressants that decrease cardiac output, while isoflurane causes peripheral vasodilation. Nitrous oxide is less likely to lower blood pressure than are other inhaled anesthetics. Blood flow to the liver and kidney is decreased by most inhaled agents. Halothane may sensitize the myocardium to the arrhythmogenic effects of endogenous catecholamines.
   3. **Respiratory effects:** Rate of respiration may be increased by inhaled anesthetics, but tidal volume and minute ventilation are decreased, leading to an increase in arterial CO_2 tension. Inhaled anesthetics decrease ventilatory response to hypoxia even at subanesthetic concentrations (eg, during recovery). Nitrous oxide has the smallest effect on respiration.
   4. **Toxicity:** Postoperative hepatitis has occurred (rarely) following halothane anesthesia in patients experiencing hypovolemic shock or other severe stress. Fluoride released by metabolism of methoxyflurane (and enflurane) may cause renal insufficiency after prolonged anesthesia. Prolonged exposure to nitrous oxide decreases methionine synthase activity and may lead to megaloblastic anemia. Susceptible patients may develop **malignant hyperthermia** when exposed to halogenated anesthetics. This rare condition of uncontrolled release of calcium by the sarcoplasmic reticulum of skeletal muscle leads to spasm, hyperthermia, and autonomic lability.

INTRAVENOUS ANESTHETICS

A. Classification, Pharmacokinetics, & Pharmacodynamics: Several different chemical classes of drugs are used as intravenous agents in anesthesia.
   1. **Barbiturates: Thiopental, thiamylal,** and **methohexital** have high lipid solubility, which promotes rapid entry into the brain and results in surgical anesthesia in one circulation time. These agents are used for induction of anesthesia and for short surgical procedures. Their anesthetic effects are terminated by redistribution from the brain to other tissues (Figure 24–4), but hepatic metabolism is required for their elimination from the body.

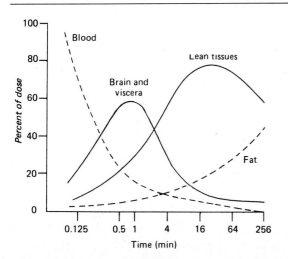

Figure 24–4. Redistribution of thiopental after an intravenous bolus administration. (Reproduced, with permission, from Katzung BG [editor]: *Basic & Clinical Pharmacology,* 6th ed. Appleton & Lange, 1995.)

They are respiratory and circulatory depressants; because they depress cerebral blood flow, they can also decrease intracranial pressure.

2. **Benzodiazepines:** **Midazolam** is used adjunctively with gaseous anesthetics and narcotics. The onset of its CNS effects is slower than thiopental, and it has a longer duration of action. Cases of severe postoperative respiratory depression have occurred. The antagonist flumazenil accelerates recovery from midazolam and other benzodiazepines.

3. **Dissociative anesthetic:** **Ketamine** produces a state called "dissociative anesthesia" in which the patient remains conscious but has marked catatonia, analgesia, and amnesia. Ketamine is an antagonist of glutamic acid, blocking the actions of this excitatory transmitter at its NMDA receptor. The drug is a cardiovascular stimulant and this action may lead to an increase in intracranial pressure. Disorientation and hallucinations, which commonly occur during recovery, can be reduced by the preoperative use of benzodiazepines.

4. **Opioids:** **Morphine** and **fentanyl** are used with other CNS depressants (nitrous oxide, benzodiazepines) in certain high-risk patients who might not survive a full general anesthetic. Intravenous opioids may cause chest wall rigidity that can impair ventilation. Respiratory depression with these drugs may be reversed postoperatively with naloxone. **Neuroleptanesthesia** is a state of analgesia and amnesia produced when fentanyl is used with droperidol and nitrous oxide.

5. **Propofol:** Propofol produces anesthesia at a rate similar to the intravenous barbiturates, and recovery is more rapid. Propofol has antiemetic actions, and recovery is not delayed after prolonged infusion. The drug is commonly used as a component of balanced anesthesia and as an anesthetic in outpatient surgery. Propofol may cause marked hypotension during induction of anesthesia, primarily through decreased peripheral resistance. Total body clearance of propofol is greater than hepatic blood flow, suggesting that its elimination includes other mechanisms in addition to metabolism by liver enzymes.

DRUG LIST

The following drugs are important members of the group discussed in this chapter. Prototypes should be learned in detail; features of the major variants should be known well enough to distinguish the variants from the prototypes and from each other.

Subclass	Prototype	Major Variants
Inhaled anesthetics Volatile liquids	Halothane	Enflurane, desflurane, isoflurane, methoxyflurane
Gas	Nitrous oxide	
Intravenous anesthetics Barbiturates	Thiopental	Thiamylal, methohexital
Opioids	Morphine	Fentanyl
Propofol	Propofol	
Benzodiazepines	Midazolam	
Dissociative agent	Ketamine	

QUESTIONS

DIRECTIONS: Each of the numbered items or incomplete statements in this section is followed by answers or by completions of the sentence. Select the ONE lettered answer or completion that is BEST in each case.

1. All of the following statements about the onset of anesthesia using inhalation agents are accurate EXCEPT
   (A) Onset of anesthesia is very fast with agents that have a high blood solubility
   (B) Onset of anesthesia is accelerated by increasing inspired anesthetic gas concentration

    (C) Changes in pulmonary blood flow have minimal effects on the rate of onset of the effects of nitrous oxide

    (D) Decreasing ventilation rate during gas inhalation will slow onset of anesthesia

    (E) Equilibrium between arterial and venous gas tension is achieved very slowly with methoxyflurane

2. All of the following effects of anesthetic agents are correct EXCEPT

    (A) Relaxation of bronchiolar smooth muscle during halothane anesthesia

    (B) Mild, generalized muscle twitching at high doses of enflurane

    (C) Muscle rigidity following administration of fentanyl

    (D) Prolongation of the postanesthesia recovery period following intravenous midazolam

    (E) Postoperative hepatitis following the use of isoflurane

3. All of the following statements concerning the anesthetic MAC are accurate EXCEPT

    (A) At a given level of anesthesia, measurement of alveolar concentrations of different anesthetics allows potency comparisons

    (B) MACs give information about the slope of the dose-response curve

    (C) The MAC value for nitrous oxide in humans is greater than 100%

    (D) MACs decrease in elderly patients

    (E) The simultaneous use of opioid analgesics lowers the MAC for inhaled anesthetics

4. All of the following statements concerning drugs used in anesthesia are correct EXCEPT

    (A) During recovery from anesthesia with inhalational agents, compensatory ventilatory responses to anoxia are reduced

    (B) Megaloblastic anemia is a common adverse effect in patients exposed to nitrous oxide for periods longer than 2 hours

    (C) Isoflurane may increase intracranial pressure in patients with head injury

    (D) High doses of opioid analgesics can be used in cardiac surgery with minimal circulatory deterioration

    (E) Intraoperative use of benzodiazepines prolongs the postanesthetic recovery period and may cause anterograde amnesia

5. John Green is a 23-year-old man with a pheochromocytoma, blood pressure 190/120, hematocrit 50%, and normal pulmonary and renal function. His catecholamines are elevated and he has a well-defined abdominal tumor on MRI. He has been scheduled for surgery. Of the agents listed below, which drug is LEAST suitable for inclusion in his anesthesia protocol?

    (A) Midazolam

    (B) Nitrous oxide

    (C) Isoflurane

    (D) Halothane

    (E) Thiopental

6. Total intravenous anesthesia with opioids has been selected for a frail 72-year-old woman about to undergo cardiac surgery. All of the following statements about intravenous opioid anesthesia are correct EXCEPT

    (A) High-dose intravenous opioids provide relatively stable hemodynamics

    (B) Opioids control the hypertensive response to surgical stimulation

    (C) Muscle rigidity may occur, especially with rapid administration of opioids

    (D) Patient awareness may occur during surgery, with recall after recovery

    (E) The patient is unlikely to experience pain during surgery

DIRECTIONS: The following section consists of a list of four to twenty-six lettered options followed by several numbered items. For each numbered item, select the ONE option that is most closely associated with it. Each answer may be selected once, more than once, or not at all.

    (A) Midazolam

    (B) Methoxyflurane

    (C) Fentanyl

    (D) Nitrous oxide

    (E) Ketamine

    (F) Isoflurane

    (G) Propofol

    (H) Halothane

    (I) Thiopental

    (J) Morphine

7. Vasopressin-resistant polyuric renal insufficiency has occurred after prolonged administration of this anesthetic
8. Use of this agent is associated with a high incidence of disorientation, sensory and perceptual illusions, and vivid dreams following anesthesia
9. Respiratory depression following use of this agent may be reversed by administration of flumazenil
10. Postoperative vomiting is uncommon with use of this intravenous agent; patients are able to ambulate sooner than those who receive other anesthetics
11. Heart rate, arterial blood pressure, and cardiac output are all increased following administration of this anesthetic agent
12. This drug decreases cerebral blood flow; redistribution from the brain to other highly-perfused tissues is responsible for termination of its anesthetic effects

ANSWERS

1. Arterial gas tension increases *slowly* following inhalation of anesthetics with high blood solubility (eg, methoxyflurane). This results in a slow rate of equilibration between blood and brain, and a slower onset of anesthesia than occurs with agents of low blood solubility (eg, nitrous oxide). The onset of the effects of nitrous oxide is not significantly altered by changes in pulmonary blood flow, since the drug has very low blood solubility. The answer is **(A)**.
2. Hepatitis following general anesthesia has been linked to use of *halothane,* although the incidence of severe hepatic necrosis is only about 1 out of 35,000 halothane administrations. The results of animal experiments suggest that halothane hepatotoxicity may be due to the formation of a toxic metabolite produced under anoxic conditions. Hepatotoxicity has not been reported following isoflurane administration; it may be relevant that this agent is the most slowly metabolized of the fluorinated hydrocarbons. All of the other statements are correct. The answer is **(E)**.
3. Dose-response characteristics of inhaled anesthetics are difficult to measure, since it is not possible to measure brain concentrations of such drugs at different stages of CNS depression. On the basis of alveolar gas concentration measurements, we can conclude that dose-response relationships are steep. Whereas a dose of 1 MAC of any agent prevents movement in response to surgical stimulation in 50% of patients (by definition), individual patients may require from 0.5 to 1.5 MACs for adequate anesthesia. The MAC gives no information about the slope of the dose-response curve. The answer is **(B)**.
4. Hematotoxicity due to nitrous oxide has *not* been reported in patients exposed to nitrous oxide anesthesia for periods up to 6 hours. However, megaloblastic anemia may be an occupational hazard for staff working in poorly ventilated dental operating rooms. The answer is **(B)**.
5. Halothane sensitizes the myocardium to catecholamines; arrhythmias may occur in patients with cardiac disease who have high circulating levels of epinephrine and norepinephrine (eg, patients with pheochromocytoma). Other modern anesthetics are considerably less arrhythmogenic. The answer is **(D)**.
6. High-dose intravenous opioids (eg, fentanyl, morphine) are widely used in cardiac anesthesia because they cause less cardiac depression than inhalational anesthetic agents. One disadvantage of this technique is patient recall, although the likelihood of patient awareness can be decreased by use of a benzodiazepine. Another disadvantage is the occurrence of hypertensive responses to surgical stimulation. The addition of vasodilators (eg, nitroprusside) or a beta-blocker (eg, esmolol) may be needed to prevent hypertension intraoperatively. The answer is **(B)**.
7. Methoxyflurane, the most potent halogenated gas anesthetic, undergoes extensive hepatic metabolism, releasing fluoride ions at levels that can be nephrotoxic. The answer is **(B)**.
8. The "emergence phenomena" described are undesirable effects of ketamine. Administration of diazepam (0.2 mg/kg) immediately prior to ketamine anesthesia reduces the incidence of these effects. The answer is **(E)**.
9. Flumazenil is a benzodiazepine receptor antagonist (see Chapter 21). It accelerates recovery from postoperative depression of the CNS due to midazolam or other benzodiazepines used in anesthesia such as diazepam and lorazepam. The short duration of action of flumazenil may necessitate multiple doses. The sedative actions of benzodiazepines are more reliably reversed by flumazenil than is respiratory depression. Use of the drug does not replace adequate monitoring of respiration and the provision of ventilatory support when needed. The answer is **(A)**.

10. Propofol is used extensively in balanced anesthesia protocols and is especially suitable for "day surgery" anesthesia. The drug's favorable properties include an antiemetic effect and a rate of recovery that is more rapid than that following use of other intravenous drugs. Propofol does not cause cumulative effects, possibly due to its short half-life (2–8 minutes) in the body. The drug is also used for prolonged sedation in critical care settings. The answer is **(G).**

11. Ketamine is the only anesthetic that routinely causes cardiovascular stimulation. This results partly from central sympathetic stimulation, and possibly from inhibition of norepinephrine reuptake at sympathetic nerve endings. The answer is **(E).**

12. Drug redistribution from brain to other body tissues may play a role in termination of CNS effects of both ketamine and thiobarbiturates. In contrast to ketamine, however, thiopental decreases cerebral blood flow. This makes thiopental a more desirable drug than inhalational anesthetics in patients with cerebral swelling. The answer is **(I).**

Local Anesthetics

25

OBJECTIVES

You should be able to:

- Describe the mechanism of blockade of the nerve impulse by local anesthetics.
- Discuss the relation between pH, pK_a, and the speed of onset of local anesthesia.
- List the factors that determine the susceptibility of nerve fibers to blockade.
- List the major toxic effects of the local anesthetics.
- Explain use-dependent blockade by local anesthetics.

CONCEPTS

Local anesthesia is the condition that results when sensory transmission from a local area of the body to the CNS is blocked. The local anesthetics constitute a group of chemically similar agents that block the sodium channels of excitable membranes. Because these drugs can be administered locally by topical application or by injection in the target area, the anesthetic effect can be restricted to a localized area, eg, the cornea or an arm. When given intravenously, these drugs have effects on other tissues. Many drugs classified in other groups, eg, antihistamines and beta-blockers, have significant local anesthetic effects.

A. Chemistry & Subclasses: Most local anesthetic drugs are esters or amides of simple benzene derivatives. Subgroups within the local anesthetics are based on this chemical characteristic and on duration of action (Figure 25–1). All of the commonly used local anesthetics carry at least one amine function and are therefore weak bases that become charged through the gain of a proton (H^+). As discussed in Chapter 1, the degree of ionization is a function of the pK_a of the drug and the pH of the medium. Because the pH of tissue may differ from the physiologic 7.4 (for example, it may be as low as 6.4 in infected tissue), the degree of ionization of the drug will vary. Because the pK_a of most local anesthetics is between 8.0 and 9.0 (benzocaine is an exception), variations in pH associated with infection can have significant effects on the proportion of ionized to nonionized drug. The question of the active form of the drug (ionized versus nonionized) is discussed below.

B. Pharmacokinetics: Many shorter-acting local anesthetics are readily absorbed from the injection site after administration. The duration of local action is therefore limited unless blood

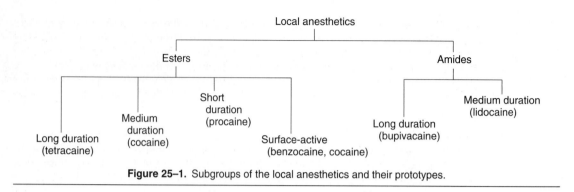

Figure 25–1. Subgroups of the local anesthetics and their prototypes.

flow to the area is reduced. This can be accomplished by administration of a vasoconstrictor (usually an alpha agonist sympathomimetic) with the local anesthetic agent. Cocaine is an important exception to this rule since it has intrinsic sympathomimetic action (because it inhibits norepinephrine reuptake into nerve terminals); cocaine does not require any additional vasoconstrictor. The longer-acting agents, eg, tetracaine and bupivacaine, are also less dependent on the coadministration of epinephrine.

Surface activity (ability to reach superficial nerves when applied to the surface of mucous membranes) is a property of only a few local anesthetics, including cocaine and benzocaine.

Metabolism of ester local anesthetics is carried out by plasma cholinesterases and may be rapid. Procaine and chloroprocaine have half-lives of only 1-2 minutes. The amides are hydrolyzed in the liver and have half-lives from 1.8 to 6 hours. Bupivacaine is a very lipid-soluble and long-acting local anesthetic. Liver dysfunction may increase the elimination half-life of amide local anesthetics.

C. Mechanism of Action: Local anesthetics block voltage-dependent sodium channels and reduce the influx of sodium ions, thereby preventing depolarization of the membrane and blocking conduction of the action potential. Local anesthetics gain access to their receptors from the cytoplasm or the membrane (Figure 25–2). Since the drug molecule must cross the lipid membrane to reach the cytoplasm, the more lipid-soluble (nonionized, uncharged) form reaches effective intracellular concentrations more rapidly than would the ionized form. On the other

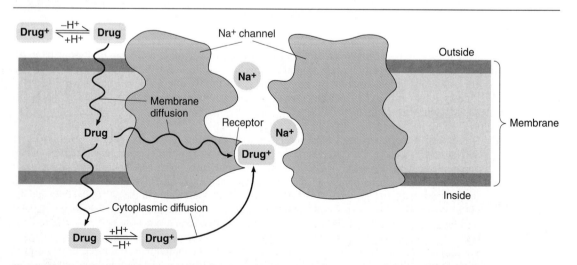

Figure 25–2. Schematic diagram of the sodium channel in an excitable membrane (eg, an axon) and the pathways by which a local anesthetic molecule *(Drug)* may reach its receptor. Sodium ions are not able to pass through the channel when the drug is bound to the receptor. The local anesthetic diffuses within the membrane in its uncharged form. In the aqueous extracellular and intracellular spaces, the charged form *(Drug⁺)* is also present.

hand, once inside the axon, the ionized (charged) form of the drug appears to be the more effective blocking entity. Thus both the nonionized and the ionized forms of the drug play important roles, the first in reaching the receptor site and the second in causing the effect. The affinity of the receptor site within the sodium channel for the local anesthetic is a function of the state of the channel—whether it is resting, open, or inactivated—and therefore follows the same rules of use-dependence and potential-dependence that were described for the sodium channel-blocking antiarrhythmic drugs (see Chapter 14).

D. **Effects:**
   1. **Nerves:** Differential sensitivity of various types of nerve fibers to local anesthetics is associated with several factors, including fiber diameter, myelination, physiologic firing rate, and anatomical location (Table 25–1). In general, smaller fibers are blocked more easily than larger ones and myelinated fibers are blocked more easily than unmyelinated ones. It is thought that activated pain fibers fire rapidly, and that pain sensation may be selectively blocked by these drugs. Fibers located in the periphery of a thick nerve bundle are blocked sooner than those in the core because they are exposed earlier to higher concentrations of the anesthetic.
   2. **Other tissues:** The effects of these drugs on the heart are discussed in Chapter 14 (see Group I antiarrhythmic agents). Most local anesthetics also have weak blocking effects on skeletal muscle neuromuscular transmission, but these actions have no clinical application. The mood elevation induced by cocaine probably reflects actions on dopamine or other amine-mediated synaptic transmission in the CNS, rather than a local anesthetic action on membranes.

E. **Clinical Use:** The local anesthetics are most commonly used for minor surgical procedures. Local anesthetics are also used in spinal anesthesia and to produce autonomic blockade in ischemic conditions. Slow epidural infusion at low concentrations has been used successfully for postoperative analgesia (in the same way as epidural opioid infusion). Repeated epidural injection in anesthetic doses may lead to tachyphylaxis, however.

F. **Interactions:** High concentrations of extracellular K^+ may enhance local anesthetic activity, while elevated extracellular Ca^{2+} may antagonize it.

G. **Toxicity:**
   1. **CNS effects:** The most important toxic effects of most local anesthetics are in the CNS. All local anesthetics are capable of producing a spectrum of central effects, including lightheadedness or sedation, restlessness, nystagmus, and tonic-clonic convulsions. Severe convulsions may be followed by coma with respiratory and cardiovascular depression.
   2. **Cardiovascular effects:** With the exception of cocaine, all local anesthetics are vasodilators. Patients with preexisting cardiovascular disease may develop heart block and other disturbances of cardiac electrical function at high plasma levels of local anesthetics. Bupi-

Table 25–1. Relative size and susceptibility to block of types of nerve fibers.[1]

Fiber Type	Function	Diameter (μm)	Myelination	Conduction Velocity (m/s)	Sensitivity to Block
Type A Alpha	Proprioception, motor	12–20	Heavy	70–120	+
Beta	Touch, pressure	5–12	Heavy	30–70	++
Gamma	Muscle spindles	3–6	Heavy	15–30	++
Delta	Pain, temperature	2–5	Heavy	12–30	+++
Type B	Preganglionic autonomic	<3	Light	3–15	++++
Type C Dorsal root	Pain	0.4–1.2	None	0.5–2.3	++++
Sympathetic	Postganglionic	0.3–1.3	None	0.7–2.3	++++

[1] Reproduced, with permission, from Katzung BG [editor]: *Basic & Clinical Pharmacology,* 6th ed. Appleton & Lange, 1995.

vacaine may produce severe cardiovascular toxicity, including arrhythmias and hypotension, if given intravenously. The ability of cocaine to block norepinephrine reuptake at sympathetic neuroeffector junctions and the drug's vasoconstricting actions contribute to cardiovascular toxicity. When used as a drug of abuse, cocaine's cardiovascular toxicity includes severe hypertension with cerebral hemorrhage, cardiac arrhythmias, and myocardial infarction.

3. **Other toxic effects:**   Prilocaine is metabolized to products that include an agent capable of causing methemoglobinemia. The ester-type local anesthetics are metabolized to products that can cause antibody formation in some patients. Allergic responses to local anesthetics are rare and can usually be avoided by using an agent from the amide subclass. In high concentrations, local anesthetics may cause a local neurotoxic action that includes histologic damage and permanent impairment of function.

4. **Treatment of toxicity:**   Severe toxicity is best treated symptomatically. Convulsions are often treated with intravenous diazepam or a short-acting barbiturate such as thiopental. Hyperventilation with oxygen is helpful. Occasionally, a neuromuscular blocking drug may be used to control violent convulsive activity. The cardiovascular toxicity of bupivacaine overdose is difficult to treat and has caused fatalities in healthy young adults.

DRUG LIST

The following drugs are important members of the group discussed in this chapter. Prototypes should be learned in detail; features of the major variants should be known well enough to distinguish the variants from prototypes and from each other; the other significant agents should be recognized as belonging to a specific subclass.

Subclass	Prototype	Major Variants	Other Significant Agents
Esters	Procaine	Cocaine, tetracaine	Benzocaine
Amides	Lidocaine	Bupivacaine	Etidocaine, prilocaine

QUESTIONS

DIRECTIONS: Each of the numbered items or incomplete statements in this section is followed by answers or by completions of the sentence. Select the ONE lettered answer or completion that is BEST in each case.

1. Properties of local anesthetics include all of the following EXCEPT
   (A) Blockade of voltage-dependent sodium channels
   (B) Preferential binding to resting channels
   (C) Slowing of axonal impulse conduction
   (D) An increase in membrane refractory period
   (E) All of the above choices are valid properties of local anesthetics

2. The pK_a of lidocaine is 7.9. In infected tissue at pH 6.9, the fraction in the ionized form will be
   (A) 1%
   (B) 10%
   (C) 50%
   (D) 90%
   (E) 99%

3. All of the following statements about nerve blockade with local anesthetics are accurate EXCEPT
   (A) Speed of onset may be reduced when injected into infected tissues
   (B) Block is faster in onset with smaller diameter fibers
   (C) Activity is use-dependent
   (D) Smaller diameter fibers recover faster
   (E) Fibers in the periphery of a nerve bundle are blocked sooner than fibers in the center of a bundle

4. The most important effect of inadvertent IV administration of a large dose of an amide local anesthetic is
   (A) Hepatic damage
   (B) Renal failure
   (C) Seizures
   (D) Gangrene
   (E) Bronchoconstriction

5. Factors that influence the action of local anesthetics include all of the following EXCEPT
   (A) Blood flow through the tissue in which the injection is made
   (B) Activity of acetylcholinesterase in the area
   (C) Use of vasoconstrictors
   (D) Amount of local anesthetic injected
   (E) Tissue pH

6. You have a vial containing 4 mL of a 2% solution of lidocaine. How much lidocaine is present in 1 mL?
   (A) 2 mg
   (B) 8 mg
   (C) 20 mg
   (D) 80 mg
   (E) 200 mg

7. All of the following statements about the toxicity of local anesthetics are accurate EXCEPT
   (A) Serious cardiovascular reactions are more likely to occur with tetracaine than with bupivacaine
   (B) Cyanosis may occur following injection of large doses of prilocaine, especially in patients with pulmonary disease
   (C) Intravenous injection of local anesthetics may depress cardiac pacemaker activity
   (D) In overdosage, hyperventilation (with oxygen) is helpful to correct acidosis and lower extracellular potassium
   (E) Most local anesthetics cause vasodilation

8. Epinephrine added to a solution of lidocaine for a peripheral nerve block will
   (A) Increase the risk of convulsions
   (B) Increase the duration of anesthetic action of the local anesthetic
   (C) Both (A) and (B)
   (D) Neither (A) nor (B)

DIRECTIONS: The following section consists of a list of four to twenty-six lettered options followed by several numbered items. For each numbered item, select the ONE option that is most closely associated with it. Each answer may be selected once, more than once, or not at all.
   (A) Benzocaine
   (B) Bupivacaine
   (C) Cocaine
   (D) Lidocaine
   (E) Procaine

9. This drug is an ester and has high surface activity. The drug's vasoconstrictor actions may be useful clinically

10. This drug has a slow onset and the longest duration of action of any local anesthetic. Its cardiac actions occur at normal heart rates

11. This drug is poorly soluble in aqueous fluids, remains at the site of its application, and is not absorbed into the systemic circulation. It has good surface activity and low toxic potential

12. This drug has very poor surface activity, a short duration, and an ester structure

ANSWERS

1. Local anesthetics bind preferentially to sodium channels in the open and inactivated states. Recovery from drug-induced block is 10–1000 times slower than recovery of channels from normal inactivation. Resting channels have a lower affinity for local anesthetics. The answer is (B).

2. Since the drug is a weak base, it will be more ionized (protonated) at pH values lower than its pK_a. Since the pH given is 1 log unit lower (more acid) than the pK_a, the ratio of ionized to nonionized drug will be approximately 90:10. The answer is **(D)**. (Recall from Chapter 1 that at a pH equal to pK_a, the ratio is 1:1; at 1 log unit difference, the ratio is [approximately] 90:10; at 2 units difference, 99:1; etc.)

3. Smaller diameter nerve fibers are more sensitive to local anesthetics and are blocked more rapidly than those of larger size. As the local concentration of drug declines during recovery from local anesthesia, smaller fibers continue to be blocked and are the last to recover. The answer is **(D)**.

4. Of the effects listed, the most important in local anesthetic overdose (of both amide and ester types) concern the CNS. Such effects can include sedation or restlessness, nystagmus, convulsions, coma, and respiratory depression. Diazepam is used for seizures caused by local anesthetics, usually without significant effects on ventilation or circulation. The answer is **(C)**.

5. The ester group of ester-type local anesthetics is hydrolyzed by plasma (and tissue) pseudocholinesterases. These drugs are poor substrates for acetylcholinesterase; the activity of this enzyme does not play a part in terminating the actions of local anesthetics. Individuals with genetically based defects in pseudocholinesterase activity are unusually sensitive to procaine and other esters. The answer is **(B)**.

6. The fact that you have 4 mL of the solution of lidocaine is irrelevant. A 2% solution of any drug contains 2 g per 100 mL. The amount of lidocaine in 1 mL of a 2% solution is 0.02 grams, or 20 mg. The answer is **(C)**. (Note: a 20 milligram-% solution contains 20 milligrams per 100 mL.)

7. Bupivacaine has the highest toxicity of the local anesthetics (other than cocaine, when used in drug abuse). The answer is **(A)**.

8. Epinephrine will increase the duration of a nerve block when it is administered with short- and medium-duration local anesthetics. As a result of the vasoconstriction that prolongs the duration of this block, less local anesthetic is required, so the risk of toxicity, eg, a convulsion, is reduced. The answer is **(B)**.

9. Cocaine is the only local anesthetic with intrinsic vasoconstrictor activity. It also has significant surface activity and is favored for head, neck, and pharyngeal surgery. Cocaine is an ester. The answer is **(C)**.

10. You should be able to identify this drug as bupivacaine from its long duration of action. Unlike lidocaine, the actions of bupivacaine on cardiac cells occur at normal heart rates. Accidental intravenous administration of bupivacaine may lead to arrhythmias and cardiovascular collapse. The answer is **(B)**.

11. Benzocaine is an ester that is used for topical anesthesia. Because of its low toxic potential, it has been used for anesthesia of large surface areas, including those within the oral cavity. The answer is **(A)**.

12. Procaine is an ester with short duration of action and negligible surface activity. The answer is **(E)**.

26   Skeletal Muscle Relaxants

OBJECTIVES

You should be able to:

- Describe the transmission process at the neuromuscular endplate and the points at which drugs can modify this process.
- List three nondepolarizing neuromuscular blockers and one depolarizing neuromuscular blocker; compare their pharmacokinetics.

- Describe the differences between depolarizing and nondepolarizing blockers from the standpoint of tetanic and posttetanic twitch strength.
- Describe the method of reversal of nondepolarizing blockade.
- List the major drugs used in the treatment of acute and chronic skeletal muscle spasticity and describe their mechanisms.

Learn the definitions that follow.

Table 26–1. Definitions.

Term	Definitions
Depolarizing blockade	Neuromuscular paralysis that results from persistent depolarization of the endplate, eg, by succinylcholine
Desensitization	A phase of blockade by a depolarizing blocker during which the endplate repolarizes but is less than normally responsive to agonists (acetylcholine or succinylcholine)
Malignant hyperthermia	Hyperthermia that results from massive release of calcium from the sarcoplasmic reticulum, leading to uncontrolled contraction and stimulation of metabolism in skeletal muscle
Nondepolarizing blockade	Neuromuscular paralysis that results from pharmacologic antagonism at the acetylcholine receptor of the endplate, eg, by tubocurarine
Spasmolytic	A drug that reduces abnormally elevated muscle tone (spasm) without paralysis, eg, baclofen, dantrolene
Stabilizing blockade	Synonym for nondepolarizing blockade

CONCEPTS

The drugs in this chapter are divided into two dissimilar groups (Figure 26–1). The **neuromuscular blocking drugs** are used to produce muscle paralysis, in order to facilitate surgery or artificial ventilation. The **spasmolytic drugs** are used to reduce abnormally elevated tone caused by neurologic or muscle disease.

NEUROMUSCULAR BLOCKING DRUGS

A. Classification & Prototypes: Skeletal muscle contraction is evoked by a nicotinic cholinergic transmission process. It is therefore subject to the same types of pharmacologic modification as autonomic ganglionic transmission. Blockade of transmission at the endplate (the postsynaptic structure bearing the nicotinic receptors) is clinically useful in producing relaxation of muscle, a requirement for surgery. The neuromuscular blockers are structurally related to acetylcholine and are either antagonists (nondepolarizing type) or agonists (depolarizing type) at the nicotinic endplate receptor. The prototype nondepolarizing agent is tubocurarine; the prototype depolarizing drug is succinylcholine.

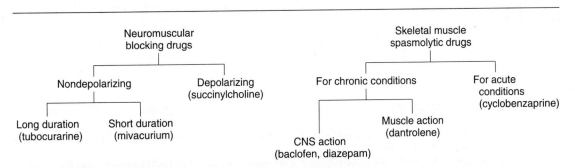

Figure 26–1. Subgroups and prototype drugs in the neuromuscular and spasmolytic drug groups.

Table 26–2. Pharmacokinetic characteristics of neuromuscular blocking drugs.

Drug	Duration of Maximum Effect	Route or Mechanism of Elimination
Nondepolarizing Atracurium	20–30 min	Spontaneous breakdown in plasma
Doxacurium	>35 min	Kidney, excreted in urine
Mivacurium	10–20 min	Hydrolysis by plasma cholinesterase
Pancuronium	60 min	Kidney, excreted in urine
Tubocurarine	60 min	Kidney, excreted in urine
Vecuronium	30 min	Liver, excreted in bile
Depolarizing Succinylcholine	5–10 min	Hydrolysis by plasma cholinesterase

B. Nondepolarizing Neuromuscular Blocking Drugs:

1. **Pharmacokinetics:** Most nondepolarizing agents have relatively long half-lives, ranging from 20 minutes to several hours. These drugs are given parenterally. Tubocurarine, pancuronium, and doxacurium depend on the kidney for elimination, and their actions are prolonged in patients with impaired renal function. See Table 26–2.

2. **Mechanism of action:** These drugs act as surmountable blockers, ie, the blockade can be overcome by increasing the amount of agonist (acetylcholine) in the synaptic cleft. Thus the drugs in this group behave as though they compete with acetylcholine at the receptor, and their effect is reversed by cholinesterase inhibitors. There is evidence, however, that some of them may also act directly to plug the ion channel operated by the acetylcholine receptor. Posttetanic potentiation is preserved in the presence of these agents, but tension during the tetanus fades rapidly. See Table 26–3 for additional details.

C. Depolarizing Neuromuscular Blocking Drugs:

1. **Pharmacokinetics:** Succinylcholine is composed of two acetylcholine molecules linked end to end. Succinylcholine is metabolized by plasma cholinesterase (butyrylcholinesterase or pseudocholinesterase) and has a duration of action of only a few minutes if given as a single dose. It is given by continuous infusion if prolonged paralysis is required. (More often paralysis is initiated with succinylcholine and then continued with a nondepolarizing agent.) Succinylcholine is not rapidly hydrolyzed by acetylcholinesterase.

2. **Mechanism of action:** Depolarizing blockers act like nicotinic agonists and depolarize the neuromuscular endplate. The initial depolarization is often accompanied by twitching and fasciculations. Because tension cannot be maintained in skeletal muscle without periodic repolarization and depolarization of the endplate, continuous depolarization results in

Table 26–3. Comparison of a typical nondepolarizing neuromuscular blocker (tubocurarine) and a depolarizing blocker (succinylcholine).[1]

	Tubocurarine	Succinylcholine Phase I	Succinylcholine Phase II
Administration of tubocurarine	Additive	Antagonistic	Augmented[2]
Administration of succinylcholine	Antagonistic	Additive	Augmented[2]
Effect of neostigmine	Antagonistic	Augmentation[2]	Antagonistic
Initial excitatory effect on skeletal muscle	None	Fasciculations	None
Response to tetanic stimulus	Unsustained ("fade")	Sustained[3]	Unsustained
Posttetanic facilitation	Yes	No	Yes

[1] Reproduced, with permission, from Katzung BG [editor]: *Basic & Clinical Pharmacology*, 6th ed. Appleton & Lange, 1995.
[2] It is not known whether this interaction is additive or synergistic (superadditive).
[3] The amplitude is decreased, but the response is sustained.

Table 26–4. Autonomic effects of neuromuscular blocking drugs.[1]

Drug	Effect on Autonomic Ganglia	Effect on Cardiac Muscarinic Receptors	Ability to Release Histamine
Nondepolarizing Atracurium	None	None	Slight
Mivacurium	None	None	Slight
Pancuronium	None	Blocks moderately	None
Tubocurarine	Blocks	None	Moderate
Vecuronium, pipecuronium, rocuronium	None	None	None
Depolarizing Succinylcholine	Stimulates	Stimulates	Slight

[1] Modified and reproduced, with permission, from Katzung BG [editor]: *Basic & Clinical Pharmacology,* 6th ed. Appleton & Lange, 1995.

muscle relaxation and paralysis. As with the nondepolarizing blockers, some evidence suggests that these drugs can also plug the endplate channel.

When given over a period of time, succinylcholine's effect changes from continuous depolarization (Phase I) to gradual repolarization with resistance to depolarization (Phase II), ie, a curare-like blockade.

D. Reversal of Blockade: The action of nondepolarizing blockers is readily reversed by increasing the concentration of normal transmitter at the receptors. This is best accomplished by administration of cholinesterase inhibitors such as neostigmine or edrophonium. In contrast, the paralysis produced by depolarizing blockers is facilitated by cholinesterase inhibitors during phase I. During phase II, the block produced by succinylcholine is reversed by cholinesterase inhibitors.

E. Toxicity:
  1. **Respiratory paralysis:** The action of full doses of neuromuscular blockers leads directly to respiratory paralysis. If mechanical ventilation is not provided, the patient will asphyxiate.
  2. **Autonomic effects and histamine release:** Some of these agents have autonomic effects or cause release of histamine, either of which can result in cardiovascular disturbances. These actions are summarized in Table 26–4.
  3. **Interactions:** Inhaled anesthetics, especially isoflurane, strongly potentiate and prolong neuromuscular blockade. Aminoglycoside antibiotics and antiarrhythmic drugs potentiate and prolong the relaxant action of neuromuscular blockers to a lesser degree.

SPASMOLYTIC DRUGS

Certain chronic diseases of the CNS (eg, cerebral palsy, multiple sclerosis, stroke) are associated with abnormally high reflex activity in the neuronal pathways that control skeletal muscle; the result is painful spasm. (Bladder and anal sphincter control are also affected in most cases and may require autonomic drugs for management.)

In other circumstances, acute injury or inflammation of muscle leads to spasm and pain. Such temporary spasm can sometimes be reduced with appropriate drug therapy.

The goal of spasmolytic therapy in both chronic and acute conditions is reduction of excessive skeletal muscle tone without reduction of strength. It is thought that reduced spasm results in reduction of pain and improved mobility.

A. Drugs for Chronic Spasm:
  1. **Classification and prototypes:** The spasmolytic drugs do not resemble acetylcholine in structure or effect. They act in the CNS or in the skeletal muscle cell rather than at the neuromuscular endplate. Three drugs are used in the treatment of the chronic conditions men-

tioned above: **diazepam,** a benzodiazepine (see Chapter 21); **baclofen,** a GABA agonist; and **dantrolene,** an agent that acts on the sarcoplasmic reticulum of skeletal muscle. All three agents are usually used by the oral route. Recent clinical studies suggest that refractory cases may respond to chronic intrathecal administration of baclofen.

2. **Mechanism of action:** The three spasmolytic drugs act by three different mechanisms. Two act in the spinal cord: diazepam facilitates GABA-mediated presynaptic inhibition, and baclofen acts as a $GABA_B$ agonist. Both reduce the tonic output of the primary spinal motoneurons.

Dantrolene acts in the skeletal muscle cell to reduce the release of activator calcium from the sarcoplasmic reticulum. Dantrolene is also effective in the treatment of malignant hyperthermia, a genetically determined disorder characterized by massive calcium release from the sarcoplasmic reticulum of skeletal muscle. Malignant hyperthermia is most often triggered by general anesthesia or neuromuscular blocking drugs. In this emergency condition dantrolene is given intravenously.

3. **Toxicity:** The sedation produced by diazepam is significant but milder than that produced by other sedative-hypnotic drugs at doses that induce equivalent muscle relaxation. Baclofen produces less sedation than diazepam. Dantrolene causes significant muscle weakness but less sedation than either diazepam or baclofen.

B. **Drugs Used for Acute Muscle Spasm:** Many drugs are promoted for the treatment of acute spasm due to muscle injury. Most of these drugs are sedatives or act in the brain stem or spinal cord. **Cyclobenzaprine,** a typical member of this group, is believed to act in the brain stem, possibly by interfering with polysynaptic reflexes that maintain skeletal muscle tone. The drug is active by the oral route and has very significant sedative and antimuscarinic actions. Cyclobenzaprine may cause confusion and visual hallucinations in some patients.

DRUG LIST

The following drugs are important members of the group discussed in this chapter. Prototypes should be learned in detail; features of the major variants should be known well enough to distinguish the variants from prototypes and from each other; the other significant agents should be recognized as belonging to a specific subclass.

Subclass	Prototype	Major Variants	Other Significant Agents
Nondepolarizing neuromuscular blockers			
Renal elimination, long duration	Tubocurarine		Pancuronium
Hepatic elimination, intermediate duration	Vecuronium		Rocuronium
Spontaneous or plasma ChE,[1] intermediate-short duration	Atracurium		Mivacurium
Depolarizing blockers	Succinylcholine		
Spasmolytic drugs	Diazepam, baclofen, dantrolene	Cyclobenzaprine	

[1] ChE: cholinesterase. (Atracurium breaks down spontaneously; mivacurium is metabolized by plasma ChE.)

QUESTIONS

DIRECTIONS: Each of the numbered items or incomplete statements in this section is followed by answers or by completions of the sentence. Select the ONE lettered answer or completion that is BEST in each case.

1. Edrophonium would facilitate the initial relaxant effect of
   (A) Tubocurarine
   (B) Pancuronium
   (C) Atracurium
   (D) Succinylcholine
   (E) Vecuronium

2. Which of the following is most often associated with hypotension caused by histamine release?
   (A) Tubocurarine
   (B) Pancuronium
   (C) Atracurium
   (D) Succinylcholine
   (E) Vecuronium

3. Characteristics of phase I depolarizing neuromuscular blockade include which of the following?
   (A) Well-sustained tension during a period of tetanic stimulation
   (B) Marked muscarinic blockade
   (C) Muscle fasciculations in the later stages of block
   (D) Reversible by pyridostigmine
   (E) Easy reversibility with pharmacologic antagonists

4. Characteristics of nondepolarizing neuromuscular blockade include which of the following?
   (A) Stimulation of autonomic ganglia
   (B) Poorly sustained tetanic tension
   (C) Block of posttetanic potentiation
   (D) Significant muscle fasciculations during onset of block
   (E) Histamine blocking action

5. Which of the following will NOT cause skeletal muscle contractions or twitching?
   (A) Nicotine
   (B) Vecuronium
   (C) Succinylcholine
   (D) Acetylcholine
   (E) Strychnine

6. Which of the following has a duration of action shorter than 10 minutes when given as a single injection?
   (A) Atracurium
   (B) Vecuronium
   (C) Pancuronium
   (D) Succinylcholine
   (E) Tubocurarine

7. Succinylcholine is associated with
   (A) Histamine release in a genetically determined population
   (B) Metabolism at the neuromuscular junction by acetylcholinesterase
   (C) Antagonism by neostigmine during the early phase of blockade
   (D) Elevated serum enzymes indicative of muscle damage, eg, CPK
   (E) Blockade of autonomic ganglia

DIRECTIONS: The following section consists of a list of four to twenty-six lettered options followed by several numbered items. For each numbered item, select the ONE option that is most closely associated with it. Each answer may be selected once, more than once, or not at all.
   (A) Atracurium
   (B) Baclofen
   (C) Cyclobenzaprine
   (D) Dantrolene
   (E) Diazepam
   (F) Isoflurane
   (G) Mivacurium
   (H) Pancuronium
   (I) Succinylcholine
   (J) Tubocurarine
   (K) Vecuronium

8. Prevents release of calcium from the sarcoplasmic reticulum
9. Depolarizes the neuromuscular endplate
10. GABA analogue (agonist at GABA$_B$ receptors) that reduces motor neuron outflow
11. Spasmolytic that is also useful in treatment of convulsions caused by local anesthetics
12. Breaks down spontaneously in plasma; no enzyme required
13. Initially potentiated by neostigmine; reversed by neostigmine in a later phase of its action
14. Nondepolarizing neuromuscular blocker that is hydrolyzed by plasma cholinesterase
15. A spasmolytic with strong sedative and muscarinic blocking properties
16. A volatile liquid that, when inhaled, potentiates nondepolarizing neuromuscular blockers

ANSWERS

1. Only depolarizing neuromuscular blockers are facilitated by edrophonium, a cholinesterase inhibitor. The answer is **(D)**.
2. The answer is **(A)**, tubocurarine.
3. Phase I depolarizing blockade is not associated with muscarinic blockade; nor is it reversible with cholinesterase inhibitors. Muscle fasciculations occur at the start of the action of succinylcholine. The answer is **(A)**.
4. Nondepolarizing blockers result in poorly sustained tetanic tension. They do not cause ganglionic stimulation or fasciculations at any time during their action (Table 26–3). The answer is **(B)**.
5. Nicotine, succinylcholine, and acetylcholine cause endplate depolarization and skeletal muscle contractions (they are nicotinic receptor agonists). Strychnine causes skeletal muscle contractions (convulsions) by blocking glycine receptors in the spinal cord. Vecuronium, a nondepolarizing blocker, does not cause contraction at any dose. The answer is **(B)**.
6. Of this list, only succinylcholine has a duration of action shorter than 10 minutes. The answer is **(D)**.
7. Succinylcholine use is associated with a rise in serum enzyme levels when muscle twitching and fasciculations are significant. The answer is **(D)**.
8. Dantrolene is the only commonly used spasmolytic that acts inside the skeletal muscle cell. The drug interferes with calcium release. The answer is **(D)**.
9. Succinylcholine is the only nicotinic agonist in the answer list. The answer is **(I)**.
10. Baclofen is a GABA$_B$ agonist. The answer is **(B)**.
11. Diazepam is useful in treating convulsions and in reducing spasm of skeletal muscle. The answer is **(E)**.
12. Atracurium breaks down spontaneously in the plasma ("Hofmann elimination"). The answer is **(A)**.
13. Only depolarizing blocking drugs are potentiated by cholinesterase inhibitors (phase I type blockade). After converting to phase II, the block may be reversed by cholinesterase inhibitors. The answer is **(I)**.
14. Mivacurium is the only nondepolarizing neuromuscular blocking drug that is eliminated by plasma cholinesterase. The answer is **(G)**.
15. Diazepam is a strong sedative, but it is not an antimuscarinic. Cyclobenzaprine has both sedative and antimuscarinic effects. The answer is **(C)**.
16. Isoflurane, a liquid that is volatilized for inhalation, strongly potentiates most nondepolarizing blocking drugs. The answer is **(F)**.

Drugs Used in Parkinsonism & Other Movement Disorders

27

OBJECTIVES

You should be able to:

- Describe the mechanisms by which levodopa, bromocriptine, amantadine, and muscarinic blocking drugs alleviate parkinsonism.
- Describe the therapeutic and toxic effects of the antiparkinsonism agents.
- List the chemical agents and drugs that cause parkinsonism symptoms.
- Identify the drugs used in management of tremor, Huntington's disease, drug-induced dyskinesias, and Wilson's disease.

CONCEPTS

Movement disorders constitute a number of heterogenous neurologic conditions with very different therapies (Figure 27–1).

PARKINSONISM

A. Pathophysiology: Parkinsonism is a common neurologic movement disorder that involves dysfunction in the basal ganglia and associated brain structures. Signs (mnemonic *raft*) include rigidity of skeletal muscles, akinesia, flat facies, and tremor at rest.

    1. Naturally occurring parkinsonism: The naturally occurring disease is of uncertain etiology and occurs with increasing frequency during aging from the fifth or sixth decade of life onward. Pathologic characteristics include a decrease in the levels of striatal dopamine and the degeneration of dopaminergic neurons in the nigrostriatal tract that normally *inhibit* the activity of striatal GABAergic neurons (Figure 27–2). Most of the postsynaptic dopamine receptors on GABAergic neurons are of the D_2 subclass (negatively coupled to adenylyl cyclase). The reduction of normal dopaminergic neurotransmission leads to excessive *excitatory* actions of cholinergic neurons on striatal GABAergic neurons; thus,

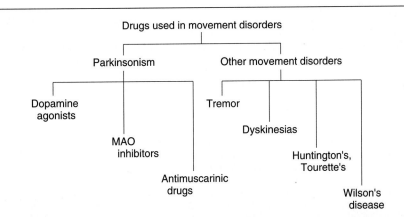

Figure 27–1. Some of the movement disorders and subgroups of drugs discussed in this chapter.

dopamine and acetylcholine activities are out of balance in parkinsonism. Huntington's chorea results from degeneration of many striatal GABAergic neurons and the loss of some cholinergic cells (Figure 27–2).

2. **Drug-induced parkinsonism:** Many drugs can *cause* parkinsonian symptoms; these effects are usually reversible. The most important of these drugs are the butyrophenone and phenothiazine **antipsychotic drugs,** which block brain dopamine receptors. At high doses, **reserpine** causes similar symptoms, presumably via the depletion of brain dopamine. MPTP (1-methyl-4-phenyl-1,2,3,6-tetrahydropyridine), a by-product of the attempted synthesis of an illicit meperidine analogue, causes irreversible parkinsonism through destruction of dopaminergic neurons in the nigrostriatal tract. Treatment with inhibitors of monoamine oxidase (MAO) type B protects against MPTP neurotoxicity in animals.

3. **Strategies:** Drug *treatment* of parkinsonism involves increasing dopamine activity in the brain or decreasing muscarinic cholinergic activity in the brain (or both).

B. **Levodopa:**
1. **Mechanisms:** Because dopamine has low bioavailability and does not readily cross the blood-brain barrier, its precursor, L-dopa (levodopa), is used. This amino acid is converted to dopamine by the enzyme aromatic L-amino acid decarboxylase (DOPA decarboxylase) which is present in many body tissues, including the brain. Levodopa is usually given with carbidopa, a drug that does not cross the blood-brain barrier but inhibits DOPA decarboxylase in peripheral tissues. With this combination, lower doses of levodopa are effective, and there are fewer peripheral side effects.

2. **Pharmacologic effects:** Levodopa ameliorates many parkinsonism signs, particularly bradykinesia; moreover, the mortality rate is decreased. However, the drug does not cure parkinsonism, and responsiveness decreases with time, which may reflect progression of the disease. Clinical response to the drug may fluctuate quite rapidly, changing from akinesia to dyskinesia over a few hours. These so-called **on-off phenomena** may be related partly to changes in levodopa levels in plasma. "Drug holidays," periods of a few weeks during which the drug is not taken, are sometimes used to reduce response fluctuations and toxic effects.

3. **Toxicity:** Most adverse effects are dose-dependent.
   a. **Gastrointestinal effects:** These effects include anorexia, nausea, and emesis. They can be reduced by taking the drug in divided doses. Tolerance to the emetic action of levodopa usually occurs after several months.
   b. **Cardiovascular effects:** Postural hypotension is common, especially in the early stage of treatment. Other cardiac effects include tachycardia, asystole, and cardiac arrhythmias (rare).

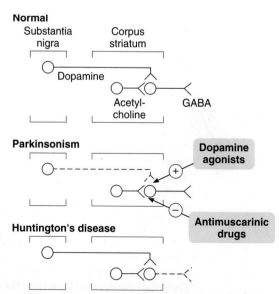

Figure 27–2. Schematic representation of the sequence of neurons involved in parkinsonism and Huntington's chorea. *Top:* Neurons in the normal brain. *Middle:* Neurons in parkinsonism. The dopaminergic neuron is lost. *Bottom:* Neurons in Huntington's disease. The GABAergic neuron is lost. (Reproduced, with permission, from Katzung BG [editor]: *Basic & Clinical Pharmacology,* 6th ed. Appleton & Lange, 1995.)

   c. **Dyskinesias:**   Choreoathetosis of the face and distal extremities occurs frequently. Individual patients may exhibit chorea, ballismus, myoclonus, tics, and tremor.
   d. **Behavioral effects:**   These can include anxiety, agitation, confusion, delusions, hallucinations, and depression.

C.   Bromocriptine:
   1. **Mechanism of action:**   Bromocriptine is an ergot alkaloid that acts as a partial agonist at certain dopamine receptors in the brain; the drug increases the functional activity of dopamine neurotransmitter pathways, including those involved in extrapyramidal functions. A similar dopamine agonist, **pergolide** is active at both D_1 and D_2 receptors. Recently approved for use in parkinsonism, pergolide may decrease response fluctuations and prolong the effectiveness of levodopa. Pergolide loses its efficacy with time.
   2. **Clinical use:**   Bromocriptine or pergolide may be used in conjunction with levodopa (and with anticholinergic drugs), and in patients who are refractory to or cannot tolerate levodopa.
   3. **Toxicity:**   **Gastrointestinal effects** include anorexia, nausea, and vomiting. **Cardiovascular effects** commonly include postural hypotension; cardiac arrhythmias may also occur. **Dyskinesias** may occur with abnormal movements similar to those caused by levodopa. **Behavioral effects** include confusion, hallucinations, and delusions; these occur more commonly than with levodopa. Like levodopa, bromocriptine and pergolide are contraindicated in patients with a history of psychosis. **Miscellaneous effects** include pulmonary infiltrates and erythromelalgia.

D.   Amantadine:
   1. **Mechanism of action:**   Amantadine enhances dopaminergic neurotransmission by mechanisms that may involve increasing synthesis or release of dopamine, or inhibition of reuptake of dopamine.
   2. **Pharmacologic effects:**   Amantadine may improve bradykinesia, rigidity, and tremor but is usually effective for only a few weeks. Amantadine also has antiviral effects.
   3. **Toxicity:**   **Behavioral effects** include restlessness, agitation, insomnia, confusion, hallucinations, and acute toxic psychosis. **Dermatologic reactions** include livedo reticularis. **Miscellaneous effects** may include gastrointestinal disturbances, urinary retention, and postural hypotension. Amantadine also causes peripheral edema that responds to diuretics.

E.   Selegiline (Deprenyl):   This drug is a selective inhibitor of MAO type B, the enzyme form that metabolizes dopamine in preference to norepinephrine and serotonin. Selegiline may increase brain dopamine levels. It is used as an adjunct to levodopa in parkinsonism.

F.   Acetylcholine-Blocking (Antimuscarinic) Drugs: Antimuscarinic drugs may improve the tremor and rigidity of parkinsonism but have little effect on bradykinesia. The available antimuscarinic agents differ in potency and in efficacy in different patients. CNS toxic effects include drowsiness, inattention, confusion, delusions, and hallucinations. Peripheral adverse effects are typical of atropine-like drugs.

DRUG THERAPY OF OTHER MOVEMENT DISORDERS

A.   Tremor: Physiologic and essential tremor are clinically similar conditions characterized by postural tremor. They may be alleviated by beta-blocking drugs such as **propranolol.** Beta-blockers should be used with caution in patients with congestive heart failure, asthma, diabetes, or hypoglycemia.

B.   Huntington's Disease and Gilles de la Tourette's Syndrome: Huntington's disease, an inherited disorder, results from a brain neurotransmitter imbalance such that GABA functions are diminished and dopaminergic functions are enhanced (Figure 27–2). There may also be a cholinergic deficit, since choline acetyltransferase is decreased in the basal ganglia of patients with this disease. Drug therapy involves the use of amine-depleting drugs (eg, **tetrabenazine**) or antipsychotic agents (eg, **haloperidol** or a **phenothiazine**) that block dopamine receptors.

Pharmacologic attempts to enhance brain GABA and acetylcholine activities have not been successful in patients with this disease.

Tourette syndrome is a disorder of unknown etiology that responds to haloperidol and similar dopamine D_2 receptor blockers.

C. Drug-Induced Dyskinesias: Parkinsonism symptoms caused by antipsychotic agents are usually reversible by lowering drug dosage, changing the therapy to a drug that is less toxic to extrapyramidal function, or using muscarinic blockers. Levodopa and bromocriptine are not useful because dopamine receptors are blocked by the antipsychotic drugs. **Tardive dyskinesias** that develop from neuroleptic therapy are possibly a form of denervation supersensitivity. They are not readily reversed; no specific drug therapy is available.

D. Wilson's Disease: This recessively inherited disorder of copper metabolism results in deposition of copper salts in the liver and other tissues. Hepatic and neurologic damage may be severe or fatal. Treatment involves use of the chelating agent penicillamine (dimethylcysteine), which removes excess copper. Toxic effects of penicillamine include gastrointestinal distress, myasthenia, optic neuropathy, and blood dyscrasias.

DRUG LIST

The following drugs are important members of the group discussed in this chapter. Prototypes should be learned in detail; features of the major variants should be known well enough to distinguish the variants from prototypes and from each other.

Subclass	Prototype	Major Variants
Drugs used in parkinsonism 　Dopamine pro-drug	Levodopa	
Levodopa adjunct (DOPA 　decarboxylase inhibitor)	Carbidopa	
Dopamine agonist	Bromocriptine	Pergolide
Indirect dopamine agonist	Amantadine	
MAO inhibitor	Selegiline	
Antimuscarinic	Benztropine	Biperiden, orphenadrine, trihexyphenidyl
Drugs used in tremor	Propranolol	
Drugs used in Huntington's disease, 　Tourette syndrome	Haloperidol	Phenothiazines
Drugs used in Wilson's disease	Penicillamine	

QUESTIONS

DIRECTIONS: Each of the numbered items or incomplete statements in this section is followed by answers or by completions of the sentence. Select the ONE lettered answer or completion that is BEST in each case.

1. All of the following statements concerning levodopa are accurate EXCEPT
    (A) Choreoathetosis of the face and distal extremities occurs commonly
    (B) Fluctuations in clinical response occur with increasing frequency as treatment continues
    (C) Levodopa effectively antagonizes the extrapyramidal adverse effects of antipsychotic drugs
    (D) Levodopa should be avoided in patients with a history of melanoma
    (E) Behavioral side effects occur more commonly if levodopa is taken in combination with carbidopa

2. Which of the following statements about carbidopa is accurate?
    (A) Carbidopa crosses the blood-brain barrier
    (B) Carbidopa inhibits monoamine oxidase type A
    (C) Carbidopa is converted to the false transmitter, carbidopamine
    (D) Carbidopa inhibits aromatic L-amino acid decarboxylase
    (E) Carbidopa inhibits monoamine oxidase type B

3. All of the following statements about bromocriptine are accurate EXCEPT
    (A) It should not be administered to patients taking antimuscarinic drugs
    (B) Bromocriptine may cause pulmonary infiltrates
    (C) The drug is contraindicated in patients with a history of psychosis
    (D) Bromocriptine is a direct-acting dopamine receptor agonist
    (E) Mental disturbances occur more commonly with bromocriptine than with levodopa

4. Concerning drugs and parkinsonism, all of the following statements are accurate EXCEPT
    (A) Levodopa causes mydriasis and can precipitate an attack of acute glaucoma
    (B) Useful therapeutic effects of amantadine may disappear after only a few weeks of treatment
    (C) The primary therapeutic benefit of antimuscarinic drugs in parkinsonism is their ability to relieve bradykinesia
    (D) The limited efficacy of pergolide may be due to down-regulation of dopamine receptors
    (E) The concomitant use of selegiline may increase the adverse effects of levodopa

5. A 72-year-old patient with parkinsonism presents with swollen feet. They are red, tender, and very painful. You could clear up these symptoms within a few days if you told the patient to stop taking
    (A) Levodopa
    (B) Selegiline
    (C) Bromocriptine
    (D) Benztropine
    (E) Amantadine

6. A patient with parkinsonism is being treated with levodopa. He suffers from irregular, involuntary muscle jerks that affect the proximal muscles of the limbs. All of the following statements about these symptoms are correct EXCEPT
    (A) The symptoms will usually be decreased if the dose of levodopa is reduced
    (B) Administration of other drugs that activate dopamine receptors will exacerbate dyskinesias
    (C) The symptoms are unlikely to be alleviated by continued treatment with levodopa
    (D) Dyskinesias are less likely to occur if levodopa is administered with carbidopa
    (E) Coadministration of muscarinic blockers does not prevent the occurrence of dyskinesias during treatment with levodopa

DIRECTIONS: The following section consists of a list of four to twenty-six lettered options followed by several numbered items. For each numbered item, select the ONE option that is most closely associated with it. Each answer may be selected once, more than once, or not at all.
    (A) Amantadine
    (B) Haloperidol
    (C) Levodopa
    (D) Pergolide
    (E) Benztropine
    (F) MPTP
    (G) Selegiline
    (H) Reserpine

7. Contraindicated in patients with prostatic hypertrophy or obstructive gastrointestinal disease

8. Potentiates dopaminergic function, possibly by increasing the release or blocking the reuptake of dopamine; livedo reticularis may occur during treatment

9. Recently approved for the treatment of parkinsonism, this drug directly stimulates both D_1 and D_2 dopamine receptors

10. A drug that selectively inhibits the metabolism of dopamine

11. This drug may cause a hypertensive crisis if given with an inhibitor of monoamine oxidase A, since it is a precursor of norepinephrine

12. Causes akinesia, rigidity, and tremor; in animal experiments, the prior administration of an inhibitor of MAO type B protects against these effects

ANSWERS

1. Levodopa, the mainstay of drug treatment of idiopathic parkinsonism, is not effective in antagonizing the akinesia, rigidity, and tremor caused by treatment with antipsychotic agents. The primary reason is that such drugs are potent blockers of dopamine receptors. Parkinsonian side effects of neuroleptics are reversible when the dose is decreased, and are attenuated by antimuscarinic agents. The answer is **(C).**

2. Carbidopa is an inhibitor of aromatic L-amino acid decarboxylase, the enzyme that converts levodopa to dopamine. Since it does not enter the CNS, the drug acts only on the enzyme present in peripheral tissues (eg, liver). Carbidopa's use in combination with levodopa decreases the dose requirement and reduces peripheral side effects of levodopa. The answer is **(D).**

3. The use of agents that promote dopaminergic transmission in combination with antimuscarinic drugs is common in the treatment of parkinsonism. Bromocriptine does not complicate treatment with antimuscarinic drugs or amantadine. If combined with levodopa, bromocriptine should be used at reduced doses to avoid intolerable adverse effects. Confusion, delusions, and hallucinations occur more frequently with bromocriptine than with levodopa. The answer is **(A).**

4. The drug most effective in relieving the bradykinesia of parkinsonism, and the disabilities arising from it, is levodopa. Antimuscarinic drugs may improve the tremor and rigidity of parkinsonism, but have little effect on bradykinesia. The answer is **(C).**

5. The symptoms described are those associated with erythromelalgia, an adverse effect of bromocriptine. The distal extremities (feet and hands) are usually involved. Arthralgia may occur along with the signs described. The answer is **(C).**

6. The form and severity of dyskinesias due to levodopa may vary widely in different patients. Dyskinesias occur in up to 80% of patients receiving levodopa for long periods. With continued treatment, dyskinesias may develop at a dose of levodopa that was previously well tolerated. They occur more commonly in patients treated with levodopa in combination with carbidopa. Carbidopa reduces the incidence of peripheral adverse effects of levodopa but often enhances the drug's CNS toxicity. The answer is **(D).**

7. Benztropine may cause urinary retention and gastrointestinal effects and should be used with caution in patients with prostatic hypertrophy or obstructive gastrointestinal disease and in those with angle-closure glaucoma. The contraindications listed are typical for drugs that block acetylcholine at muscarinic receptors. The answer is **(E).**

8. The antiviral agent, amantadine, has antiparkinsonism activity, possibly by promoting dopaminergic neurotransmission. The benefits of the drug are usually short-lived, disappearing after only a few weeks of treatment. Its adverse effects include CNS excitation, peripheral edema, and dermatologic reactions. The answer is **(A).**

9. Pergolide is approved for use in the treatment of parkinsonism. It is a dopamine receptor agonist similar to bromocriptine in its actions. The drug loses its efficacy with time, perhaps because of down-regulation of dopamine receptors. The answer is **(D).**

10. Selegiline inhibits monoamine oxidase type B, the enzyme that metabolizes dopamine. The drug appears to be useful as an adjunct to levodopa in parkinsonism. Because selegiline is selective for the MAO-B isoform, adverse reactions with tyramine (which is metabolized by monoamine oxidase type A) are uncommon. (Unselective MAO inhibitors, such as those used in depression [Chapter 29], are subject to dangerous interactions with tyramine.) The answer is **(G).**

11. The only catecholamine precursor listed is levodopa. Remember that levodopa is a precursor of norepinephrine and epinephrine as well as dopamine, and that norepinephrine and epinephrine are metabolized primarily by monoamine oxidase type A. The answer is **(C).**

12. MPTP causes parkinsonlike extrapyramidal dysfunction by destroying dopaminergic neurons in the nigrostriatal tract. This neurotoxic action requires the formation of toxic metabolites from the metabolism of MPTP by monoamine oxidase type B. MPTP is used as an experimental tool in animal models of parkinsonism. Antipsychotic drugs (eg, haloperidol) and reserpine also cause parkinson-like adverse effects, but these are not prevented by the administration of inhibitors of MAO type B. The answer is **(F).**

Antipsychotic Drugs & Lithium   28

OBJECTIVES

You should be able to:

- Describe the dopamine hypothesis of schizophrenia.
- List the major receptors blocked by antipsychotic drugs.
- Describe the pharmacodynamics of antipsychotic drugs in normal and schizophrenic individuals and relate these pharmacodynamics to their clinical uses.
- List the adverse effects of the major antipsychotic drugs.
- Describe the pharmacokinetics and pharmacodynamics of lithium.

CONCEPTS

ANTIPSYCHOTIC DRUGS

The antipsychotic drugs (**neuroleptics**) are effective in controlling many of the manifestations of psychotic illness. Though not cured by drug therapy, the symptoms of schizophrenia (thought disorder, emotional withdrawal, and hallucinations or delusions) may be markedly reduced by antipsychotic drugs. Unfortunately, prolonged therapy (years) is often needed and can result in severe toxicity in some patients.

A. Classification: The major chemical subgroups of antipsychotic drugs are the **phenothiazines** (eg, chlorpromazine, thioridazine, fluphenazine); the **thioxanthenes** (eg, thiothixene); and the **butyrophenones** (eg, haloperidol).

    Several newer heterocyclic drugs (clozapine, loxapine, molindone, risperidone) appear to be effective in schizophrenia; clozapine and risperidone may have a lower incidence of extrapyramidal effects than standard drugs.

B. Pharmacokinetics: The antipsychotic drugs are well absorbed when given orally and, because they are lipid-soluble, readily enter the CNS and most other body tissues. Many are bound extensively to plasma proteins. These agents require metabolism by liver enzymes prior to elimination and have long plasma half-lives that permit once-daily dosage. Parenteral forms of fluphenazine, thioridazine, and haloperidol are used for rapid initiation of therapy.

C. Mechanism of Action: The **dopamine hypothesis of schizophrenia** proposes that this disorder is caused by a relative excess of functional activity of the neurotransmitter dopamine in specific neuronal tracts in the brain. This hypothesis is based on the following observations (1) Most antipsychotic drugs block brain dopamine receptors (especially D_2 receptors). (2) Dopamine agonist drugs (eg, amphetamine, levodopa)) exacerbate schizophrenia. (3) An increased density of dopamine receptors has been detected in certain brain regions of untreated schizophrenics. The dopamine hypothesis of schizophrenia is not fully satisfactory because antipsychotic drugs are only partly effective in most patients, and some effective drugs have much higher affinity for other receptors (eg, D_4, 5-HT, alpha adrenoceptors) than for D_2.

    Blockade of dopamine receptors in the mesocortical and mesolimbic pathways of the CNS is generally considered to be the mechanism of action of conventional antipsychotics. Binding affinity to the D_2 subclass of dopamine receptors (negatively coupled to adenylyl cyclase) correlates well with clinical antipsychotic potency. Some of these agents exert blocking actions on other brain neurotransmitter receptors, including serotonergic and alpha adrenoceptors. Alpha adrenoceptor-blocking action also correlates well with antipsychotic effect for many of the drugs. The atypical drug, clozapine, has a much higher affinity for D_4 and 5-HT$_{2a}$ receptors than for D_2 receptors.

D. Effects: Dopamine receptor blockade is the major effect that correlates with therapeutic benefit. Dopaminergic tracts in the brain include the mesocortical-mesolimbic pathways (regulating mentation, mood), the nigrostriatal tract (extrapyramidal function), the tuberoinfundibular pathways (prolactin release), and the chemoreceptor trigger zone (emesis). Mesocortical-mesolimbic dopamine receptor blockade presumably underlies antipsychotic effects, and a similar action on the chemoreceptor trigger zone leads to the useful antiemetic properties of some antipsychotic drugs. Adverse effects resulting from dopamine receptor blockade include extrapyramidal dysfunction and hyperprolactinemia (see below). The relative receptor blocking actions of different antipsychotic drugs is shown in Table 28–1.

The role of other receptors in the therapeutic effects of these drugs is unclear. As noted in Table 28–1, newer antipsychotic agents have higher affinities for receptors other than the D_2 receptor. Clozapine, the first antipsychotic drug with significant D_4 receptor-blocking action, has been claimed to be effective in some patients who are unresponsive to the traditional phenothiazines and haloperidol. Clozapine and risperidone both have significant affinity for 5-HT$_{2a}$ receptors and both appear to have a lower incidence of extrapyramidal toxicity than older agents.

E. Clinical Use:

1. **Treatment of schizophrenia:** Antipsychotic drugs can reduce hyperactivity, bizarre ideation, hallucinations, and delusions and thus facilitate the patient's functioning in an outpatient environment. Beneficial effects may take several weeks to develop. There is no evidence that the different drugs have differing efficacies as antischizophrenic agents, but individual patients may respond more favorably to a particular drug. Clozapine is effective in some patients who are refractory to standard antipsychotic drugs.

2. **Other psychiatric and neurologic indications:** Antipsychotic drugs may be useful in the initial treatment of mania, in the management of psychotic symptoms of schizoaffective disorders, in Tourette syndrome, and for management of toxic psychoses caused by overdosage of certain CNS stimulants. Molindone is used mainly in Tourette syndrome; it is rarely used in schizophrenia.

3. **Nonpsychiatric indications:** With the exception of thioridazine, most phenothiazines have antiemetic actions; prochlorperazine is promoted solely for this indication. The antihistaminic action of phenothiazines is used in the treatment of pruritus and for preoperative sedation (eg, promethazine). H_1 receptor blockade, most often seen with short side-chain phenothiazines, provides the basis for their use as antipruritics and antiemetics.

F. Toxicity:

1. **Neurologic effects:** Dose-dependent extrapyramidal effects include a parkinson-like syndrome (with akinesia, rigidity, and tremor). This toxicity can be reversed with a decrease in dose and can be antagonized by atropine-like drugs. Extrapyramidal toxicity occurs most

Table 28–1. Relative receptor blocking actions of neuroleptic drugs.[1]

Drug	D_2 Block	D_4 Block	Alpha$_1$ Block	5-HT$_2$ Block	Muscarinic Block	H$_1$ Block
Most phenothiazines & thioxanthenes	++	–	++	+	+	+
Thioridazine	++	–	++	+	+++	+
Haloperidol	+++	–	+	–	–	–
Clozapine	–	++	++	++	+	–
Molindone	++	–	+	–	+	+

[1] +, blockade; –, no effect. The number of plus signs indicates the intensity of receptor blockade.

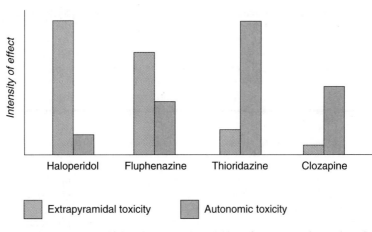

Figure 28–1. Relative extrapyramidal and autonomic toxicities of representative antipsychotic drugs. Extrapyramidal toxicities take the form of parkinsonism, akathisias, and dystonias. Autonomic toxicities are manifest as alpha adrenoceptor blockade (orthostatic hypotension) or muscarinic blockade (dry mouth, blurred vision, urinary retention).

frequently with haloperidol (Figure 28–1) and the more potent piperazine side-chain phenothiazines (eg, fluphenazine, trifluoperazine). Parkinsonism occurs very infrequently with clozapine. Other extrapyramidal dysfunctions include akathisia and dystonias, which usually respond to treatment with diphenhydramine. **Tardive dyskinesia** may develop late in therapy (ie, after 6 months to several years of treatment). This important toxicity includes choreoathetoid movements of muscles of lips and buccal cavity and may be irreversible. Antimuscarinic drugs that usually ameliorate other extrapyramidal effects generally *increase* the severity of tardive dyskinesia symptoms. There is no effective drug treatment for tardive dyskinesia at present. Changing drug therapy of the patient to clozapine does not exacerbate the condition. Tardive dyskinesia may be attenuated *temporarily* by increasing neuroleptic dosage; this has led to the suggestion that tardive dyskinesia is caused by dopamine receptor sensitization.

2. **Autonomic effects:** These include blockade of peripheral muscarinic receptors and alpha adrenoceptors. These effects may be more difficult to manage in elderly patients. Tolerance to some of the autonomic effects occurs with continued therapy. As shown in Figure 28–1, thioridazine has the strongest autonomic effects and haloperidol the weakest. Clozapine is intermediate.

   a. **Muscarinic receptor blockade:** Atropine-like effects (dry mouth, constipation, urinary retention and visual problems) are often pronounced during use of thioridazine and phenothiazines with aliphatic side chains (eg, chlorpromazine). Antimuscarinic CNS effects may include a toxic confusional state similar to that produced by atropine and the tricyclic antidepressants.

   b. **Alpha receptor blockade:** Postural hypotension is a common manifestation of alpha blockade, especially with phenothiazines. In the elderly, measures must be taken to avoid falls due to postural fainting. Failure to ejaculate is common in men treated with the phenothiazines.

3. **Endocrine and metabolic effects:** These include weight gain, gynecomastia, the amenorrhea-galactorrhea syndrome, and infertility. These effects are predictable manifestations of dopamine receptor blockade in the pituitary: dopamine is the normal inhibitory regulator of prolactin secretion.

4. **Neuroleptic malignant syndrome:** Patients who are particularly sensitive to the extrapyramidal effects of antipsychotic drugs may develop a malignant syndrome. The symptoms include muscle rigidity, impairment of sweating, hyperpyrexia, and autonomic instability that may be life-threatening. Drug treatment involves the prompt use of dantrolene and dopamine agonists.

5. **Sedation:** Sedation is more marked with phenothiazines than with other antipsychotics; this effect is normally perceived as unpleasant by nonpsychotic individuals.

6. **Miscellaneous toxicities:** Visual impairment caused by retinal deposits has occurred with **thioridazine**; at high doses this drug may also cause severe conduction defects in the heart that result in fatal ventricular arrhythmias. **Clozapine** causes a small but important (1–2%) incidence of agranulocytosis. At high doses clozapine may cause seizures.

7. **Overdosage toxicity:** Poisoning with antipsychotics other than thioridazine is not usually fatal. Hypotension often responds to fluid replacement. Neuroleptics lower the convulsive threshold and may cause seizures, which are usually managed with diazepam or phenytoin. Thioridazine overdose, because of cardiotoxicity, is more difficult to treat.

LITHIUM & OTHER DRUGS USED IN BIPOLAR (MANIC-DEPRESSIVE) DISORDER

A. **Pharmacokinetics:** Lithium is absorbed rapidly and completely from the gut. The drug is distributed throughout the body water and excreted by the kidneys with a half-life of about 20 hours. Plasma levels should be monitored, especially during the first weeks of therapy, to establish an effective and safe dosage regimen. Plasma levels of the drug may be altered by changes in the efficiency of proximal tubular reabsorption of cations. Thus, chronic treatment with diuretics (thiazides), which stimulates proximal tubule cation reabsorption, may result in increasing plasma lithium to toxic levels. Theophylline increases the renal clearance of lithium.

B. **Mechanism of Action:** The mechanism of action of lithium is not well defined. The drug inhibits the recycling of neuronal membrane phosphoinositides involved in the generation of inositol trisphosphate (IP_3) and diacylglycerol (DAG), which act as second messengers in both alpha adrenoceptor and muscarinic neurotransmission (Figure 28–2).

C. **Clinical Use:** Lithium carbonate is used in the treatment of bipolar affective disorder (manic-depressive disease). Maintenance therapy with lithium decreases manic behavior and modulates both the frequency and the magnitude of mood swings. Antipsychotic drug therapy may also be required, especially at the initiation of lithium treatment. Other drugs are of value in bipolar affective disorder. The tricyclic antiepileptic drug, carbamazepine, has been used to treat mania in patients who respond inadequately to lithium. The antiseizure drug, clonazepam, has also been used.

D. **Toxicity:** Adverse neurologic effects of lithium include tremor, sedation, ataxia, and aphasia. Thyroid enlargement may occur, but thyroid dysfunction is rare. Reversible nephrogenic diabetes insipidus commonly occurs at therapeutic drug levels. Edema is a frequent adverse effect of lithium therapy, and leucocytosis is always present. The use of lithium during pregnancy may increase the incidence of congenital cardiac anomalies.

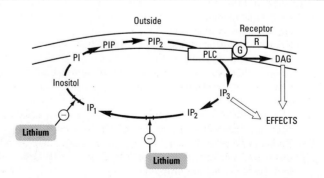

Figure 28–2. Postulated effect of lithium on the IP_3 and DAG second messenger system. The schematic diagram shows the synaptic membrane of a neuron in the brain. PLC, phospholipase-C; G, coupling protein; R, receptor; PI, PIP, PIP_2, IP_2, IP_1, intermediates in the production of IP_3. By interfering with this cycle, lithium may cause a use-dependent reduction of synaptic transmission. (Modified and reproduced, with permission, from Katzung BG [editor]: *Basic & Clinical Pharmacology*, 6th ed. Appleton & Lange, 1995.)

DRUG LIST

The following drugs are important members of the drug groups discussed in this chapter. Prototypes should be learned in detail; the other significant agents should be recognized as belonging to a specific subclass.

Subclass	Prototype	Other Significant Agents
Phenothiazines		
Aliphatic	Chlorpromazine[1]	
Piperidine	Thioridazine	Mesoridazine
Piperazine	Trifluoperazine	Perphenazine, fluphenazine
Thioxanthenes	Thiothixene	
Butyrophenones	Haloperidol	
Heterocyclics	Clozapine, molindone, pimozide	Loxapine, risperidone
Antimanic drugs	Lithium	Carbamazepine, clonazepam

[1] **NOTE:** Some authorities consider chlorpromazine obsolete because of its high incidence of toxic effects.

QUESTIONS

DIRECTIONS: Each of the numbered items or incomplete statements in this section is followed by answers or by completions of the sentence. Select the ONE lettered answer or completion that is BEST in each case.

1. Concerning hypotheses for the pathophysiologic basis of schizophrenia, all of the following statements are accurate EXCEPT
   (A) Positron emission tomography has shown increased dopamine receptors in the brains of both untreated and drug-treated schizophrenics
   (B) In a patient with parkinsonism, psychotic effects may occur during treatment with dopamine receptor agonists
   (C) The clinical potency of many antipsychotic drugs correlates well with their alpha adrenoceptor-blocking actions
   (D) All effective antipsychotic drugs have high affinity for dopamine D_2 receptors
   (E) Drug treatment of schizophrenics sometimes results in changes in the cerebrospinal fluid levels of the dopamine metabolite, homovanillic acid

2. Fluphenazine has been prescribed for a 20-year-old male patient. His schizophrenic symptoms have improved enough for him to reside in a "halfway house" in the community. He visits his physician with a list of complaints about his medication. Which one of the following is LEAST likely to be on his list?
   (A) He is constipated
   (B) His sex drive has decreased
   (C) He gets dizzy if he stands up too quickly
   (D) He salivates excessively
   (E) He has difficulty reading the newspaper

3. The following statements concerning adverse effects of antipsychotic drugs are all accurate EXCEPT
   (A) The late-occurring choreoathetoid movements caused by conventional antipsychotic drugs are exacerbated by antimuscarinic agents
   (B) Retinal pigmentation is a dose-dependent toxic effect of thioridazine
   (C) Uncontrollable restlessness in a patient on antipsychotic medications is usually alleviated by increasing the drug dose
   (D) Acute dystonic reactions usually respond to diphenhydramine
   (E) Blurring of vision and urinary retention are likely side effects of chlorpromazine

4. Clinical uses of antipsychotic drugs include all of the following EXCEPT
   (A) Management of psychosis caused by phencyclidine intoxication
   (B) Treatment of schizoaffective disorders

    (C) Management of Tourette syndrome
    (D) Treatment of the amenorrhea-galactorrhea syndrome
    (E) Acute management of the manic phase of bipolar disorder

5. Akinesia, rigidity, and tremor occur more frequently during treatment with haloperidol than with thioridazine. The most likely explanation is that
    (A) Haloperidol has a low affinity for D_2 receptors
    (B) Thioridazine has greater alpha adrenoceptor- blocking actions
    (C) Haloperidol activates GABAergic neurons in the striatum
    (D) Thioridazine has greater blocking actions on brain muscarinic receptors
    (E) Haloperidol acts presynaptically to block dopamine release

6. All of the following statements concerning drug treatment of manic-depressive (bipolar) affective disorder are accurate EXCEPT
    (A) During pregnancy lithium dosage must be increased because volume of distribution and clearance are both increased
    (B) Excessive intake of sodium chloride is likely to enhance the toxicity of lithium
    (C) Lithium dosage may need to be lowered in patients taking oral diuretics
    (D) Patients unable to tolerate lithium may respond favorably to clonazepam
    (E) Theophylline increases the dose requirement in patients taking lithium

7. A 30-year-old male patient is on drug therapy for a psychiatric problem. He complains that he feels "flat" and that he gets confused at times. He has been gaining weight and has lost his sex drive. As he moves his hands you notice a slight tremor. He tells you that since he has been on medication he is always thirsty and frequently has to urinate. The drug he is most likely to be taking is:
    (A) Fluphenazine hydrochloride
    (B) Clozapine
    (C) Thioridazine hydrochloride
    (D) Lithium carbonate
    (E) Clonazepam

DIRECTIONS: The following section consists of a list of four to twenty-six lettered options followed by several numbered items. For each numbered item, select the ONE option that is most closely associated with it. Each answer may be selected once, more than once, or not at all.
    (A) Bromocriptine
    (B) Promethazine
    (C) Lithium
    (D) Trifluoperazine
    (E) Thioridazine
    (F) Clozapine
    (G) Haloperidol
    (H) Clonazepam
    (I) Carbamazepine
    (J) Chlorpromazine

8. The calming and antiemetic properties of this phenothiazine, together with its atropine-like properties, form the basis for its nonpsychiatric use in preoperative sedation

9. Weekly blood counts are mandatory for patients who are taking this drug

10. This drug may cause abnormal electrocardiograms at therapeutic doses; cardiotoxicity is enhanced if the agent is administered with drugs that have quinidine-like actions

11. Although it can exacerbate the symptoms of schizophrenia, this drug may be useful in the management of the neuroleptic malignant syndrome

12. Useful as a mood stabilizer in patients with bipolar affective disorders who are intolerant to lithium; this drug has hematotoxic potential

13. Used as an anticonvulsant, this agent is also valuable in some patients with bipolar disorder

14. This drug is notable for causing retinal deposits and damage, and for having strong antimuscarinic effects

ANSWERS

1. Although positive correlations have been made between antipsychotic efficacy and the abilities of drugs to block D_2 receptors, similar correlations also have been made with respect to their

alpha adrenoceptor-blocking actions. Most conventional antipsychotic drugs block D_2 receptors. However, such an action does not appear to be an absolute requirement for antipsychotic action, since clozapine has a very low affinity for such receptors. All of the other statements are accurate. The answer is **(D)**.

2. Sedative effects occur with most of the phenothiazines; these drugs also act as antagonists at muscarinic and alpha adrenoceptors. Postural hypotension, blurring of vision, and constipation are common autonomic side effects, as is *dry* mouth. Effects on the male libido may result from increases in prolactin or from increased peripheral conversion of androgens to estrogens. The answer is **(D)**.

3. Uncontrollable restlessness (akathisia) is an extrapyramidal side effect of antipsychotic medications. In some patients, akathisias may be difficult to distinguish from the expression of the positive symptoms of schizophrenia. Akathisias are managed by *decreasing* the antipsychotic drug dose or by treatment with drugs that have anticholinergic actions. The answer is **(C)**.

4. Hyperprolactinemia and the amenorrhea-galactorrhea syndrome may occur as an adverse effect during treatment with antipsychotic drugs that block dopamine receptors in the tuberoinfundibular tract. This prevents the normal inhibitory action of dopamine on release of prolactin from the anterior pituitary gland. The answer is **(D)**.

5. Parkinsonian adverse effects occur more commonly with haloperidol than with thioridazine. One possible explanation is that thioridazine exerts more pronounced blocking actions at brain muscarinic receptors. This action partly compensates for dopamine receptor blockade in the nigrostriatal tract, so that extrapyramidal function is more effectively maintained. A second possibility (not listed) is that haloperidol has a higher affinity for dopamine D_2 receptors than does thioridazine. The answer is **(D)**.

6. Reliance is placed on measurements of serum lithium concentrations for optimal dosage regimens. Lithium clearance is influenced by many factors including renal function, serum sodium concentration, hydration state, pregnancy, and the presence of other drugs. High urinary levels of sodium inhibit renal tubular reabsorption of lithium, thus *decreasing* its plasma levels. By decreasing blood volume, thiazides may increase lithium plasma levels. The answer is **(B)**.

7. Confusion, mood changes, decreased sexual interest, and weight gain are symptoms that may be unrelated to drug administration. On the other hand, psychiatric drugs, including those used in the treatment of psychotic and affective disorders, may be responsible for such symptoms. Tremor and symptoms of nephrogenic diabetes insipidus are characteristic adverse effects of lithium that may occur at therapeutic blood levels of the drug. The answer is **(D)**.

8. With the exception of thioridazine, phenothiazines exert strong antiemetic effects. Phenothiazines with short side chains have marked histamine H_1 receptor blocking action and are used for relief of pruritus or, in the case of promethazine, as preoperative sedatives. The answer is **(B)**.

9. Agranulocytosis occurs in a small percentage of patients on clozapine. This potentially fatal abnormality can develop rapidly, usually between the 6th and 18th week of therapy. Hematotoxicity is reversible if clozapine is discontinued immediately following a significant decrease in WBCs. The answer is **(F)**.

10. Thioridazine has several distinctive toxicities. The drug has quinidine-like actions on the heart and, in overdose, may cause arrhythmias and cardiac conduction block. The answer is **(E)**.

11. The neuroleptic malignant syndrome is characterized by muscle rigidity, high fever, and autonomic instability. The syndrome may result from a too-rapid block of dopamine receptors in patients who are highly sensitive to the extrapyramidal effects of antipsychotic drugs. Management involves the physical control of fever, the use of muscle relaxants (eg, dantrolene or diazepam), and administration of the dopamine receptor agonist, bromocriptine. Like most drugs that increase brain dopaminergic activity, bromocriptine may exacerbate psychotic symptoms. The answer is **(A)**.

12. Carbamazepine can be used to treat mania and for prophylaxis in patients with bipolar affective disorders. A low incidence of agranulocytosis occurs when the drug is employed for treatment of trigeminal neuralgia in older patients. The answer is **(I)**.

13. Clonazepam is of value in some patients with bipolar disorder but is used primarily in the treatment of petit mal and myoclonic epilepsy. The answer is **(H)**.

14. In addition to causing significant cardiac toxicity, thioridazine is a strong antimuscarinic agent and may cause retinal damage. Atropine-like side effects are more prominent than those

caused by other phenothiazines, but the drug is less likely to cause extrapyramidal dysfunction. At high doses, thioridazine causes retinal deposits which, in advanced cases, resemble retinitis pigmentosa. The patient may complain of "browning of vision." The answer is **(E).**

29

Antidepressants

OBJECTIVES

You should be able to:

- Describe the probable mechanisms and the major pharmacodynamic properties of tricyclic antidepressants.
- List the toxic effects that occur during chronic therapy and after an overdose of tricyclic antidepressants.
- Describe the therapeutic use and toxic effects of MAO inhibitors.
- Identify the second-generation antidepressants and their distinctive properties.
- Identify the prototype selective serotonin reuptake inhibitor and list its major characteristics.
- Identify the major drug interactions associated with the use of antidepressant drugs.

Learn the definitions that follow.

Table 29–1. Definitions.

Term	Definition
Tricyclics	A group of structurally related drugs containing a three-ring nucleus; these drugs resemble phenothiazines chemically
MAO inhibitors	Drugs that inhibit monoamine oxidase type A, which metabolizes norepinephrine and serotonin, or monoamine oxidase B, which metabolizes dopamine
Second-generation antidepressants	A group of more recently introduced antidepressant drugs of varied chemical structures; several have actions different from those of tricyclic antidepressants
Amine hypothesis of mood	The hypothesis that major depressive disorders result from a functional deficiency of norepinephrine or serotonin at synapses in the central nervous system

CONCEPTS

Depression is a common condition with both psychologic and physical manifestations. The three major types of depression are (1) **reactive depression,** a response to external events; (2) **bipolar affective (manic-depressive) disorder,** discussed in Chapter 28; and (3) **major depressive disorder,** or **endogenous depression,** a depression of mood without any obvious medical or situational causes. The drugs used in endogenous depression are the subject of this chapter.

The **amine hypothesis of mood** postulates that brain amines, particularly norepinephrine and serotonin, are neurotransmitters in pathways that function in the expression of mood states. According to the amine hypothesis, a functional decrease in the activity of such amines would result in depression; a functional increase of activity would result in mood elevation. Difficulties with this hypothesis include the facts that (1) antidepressant drugs cause a change in amine activity within hours but require weeks to achieve clinical effects; and (2) these drugs cause a slow *down*-regulation of amine receptors.

A. Classification & Pharmacokinetics: Four groups of drugs are used to treat endogenous depression (Figure 29–1): the **tricyclic antidepressants;** the **second-generation agents,** some of which are related to the tricyclic agents; the **selective serotonin reuptake inhibitors (SSRI),** and the **monoamine oxidase inhibitors.**

1. Tricyclics: The tricyclic drugs (eg, imipramine, amitriptyline) are structurally related to the phenothiazine antipsychotics and share certain of their pharmacologic effects. The tricyclics are well absorbed orally but may undergo first-pass metabolism. Extensive hepatic metabolism is required prior to their elimination; plasma half-lives of 8–36 hours usually permit once-daily dosing. Some tricyclics form active metabolites.

2. Second-generation drugs: The second-generation antidepressants (eg, amoxapine, bupropion, maprotiline, trazodone) have varied chemical structures. The pharmacokinetics of these agents are similar to those of the tricyclic drugs, except for trazodone, which has a shorter half-life and often requires administration twice or three times daily.

3. Selective serotonin reuptake inhibitors: Fluoxetine was originally considered another member of the second-generation antidepressants, but it now appears to be the initial member of a new subgroup, the selective serotonin reuptake inhibitors (SSRI). Fluoxetine forms an active metabolite with a long half-life. Sertraline and paroxetine, newer members of this subgroup, have long half-lives and are given orally once a day.

4. MAO inhibitors: These drugs (eg, phenelzine, tranylcypromine, isocarboxazid) are structurally related to amphetamines and are orally active. Tranylcypromine inhibits monoamine oxidase reversibly; the others do so irreversibly. Tranylcypromine is faster in onset but has a shorter duration of action (about a week) than do other MAO inhibitors (with durations of 2–3 weeks). In spite of these prolonged actions, the MAO inhibitors are given daily. As inhibitors of hepatic drug-metabolizing enzymes, these drugs cause many drug interactions.

Moclobemide is a newer MAO inhibitor that is currently in clinical trials. It is of considerable interest because it differs in several respects from the older agents: moclobemide is selective for MAO-A, the serotonin- and norepinephrine-selective form of the enzyme; also, moclobemide is readily displaced from the enzyme by tyramine and has a much shorter duration of action than other drugs in this group.

B. Mechanism of Action:

1. Acute action: Potential sites of action of antidepressants in central nervous system synapses are shown in Figure 29–2. The acute effect of tricyclic drugs is to inhibit the uptake mechanisms responsible for the termination of the synaptic actions of both norepinephrine and serotonin in the brain. This is thought to result in potentiation of their neurotransmitter actions.

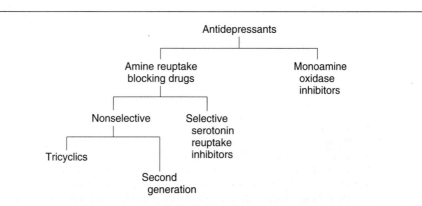

Figure 29–1. Major classes of antidepressant drugs.

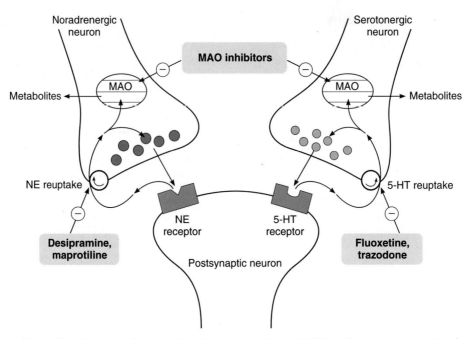

Figure 29–2. Possible sites of action of antidepressant drugs. Inhibition of neuronal reuptake of norepinephrine and serotonin increases the synaptic activities of these neurotransmitters. Inhibition of MAO increases the presynaptic stores of both norepinephrine and serotonin, which leads to increased neurotransmitter effects. **NOTE:** these are acute actions of antidepressants; chronic therapy may lead to down-regulation of brain beta receptors.

The acute actions of some second-generation drugs appear to result from selective blockade of reuptake of norepinephrine (eg, with maprotiline); for other drugs in this group, inhibition of serotonin reuptake dominates (eg, trazodone, Table 29–2). The acute effect of the selective serotonin reuptake inhibitors is, as the name indicates, an even more selective action on the 5-HT reuptake carrier.

The MAO inhibitors increase brain amine levels by interfering with their metabolism in the nerve endings, resulting in an increase in the vesicular stores of norepinephrine and serotonin. When neuronal activity discharges these vesicles, increased amounts of the amines are released, enhancing the actions of the neurotransmitters.

2. **Chronic actions:** Our understanding of the mechanisms of these drugs is complicated by the fact that chronic treatment of animals with antidepressant drugs consistently causes down-regulation of brain norepinephrine receptors, especially beta adrenoceptors. Down-regulation of beta receptors occurs during chronic treatment with tricyclics, second-generation drugs, selective serotonin reuptake inhibitors, and MAO inhibitors. This change in adrenoceptor number may reflect a decrease in the neurotransmitter actions of norepinephrine, an action that is not in simple accord with the amine hypothesis of mood.

C. **Effects:**
1. **Amine uptake blockade:** Block of amine reuptake carriers is the major CNS effect of tricyclics and most second-generation drugs. Block of norepinephrine reuptake occurs in the peripheral autonomic nervous system as well as the CNS, and may lead to sympathomimetic effects. It is not known what role peripheral blockade of serotonin uptake may play.
2. **Sedation:** Sedation is a common CNS effect of tricyclic drugs (although less so with protriptyline and desipramine) and of most second-generation drugs (Table 29–2). MAO inhibitors, selective serotonin reuptake inhibitors, and bupropion may be mildly stimulating.
3. **Muscarinic receptor blockade:** Muscarinic blockade occurs with all tricyclics and is particularly marked with amitriptyline and doxepin (Table 29–2). The newer agents appear

Table 29–2. Pharmacodynamics of common tricyclic antidepressants, second-generation agents, and selective serotonin reuptake inhibitors.[1,2]

Drug	Sedation	Muscarinic Receptor Blockade	NE Reuptake Blockade	5-HT Reuptake Blockade
Tricyclic antidepressants Amitriptyline, doxepin	+++	+++	++	+++
Desipramine, protriptyline	+	+	+++	–
Imipramine, nortriptyline	++	+	+	++
Second-generation antidepressants Amoxapine	++	+	++	+
Bupropion	–	–	–	–
Trazodone	+++	–	–	+
Maprotiline	++	+	+++	–
Selective serotonin reuptake inhibitors (SSRI) (Fluoxetine)	–	+	–	+++

[1] For study purposes, similar drugs have been grouped, even though they may not be identical in their actions.
[2] Key: – = none; + = slight; ++ = moderate; +++ = marked

to be less potent antimuscarinics; atropine-like effects are minimal with selective serotonin reuptake inhibitors, bupropion, and trazodone.

4. **Cardiovascular effects:** Cardiovascular effects include hypotension from alpha adrenoceptor blockade and depression of cardiac conduction. The latter effect may lead to arrhythmias.

5. **Seizures:** Because convulsive threshold is lowered by tricyclic drugs, seizures may occur with overdoses of these agents. Overdoses of MAO inhibitors may also cause seizures.

D. Clinical Use:

1. **Major depressive disorders:** Endogenous depression is the major clinical indication for the antidepressant drugs. Patients typically vary in their responsiveness to individual agents. Tricyclic drugs are thought to be most useful in patients with psychomotor retardation, sleep disturbances, poor appetite, weight loss, and decreased libido. Selective serotonin reuptake inhibitors may decrease appetite; overweight patients often lose weight on these drugs. MAO inhibitors may be most useful in patients with significant anxiety, phobic features, and hypochondriasis.

Most second-generation drugs have proved to be as effective as tricyclics, and in some cases, second-generation agents may have a more favorable adverse effect profile. The selective serotonin reuptake blockers are usually accepted better by patients; these drugs have also proved to be effective in some patients who are refractory to tricyclic drugs.

2. **Other clinical uses:** Tricyclic drugs are also used in the treatment of manic-depressive disorders, acute panic attacks and phobic disorders (compare with alprazolam), enuresis, and chronic pain states. Clomipramine and the selective serotonin reuptake inhibitors are effective in obsessive compulsive disorders. *Tricyclic antidepressants are not recommended for routine use as anxiolytics.*

E. Toxicity:

1. **Tricyclic adverse effects:** The adverse effects of tricyclic antidepressants, in large part predictable from their pharmacodynamic actions (see Effects, above), include (1) excessive sedation, lassitude, fatigue, and, sometimes, confusion; (2) sympathomimetic effects, including tachycardia, agitation, sweating, and insomnia; (3) atropine-like effects; (4) orthostatic hypotension, ECG abnormalities, and cardiomyopathies; and (5) tremor and paresthesias.

2. **Tricyclic drug interactions:** Interactions include additive depression of the CNS with other central depressants, including ethanol, barbiturates, benzodiazepines, and opioids. Tricyclics may also cause reversal of the antihypertensive action of guanethidine by block-

ade of active guanethidine accumulation into sympathetic nerve endings. Methyldopa accumulation in central neurons may be similarly blocked. Less commonly, tricyclics may interfere with the action of methylnorepinephrine (the active metabolite of methyldopa) and clonidine by blocking their central alpha receptors.

3. **Tricyclic overdosage:** Overdosage with these drugs (often with suicidal intent) is extremely hazardous; manifestations include (1) agitation, delirium, neuromuscular irritability, convulsions, and coma; (2) respiratory depression and circulatory collapse; (3) hyperpyrexia; and (4) cardiac conduction defects and severe arrhythmias.

4. **Second-generation drugs and selective serotonin reuptake inhibitors:** With the exception of trazodone, these drugs usually cause less sedative effects than conventional tricyclics. Except for amoxapine and maprotiline, these drugs cause less autonomic dysfunction than do the tricyclics. Amoxapine is also a dopamine receptor blocker and may cause akathisia, parkinsonism and the amenorrhea-galactorrhea syndrome. Adverse effects of bupropion include dizziness, dry mouth, aggravation of psychosis, and at high doses, seizures. Fluoxetine and the newer SSRI may cause anxiety, agitation, and insomnia. Reports that the use of fluoxetine increases suicidal ideation or violence in some patients have not been substantiated. Seizures are a prominent feature of overdosage with amoxapine, fluoxetine, and maprotiline. Amoxapine and maprotiline also have cardiotoxic potential.

5. **MAO inhibitors:** Adverse effects of the MAO inhibitors include hypertensive reactions in response to indirectly acting sympathomimetics, hyperthermia, and CNS stimulation leading to agitation and convulsions. In particular, hypertensive crisis may occur in patients taking MAO inhibitors who consume food that contains high concentrations of the indirect sympathomimetic tyramine (eg, fermented food). In the absence of indirect sympathomimetics, MAO inhibitors typically lower blood pressure; overdosage with these drugs may result in shock, hyperthermia, and seizures. MAO inhibitors should not be administered together with fluoxetine or other selective serotonin reuptake inhibitors because their combined use may cause a **"serotonin syndrome"** characterized by hyperthermia, muscle rigidity, myoclonus, and rapid changes in mental status and vital signs.

DRUG LIST

The following drugs are important members of the group discussed in this chapter. Prototypes should be learned in detail; features of the major variants should be known well enough to distinguish the variants from prototypes and from each other; the other significant agents should be recognized as belonging to a specific subclass.

Subclass	Prototype	Major Variants	Other Significant Agents
Tricyclic drugs	Imipramine, amitriptyline	Desipramine, nortriptyline	Doxepin, protriptyline
Second-generation drugs	Amoxapine, bupropion, maprotiline, trazodone		
Selective serotonin reuptake inhibitors	Fluoxetine		Paroxetine, sertraline
MAO inhibitors	Phenelzine, moclobemide	Tranylcypromine	Isocarboxazid

QUESTIONS

DIRECTIONS: Each of the numbered items or incomplete statements in this section is followed by answers or by completions of the sentence. Select the ONE lettered answer or completion that is BEST in each case.

1. Concerning the proposed mechanisms of action of antidepressant drugs, all of the following statements are accurate EXCEPT
   (A) The acute effect of most tricyclic drugs is to block the neuronal reuptake of norepinephrine and serotonin in the CNS

    (B) Endogenous depression has been postulated to result from decreased functional activity at certain central noradrenergic or serotonergic synapses

    (C) Chronic treatment with selective serotonin reuptake inhibitors leads to a down-regulation of adrenoceptors

    (D) MAO inhibitors decrease the metabolism of norepinephrine, serotonin, and dopamine

    (E) Elevation in the cerebrospinal fluid levels of amine metabolites prior to drug therapy occurs in most depressed patients

2. Effects of the tricyclic antidepressant drugs include all of the following EXCEPT

    (A) Sympathomimetic actions

    (B) Alpha adrenoceptor blockade

    (C) Elevation of the seizure threshold

    (D) Sedation

    (E) Muscarinic receptor-blocking action

3. Regarding the clinical use of antidepressant drugs, all of the following statements are accurate EXCEPT

    (A) Antidepressant drugs may have to be administered for several weeks before a noticeable improvement in depressive symptoms occurs

    (B) In selecting an appropriate drug for treatment of depression, the past history of patient response to specific drugs is a valuable guide

    (C) In the treatment of depressions characterized by psychomotor retardation, poor appetite, and weight loss, amitriptyline is usually more effective than imipramine

    (D) MAO inhibitors are more likely to be effective in depressions with attendant anxiety, phobic features, and hypochondriasis

    (E) Fluoxetine may be effective in depressions refractory to tricyclic drugs

4. Drug interactions involving antidepressants include all of the following EXCEPT

    (A) Increased antihypertensive effects of methyldopa when tricyclics are administered

    (B) Hypertensive crisis in patients on MAO inhibitors when foods containing tyramine are ingested

    (C) Behavioral excitation and hypertension in patients taking MAO inhibitors when meperidine is administered

    (D) Additive impairment of driving ability in patients taking a tricyclic antidepressant when ethanol is ingested

    (E) Prolongation of tricyclic drug half-life in patients when cimetidine is administered

Items 5–6: A patient under treatment for a major depressive disorder is brought to the emergency room after ingesting 50 times the normal therapeutic dose of amitriptyline.

5. Signs and symptoms in this patient are likely to include all of the following EXCEPT

    (A) Pinpoint pupils

    (B) Hypotension

    (C) Coma and shock

    (D) Hot dry skin

    (E) Acidosis

6. During the course of treatment of this patient, it would be reasonable to institute all of the following measures EXCEPT

    (A) Administration of lidocaine (to control cardiac arrhythmias)

    (B) Hemodialysis (to hasten drug elimination)

    (C) Administration of bicarbonate and KCl (to correct acidosis and hypokalemia)

    (D) Intravenous administration of diazepam (to control seizures)

    (E) Electrical pacing (to maintain the rhythm of the heart)

DIRECTIONS: The following section consists of a list of four to twenty-six lettered options followed by several numbered items. For each numbered item, select the ONE option that is most closely associated with it. Each answer may be selected once, more than once, or not at all.

    (A) Amoxapine

    (B) Amitriptyline

    (C) Isocarboxazid

    (D) Maprotiline

    (E) Fluoxetine

    (F) Bupropion
    (G) Desipramine
    (H) Clomipramine
    (I)   Sertraline
    (J) Moclobemide

7. A selective inhibitor of norepinephrine reuptake with four rings in its structure; seizures may occur at the top of the therapeutic dose range of this drug

8. A selective blocker of neuronal reuptake of serotonin; metabolized to an active metabolite with a prolonged half-life

9. This drug binds nonselectively to MAO A and B

10. This second-generation antidepressant has a marked ability to block dopamine receptors. The drug may cause dangerous neurotoxicity in overdose

11. This tricyclic antidepressant is used primarily in the management of obsessive-compulsive disorders; the mechanism of action is not defined

12. The antidepressant actions of this drug do not appear to occur via effects on MAO or on the re-uptake systems for norepinephrine or serotonin

13. A selective MAO inhibitor with a short half-life of less than 12 hours

14. MAO inhibitor with a prolonged (2–3 weeks) duration of action

ANSWERS

1. Concentrations of norepinephrine and serotonin metabolites in the cerebrospinal fluid of depressed patients prior to drug treatment are not higher than normal. Some studies have reported *decreased* levels of these metabolites. Down-regulation of adrenoceptors appears to be a common feature of all modes of chronic drug treatment of depression, including the use of drugs that have no direct actions on catecholamine receptors. The answer is **(E)**.

2. Tricyclics modify peripheral sympathetic effects in two ways: through blockade of norepinephrine reuptake at neuroeffector junctions and through alpha adrenoceptor blockade. Sedation and atropine-like side effects are common. In contrast to sedative-hypnotics, tricyclics lower the threshold to seizures. The answer is **(C)**.

3. There is no evidence that any tricyclic drug is more effective than another in antidepressant efficacy. While an individual patient may respond more favorably to a specific drug, controlled studies show that the tricyclic drugs are equivalent in their effectiveness as antidepressants. The answer is **(C)**.

4. Tricyclic drugs block neuronal uptake of several antihypertensive medications (including guanethidine), thus reversing beneficial effects on blood pressure. While the precise mechanism is not defined, the tricyclics may also block the antihypertensive effects of clonidine and methyldopa. The H_2 blocker cimetidine, a potent inhibitor of liver drug-metabolizing enzymes, has been implicated in many drug interactions. The answer is **(A)**.

5. Anticholinergic effects common in tricyclic drug overdosage include hot dry skin, decreased bowel sounds, tachycardia, and *dilated* pupils. Hypotension occurs frequently, due to marked blockade at alpha adrenoceptors. The answer is **(A)**.

6. Tricyclic antidepressant overdose is a medical emergency. The "three Cs"—coma, convulsions, and cardiac problems—are the most common causes of death. Widening of the QRS complex on the ECG is a major diagnostic feature of cardiac toxicity. Arrhythmias resulting from cardiac toxicity are difficult to manage; they require the use of drugs with the least effect on cardiac conductivity (eg, lidocaine, phenytoin). There is no evidence that hemodialysis (or hemoperfusion) increases the rate of elimination of tricyclic antidepressants, presumably because of their large volume of distribution and their binding to tissue components. The answer is **(B)**.

7. Maprotiline is chemically similar to the tricyclic drug desipramine, except that it has a tetracyclic structure. Maprotiline is almost equivalent to desipramine in terms of its sedative and muscarinic receptor blocking actions, but has caused seizures at the top of its recommended dose range. Both drugs act selectively to block the reuptake of norepinephrine. The answer is **(D)**.

8. Fluoxetine and sertraline are selective serotonin reuptake inhibitors. Fluoxetine is metabolized to the active metabolite norfluoxetine, which has a half-life of 7 to 9 days. This characteristic of fluoxetine has caused dosing problems due to the cumulation of its metabolite. The answer is **(E)**.

9. Isocarboxazid binds irreversibly to both types of MAO; inhibition may persist after the drug is no longer detectable in the plasma. The answer is **(C).**

10. Amoxapine, a metabolite of the antipsychotic drug, loxapine, retains dopamine receptor-blocking action. This results in some of the adverse effects commonly associated with antipsychotic drug use, including akathisia, parkinsonian symptoms, and hyperprolactinemia. The answer is **(A).**

11. Clomipramine appears to have selective activity in the treatment of obsessive-compulsive disorder (OCD). Clomipramine may act via blockade of serotonin reuptake, since OCD is also responsive to sertraline and other selective serotonin reuptake inhibitors. The answer is **(H).**

12. Bupropion has no actions on the reuptake or metabolism of norepinephrine or serotonin. The chemical structure of bupropion is similar to that of the central stimulant, amphetamine. Effects on dopaminergic transmission may underlie its antidepressant actions. The answer is **(F).**

13. Older MAO inhibitors have very long durations of action (weeks). The newer agent, moclobemide, is almost completely excreted within 12 hours and acts selectively on MAO-A, the form of the enzyme that selectively metabolizes norepinephrine and serotonin. The drug is readily displaced from MAO by tyramine and is less likely than the older drugs to contribute to a tyramine-induced hypertensive crisis. The answer is **(J).**

14. Isocarboxazid is the other MAO inhibitor on this list; its action is prolonged because it binds irreversibly to the enzyme. The answer is **(C).**

Opioid Analgesics & Antagonists

30

OBJECTIVES

You should be able to:

- List the receptors affected by opioid analgesics and the endogenous opioid peptides.
- Given a list of major opioid agonists, rank them in analgesic efficacy.
- Identify opioid receptor antagonists and mixed agonist-antagonists.
- Describe the main pharmacodynamic and pharmacokinetic properties of agonist opioid analgesics and list their clinical uses.
- List the main adverse effects of acute and chronic use of opioid analgesics.
- Describe the clinical uses of the opioid receptor antagonists.
- List two opioids used for antitussive effects and one used for antidiarrheal effects.

Learn the definitions that follow.

Table 30–1. Definitions.

Term	Definition
Opiate	A drug derived from alkaloids of the opium poppy
Opioid	The class of drugs that includes opiates, opiopeptins, and all synthetic and semi-synthetic drugs that mimic the actions of the opiates
Opiopeptins	Endogenous peptides that act on opioid receptors
Opioid agonist	A drug that activates some or all opioid receptor subtypes and does not block any
Opioid antagonist	A drug that blocks some or all opioid receptor subtypes
Mixed agonist-antagonist	A drug that activates some opioid receptor subtypes and blocks other subtypes

CONCEPTS

A. Classification: Morphine and other natural derivatives of the opium poppy are **opiates.** Opiates, synthetic drugs, and the endogenous compounds that produce morphine-like effects comprise the **opioids.** The opioids derive from several chemical subgroups, including phenanthrenes, phenylheptylamines, phenylpiperidines, morphinans, and benzomorphans.

Λ useful subdivision of the opioids appears in Figure 30 1.

  1. Spectrum of clinical uses: Opioid drugs are subdivided on the basis of their major therapeutic uses (eg, as analgesics, antitussives, and antidiarrheal drugs).

  2. Strength of analgesia: On the basis of their relative abilities to relieve pain, the analgesic opioids may be classified as strong, moderate, and weak agonists.

  3. Ratio of agonist to antagonist effects: These drugs may be classified as agonists (receptor activators), antagonists (receptor blockers), or mixed agonist-antagonists.

B. Pharmacokinetics: Most drugs in this class are well absorbed, but morphine, hydromorphone, and oxymorphone undergo extensive first-pass metabolism when taken orally. Opioid drugs cross the placental barrier and exert effects on the fetus that can result in both respiratory depression and (with continuous exposure) physical dependence in neonates. The drugs undergo metabolism by hepatic enzymes, usually to glucuronide conjugates, prior to their elimination by the kidney. Depending on the specific drug, the duration of their analgesic effects ranges from 2 to 7 hours; this may increase in patients with liver disease. Certain glucuronide metabolites retain analgesic activity (eg, morphine-6-glucuronide); prolonged analgesia may occur in renal failure because of accumulation of active metabolites.

C. Mechanism of Action:

  1. Receptor mechanisms: The effects of opioid analgesics are usually explained in terms of their interactions with specific opioid receptors in the CNS and peripheral tissues. Some opioid receptors are located on primary afferents and spinal cord pain transmission neurons (ascending pathways) and on neurons in the midbrain and medulla (descending pathways) that function in pain modulation (Figure 30–2). Other opioid receptors, which may be involved in altering reactivity to pain, are located on neurons in the basal ganglia, hypothalamus, limbic structures and the cerebral cortex. Several receptor subtypes are selectively involved in opioid drug actions.

    a. Mu (μ) and delta (δ) receptors: Activation of mu and delta receptors appears to be responsible for supraspinal analgesia, euphoria, and respiratory and physical dependence effects.

    b. Kappa (κ) receptors: Kappa receptors appear to mediate spinal analgesia and sedative effects.

    c. Sigma (σ) receptors: Sigma receptors may be responsible for dysphoric effects, and for the hallucinogenic and cardiac stimulant properties of certain opioids.

  2. Opioid peptides: Opioid receptors are thought to be activated by endogenous chemicals under physiologic conditions. Several naturally occurring peptides (opiopeptins) that produce morphine-like effects have been identified; these include 2 pentapeptides (leu-enkephalin and met-enkephalin), a 17-amino-acid peptide (dynorphin), and a 31-amino-acid peptide (beta-endorphin). These peptides bind to opioid receptors and can be displaced from binding by opioid antagonists. Although it remains unclear if these peptides function as classical neurotransmitters, they appear to modulate transmission at many sites in the brain and spinal cord, and in primary afferents.

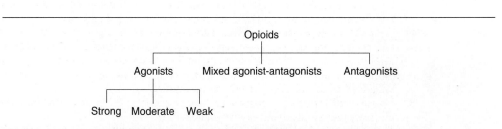

Figure 30–1. Subgroups of drugs that act on opioid receptors.

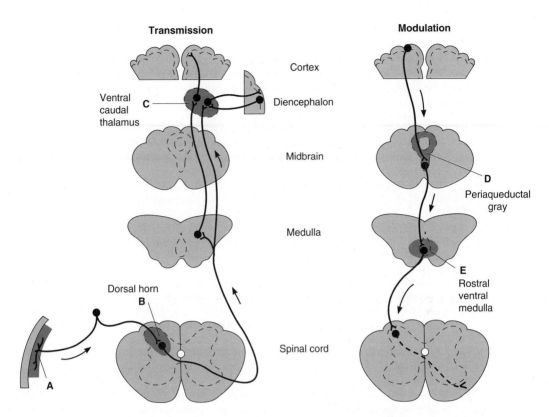

Figure 30–2. Putative sites of action (darker color) of opioid analgesics. On the left, sites of action on the pain transmission pathway from the periphery to the higher centers are shown. At **A,** possible direct action of opioids on painful peripheral tissues. **B:** Inhibition occurs in the spinal cord. **C:** Possible site of action in the thalamus. On the right, actions on pain-modulating neurons in the midbrain (site **D**) and the medulla (site **E**); these actions secondarily affect pain transmission pathways. (Reproduced, with permission, from Katzung BG [editor]: *Basic & Clinical Pharmacology,* 6th ed. Appleton & Lange, 1995.)

    3. Second messengers: In general, opioids *inhibit* synaptic activity; the mechanisms involved are not fully understood. Certain opioid receptors are coupled to adenylyl cyclase and modulate the functions of cyclic AMP. The acute actions of opioids also include inhibition of calcium entry into neurons and an increase in potassium ion conductance. These actions may be relevant to the observed inhibitory effects of exogenous opioids and opiopeptins on the electrical activity of neurons in many regions of the CNS.

D. Acute Effects: The acute effects of opioids include the following:
    1. Analgesia: The opioids are the most powerful drugs available for the relief of pain. Strong agonists (ie, those with the highest analgesic efficacy) include morphine, methadone, meperidine, and fentanyl. Codeine, hydrocodone, and oxycodone are mild-to-moderate agonists. Propoxyphene is a very weak agonist drug.
    2. Sedation and euphoria: These central effects may occur at doses below those required for maximal analgesia. Some patients experience dysphoria. At higher doses, the drugs may cause mental clouding and result in a stuporous state called narcosis.
    3. Respiratory depression: Opioid actions in the medulla lead to inhibition of the respiratory center, with decreased response to carbon dioxide challenge. Increased P_{CO_2} may cause cerebral vascular dilation, increased blood flow, and increased intracranial pressure.
    4. Antitussive actions: Suppression of the cough reflex, by unknown mechanisms, is the basis for the clinical use of opioids as antitussives.
    5. Nausea and vomiting: Nausea and vomiting are caused by activation of the chemoreceptor trigger zone and are increased by ambulation.
    6. Gastrointestinal effects: Constipation occurs through decreased intestinal peristalsis,

which is probably mediated by effects on opioid receptors in the enteric nervous system. This powerful action is the basis for the clinical use of these drugs as antidiarrheal agents.

7. **Smooth muscle:** Opioids cause contraction of biliary tract smooth muscle (which may cause biliary colic), increased ureteral and bladder sphincter tone, and a reduction in uterine tone that may contribute to a prolongation of labor.

8. **Miosis:** Pupillary constriction is a characteristic effect of opioids.

E. Chronic Effects: The results of chronic use of opioid analgesics include the following:

1. **Tolerance:** Marked tolerance develops to the above acute pharmacologic effects, with the exception of miosis and constipation. There is **cross-tolerance** between different opioid agonists.

2. **Dependence:** Psychologic and physical dependence is part of the basis for the abuse liability of many drugs in this group, particularly the strong agonists. Physical dependence is revealed on abrupt discontinuance as an **abstinence syndrome,** which includes rhinorrhea, lacrimation, chills, gooseflesh, muscle aches, diarrhea, anxiety, and hostility. A more intense state of **precipitated withdrawal** results when an opioid antagonist is administered to a physically dependent individual.

F. Clinical Uses: The most important clinical uses of these drugs are as follows:

1. **Analgesia:** Treatment of relatively constant moderate-to-severe pain. (See the Drug List for examples in each category.) Prolonged analgesia, with some reduction in adverse effects, can be achieved with epidural administration of certain strong agonist drugs, eg, morphine.

2. **Cough suppression:** Useful antitussive drugs include codeine and dextromethorphan.

3. **Treatment of diarrhea:** Selective antidiarrheal opioids include diphenoxylate and loperamide.

4. **Management of acute pulmonary edema:** Although largely replaced by furosemide, morphine is an effective agent in acute pulmonary edema (and was a drug of choice for many years).

5. **Anesthesia:** Opioids are used as preoperative medications and as intraoperative adjunctive agents in balanced anesthesia protocols. High dose intravenous opioids (eg, morphine, fentanyl) are often the major component of anesthesia for cardiac surgery.

6. **Opioid dependence:** Methadone, one of the longest-acting opioids, is used in the management of opioid withdrawal states and in maintenance programs for addicts. In withdrawal states, methadone permits a slow tapering of opioid effect, which diminishes the intensity of abstinence symptoms. In maintenance programs, the drug's prolonged action blocks the euphoria-inducing effects of doses of shorter-acting opioids (eg, heroin, morphine).

G. Toxicity: Most of the adverse effects of the opioid analgesics are predictable from their pharmacologic effects.

1. **Overdosage:** Coma, with marked respiratory depression and hypotension, may be fatal if untreated. Suspected overdosage is confirmed if intravenous injection of the antagonist drug, naloxone, results in prompt signs of recovery. Treatment involves the use of antagonists such as naloxone and other therapeutic measures, especially respiratory support.

2. **Drug interactions:** The most important drug interactions involving opioid analgesics are additive CNS depression with ethanol, sedative-hypnotics, anesthetics, antipsychotic drugs, tricyclic antidepressants, and antihistamines. Concomitant use of certain opioids (eg, meperidine) with MAO inhibitors increases the incidence of hyperpyrexic coma.

H. Agonist-Antagonist Drugs:

1. **Analgesic activity:** The analgesic activity of some mixed agonist-antagonists (eg, buprenorphine, butorphanol, nalbuphine) may be equivalent to that of strong agonists; others (eg, pentazocine) have only moderate efficacy.

2. **Receptors:** Butorphanol, nalbuphine, and pentazocine are kappa agonists. They have weak mu receptor activity (nalbuphine is a mu-receptor antagonist), which leads to unpredictable results if these drugs are used together with pure agonists. Buprenorphine, a partial agonist at mu receptors, has a long duration of effect since it binds strongly to such receptors; this property renders its effects resistant to naloxone reversal.

3. **Effects:** The mixed agonist-antagonist drugs usually cause sedation at analgesic doses; dizziness, sweating, and nausea may also occur. Anxiety, hallucinations, and nightmares are possible adverse effects. Respiratory depression may be less common than with pure agonists. Tolerance develops with chronic use but is less than the tolerance that develops to the pure agonists; there is minimal cross-tolerance. Physical dependence occurs, but the abuse liability of mixed agonist-antagonists drugs is less than that of morphine and meperidine.

I. **Opioid Antagonists:** Naloxone and naltrexone are pure opioid receptor antagonists that have few other effects at doses which produce marked antagonism of agonist effects. The major clinical use of the opioid antagonists is in the management of acute opioid overdose. At higher doses, naloxone may be useful in the treatment of shock and spinal cord injury, although the evidence for this is controversial. Naloxone has a short duration of action (1–2 hours). Naltrexone has a duration of action of 24–48 hours and is only available for oral use.

DRUG LIST

The following drugs are important members of the group discussed in this chapter. Prototypes should be learned in detail; features of the major variants should be known well enough to distinguish the variants from prototypes and from each other; the other significant agents should be recognized as belonging to a specific subclass.

Subclass	Prototypes	Major Variants	Other Significant Agents
Strong agonists	Morphine	Heroin, meperidine, methadone	Fentanyl
Moderate agonists	Codeine		Oxycodone, hydrocodone
Weak agonist	Propoxyphene		
Mixed agonist-antagonists	Pentazocine	Nalbuphine	Buprenorphine, butorphanol
Antagonists	Naloxone	Naltrexone	
Antitussives	Dextromethorphan		Codeine
Antidiarrheal	Diphenoxylate		

QUESTIONS

DIRECTIONS: Each of the numbered items or incomplete statements in this section is followed by answers or by completions of the sentence. Select the ONE lettered answer or completion that is BEST in each case.

1. All of the following statements about opioid analgesics are accurate EXCEPT
   (A) Opioid analgesics have no significant direct effects on the heart
   (B) Opioid analgesics stimulate the chemoreceptor trigger zone
   (C) Opioid analgesics relax smooth muscle of the bladder
   (D) Opioid analgesics decrease intestinal peristalsis
   (E) Opioid analgesics cross the placental barrier
2. Which ONE of the following actions of opioid analgesics is mediated via kappa receptors?
   (A) Supraspinal analgesia
   (B) Cerebral vascular dilation
   (C) Spinal analgesia
   (D) Euphoria
   (E) Physical dependence
3. Opiopeptins (opioid peptides) are released from larger precursor peptides. Which ONE of the following is released from pro-opiomelanocortin (POMC)?
   (A) Beta-endorphin
   (B) Leu-enkephalin

    (C) Somatostatin
    (D) Dynorphin
    (E) Substance P

4. With continued use of strong opioid analgesics, tolerance develops to all of the following effects EXCEPT
    (A) Sedation
    (B) Analgesia
    (C) Pupillary constriction
    (D) Decreased response to carbon dioxide challenge
    (E) Euphoria

5. Which ONE of the following is LEAST likely to be a contraindication to the use of morphine?
    (A) Head injury
    (B) Borderline respiratory reserve
    (C) Adrenal insufficiency
    (D) Pregnancy
    (E) Pulmonary edema

Items 6–7: A heroin addict comes to the emergency room in an anxious and agitated state. He complains of chills, muscle aches, and diarrhea; he has also been vomiting. His symptoms include hyperventilation and hyperthermia. He claims to have had an intravenous "fix" approximately 12 hours ago. The physician notes that pupil size is greater than normal.

6. What is the most likely cause of these signs and symptoms?
    (A) The patient has overdosed with an opioid
    (B) These are early signs of the toxicity of MPTP, a contaminant in "street heroin"
    (C) The signs and symptoms are those of the abstinence syndrome
    (D) In addition to opioids, the patient has been taking barbiturates
    (E) The patient has hepatitis B

7. Which of the following will be most effective in alleviating the symptoms experienced by this patient?
    (A) Naloxone
    (B) Codeine
    (C) Acetaminophen
    (D) Methadone
    (E) Diazepam

DIRECTIONS: The following section consists of a list of four to twenty-six lettered options followed by several numbered items. For each numbered item, select the ONE option that is most closely associated with it. Each answer may be selected once, more than once, or not at all.
    (A) Dextromethorphan
    (B) Nalbuphine
    (C) Oxycodone
    (D) Codeine
    (E) Naltrexone
    (F) Fentanyl
    (G) Propoxyphene
    (H) Methadone
    (I) Diphenoxylate
    (J) Meperidine

8. This drug has analgesic efficacy equivalent to that of morphine; the agent is an antagonist at mu receptors

9. This antagonist drug has been proposed as a maintenance drug in treatment programs for opioid addicts; a single oral dose will block the effects of injected heroin for up to 48 hours

10. This drug is an effective antitussive; it is free of analgesic and addictive properties and only rarely causes constipation

11. This drug is a full agonist at opioid receptors. It has analgesic activity equivalent to that of morphine, but with a longer duration of action. Withdrawal signs on abrupt discontinuance are milder than those with morphine

12. In some studies, this opioid agonist is reported to have analgesic efficacy no greater than that of a placebo; the drug may cause seizures in overdosage

ANSWERS

1. The opioids commonly cause contraction of smooth muscle. They constrict biliary ducts and increase both ureteral and bladder tone. Increased urethral sphincter tone may precipitate urinary retention. Although opioids increase intestinal smooth muscle tone, they reduce propulsive movements (peristalsis). In contrast, opioids decrease uterine tone—probably via central mechanisms—and may prolong labor. The answer is **(C)**.

2. Kappa receptor activation does not appear to be responsible for supraspinal analgesia, dependence, euphoria, or respiratory depression. Increases in cerebral blood flow and (possibly) increased intracranial pressure result from the respiratory depressant actions of opioid analgesics. The latter effects are due to increased arterial P_{CO_2}, which results from mu receptor inhibition of the medullary respiratory center. However, the activation of kappa receptors contributes to analgesia at the spinal level and is probably responsible for sedative actions of the opioids. The answer is **(C)**.

3. Pro-opiomelanocortin (POMC) contains both beta-endorphin and met-enkephalin, in addition to ACTH and a melanocyte stimulating peptide. The answer is **(A)**.

4. Tolerance develops most readily when large doses of opioid agonists are given at short intervals. Marked tolerance may develop to the analgesic, sedative, euphoriant, emetic, and respiratory depressant effects of these drugs. Tolerance does not develop to the miotic action and the constipating effects of opioid agonists. The answer is **(C)**.

5. Intravenous morphine effectively relieves dyspnea from pulmonary edema associated with left ventricular failure. The mechanism is not clear but may involve a decrease in perception of shortness of breath, relief of anxiety, and reductions in cardiac preload (decreased venous tone) and afterload (decreased peripheral resistance). The answer is **(E)**.

6. The signs and symptoms are those of withdrawal in a patient physically dependent on an opioid agonist. Such signs and symptoms usually start within 6–10 hours after the last dose; their intensity depends on the degree of physical dependence that has developed. Peak effects usually occur at 36–48 hours. Mydriasis is a prominent feature of the abstinence syndrome; other symptoms include rhinorrhea, lacrimation, piloerection, and yawning. The answer is **(C)**.

7. Prevention of signs and symptoms of withdrawal after chronic use of a strong opiate like heroin requires replacement with another strong opioid analgesic drug. Codeine will not be effective. The antagonist, naloxone, will actually precipitate a severe abstinence syndrome in a person who is physically dependent on opioids. Potential beneficial effects of diazepam are restricted to relief of anxiety and agitation. The answer is **(D)**.

8. Mixed agonist-antagonist drugs may have analgesic efficacy equivalent to that of strong agonists. This is true for nalbuphine despite its antagonist action at mu receptors. Use of drugs in the agonist-antagonist subclass may lead to unpredictable results if combined with full agonists; agonist-antagonist drugs may precipitate an abstinence syndrome by blocking opioid receptors. These drugs are less likely to cause respiratory depression than full agonist opioid analgesics. When such depression occurs, it may be difficult to reverse with opioid antagonists. The answer is **(B)**.

9. The opioid antagonist, naltrexone, has a much longer half-life than naloxone, with effects that may last as long as 2 days. A high degree of client compliance would be required for naltrexone to be of value in treatment programs. The answer is **(E)**.

10. Dextromethorphan, an effective antitussive drug, is the dextrorotatory stereoisomer of levorphanol. Dextromethorphan has no appreciable analgesic activity and minimal abuse liability. In comparison with codeine, also an effective antitussive, dextromethorphan causes less constipation. The answer is **(A)**.

11. The full agonists—fentanyl, hydromorphone, meperidine, methadone and oxymorphone—are all equivalent to morphine in analgesic efficacy. Methadone has the greatest bioavailability of the drugs used orally, and its effects are more prolonged. Tolerance and physical dependence develop and dissipate more slowly with methadone than with morphine. These properties underlie the use of methadone for detoxification and in maintenance programs. The answer is **(H)**.

12. Propoxyphene is chemically related to methadone but has very low analgesic activity. Propoxyphene causes a small additive analgesic effect when used in combination with aspirin or acetaminophen. Overdosage of propoxyphene results in severe toxicity, including respiratory depression, circulatory collapse, pulmonary edema, and seizures. The answer is **(G)**.

31

Drugs of Abuse

OBJECTIVES

You should be able to:

- List the most important factors that contribute to drug abuse.
- Describe the major actions of drugs that are commonly abused in the USA.
- Describe the major signs and symptoms of withdrawal from opioid analgesics and from sedative-hypnotics, including ethanol.
- Identify the most likely causes of fatalities from commonly abused agents.

Learn the definitions that follow.

Table 31–1. Definitions.	
Term	**Definition**
Tolerance	A decreased response to a drug, necessitating larger doses to achieve the same effect. This can result from increased disposition of the drug (metabolic tolerance), an ability to compensate for the effects of a drug (behavioral tolerance), or changes in receptor or effector systems involved in drug actions (functional tolerance)
Psychologic dependence	Compulsive drug-using behavior in which the individual uses the drug for personal satisfaction, often in the face of known risks to health
Physical dependence	A state characterized by signs and symptoms, frequently the opposite of those caused by a drug, when it is withdrawn from chronic use or when the dose is abruptly lowered. Psychologic dependence usually precedes physical dependence
Abstinence syndrome	A term used to describe the signs and symptoms that occur on withdrawal of a drug in a physically-dependent person
Controlled substance	A drug deemed to have abuse liability that is listed on governmental Schedules of Controlled Substances[1]. Such schedules categorize illicit drugs, control prescribing practices, and mandate penalties for illegal possession, manufacture, and sale of listed drugs. Controlled substance schedules are presumed to reflect current attitudes toward substance abuse; therefore, which drugs are regulated depends on a social judgment
Designer drug	A synthetic derivative of a drug, with slightly modified structure but no major change in pharmacodynamic action. Circumvention of the Schedules of Controlled Drugs is a motivation for the illicit synthesis of designer drugs

[1] An example of such a schedule promulgated by the United States Drug Enforcement Agency is shown in Table 31–2. Note that the criteria given by the agency do not always reflect the actual pharmacologic properties of the drugs.

CONCEPTS

Drug abuse is usually taken to mean the use of an illicit drug, or the excessive or nonmedical use of a licit drug. It also denotes the deliberate use of chemicals that generally are not considered drugs by the lay public but may be harmful to the user. The motivation for drug abuse appears to be the anticipated feeling of pleasure derived from the CNS effects of the drug. If physical dependence is present, prevention of an abstinence syndrome acts as a reinforcement to continued drug abuse.

MAJOR CATEGORIES OF DRUGS OF ABUSE

A. Sedative-Hypnotics:

The sedative-hypnotic drugs are responsible for many cases of drug abuse in the United States, Europe, and Japan. The group includes **ethanol, barbiturates,** and **benzodiazepines,** all of which are more readily available to the general public than are opioids, cocaine, or hallucinogens. Benzodiazepines are the most commonly prescribed drugs for anxiety and, as Schedule IV drugs, are judged by the U.S. government to have low abuse liability (Table 31–2). Ethanol is not listed in schedules of controlled substances with abuse liability because it is rarely prescribed and the schedules apply to prescription drugs.

1. **Effects:** Sedative-hypnotics are CNS depressants, and their effects are enhanced by concomitant use of opioid analgesics, antipsychotic agents, and antihistamines with sedative properties. Acute overdoses commonly result in death through depression of the medullary respiratory and cardiovascular centers. Sedative-hypnotics reduce inhibitions, suppress anxiety, and produce relaxation. All of these actions are thought to induce development of psychologic dependence.

2. **Withdrawal:** Physical dependence occurs with continued use of sedative-hypnotics; the signs and symptoms of the abstinence syndrome are most pronounced with drugs that have a half-life of less than 24 hours (eg, ethanol, secobarbital, methaqualone). However, physical dependence may occur with any sedative-hypnotic, including the longer-acting benzodiazepines. The most important signs of withdrawal derive from excessive **CNS stimulation,** and include anxiety, tremor, nausea and vomiting, delirium, and hallucinations. **Convulsions** are not uncommon and may be life-threatening. Treatment involves substitution with a long-acting sedative-hypnotic (eg, diazepam) to suppress the acute withdrawal syndrome, followed by a gradual decrease in dosage. Clonidine or propranolol may also be of value. A syndrome of **therapeutic withdrawal** has occurred on discontinuance of sedative-hypnotics after long-term treatment. In addition to the symptoms of classic withdrawal listed above, this syndrome includes weight loss, paresthesias, and headache. (See Chapters 21 and 22 for additional details.)

B. **Opioid Analgesics:**

1. **Effects:** The most commonly abused drugs in this group are **heroin, morphine, oxycodone,** and—among health professionals—**meperidine** and **fentanyl.** The effects of intravenous heroin are described by abusers as a "rush" or orgasmic feeling followed by euphoria and then sedation. Intravenous administration of opioid analgesics is associated with rapid development of tolerance and psychologic and physical dependence. Oral administration or smoking of opioids causes milder effects, with a slower onset of tolerance and dependence. Death from illicit use of opioids is usually caused by respiratory depression; such overdosage is often the result of obtaining an unusually potent (ie, purer) batch of the drug.

2. **Withdrawal:** Deprivation of opioids in physically dependent individuals leads to an abstinence syndrome that includes lacrimation, rhinorrhea, yawning, sweating, weakness, gooseflesh ("cold turkey"), nausea and vomiting, tremor, and hyperpnea. Although extremely unpleasant, withdrawal from opioids is rarely fatal (unlike withdrawal from sedative-hypnotics). Treatment involves replacement of the illicit drug with a pharmacologically equivalent agent (eg, methadone), followed by slow "tapering off."

C. **Stimulants:** A chemically heterogeneous subgroup, the stimulants include caffeine, nicotine, amphetamines, and cocaine.

Table 31–2. Illustrations from Schedules of Controlled Drugs.[1]

Schedule	Criteria	Examples
I	No medical use; high addiction potential	Heroin, LSD, mescaline, methaqualone, PCP, DOM, MDMA
II	Medical use; high addiction potential	Strong opioid agonists, cocaine, short half-life barbiturates, amphetamines, cannabinols
III	Medical use; moderate potential for dependence	Moderate opioid agonists (codeine), thiopental
IV	Medical use; low abuse potential	Benzodiazepines, chloral hydrate, meprobamate, weak opioid agonists

[1] Adapted, with permission, from Katzung BG (editor): *Basic & Clinical Pharmacology*, 6th ed. Appleton & Lange, 1995)

1. **Caffeine and nicotine:**
   a. **Effects:** Caffeine (in beverages) and nicotine (in tobacco products) are legal in most Western cultures, even though they have adverse medical effects. In the USA, cigarette smoking is now the major preventable cause of death; tobacco use is associated with a high incidence of cardiovascular, respiratory, and neoplastic disease. Psychologic dependence on caffeine and nicotine has been recognized for some time. More recently, demonstration of abstinence signs and symptoms has provided evidence for physical dependence.
   b. **Withdrawal:** Withdrawal from caffeine is accompanied by lethargy, irritability, and headache. The anxiety and mental discomfort experienced on discontinuing nicotine are major impediments to "kicking the habit."
   c. **Toxicity:** Acute toxicity from overdosage of caffeine and nicotine is rare when they are used in their usual forms but includes excessive CNS stimulation with tremor, insomnia, and nervousness; cardiac stimulation and arrhythmias; and, in the case of nicotine, prominent autonomic signs (Chapters 6 and 7).

2. **Amphetamines:**
   a. **Effects:** Amphetamines cause a feeling of euphoria and self-confidence that contributes to the rapid development of psychologic dependence. Drugs in this class include **dextroamphetamine** and **methamphetamine** ("speed"), a crystal form of which ("ice") can be smoked. Chronic high-dose abuse leads to a psychotic state (with delusions and paranoia) that is difficult to differentiate from schizophrenia.
   b. **Tolerance and withdrawal:** Tolerance can be marked, and an abstinence syndrome, characterized by increased appetite, sleepiness, exhaustion, and mental depression, can occur upon withdrawal.
   c. **Congeners of amphetamines:** Several chemical congeners of amphetamines have hallucinogenic properties. These include 2,5-dimethoxy-4-methylamphetamine (**DOM, STP**), methylene dioxyamphetamine (**MDA**), and methylene dioxymethamphetamine (**MDMA, "Ecstasy"**). The last compound is purported to facilitate communication in psychotherapy. These derivatives have been reported to be neurotoxic to serotonergic neurons in the brains of animals, with uncertain toxic consequences in humans.

3. **Cocaine:** Cocaine has marked amphetamine-like effects ("super-speed"). Its abuse has reached epidemic proportions in the USA, partly because of the availability of a free-base form ("crack") that can be smoked. The euphoria, self-confidence, and mental alertness produced by cocaine are short lasting and positively reinforce its continued use.
   a. **Effects:** Overdoses with cocaine commonly result in fatalities from arrhythmias, seizures, or respiratory depression. Cardiac toxicity is due partly to blockade of norepinephrine reuptake by cocaine; its local anesthetic action contributes to the production of seizures. In addition, the powerful vasoconstrictive action of cocaine may lead to severe hypertensive episodes, resulting in myocardial infarcts and strokes.
   b. **Withdrawal:** The abstinence syndrome following withdrawal from cocaine is similar to that following amphetamine discontinuance. Severe depression of mood is common and strongly reinforces the compulsion to use the drug.

D. **Hallucinogens:**
   1. **Phencyclidine:** The arylcyclohexylamine drug **phencyclidine** (PCP, "angel dust") is probably the most dangerous of the currently popular hallucinogenic agents. Psychotic reactions are common with PCP, and impaired judgment often leads to reckless behavior. This drug should be classified as a **psychotomimetic**. Effects of overdosage with PCP include marked hypertension and seizures, which may be fatal.
   2. **Miscellaneous hallucinogenic agents:** Several drugs with hallucinogenic effects have been classified as having abuse liability; these drugs include **lysergic acid diethylamide** (LSD), **mescaline,** and **psilocybin.** Hallucinogenic effects may also occur with scopolamine. Terms used to describe the CNS effects of such drugs include "psychedelic" and "mind-revealing." The perceptual and psychologic effects of such drugs are usually accompanied by marked somatic effects, particularly nausea, weakness, and paresthesias. Panic reactions ("bad trips") may also occur. There is little evidence that use of these agents leads to the development of physical dependence.

E. **Marijuana:**
1. **Classification:**   Marijuana ("grass") is a collective term for the psychoactive constituents present in crude extracts of the plant *Cannabis sativa* (hemp), the active principles of which include the compounds **tetrahydrocannabinol (THC),** cannabidiol (CBD), and cannabinol (CBN). **Hashish** is a partially purified material that is more potent.
2. **Effects:**   CNS effects of marijuana include a feeling of being "high," with euphoria, disinhibition, uncontrollable laughter, changes in perception, and achievement of a dreamlike state. Mental concentration may be difficult. Vasodilation occurs and pulse rate is characteristically increased. Habitual users show a reddened conjunctiva. A mild withdrawal state has been noted only in heavy long-term users of marijuana. The dangers of marijuana use concern its impairment of judgment and reflexes, effects that are potentiated by concomitant use of sedative-hypnotics, including ethanol. The specific hazards of long-term use are unknown. Potential therapeutic effects of marijuana include its ability to decrease intraocular pressure and its antiemetic actions. **Dronabinol** (a controlled-substance pharmaceutical form of THC) is used to combat nausea in cancer chemotherapy.

F. **Inhalants:**   Certain gases or volatile liquids are abused because they provide a feeling of euphoria or disinhibition. This class includes the following agents:
1. **Anesthetics:**   This group includes nitrous oxide, chloroform, and diethylether. These agents are hazardous because they affect judgment and induce loss of consciousness. Inhalation of nitrous oxide as the pure gas (no oxygen) has caused asphyxia and death. Ether is highly flammable.
2. **Industrial solvents:**   Solvents and a wide range of volatile compounds are present in commercial products such as gasoline, paint thinners, aerosol propellants, glues, rubber cements, and shoe polish. Because of their ready availability, these substances are most frequently abused by children in their early adolescence. Active ingredients that have been identified include benzene, hexane, methylethylketone, toluene, and trichloroethylene. Many of these are toxic to the liver, kidney, lungs, bone marrow, and peripheral nerves, and cause brain damage in animals.
3. **Organic nitrites:**   Amyl nitrite, isobutylnitrite, and other organic nitrites are referred to as "poppers" and are alleged to be sex enhancers. Inhalation of the nitrites causes dizziness, tachycardia, hypotension, and flushing. With the exception of methemoglobinemia, few serious adverse effects have been reported.

DRUG LIST

The following drugs are important members of the group discussed in this chapter. Prototypes should be learned in detail; features of the major variants should be known well enough to distinguish the variants from prototypes and from each other; the other significant agents should be recognized as belonging to a specific subclass.

Subclass	Prototype	Major Variants	Other Significant Agents
Sedative-hypnotics	Ethanol, phenobarbital, chlordiazepoxide	Secobarbital, diazepam	Methaqualone, meprobamate
Opioids	Heroin	Meperidine	Strong agonist opioid analgesics
Stimulants	Amphetamine	Methamphetamine, phenmetrazine	DOM, MDA, MDMA
	Cocaine, caffeine, nicotine		
Hallucinogens	LSD, phencyclidine	Mescaline	Scopolamine
Marijuana	"Grass"	Hashish	Dronabinol
Inhalants	Nitrous oxide, toluene	Ether	Chloroform, benzene
	Amyl nitrite	Isobutylnitrite	

QUESTIONS

DIRECTIONS: Each of the numbered items or incomplete statements in this section is followed by answers or by completions of the sentence. Select the ONE lettered answer or completion that is BEST in each case.

1. Which one of the following statements about the abuse of sedative-hypnotics is MOST correct?
   (A) Discontinuance of normal therapeutic doses of benzodiazepines is not followed by withdrawal signs
   (B) The abstinence syndrome is less severe following withdrawal from short-acting barbiturates than from phenobarbital
   (C) Chlordiazepoxide is commonly used in the detoxification of alcoholic patients
   (D) With chronic use, tolerance to the respiratory depressant effects of barbiturates is less complete than tolerance to their sedative effects
   (E) Flumazenil is useful in overdoses of benzodiazepines, ethanol, or barbiturates

2. All of the following statements about abuse of the opioid analgesics are accurate EXCEPT
   (A) A patient experiencing withdrawal from heroin is free of the symptoms of abstinence in 5–7 days
   (B) In withdrawal from opioids, clonidine may be useful in reducing symptoms caused by sympathetic overactivity
   (C) Lacrimation, rhinorrhea, yawning, and sweating are early signs of withdrawal from opioid analgesics
   (D) Naloxone may precipitate a severe withdrawal state in abusers of opioid analgesics
   (E) Methadone alleviates most of the symptoms of heroin withdrawal

3. All of the following statements about the CNS stimulants are accurate EXCEPT
   (A) A paranoid schizophrenic state is characteristic of high dose amphetamine abuse
   (B) Cocaine has potent vasoconstrictor and local anesthetic actions
   (C) MDMA is reported to be neurotoxic to brain serotonergic systems
   (D) While psychologic dependence to amphetamines is strong, physical dependence does not occur
   (E) Treatment of cocaine overdose includes the use of diazepam and propranolol

4. All of the following statements about hallucinogens are accurate EXCEPT
   (A) Mescaline and related hallucinogens are thought to exert their CNS actions through serotonergic systems in the brain
   (B) Acute psychotic reactions occur commonly with the use of LSD
   (C) Phencyclidine is unique among hallucinogens in that animals will self-administer it
   (D) Dilated pupils, tachycardia, tremor, and alertness are characteristic effects of psilocybin
   (E) Scopolamine can be anticipated to cause ocular dysfunction, dry mouth, and urinary retention

5. Pharmacologic effects of marijuana include all of the following EXCEPT
   (A) Increased pulse rate
   (B) Pupillary constriction
   (C) Hypotension
   (D) Conjunctival reddening
   (E) Decreased psychomotor performance

6. All of the following statements about inhalants are accurate EXCEPT
   (A) Fluorocarbons may cause sudden death due to cardiac arrhythmias
   (B) Dizziness, hypotension, tachycardia and flushing last only a few minutes following isobutyl nitrite inhalation
   (C) Methemoglobinemia is a common toxicologic problem following repetitive inhalation of industrial solvents
   (D) Euphoria, numbness, tingling sensations, with visual and auditory disturbances occur in most persons who inhale 35% nitrous oxide
   (E) Abuse of diethylether can be a "disinhibiting" experience

Items 7–8: A college student is brought to the emergency room by friends. The physician is informed that he had taken "a drug" and that he "went crazy." The patient is agitated and delirious. Several persons are required to hold him down. His skin is warm and sweaty, and his pupils are dilated. Bowel sounds are normal. Signs and symptoms include tachycardia, marked hypertension, hyperthermia, increased muscle tone, and both horizontal and vertical nystagmus.

7. The most likely cause of these signs and symptoms is intoxication due to
   (A) Scopolamine
   (B) Heroin
   (C) Hashish
   (D) Phencyclidine
   (E) Secobarbital

8. The management of this patient is likely to include all of the following EXCEPT
   (A) Control of hyperthermia with cooling measures
   (B) Alkalinization of the urine to increase drug elimination
   (C) Administration of benzodiazepines
   (D) Nasogastric suction
   (E) Administration of haloperidol if the patient develops psychotic symptoms

ANSWERS

1. Even normal doses of sedative hypnotics (including benzodiazepines) can lead to physical dependence. The abstinence syndrome is more severe with short-acting sedative-hypnotics. Diazepam is the drug of choice in sedative-hypnotic detoxification. Only a minor degree of tolerance develops to respiratory depressant actions of barbiturates, compared to that for sedative effects. Flumazenil is only useful in antagonizing benzodiazepines. The answer is **(D)**.

2. A secondary phase of heroin withdrawal may last 26–30 weeks. Methadone is commonly used in detoxification of the heroin addict because it is a strong agonist, has high oral bioavailability, and has a relatively long half-life. The answer is **(A)**.

3. Abuse of amphetamines results in marked tolerance and both psychologic and physical dependence. Withdrawal is manifested by signs and symptoms opposite to those produced by such drugs. The answer is **(D)**.

4. Psilocybin, mescaline, and LSD have similar central and peripheral effects. While adverse psychologic effects are common, acute psychotic reactions occur *infrequently*, usually in persons with a past history of psychotic disorders. Unlike most hallucinogens, phencyclidine acts as a positive reinforcer of self-administration in animals. The answer is **(B)**.

5. Two of the most characteristic signs of marijuana use are increased pulse rate and reddening of the conjunctiva. Pupil size is *not changed* by marijuana. The answer is **(B)**.

6. Toxic inhalants including heptane, hexane, methylethylketone, toluene, and trichloroethylene may result in central and peripheral neurotoxicity, liver and kidney damage, and pulmonary disease. Industrial solvents *rarely* cause methemoglobinemia, but this may occur following excessive use of nitrites. The answer is **(C)**.

7. The signs and symptoms point to phencyclidine intoxication. The presence of both horizontal and vertical nystagmus is pathognomonic. The answer is **(D)**.

8. Overdose with phencyclidine is dangerous. The basic principles of treatment are to maintain ventilation and to control seizures, blood pressure, and hyperthermia. Phencyclidine is secreted into the stomach, so removal of the drug may be hastened by continual nasogastric suction. Phencyclidine is a weak base, and its renal elimination is accelerated by urinary *acidification*. Treatment with antipsychotic drugs may be appropriate if psychotic symptoms follow the acute intoxication. The answer is **(B)**.

Part VI. Drugs with Important Actions on Blood, Inflammation, & Gout

32 Agents Used in Anemias

OBJECTIVES

You should be able to:

- Describe the normal mechanism of regulation of iron storage in the body.
- List the major forms of iron used in the therapy of anemias.
- List the anemias for which iron supplementation is indicated and those for which it is contraindicated.
- Describe the acute and chronic toxicity of iron.
- Describe the clinical applications of Vitamin B_{12} and folic acid.
- Describe the major hazard involved in the use of folic acid as sole therapy for megaloblastic anemia.
- Describe the major bone marrow colony-stimulating factors.

CONCEPTS

TYPES OF ANEMIAS

A. Iron & Vitamin Deficiency Anemias: Microcytic hypochromic anemia, caused by iron deficiency, is the most common type of anemia. Megaloblastic anemias are caused by a deficiency of vitamin B_{12} or folic acid, cofactors required for the normal maturation of red blood cells. Pernicious anemia, the most common type of vitamin B_{12}-deficiency anemia, is caused by a defect in the synthesis of intrinsic factor, a protein required for efficient absorption of dietary vitamin B_{12}.

B. Other Anemias: Anemias caused by radiation or cancer chemotherapy involve suppression of bone marrow stem cells. Development of techniques for recombinant DNA-directed synthesis of marrow growth factors (erythropoietin and the white cell colony-stimulating factors, filgrastim and sargramostim) now make possible the treatment of more patients with depressed marrow activity. Anemias due to marrow depression have also been treated—in special cases—by marrow transplantation.

C. Prototypes: Figure 32–1 illustrates the major drugs discussed in this chapter.

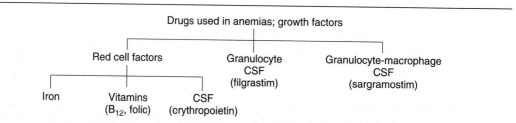

Figure 32–1. Drugs used in the treatment of anemias and bone marrow depression. CSF, colony-stimulating factor.

IRON

A. Role of Iron: Iron is the essential metallic component of heme, the molecule responsible for the bulk of oxygen transport in the blood. Although most of the iron in the body is present in hemoglobin (heme plus globin), an important fraction is bound to transferrin, a transport protein, and to ferritin and hemosiderin, two storage proteins. Deficiency of iron occurs most often in women because of menstrual blood loss and in vegetarians or malnourished individuals because of inadequate dietary iron intake.

B. Regulation of Iron Stores: Regulation of body iron content occurs through modulation of absorption in the intestine. There is no mechanism for the efficient excretion of iron. As a result, failure of gastrointestinal regulation of iron absorption is one cause of diseases associated with excess iron stores, eg, hemochromatosis.

   1. Absorption: Iron is absorbed as the ferrous ion and oxidized in the mucosal cell to the ferric form.

   2. Storage: Trivalent ferric iron can be stored in the mucosa (bound to ferritin) or carried elsewhere in the body (bound to transferrin). Excess iron is stored in protein-bound form as hemosiderin in the reticuloendothelial system. An accumulation of hemosiderin occurs in hemolytic anemias (anemias caused by excess destruction of red blood cells), and in hemochromatosis.

   3. Elimination: Minimal amounts of iron are lost from the body with sweat and saliva and in exfoliated skin and intestinal mucosal cells, but as noted above, there is no efficient method for excretion of excess iron.

C. Clinical Use: Iron deficiency anemia is the only indication for the use of iron. Iron deficiency can be diagnosed from red blood cell changes (microcytic cell size, diminished hemoglobin content of blood) and from measurements of serum and bone marrow iron stores. The disease is treated by dietary ferrous iron supplementation and, in special cases, by parenteral administration of the metal (see Drug List). Iron should *not* be given in hemolytic anemia because iron stores are elevated, not depressed, in this type of anemia.

D. Toxicity of Iron:

   1. Signs and symptoms: Acute iron intoxication is most common in children and usually occurs as a result of accidental ingestion of iron supplementation tablets. Depending on the dose, necrotizing gastroenteritis, shock, metabolic acidosis, coma, and death may result. Chronic toxicity occurs most often in individuals who must receive frequent transfusions (eg, patients with sickle cell anemia) and in those with hemochromatosis, an inherited abnormality of iron absorption.

   2. Treatment of acute iron intoxication: Immediate treatment is necessary and usually consists of removal of unabsorbed tablets from the gut, correction of acid-base and electrolyte abnormalities, and administration of iron-complexing agents. The latter agents include oral phosphate or carbonate salts (to precipitate unabsorbed iron) and parenteral deferoxamine, which chelates circulating iron.

   3. Treatment of chronic iron toxicity: Treatment of hemochromatosis is usually by phlebotomy, which efficiently removes approximately 250 mg iron with each unit of blood removed.

VITAMIN B$_{12}$

A. Role of Vitamin B$_{12}$: Vitamin B$_{12}$ (cobalamin), a cobalt-containing molecule, is (along with folic acid) a cofactor in the transfer of one-carbon units, a step necessary for the synthesis of DNA. Impairment of DNA synthesis affects all cells, but because red blood cells must be produced continuously, deficiency of either B$_{12}$ or folic acid usually manifests first as anemia.

B. Pharmacokinetics: Vitamin B$_{12}$ is produced only by bacteria; this vitamin cannot be synthesized by multicellular organisms. It is absorbed from the gastrointestinal tract in the presence of intrinsic factor, a product of the parietal cells of the stomach. Vitamin B$_{12}$ is stored in the liver in large amounts; a normal individual has enough to last 5 years. Plasma transport is accomplished by binding to transcobalamin II, a glycoprotein. When parenteral vitamin B_{12} is given, any in excess of the transport protein binding capacity (about 50–100 µg) is excreted. The two available forms of vitamin B_{12}, cyanocobalamin and hydroxocobalamin, have similar pharmacokinetics, but hydroxocobalamin is somewhat more firmly bound to plasma proteins and has a longer circulating half-life.

C. **Pharmacodynamics:** Vitamin B_{12} is essential in two reactions: conversion of methyl-malonyl-CoA to succinyl-CoA and conversion of homocysteine to methionine. The first of these reactions appears to be essential for lipid metabolism; a deficiency of vitamin B_{12} results in abnormalities of the lipids essential for normal neuronal function. The second reaction, conversion of homocysteine to methionine, is linked to folic acid metabolism and DNA synthesis. This reaction is essential for normal production of red blood cells.

D. **Clinical Use & Toxicity:** Vitamin B_{12} is available as hydroxocobalamin and cyanocobalamin, which have equivalent effects. The major application is in the treatment of naturally occurring pernicious anemia and anemia caused by gastric resection. Because B_{12}-deficiency anemia is almost always caused by inadequate absorption, therapy should be parenteral. Although oral therapy may suffice for maintenance, massive doses must be used. In addition to anemia, an important manifestation of vitamin B_{12} deficiency is the development of neurologic defects, which may become irreversible if not treated promptly. Treatment is by replacement of vitamin B_{12}, using parenteral therapy.

Because hydroxocobalamin binds cyanide ion to form cyanocobalamin, hydroxocobalamin has also been used successfully to treat cyanide toxicity caused by nitroprusside. Neither form of vitamin B_{12} has significant toxicity.

FOLIC ACID

A. **Role of Folic Acid:** Folic acid is necessary for the synthesis of purines and for the formation of thymidylic acid. Because of the need for continuous production of red cells, anemia is usually the first sign of folic acid deficiency. Recent studies indicate that deficiency of folic acid during pregnancy increases the risk of neural tube defects in the fetus.

B. **Pharmacokinetics:** Folic acid is also known as pteroylglutamic acid. It is readily absorbed from the gastrointestinal tract. Only modest amounts are stored in the body, so a decrease in dietary intake is followed by anemia within a few months.

C. **Pharmacodynamics:** Folic acid is necessary for the transfer of one-carbon fragments in the synthesis of purine and pyrimidine bases. Therefore it is most important in the health of rapidly dividing cells, in which DNA must be rapidly synthesized. (For the same reason, *anti*folate drugs are useful in the treatment of various infections and neoplasms.)

D. **Clinical Use & Toxicity:** Folic acid deficiency is most often caused by dietary insufficiency or by malabsorption. Anemia due to folic acid deficiency is readily treated by oral folic acid supplementation. Folic acid supplements will also correct the anemia but not the neurologic deficits of vitamin B_{12} deficiency. Therefore, vitamin B_{12} deficiency must be ruled out before selecting folic acid as the sole therapeutic agent in megaloblastic anemia. Folic acid has no recognized toxicity.

ERYTHROPOIETIN & COLONY-STIMULATING FACTORS

Almost a dozen glycoprotein hormones have been discovered that regulate the differentiation and maturation of stem cells within the bone marrow. Three substances are now available, through recombinant DNA technology, for the treatment of various conditions associated with bone marrow depression. Other members of this group are under study.

A. **Erythropoietin:** Erythropoietin is produced by the kidney; suppression of its synthesis is responsible for the anemia of renal failure. The substance stimulates the production of red cells by combination with specific receptors on erythroid progenitors in the bone marrow.

Erythropoietin is used for the treatment of anemias associated with renal failure and with bone marrow failure, eg, following transplantation or treatment with drugs that are toxic to the bone marrow. The drug has also been used to accelerate the replacement of red cells removed through phlebotomy. Toxicity is minimal and usually the result of excessive increase in hematocrit.

B. Sargramostim: Sargramostim (granulocyte-macrophage colony-stimulating factor, GM-CSF) stimulates the production of granulocytes and macrophages. The drug is used to accelerate the recovery of granulocytes after cancer chemotherapy and other marrow-suppressing therapies. This agent reduces the incidence of infection following bone marrow suppression, presumably by strengthening natural defense mechanisms. Sargramostim also stimulates production of red cells and platelets, although these effects are of far less importance. Toxicities include fever, arthralgias, and capillary damage with edema.

C. Filgrastim: Filgrastim (granulocyte colony-stimulating factor, G-CSF) stimulates the production of neutrophils. This agent is much more selective than sargramostim, having no detectable effect on cell lines other than granulocytes. However, filgrastim's clinical applications duplicate those of sargramostim. Toxicity is minimal but can include bone pain.

DRUG LIST

The following drugs are important members of the group discussed in this chapter. Prototypes should be learned in detail; features of the major variants should be known well enough to distinguish the variants from prototypes and from each other; the other significant agents should be recognized as belonging to a specific subclass.

Subclass	Prototype	Major Variants	Other Significant Agents
Oral iron supplements	Ferrous sulfate		Ferrous gluconate, ferrous fumarate
Parenteral iron	Iron dextran		
Vitamin B_{12}	Cyanocobalamin	Hydroxocobalamin	
Folic acid	Pteroylglutamic acid		
Erythropoietin	Erythropoietin		
Granulocyte-macrophage colony-stimulating factor	Sargramostim		
Granulocyte colony-stimulating factor	Filgrastim		

QUESTIONS

DIRECTIONS: Each of the numbered items or incomplete statements in this section is followed by answers or by completions of the sentence. Select the ONE lettered answer or completion that is BEST in each case.

Items 1–2: A 23-year-old pregnant woman is referred by her obstetrician for evaluation of anemia. She is in her fourth month of pregnancy and has no previous history of anemia; her grandfather had pernicious anemia. Her hemoglobin is 10 gm/dL.

1. Each of the following statements about factors important in anemias is correct EXCEPT
   (A) Pernicious anemia is associated with both neurologic abnormalities and anemia; only the anemia of pernicious anemia responds to folic acid
   (B) Efficient absorption of vitamin B_{12} requires complexation with a protein that is secreted by the stomach
   (C) Megaloblastic anemias usually respond to folic acid or vitamin B_{12}
   (D) Vitamin B_{12} supplements are important in pregnancy to reduce the risk of neural tube defects
   (E) Ordinary nutritional iron deficiencies should be treated with oral iron supplements

2. The lab data for your pregnant patient indicate that she does not have a macrocytic anemia but instead has a typical microcytic anemia of pregnancy. Optimal treatment of normocytic or mild microcytic anemia associated with pregnancy utilizes
   (A) A high fiber diet
   (B) Parenteral iron dextran injections
   (C) Iron dextran tablets
   (D) Ferrous sulfate tablets
   (E) Folic acid supplements

3. Syndromes of toxicity associated with iron include all of the following EXCEPT
   (A) Acute oral ingestion of a large overdose causes constipation
   (B) Chronic iron overload, as in hemochromatosis, causes liver disease
   (C) Acute overdose may cause metabolic acidosis
   (D) Hemolytic anemia may cause chronic iron toxicity
   (E) Overdoses of iron are usually treated medically, since the body does not have a natural means of excreting this element

DIRECTIONS: The following section consists of a list of four to twenty-six lettered options followed by several numbered items. For each numbered item, select the ONE option that is most closely associated with it. Each answer may be selected once, more than once, or not at all.
   (A) Folic acid
   (B) Cyanocobalamin
   (C) Ferrous sulfate
   (D) Iron dextran
   (E) Deferoxamine

4. Essential for the therapy of neurologic defects in pernicious anemia
5. Used primarily in severe iron deficiency and iron malabsorption syndromes
6. Used in the emergency treatment of acute iron intoxication
7. Stored in the liver in an amount sufficient for approximately 5 years

DIRECTIONS: The following section consists of a list of four to twenty-six lettered options followed by several numbered items. For each numbered item, select the ONE option that is most closely associated with it. Each answer may be selected once, more than once, or not at all.
   (A) Erythropoietin
   (B) Transferrin
   (C) Filgrastim
   (D) Sargramostim
   (E) Hemosiderin
   (F) Interleukin-9
   (G) Folic acid

8. Greatly increased in tissues of patients with hemochromatosis
9. Granulocyte-macrophage colony-stimulating factor
10. Most useful in patients with red cell deficiency caused by renal disease or depression of the bone marrow
11. Essential for the endocytosis of iron into red cell progenitors
12. Deficiency during pregnancy increases the risk of neural tube defects in the newborn

ANSWERS

1. Folic acid deficiency in pregnancy, not vitamin B_{12} deficiency, is associated with neural tube defects. The answer is **(D).**
2. The anemia usually associated with pregnancy is a simple iron deficiency anemia. In this condition, only oral iron supplementation is indicated. The answer is **(D).**
3. Intolerance to normal oral doses of iron is sometimes associated with constipation. Acute iron overdose, however, causes severe necrotizing gastroenteritis, not constipation. The answer is **(A).**

4. Only vitamin B_{12} reverses the neurologic deficits of pernicious anemia—and only if used early in the course of the disease. The answer is **(B)**.
5. Iron dextran, which can be given parenterally, is useful if iron stores must be replenished rapidly. The answer is **(D)**.
6. Deferoxamine, a chelator of iron, is useful in acute iron intoxication. The answer is **(E)**.
7. Vitamin B_{12} is stored in the liver in amounts sufficient for about 5 years of red cell production. The answer is **(B)**.
8. Hemosiderin is one of the major storage forms of iron. Deposits in the liver, heart, and other tissues cause clinical abnormalities in hemochromatosis. The answer is **(E)**.
9. Sargramostim is GM-CSF. The answer is **(D)**.
10. Erythropoietin is now used in patients with severe anemia caused by renal disease (in which erythropoietin is reduced) and by other causes of marrow depression, eg, chemotherapy or radiation. The answer is **(A)**.
11. Iron must be complexed with transferrin for endocytosis into red cell progenitors. The answer is **(B)**.
12. In adults, folate deficiency does not have major neurologic toxicity, whereas B_{12} deficiency does. On the other hand, deficiency of folic acid during pregnancy has been recognized as a teratogenic factor in neural tube defects in the fetus. The answer is **(G)**.

Drugs Used in Coagulation Disorders

33

OBJECTIVES

You should be able to:

- Compare the oral anticoagulants with heparin in terms of their pharmacokinetics, mechanisms, and toxicities.
- Compare the four thrombolytic preparations.
- Compare the antiplatelet drugs.
- List three different drugs used to treat disorders of excessive bleeding.

Learn the definitions that follow.

Table 33–1. Definitions.

Term	Definition
Clotting cascade	System of serine proteases and substrates in the plasma and tissues that provides for very rapid generation of clotting factors to prevent loss of blood when damage occurs to a vessel
Extrinsic pathway	Factors in tissues that are important in triggering the clotting process
Intrinsic pathway	Factors in the plasma that are activated for clotting, eg, II, VII, IX, X
Low molecular weight heparin	Preparation of heparin fractions of molecular molecular weight 2000–6000. Regular heparin has a molecular weight weight range of 2000–30,000
Partial thromboplastin time (PTT)	Laboratory test for heparin effect; prolonged when drug effect is adequate
Prothrombin time test (PT)	Laboratory test for warfarin (and other oral anticoagulant) effect; prolonged when drug effect is adequate

CONCEPTS

The drugs used in clotting and bleeding disorders fall into two primary groups: drugs used to decrease clotting or dissolve clots already present, and drugs used to increase clotting in patients with clotting deficiencies (Figure 33–1). All of these drugs interact at some point with the clotting process or cascade (as shown in Figure 33–2), a series of enzyme activation steps that originate within the blood itself (intrinsic system) or in tissues (extrinsic system).

ANTICOAGULANTS

A. Classification & Prototypes: Anticoagulants reduce the formation of fibrin clots. Two major types of anticoagulants are available: heparin, which must be used parenterally, and the orally active coumarin derivatives. Whereas heparin is the only member of its group, warfarin is one of several coumarin agents. The two groups differ in their chemistry, pharmacokinetics, and pharmacodynamics (Table 33–2).

B. Heparin:
1. Chemistry: Heparin is a large sulfated polysaccharide polymer. Each batch contains molecules of varying size with an average molecular weight (in the regular, high molecular weight [HMW] formulation) of about 15,000. Heparin is highly acidic and can be neutralized by basic molecules (eg, protamine). The drug must be given parenterally (intravenously or subcutaneously). Intramuscular injection is avoided because of the risk of hematoma formation.

   Low molecular weight (LMW) fractions of heparin have been developed. One of these, **enoxaparin,** has a molecular weight range of 2000 to 6000. Like HMW heparin, it is given intravenously or subcutaneously. **Hirudin,** an anticoagulant protein extracted from the saliva of the leech, is a powerful and selective thrombin inhibitor that can inactivate thrombin within a developing clot. The drug is relatively free of effects on bleeding time and platelets. A recombinant preparation is in clinical trials.

2. Mechanism and effects: Regular (high molecular weight) heparin catalyzes the activation of **antithrombin III,** a factor normally present in blood in inactive form. Antithrombin III combines with and inactivates thrombin (activated factor II) and activated factors IX, X, XI, and XIII. Low doses of heparin also coat the endothelial wall of vessels and reduce the activation of clotting elements by these cells. Because it acts on preformed blood components, heparin is active in vitro—almost instantaneously. The action of heparin is monitored with the activated partial thromboplastin time (aPTT or PTT).

   Low molecular weight heparin has a greater effect on activated factor IX than on the other factors listed above.

3. Clinical use: Because of its rapid effect, heparin is used when anticoagulation is needed immediately, (eg, when starting therapy). The drug is often used for 1 to 2 weeks immediately following a myocardial infarction. Because it does not pass the placenta, it is the drug of choice when an anticoagulant must be used in pregnancy.

4. Toxicity: Increased bleeding is the most common adverse effect and may cause hemorrhagic stroke. Additive interactions with other anticoagulants often occur. The drug causes moderate transient thrombocytopenia in many patients and severe thrombocytopenia in a small percentage of users. Prolonged use is associated with osteoporosis.

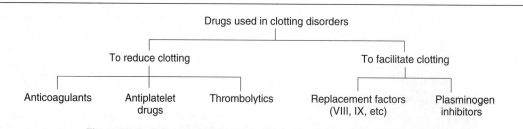

Figure 33–1. Subclasses of drugs used in the treatment of clotting disorders.

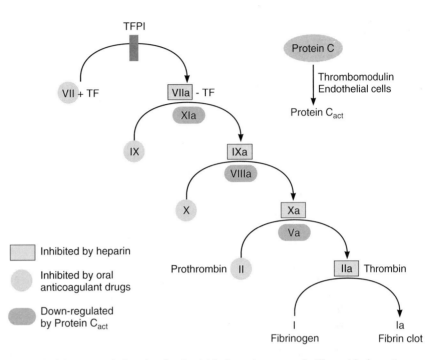

Figure 33–2. A model of drug coagulation showing the intrinsic system cascade. The extrinsic system generates tissue factor (TF), which is important in maintaining the velocity of the intrinsic system cascade. TFPI, tissue factor pathway inhibitor. (Reproduced, with permission, from Katzung BG [editor]: *Basic & Clinical Pharmacology*, 6th ed. Appleton & Lange, 1995.)

Low molecular weight heparin appears to cause less bleeding than the regular high molecular weight product; thus, less monitoring is necessary and doses can be given less frequently, eg, once or twice a day.

C. Coumarin Anticoagulants:

1. **Chemistry and pharmacokinetics:** The coumarin anticoagulants are small, lipid-soluble molecules. They are readily absorbed after oral administration (and therefore are commonly called "oral anticoagulants" to distinguish them from heparin). They also pass the placental barrier readily and are therefore potentially dangerous to the fetus. Warfarin is the only member of this group with clinical importance in the USA.

2. **Mechanism and effects:** Coumarins interfere with the normal synthesis of clotting factors in the liver, a process that depends on vitamin K. These cofactors include II, VII, IX, and X. Because these factors have half-lives of 8 to 60 hours in the plasma, an anticoagulant effect is observed only after sufficient time has passed for the preformed normal factors to be eliminated. Warfarin has no effect on blood clotting in vitro. The action of warfarin can be reversed with vitamin K, but recovery requires the synthesis of new normal clotting

Table 33–2. Properties of heparin and warfarin.

Property	Heparin	Warfarin
Structure	Large polymer, acidic	Small lipid-soluble molecule
Route of administration	Parenteral	Oral
Site of action	Blood	Liver
Onset of action	Rapid (seconds)	Slow, limited by half-lives of factors being replaced
Mechanism of action	Activates antithrombin III	Impairs synthesis of factors II, VII, IX, X
Antidote	Protamine	Vitamin K, plasma
Use	Acute, over days	Chronic, over weeks to months

factors and is therefore very slow (2 to 3 days). More rapid reversal can be achieved by transfusion with fresh or frozen plasma that contains normal clotting factors. The effect of warfarin is monitored by means of the prothrombin time (PT or "pro time") test.

3. **Clinical use:** Warfarin is used for chronic anticoagulation except in pregnant women (heparin must be used during pregnancy). Warfarin is indicated in established venous thrombosis and is often used for 2 to 6 months following a myocardial infarction.

4. **Toxicity:** Bleeding is the most important adverse effect of warfarin. Like heparin, it interacts with other anticlotting drugs. Warfarin also causes bone defects in the developing fetus and therefore is contraindicated in pregnancy. Because it acts in and is metabolized in the liver, warfarin interacts with drugs that influence hepatic drug metabolism.

THROMBOLYTIC AGENTS

A. **Classification & Prototypes (Table 33–3):** The thrombolytic drugs currently available are alteplase (tissue plasminogen activator, tPA), anistreplase, urokinase, and streptokinase. All are given intravenously.

B. **Mechanism of Action:** Plasmin is the normal endogenous fibrinolytic enzyme. It splits fibrin into fragments, promoting the breakdown and dissolution of the clot (Figure 33–3). The thrombolytic enzymes catalyze the activation of the inactive precursor, plasminogen, to plasmin.

1. **Tissue plasminogen activator:** tPA is a large human protein (molecular weight > 50,000) produced in bacteria through recombinant DNA techniques. tPA directly converts fibrin-bound plasminogen to plasmin. In theory, the drug's selectivity for plasminogen that has already bound to fibrin (ie, a clot) should result in greater selectivity and less danger of spontaneous bleeding. In fact, tPA's selectivity appears to be quite limited.

2. **Anistreplase:** This anisoylated plasminogen-streptokinase activator complex (APSAC) is a pro-drug. As the anisoyl group is hydrolyzed in vivo (a slow, spontaneous process), the streptokinase-activated plasminogen is released and converts endogenous plasminogen to plasmin. This slow release provides for the long half-life of this drug. The human plasminogen in this product is obtained through recombinant bacterial synthesis.

3. **Streptokinase:** Obtained from bacterial cultures, streptokinase forms a complex with endogenous plasminogen that catalyzes the rapid conversion of plasminogen to plasmin.

4. **Urokinase:** Urokinase is extracted from cultured human kidney cells. This enzyme directly converts plasminogen to plasmin.

C. **Clinical Use:** At the present time, the major application of the thrombolytic agents is in the emergency treatment of coronary artery thrombosis. Under ideal conditions (ie, treatment within 1 to 3 hours), these agents may cause prompt recanalization of the occluded vessel. They have been used by the intra-arterial route in coronary thrombosis, but this route does not seem to have a significant advantage over the intravenous route. The thrombolytic agents are also used in cases of multiple pulmonary emboli and deep venous thrombosis.

Table 33–3. Properties of thrombolytic enzymes.

Agent	Source	Duration of Action	Comments
Alteplase (tPA)	Recombinant human protein	2–10 min	Active plasminogen activator (converts plasminogen to plasmin); IV infusion required. Most expensive (> $2000 per treatment)
Anistreplase	Pro-drug: streptokinase plus recombinant human plasminogen	1–2 hours	Slowly releases streptokinase-activated plasminogen; single bolus administration provides long duration of action. Second most expensive (> $1800 per treatment)
Streptokinase	Bacterial product	20–25 min	Streptokinase combines with plasminogen; the combination activates plasminogen to plasmin; IV infusion required. Least expensive ($200 per treatment)
Urokinase	Human kidney cell culture	<20 min	Active plasminogen activator

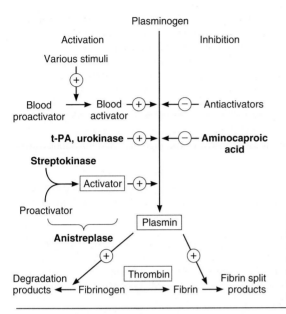

Figure 33–3. Diagram of the fibrinolytic system. The useful thrombolytic drugs are shown on the left in **bold** type. These drugs increase the formation of plasmin, the major fibrinolytic enzyme. Aminocaproic acid, a useful inhibitor of fibrinolysis, is shown on the right. (Reproduced, with permission, from Katzung BG [editor]: *Basic & Clinical Pharmacology,* 6th ed. Appleton & Lange, 1995.)

D. Toxicity: Bleeding is the most important hazard of these drugs. Even tPA, which should be somewhat more selective for preformed clots, causes a significant increase in cerebral hemorrhage and other serious bleeding. Because it is a foreign protein, streptokinase may evoke the production of antibodies and lose its effectiveness or even induce severe allergic reactions upon subsequent therapy. Patients who have had streptococcal infections may have preformed antibodies to the drug. Because they are human proteins, urokinase and tPA are not subject to this problem. However, they are much more expensive than streptokinase and not much more effective.

ANTIPLATELET DRUGS

Platelets play a central role in the clotting process and are especially important in clots that form in the arterial circulation. Therefore, platelets are believed to be especially important in coronary and cerebral artery occlusion.

A. Classification & Prototypes: Antiplatelet drugs include aspirin and other nonsteroidal antiinflammatory drugs (NSAIDs), ticlopidine, dipyridamole, and sulfinpyrazone. These drugs increase bleeding time.

B. Mechanism of Action: Aspirin and other NSAIDs inhibit thromboxane synthesis by blocking the enzyme cyclooxygenase. Aspirin is particularly effective because it irreversibly inactivates the enzyme. Because the platelet lacks the machinery for synthesis of new protein, inhibition by aspirin persists until new platelets are formed. Other NSAIDs cause a less persistent antiplatelet effect.

Ticlopidine's mechanism of action is not understood but involves the inhibition of ADP, a powerful stimulant of platelet aggregation.

The mechanisms of dipyridamole and sulfinpyrazone are not well understood. Some evidence suggests that dipyridamole increases the concentration of cAMP in the platelet by inhibiting phosphodiesterase.

C. Clinical Use: Aspirin is used in individuals who have had one or more myocardial infarcts to prevent further infarcts. A large recent study suggested that the drug also reduces the incidence of first infarcts. The drug is also being used extensively to prevent transient ischemic attacks ("TIAs") and other thrombotic events.

Ticlopidine is effective in preventing TIAs and is particularly valuable for patients who cannot tolerate aspirin. Dipyridamole is limited to use for the prevention of thrombosis in patients with an artificial heart valve. Sulfinpyrazone is rarely used.

D. Toxicity: Aspirin and other NSAIDs cause gastrointestinal and CNS effects (see Chapter 35). All antiplatelet drugs significantly enhance the effects of other anticlotting agents. The toxicity of ticlopidine includes gastrointestinal upset, bleeding in up to 5% of patients, and leukopenia in about 1%.

DRUGS USED IN BLEEDING DISORDERS

Inadequate blood clotting may result from vitamin K deficiency, genetically determined errors of clotting factor synthesis (eg, hemophilia), a variety of drug-induced conditions, and thrombocytopenia.

A. Vitamin K: Vitamin K deficiency is particularly common in newborns and in older individuals with abnormalities of fat absorption. The deficiency is readily treated with oral or parenteral vitamin K supplements using phytonadione (K_1) or menadione (K_2).

B. Clotting Factors: The most important agents used to treat hemophilia are fresh plasma and purified human blood clotting factors, especially **factor VIII** and **factor IX.** These products are extremely expensive and carry a risk of infection and immunologic reactions. The factors have been produced by recombinant synthesis, but this process is more expensive than purifying them from whole blood.

C. Antifibrinolysin Agents: Antifibrinolysin agents are valuable for the management of acute bleeding episodes in hemophiliacs and others with bleeding disorders. **Aminocaproic acid** and **tranexamic acid** are orally active agents that inhibit fibrinolysis by inhibiting plasminogen activation.

DRUG LIST

The following drugs are important members of the group discussed in this chapter. Prototypes should be learned in detail; features of the major variants should be known well enough to distinguish the variants from prototypes and from each other; the other significant agents should be recognized as belonging to a specific subclass.

Subclass	Prototype	Major Variants	Other Significant Agents
Anticoagulants Parenteral	Heparin	Enoxaparin	
Oral	Warfarin		
Antiplatelet drugs	Aspirin	Ticlopidine	Dipyridamole
Thrombolytic drugs	Streptokinase, alteplase		Anistreplase, urokinase
Clotting factors	Factor VIII	Factor IX	
Vitamin K	Phytonadione (K_1)		Menadione (K_2)
Antifibrinolysin drugs	Aminocaproic acid		Tranexamic acid

QUESTIONS

DIRECTIONS: Each of the numbered items or incomplete statements in this section is followed by answers or by completions of the sentence. Select the ONE lettered answer or completion that is BEST in each case.

Items 1–3: A 58-year-old business executive is brought to the emergency room two hours after the onset of severe chest pain during a vigorous tennis game. He has a history of poorly controlled mild hypertension and elevated blood cholesterol but does not smoke. ECG changes confirm the diagnosis of myocardial infarction. The decision is made to reduce clotting and attempt to open his occluded artery.

1. Activation of plasminogen to plasmin
   (A) Is brought about by heparin
   (B) Is brought about by warfarin
   (C) Is brought about by anistreplase
   (D) Is used preoperatively and during surgery in patients at risk of deep vein thromboses
   (E) Can be reversed by administration of vitamin K_1 oxide

2. Concerning antithrombotic drugs,
   (A) Aspirin's antiplatelet activity is due to the inhibition of prostacyclin production
   (B) Large doses of aspirin are generally more effective than smaller doses in producing antiplatelet effects
   (C) Thrombolytic agents are usually administered intramuscularly
   (D) A selective fibrinolysin inhibitor should be an effective antiplatelet agent
   (E) Thromboxane is the primary platelet-active agent produced in platelets

3. Aspirin should be used cautiously in a patient receiving heparin because aspirin
   (A) Inhibits vitamin K absorption
   (B) Has antithrombin activity
   (C) Inhibits metabolism of heparin
   (D) Inhibits platelet aggregation
   (E) All of the above

4. The following changes in plasma concentration of warfarin were observed in a patient when two other agents, drugs B and C, were given on a daily basis at constant dosage starting at the times shown. Which of the following statements most accurately describes what is shown in the graph below?

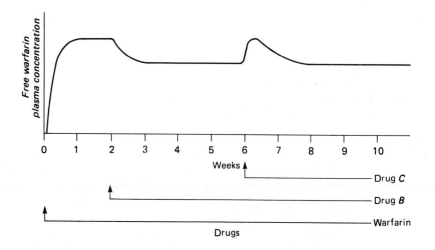

   (A) Drug B displaces warfarin from plasma proteins; drug C displaces warfarin from tissue binding sites
   (B) Drug B stimulates liver metabolism of warfarin; drug C displaces warfarin from plasma protein
   (C) Drug B stimulates renal clearance of warfarin; drug C inhibits hepatic metabolism of drug B
   (D) Drug B stimulates hepatic metabolism of warfarin; drug C displaces drug B from tissue binding sites
   (E) None of the above

5. Which of the following may be of value in the treatment of multiple small pulmonary emboli?
   (A) Heparin
   (B) Warfarin
   (C) Urokinase
   (D) Streptokinase
   (E) All of the above

6. Concerning anticoagulants, all of the following are correct EXCEPT
    (A) Parenteral administration of heparin provides immediate anticoagulation
    (B) Oral administration of warfarin provides delayed anticoagulation
    (C) The anticoagulant action of regular heparin requires the presence of antithrombin III
    (D) Warfarin is the preferred anticoagulant in pregnant women
    (E) Heparin overdose can be reversed with the basic protein, protamine

DIRECTIONS: The following section consists a list of four to twenty-six lettered options followed by several numbered items. For each numbered item, select the ONE option that is most closely associated with it. Each answer may be selected once, more than once, or not at all.
    (A) Dipyridamole
    (B) Aminocaproic acid
    (C) Heparin
    (D) Factor IX
    (E) Whole plasma
    (F) Protamine
    (G) Warfarin
    (H) Alteplase
    (I) Anistreplase
    (J) Ticlopidine

7. Used for rapid reversal of effects of warfarin
8. Synthetic chemical used for the treatment of an acute bleeding episode in a hemophiliac
9. Restricted to prevention of clotting associated with an artificial heart valve
10. Small, lipid-soluble molecule that acts in the liver
11. Used for the treatment of bleeding due to excess heparin
12. Human protein used in hemophiliacs to prevent or treat bleeding

ANSWERS

1. The answer is **(C)**, anistreplase. Thrombolytic drugs are not used in patients scheduled for surgery or in those with neoplasms because of the risk of drug-induced bleeding.
2. Prostacyclin is the major *anti*aggregation platelet-active product of the endothelium. Large doses of aspirin inhibit prostacyclin as well as thromboxane synthesis; therefore, low doses are thought to be more effective. Thromboxane, an important contributor to the platelet aggregation process, is produced mainly in platelets. The answer is **(E)**.
3. Because aspirin interferes with clotting by a different mechanism (inhibition of platelet aggregation), the drug has the potential to interact synergistically with heparin. The answer is **(D)**.
4. A drug that increases metabolism (clearance) of the anticoagulant will lower the steady-state plasma concentration (both free and bound forms), whereas one that displaces the anticoagulant will increase the plasma level of the free form only until elimination of the drug has again lowered it to the steady-state level. The answer is **(B)**.
5. Urokinase and streptokinase may be useful in the removal of a clot that is already present; heparin (immediately) and warfarin (more slowly) act to prevent the extension of the clot and the formation of new ones. The answer is **(E)**.
6. Warfarin is avoided in pregnant women because it crosses the placental barrier and causes teratogenic effects. The answer is **(D)**.
7. Only a full complement of normal clotting factors can reverse warfarin's effects rapidly. The answer is **(E)**.
8. Aminocaproic acid is a small, synthetic molecule that inhibits thrombolysis and is useful in bleeding episodes in hemophilia. The answer is **(B)**.
9. Dipyridamole is an antiplatelet agent that has proven useful only in patients with artificial heart valves. The answer is **(A)**.
10. Warfarin is the small, lipid soluble agent that acts in the liver to inhibit the synthesis of clotting factors II, VII, IX, and X. The answer is **(G)**.
11. Heparin is a very acidic molecule that binds firmly to basic polymers such as protamine. Such binding prevents the action of heparin. The answer is **(F)**.
12. Factor VIII and factor IX are human proteins used to treat hemophilia. The answer is **(D)**.

Drugs Used in the Treatment of Hyperlipidemias

34

OBJECTIVES

You should be able to:

- Describe the dietary management of hyperlipoproteinemia.
- Describe the mechanism of action and toxic effects of nicotinic acid, HMG-CoA reductase inhibitors, gemfibrozil, probucol, and bile acid-binding resins.

Learn the definitions that follow.

Table 34–1. Definitions.

Term	Definition
Chylomicrons	Largest of the lipoproteins; carry fat from the gut to the other tissues
FFA	Free fatty acids; products of triglyceride hydrolysis
HDL	High-density lipoproteins; formed in the tissues, a mechanism for cholesterol transport from the periphery to the liver
HMG-CoA	3-Hydroxy-3-methylglutaryl-coenzyme A; a precursor of cholesterol
IDL	Intermediate-density lipoproteins; remnants of LDL particles that have been depleted of FFA by lipoprotein lipase
LDL	Low-density lipoproteins; major form in which lipid is recaptured by the liver; requires functional LDL receptors for normal endocytosis into hepatocytes
Lipoproteins	Macromolecular complexes in which lipids are transported in the blood, eg, LDL, IDL
LPL	Lipoprotein lipase; an enzyme found in the peripheral tissues that hydrolyzes lipoproteins and depletes triglycerides in the lipoprotein complexes
Triglyceride	Ester of 3 fatty acids with glycerol; a major form of fat storage
VLDL	Very-low-density lipoproteins; secreted by the liver; the initial transporter of cholesterol and other lipids from the liver to the periphery

CONCEPTS

HYPERLIPOPROTEINEMIA

A. Pathogenesis: Premature or accelerated development of atherosclerosis is strongly associated with elevated levels (above 200 mg/dL) of certain plasma lipoproteins, especially the lipoproteins associated with cholesterol transport. Elevations of low-density lipoproteins (LDL), intermediate-density lipoproteins (IDL), or very-low-density lipoproteins (VLDL) constitute hyperlipoproteinemias. A *depressed* level of high-density lipoproteins (HDL) is also associated with increased risk of atherosclerosis. In some families, hyperlipemia, an elevation of triglycerides, is similarly correlated with atherosclerosis. Chylomicronemia, the occurrence of chylomicrons in the serum while fasting, is a recessive trait correlated with acute pancreatitis and can be managed by restriction of total fat intake. See Table 34–2.

Regulation of plasma lipoprotein levels involves a balance between dietary fat intake, hepatic processing, and utilization in peripheral tissues. Primary disturbances in regulation occur in various familial diseases. Secondary disturbances are associated with many endocrine conditions and diseases of the liver or kidneys.

Table 34–2. The primary hyperlipoproteinemias and their drug treatment.[1]

Condition	Single Drug	Drug Combination
Primary chylomicronemia (familial lipoprotein lipase or cofactor deficiency)	Dietary management	
Familial hypertriglyceridemia		
Severe	Niacin, gemfibrozil	Niacin plus gemfibrozil
Moderate	Gemfibrozil, niacin	
Familial combined hyperlipidemia		
VLDL increased	Niacin, gemfibrozil	
LDL increased	Resin, niacin, reductase inhibitor	Niacin plus resin or reductase inhibitor
VLDL, LDL increased	Niacin	Niacin plus resin or reductase inhibitor
Familial dysbetalipoproteinemia	Niacin, gemfibrozil	Gemfibrozil plus niacin or niacin plus reductase inhibitor
Familial hypercholesterolemia		
Heterozygous	Resin, reductase inhibitor, niacin	Two or three of the individual drugs
Homozygous	Probucol, niacin	Resin plus niacin plus reductase inhibitor; probucol plus agents above
$LP_{(a)}$ hyperlipoproteinemia	Niacin	Niacin plus reductase inhibitor
Unclassified hypercholesterolemia	Resin, niacin, reductase inhibitor	

[1] Reproduced, with permission, from Katzung BG (editor): *Basic & Clinical Pharmacology,* 6th ed. Appleton & Lange, 1995.

Major enzymes involved in lipoprotein regulation include: (1) Acyl-CoA:cholesterol acyltransferase (ACAT), which esterifies some cholesterol in the core of chylomicrons; (2) Lecithin:cholesterol acyltransferase (LCAT), which esterifies cholesterol and helps transfer it to LDL; (3) Lipoprotein lipase (LPL), which hydrolyzes triglycerides to free fatty acids (FFA) and glycerol; and (4) 3-Hydroxy-3-methylglutaryl-coenzyme A (HMG-CoA) reductase, which is essential in the synthesis of cholesterol and other steroids in the liver.

B. Treatment Strategies: Treatment always includes dietary management. Drug therapy is added if necessary.

  1. Diet: Dietary measures are the first method of management and may be sufficient to reduce lipoprotein levels to a safe range. Cholesterol and saturated fats are the primary dietary factors that contribute to elevated levels of plasma lipoproteins. Alcohol intake raises VLDL levels. Diets are designed to reduce the total intake of these substances.

  2. Drugs: Drug therapy can reduce fat absorption from the intestine (resins), modify hepatic synthesis (HMG-CoA reductase inhibitors) or release of lipoproteins (niacin), increase peripheral clearance of lipoproteins (gemfibrozil group), and possibly exert other effects (probucol). These drugs are all given orally. See Figure 34–1.

RESINS

A. Mechanism & Effects: Bile acid-binding resins (cholestyramine and colestipol) are large nonabsorbable polymers that bind bile acids and similar steroids in the intestine. Neomycin, though not a resin, also causes a reduction in bile acid reabsorption.

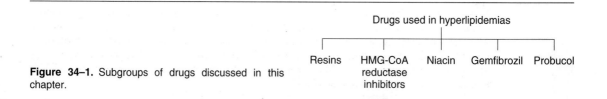

Figure 34–1. Subgroups of drugs discussed in this chapter.

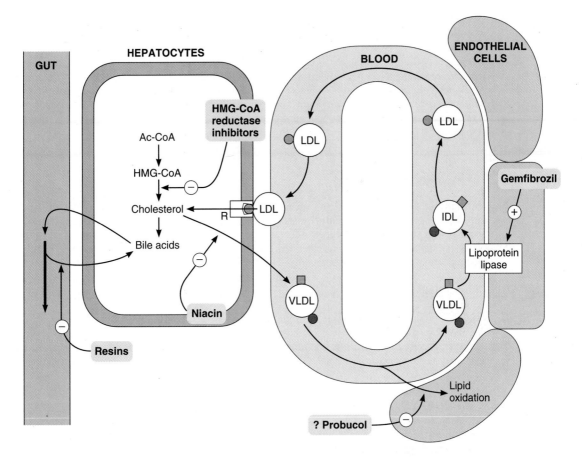

Figure 34–2. Schematic diagram of lipoprotein handling by the liver hepatocytes and by vascular endothelial cells in vessels in peripheral tissues. The sites of action of the drugs are shown (+, stimulation; -, inhibition). R = LDL receptor.

By preventing absorption of dietary cholesterol and reducing reabsorption of bile acids secreted by the liver, these agents greatly enhance the diversion of hepatic cholesterol synthesis to new bile acids, thereby reducing the availability of cholesterol for the production of plasma lipids (Figure 34–2). A compensatory increase in high-affinity LDL receptors often occurs in the liver.

B. Clinical Use: See Table 34–2.

C. Toxicity: Adverse effects include bloating, constipation, and impaired absorption of some cationic or neutral drugs. Neomycin is rarely used because it is associated with a higher incidence of adverse effects than are the resins.

HMG-CoA REDUCTASE INHIBITORS

A. Mechanism & Effects: Lovastatin (mevinolin) and simvastatin are pro-drug lactones. Pravastatin and fluvastatin are active as given. In the body, the active drugs are structural analogues that competitively inhibit mevalonate synthesis by HMG-CoA reductase, a process essential for cholesterol biosynthesis in the liver (Figure 34–2). The liver compensates by increasing the number of high-affinity LDL receptors and this results in increased clearance of VLDL remnants (IDL) and LDL from the blood.

B. **Clinical Use:** See Table 34–2. These drugs often reduce LDL levels dramatically, especially when used in combination with other drugs.

C. **Toxicity:** Mild elevations of serum transaminase are common but are not often associated with hepatic damage. Patients with preexisting liver disease may have more severe reactions. An increase in creatine kinase (released from skeletal muscle) is noted in about 10% of patients; in a few, severe muscle pain and even rhabdomyolysis may occur. Progression of cataracts was reported in a few patients in early studies but has not been found in more extensive trials.

NIACIN (NICOTINIC ACID)

A. **Mechanism & Effects:** Niacin (but not nicotinamide) reduces the secretion of VLDL from the liver (Figure 34–2), possibly by inhibiting hepatic synthesis of apolipoproteins. Consequently, LDL formation is reduced. Increased clearance of VLDL by lipoprotein lipase in the periphery has also been demonstrated. In addition, the levels of HDL may increase. Finally, niacin decreases circulating fibrinogen and increases tissue plasminogen activator.

B. **Clinical Use:** See Table 34–2.

C. **Toxicity:** Cutaneous flushing is a common adverse effect. Aspirin may reduce the intensity of this flushing, suggesting that it is mediated by prostaglandin release. Tolerance usually develops within a few days. Pruritus and other skin conditions are reported. Moderate elevations of liver enzymes may occur.

GEMFIBROZIL & RELATED DRUGS

A. **Mechanism & Effects:** Gemfibrozil, fenofibrate, and clofibrate cause a decrease in VLDL levels through a peripheral effect. This effect is probably stimulation of lipoprotein lipase (Figure 34–2), resulting in an increase in the clearance of triglyceride-rich lipoproteins. Cholesterol biosynthesis in the liver is secondarily reduced. There may be an increase in HDL levels.

B. **Clinical Use:** See Table 34–2. Clofibrate is less widely used than gemfibrozil and other newer analogues because of the greater toxicity associated with clofibrate.

C. **Toxicity:** Nausea is the most common adverse effect with all members of this subgroup. Skin rashes are common with gemfibrozil. Myalgia is reported in patients taking clofibrate; an antiplatelet effect may cause an interaction between this drug and anticoagulants. Most importantly, clofibrate has been associated with an increase in the incidence of gastrointestinal and hepatobiliary neoplasms.

PROBUCOL

A. **Mechanism & Effects:** Probucol reduces LDL cholesterol levels by an unknown mechanism. Unfortunately, this drug often reduces HDL levels as well, which limits its usefulness. However, some evidence suggests that the drug may inhibit atherogenesis by other mechanisms in addition to its effect on plasma lipids, possibly by an antioxidant effect (Figure 34–2). Probucol distributes into adipose tissue and has a very long half-life.

B. **Clinical Use:** See Table 34–2. Probucol is particularly important in the treatment of homozygous familial hypercholesterolemia, because the drug's actions do not require functioning hepatic LDL receptors.

C. **Toxicity:** Probucol frequently causes gastrointestinal symptoms. The drug also causes ECG changes and may precipitate dangerous cardiac arrhythmias.

COMBINATION THERAPY

All patients with hyperlipidemia are treated first with dietary modification, but this is often insufficient and drugs must be added. Because of the difficulty of lowering serum lipids with a single drug, combinations of drugs are often required to achieve the maximum lowering possible with minimum toxicity. The most common combinations are listed in Table 34–2.

DRUG LIST

The following drugs are important members of the group discussed in this chapter. Prototypes should be learned in detail; features of the major variants should be known well enough to distinguish the variants from prototypes and from each other; the other significant agents should be recognized as belonging to a specific subclass.

Subclass	Prototype	Major Variants	Other Significant Agents
Bile acid-binding resins	Cholestyramine		Colestipol
Cholesterol synthesis inhibitor	Lovastatin	Pravastatin	Simvastatin, fluvastatin
VLDL secretion inhibitor	Niacin		
Lipoprotein lipase stimulants	Gemfibrozil		Fenofibrate, clofibrate
Mechanism uncertain (antioxidant?)	Probucol		

QUESTIONS

DIRECTIONS: Each of the numbered items or incomplete statements in this section is followed by answers or by completions of the sentence. Select the ONE lettered answer or completion that is BEST in each case.

1. Increased levels of which of the following may be associated with a decreased risk of atherosclerosis?
   (A) Very-low-density lipoproteins (VLDL)
   (B) Low-density lipoproteins (LDL)
   (C) Intermediate-density lipoproteins (IDL)
   (D) High-density lipoproteins (HDL)
   (E) Cholesterol
2. Lovastatin has all of the following effects EXCEPT
   (A) Results in increased synthesis of high affinity LDL receptors
   (B) Decreases LDL and VLDL plasma levels
   (C) Increases serum transaminase levels
   (D) May cause skeletal muscle pain and rhabdomyolysis
   (E) Stimulates lipoprotein lipase
3. Which of the following cause(s) a reduction in absorption of bile acids from the gastrointestinal tract?
   (A) HMG-CoA reductase inhibitors
   (B) Colestipol
   (C) Niacin
   (D) Probucol
   (E) All of the above
4. The major recognized mechanism of action of niacin is
   (A) Reduction of secretion of HDL by the liver
   (B) Reduction of secretion of VLDL by the liver
   (C) Increased lipid hydrolysis by lipoprotein lipase
   (D) Decreased lipid hydrolysis by lipoprotein lipase
   (E) Reduced oxidation of lipids in endothelial cells

5. The major mechanism of action of gemfibrozil is
   (A) Reduction of secretion of HDL by the liver
   (B) Reduction of secretion of VLDL by the liver
   (C) Increased lipid hydrolysis by lipoprotein lipase
   (D) Decreased lipid hydrolysis by lipoprotein lipase
   (E) Reduced oxidation of lipids in endothelial cells
6. The major toxicity of HMG-CoA reductase inhibitors is
   (A) Severe cardiac arrhythmias
   (B) Tissue injury with elevated liver and muscle enzymes
   (C) Gallstones
   (D) Acute pancreatitis
   (E) Gastrointestinal and hepatobiliary neoplasms
7. The major toxicity of gemfibrozil is
   (A) Liver damage
   (B) Severe cardiac arrhythmias
   (C) Nausea, vomiting, and skin rashes
   (D) Flushing of the skin
   (E) Gastrointestinal and hepatobiliary neoplasms

DIRECTIONS: The following section consists of a list of four to twenty-six lettered options followed by several numbered items. For each numbered item, select the ONE option that is most closely associated with it. Each answer may be selected once, more than once, or not at all.
   (A) Gemfibrozil
   (B) Nicotinic acid
   (C) Cholestyramine
   (D) Probucol
   (E) Pravastatin
   (F) Neomycin

8. Associated with cardiac arrhythmias
9. Causes cutaneous vasodilation and reduces VLDL and LDL levels
10. Nonabsorbable synthetic polymer; acts entirely within the intestine
11. Structural analogue of a steroid precursor that competitively inhibits cholesterol synthesis in the liver
12. Activates lipoprotein lipase and increases hydrolysis of triglycerides

ANSWERS

1. Increase of most of the lipoproteins is associated with increased risk of atherosclerosis. HDL ("good cholesterol"), however, is associated with a decrease in risk. The answer is **(D)**.
2. Lovastatin can cause all of the effects except stimulation of lipoprotein lipase, a peripheral (not hepatic) enzyme. The answer is **(E)**.
3. Colestipol (a resin) reduces absorption of bile acids (see Figure 34–2). The answer is **(B)**.
4. The major recognized effect of niacin is reduction of VLDL secretion by the liver (Figure 34–2). The answer is **(B)**.
5. The major mechanism recognized for gemfibrozil is stimulation of lipoprotein lipase. The answer is **(C)**.
6. The major toxicity of the HMG-CoA reductase inhibitors is tissue damage with resulting elevation of enzymes of liver and muscle. The answer is **(B)**.
7. The major toxicity of gemfibrozil (and fenofibrate) is gastrointestinal upset and skin rash. The answer is **(C)**.
8. Probucol has been associated with serious arrhythmias. Nicotinic acid may also occasionally cause arrhythmias, but this is uncommon. The answer is **(D)**.
9. The answer is **(B)**, nicotinic acid (niacin).
10. Cholestyramine and neomycin both slow the absorption of bile acids from the gut. However, neomycin is a natural product and not a polymer (see Chapter 45). The answer is **(C)**.
11. HMG-CoA reductase inhibitors are structural analogues. The answer is **(E)**, pravastatin.
12. Gemfibrozil activates lipoprotein lipase. The answer is **(A)**.

Nonsteroidal Anti-Inflammatory Drugs, Acetaminophen, & Drugs Used in Gout

35

OBJECTIVES

You should be able to:

- Describe the effects of aspirin on prostaglandin synthesis.
- List the toxic effects of aspirin.
- Contrast the actions of aspirin and the newer NSAIDs.
- Describe the mechanisms of action of three different drug groups used in gout.
- Describe the effects and the major toxicity of acetaminophen.

CONCEPTS

ANTI-INFLAMMATORY DRUGS

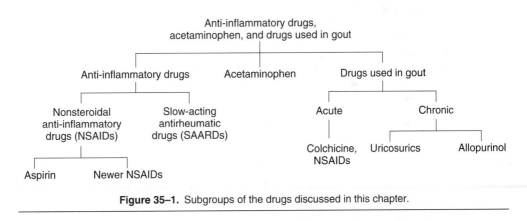

Figure 35–1. Subgroups of the drugs discussed in this chapter.

ASPIRIN & NEWER NONSTEROIDAL ANTI-INFLAMMATORY DRUGS (NSAIDs)

A. Classification & Prototypes: Aspirin (acetylsalicylic acid) and the salicylates are traditionally used in the treatment of pain, inflammation, and fever. Aspirin is the prototypical salicylate. The newer NSAIDs (ibuprofen, indomethacin, many others) vary primarily in their potency and duration of action. Ibuprofen is the lower potency, shorter-acting NSAID prototype. Naproxen is a longer-acting agent. Indomethacin is the prototypical high potency NSAID.

B. Mechanism of Action: As noted in Chapter 18, cyclooxygenase, the enzyme that converts arachidonic acid into the endoperoxide precursors of prostaglandin, has been found to have at least two different isoforms: Cox I and Cox II. Cox I is present in noninflammatory cells, whereas Cox II is present in lymphocytes, polymorphonuclear cells, and other inflammatory cells.

Aspirin and all newer NSAIDs inhibit cyclooxygenase. As a result, synthesis of prostaglandins and thromboxane is reduced. Because available NSAIDs inhibit Cox I as much as or more than Cox II, these drugs deplete prostaglandins necessary for normal cell function (eg, cytoprotection in the stomach), as well as prostaglandins involved in inflammation. The major difference between the mechanisms of aspirin and the newer NSAIDs is that aspirin (but not its active metabolite, salicylate) acetylates and thereby irreversibly inhibits cyclooxygenase, whereas the inhibition produced by newer agents is reversible. The irreversible action of aspirin results in a longer duration of its antiplatelet effect.

C. Effects: Arachidonic acid derivatives are important mediators of inflammation; cyclooxygenase inhibitors reduce the manifestations of inflammation, although they have no effect on underlying tissue damage or immunologic reactions. Prostaglandin synthesis in the CNS in response to pyrogenic substances is similarly suppressed by NSAIDs, resulting in reduction of fever (antipyretic action). The analgesic mechanism of these agents is less well understood. Activation of peripheral pain sensors may be diminished as a result of reduced production of prostaglandins in injured tissue; in addition, a central mechanism is operative.

D. Pharmacokinetics & Clinical Use:
1. **Aspirin:** Aspirin has three therapeutic dose ranges: the low range (<300 mg/day) is effective in reducing platelet aggregation; intermediate doses (300 to 2400 mg/day) have antipyretic and analgesic effects; and high doses (2400 to 4000 mg/day) are used for their anti-inflammatory effect. Aspirin is readily absorbed and is hydrolyzed in blood and tissues to acetate and salicylic acid. Salicylate is probably the major active molecule in the anti-inflammatory action of aspirin. Elimination of salicylate is first order at low doses, with a half-life of 3–5 hours. At high (anti-inflammatory) doses, half-life increases to 15 hours or more and elimination becomes zero order. Excretion is via the kidney.
2. **Newer NSAIDs:** The newer cyclooxygenase inhibitors are well absorbed after oral administration and are excreted via the kidney. Ibuprofen has a half-life of about 2 hours, is relatively safe, and is the least expensive of the newer NSAIDs. Indomethacin is a potent NSAID with increased toxicity. Naproxen and piroxicam are noteworthy because of their longer half-lives (12–24 hours), which permit less frequent dosing. Newer NSAIDs are used for pain of dysmenorrhea, inflammation (especially that of rheumatoid arthritis and gout), and patent ductus arteriosus in premature infants. Both ibuprofen and naproxen are now available in low-dose, over-the-counter formulations.

E. Toxicity:
1. **Aspirin:** Possible adverse effects from therapeutic anti-inflammatory doses of aspirin are gastrointestinal disturbances and increased risk of bleeding. Chronic aspirin overdosage is associated with reduced synthesis of prothrombin. When prostaglandin synthesis is inhibited by even small doses of aspirin, persons with aspirin hypersensitivity (especially associated with nasal polyps) may experience asthma from the increased synthesis of leukotrienes. At higher doses, tinnitus, vertigo, hyperventilation, and respiratory alkalosis are observed. At very high doses, the drug causes metabolic acidosis, dehydration, hyperthermia, collapse, coma, and death. If given aspirin, children with viral infections are at increased risk of developing Reye's syndrome (hepatic fatty degeneration and encephalopathy). Dialysis is effective in removing salicylates.
2. **Newer NSAIDs:** Like aspirin, these agents may cause significant gastrointestinal disturbance, but the incidence is lower than with aspirin. At high therapeutic dosage, however, there is a significant risk of renal damage with all the newer NSAIDs, especially in patients with pre-existing renal disease. Since these drugs are cleared by the kidney, renal damage results in higher, more toxic, serum concentrations. Phenylbutazone should not be used chronically because it causes aplastic anemia and agranulocytosis.

SLOW-ACTING ANTIRHEUMATIC DRUGS (SAARDs)

A. Classification & Prototypes: This heterogeneous group of agents has anti-inflammatory actions in several connective tissue diseases. These agents are considered "slow acting" because it may take months for their benefits to become apparent. The major members of the group are cytotoxic agents, especially **methotrexate;** the **gold compounds,** which are used only as anti-inflammatory agents; **hydroxychloroquine** (an antimalarial drug); and **penicil-**

lamine, which is also used as a chelating agent. **Corticosteroids** may be considered anti-inflammatory drugs with an intermediate rate of action, ie, slower than NSAIDs but faster than the SAARDs. However, the corticosteroids are too toxic for chronic use (see Chapter 38) and are reserved for temporary control of severe exacerbations of inflammatory joint conditions.

B. Mechanisms of Action: The mechanisms of these drugs are poorly understood. Methotrexate, a cytotoxic immunosuppressant drug, probably acts by reducing the numbers of immune cells available to maintain the inflammatory response. Organic gold compounds alter the activity of macrophages, cells that play a central role in inflammation, especially that of arthritis. Gold compounds also inhibit lysosomal enzyme activity, reduce histamine release, and suppress phagocytic activity by polymorphonuclear leukocytes. Hydroxychloroquine may interfere with the activity of T lymphocytes, decrease leukocyte chemotaxis, stabilize lysosomal membranes, interfere with DNA and RNA synthesis, and trap free radicals. Penicillamine appears to have anti-inflammatory effects similar to those of hydroxychloroquine.

C. Effects: These agents have a slow onset of anti-inflammatory action in patients with rheumatoid or other immune complexes in their serum. Benefits may require several months to become manifest. It has been claimed that these drugs may slow or arrest the underlying joint destruction in rheumatoid arthritis, but this is controversial.

D. Pharmacokinetics & Clinical Use: Slow-acting anti-inflammatory drugs are used in patients with rheumatoid arthritis who do not respond to other agents. Methotrexate, hydroxychloroquine, and penicillamine are given orally. Gold compounds are available for parenteral use (gold sodium thiomalate and aurothioglucose) and for oral administration (auranofin). Many patients do not respond to the SAARDs (especially gold) and there is continuing controversy about the efficacy of these drugs in the therapy of arthritis.

E. Toxicity: All slow-acting agents can cause severe or fatal toxicities. Careful monitoring of patients who take these drugs is mandatory. Methotrexate causes bone marrow depression, hepatotoxicity, and teratogenic fetal damage or abortion. The major toxicities of gold include potentially fatal dermatitis and bone marrow depression. Oral gold causes a high incidence of severe gastrointestinal disturbances. Hydroxychloroquine causes dermatitis, bone marrow depression, and retinal degeneration. Penicillamine causes renal damage and aplastic anemia.

ACETAMINOPHEN

A. Classification & Prototypes: Acetaminophen is the only over-the-counter, non-anti-inflammatory analgesic commonly available in the USA. Phenacetin, a toxic pro-drug that is metabolized to acetaminophen, is still available in some other countries.

B. Mechanism of Action: The mechanism of analgesic action of acetaminophen is unclear. The drug is a weak cyclooxygenase inhibitor in peripheral tissues, thus accounting for its lack of anti-inflammatory effect. Acetaminophen may be a more effective inhibitor of prostaglandin synthesis in the CNS, resulting in analgesic and antipyretic action.

C. Effects: As noted above, acetaminophen is an analgesic and antipyretic agent that lacks the anti-inflammatory effects of NSAIDs. This drug does not have significant antiplatelet effects.

D. Pharmacokinetics & Clinical Use: Acetaminophen is effective for the same indications as intermediate-dose aspirin. Acetaminophen is therefore useful as an aspirin substitute, especially in children with viral infections (who are at risk for Reye's syndrome if they take aspirin) and in individuals with any type of aspirin intolerance. Acetaminophen is well absorbed and metabolized in the liver. Its half-life, which is 2–3 hours in persons with normal hepatic function, is unaffected by renal disease.

E. Toxicity: In therapeutic dosages, acetaminophen has negligible toxicity. When taken in overdose, however, the drug is a very dangerous hepatotoxin. The mechanism of toxicity requires oxidation to cytotoxic intermediates by phase I P450 enzymes. This occurs if substrates for phase II conjugation reactions (acetate and glucuronide) are lacking (see Chapter 4).

DRUGS USED IN GOUT

A. Classification & Prototypes: Gout is associated with increased body stores of uric acid. Acute attacks involve joint inflammation caused by precipitation of uric acid crystals. Treatment strategies include (1) reducing inflammation during acute attacks (with colchicine or NSAIDs, Figure 35–2); (2) accelerating renal excretion of uric acid with uricosuric drugs (probenecid or sulfinpyrazone); and (3) reducing the conversion of purines to uric acid by xanthine oxidase (with allopurinol).

B. Colchicine & Other Drugs Used for Acute Gout:

1. **Mechanism:** Colchicine, a selective inhibitor of microtubule assembly, reduces leukocyte migration and phagocytosis; the drug may also reduce production of leukotriene B_4. Potent NSAIDs such as indomethacin are also effective (but not as selective) in inhibiting the inflammation of acute gouty arthritis. These agents act through the reduction of prostaglandin formation (see the discussion at the beginning of this chapter and Chapter 18) and through the inhibition of crystal phagocytosis by macrophages (Figure 35–2).

2. **Effects:** Because it reacts with tubulin and interferes with microtubule assembly, colchicine is a general mitotic poison. Tubulin is necessary for normal cell division, motility, and many other processes; therefore, colchicine has systemic toxicity if used in excess. NSAIDs reduce the synthesis of mediators of inflammation by inflammatory cells in the gouty joint.

3. **Pharmacokinetics and clinical use:** Indomethacin or colchicine is preferred for the treatment of acute gouty arthritis. Colchicine is also of value in the management of "Mediterranean fever," a disease of unknown etiology characterized by fever, hepatitis, peritonitis, pleuritis, arthritis, and, occasionally, amyloidosis. Phenylbutazone, a dangerous NSAID when used chronically, is still sometimes used for short-term management of gouty arthritis. Indomethacin and colchicine are used orally, although a parenteral preparation of colchicine is available.

4. **Toxicity:** Because colchicine can severely damage the liver and kidney, dosage must be carefully limited and monitored. Therapeutic doses are often associated with gastrointesti-

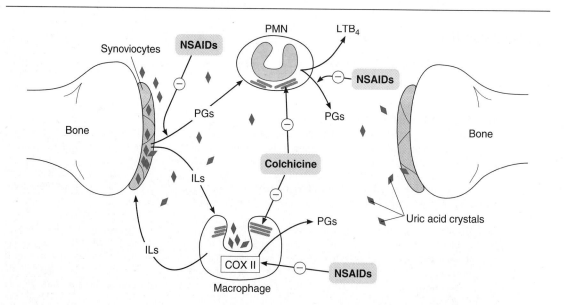

Figure 35–2. Sites of action of some anti-inflammatory drugs in a gouty joint. Damaged synoviocytes release prostaglandins (PGs), interleukins (ILs), and other mediators of inflammation. Polymorphonuclear leukocytes (PMNs), macrophages, and other inflammatory cells enter the joint and also release inflammatory substances, including leukotrienes (eg, LTB_4) that attract additional inflammatory cells. Colchicine acts on microtubules in the inflammatory cells. NSAIDs act on cyclooxygenase II in all of the cells of the joint.

nal upset, especially diarrhea. Indomethacin may cause renal damage or bone marrow depression. Phenylbutazone has caused many cases of aplastic anemia.

C. Uricosuric Agents:
1. **Mechanism:** Uricosuric agents (**probenecid, sulfinpyrazone**) are weak acids that compete with uric acid in the renal tubule for reabsorption by the weak acid carrier mechanism. At low doses, these agents may also compete with uric acid for secretion by the tubule and (occasionally) can even elevate serum uric acid concentration. Elevation of uric acid levels by this mechanism occurs with aspirin (another weak acid) over much of its dose range.
2. **Effects:** Uricosuric drugs act primarily in the kidney and inhibit the secretion of other weak acids (eg, penicillin) in addition to inhibiting the reabsorption of uric acid.
3. **Pharmacokinetics and clinical use:** Chronic gout is treated orally with a uricosuric or allopurinol. These drugs are of no value in acute gouty arthritis and are best withheld for 1–2 weeks after an acute episode.
4. **Toxicity:** Uricosuric drugs may precipitate an attack of acute gouty arthritis during the early phase of their action. This can be avoided by simultaneously administering colchicine or indomethacin. Because they are sulfonamides, the uricosuric drugs share allergies with the other classes of sulfa drugs (diuretics, antimicrobials, hypoglycemic drugs).

D. Allopurinol:
1. **Mechanism:** Allopurinol is converted to oxipurinol (alloxanthine) by xanthine oxidase, the enzyme that converts hypoxanthine to xanthine and xanthine to uric acid. Allopurinol and oxipurinol are inhibitors of this enzyme. Allopurinol is relatively selective in humans but can severely impair purine metabolism of some protozoa; the drug has also been used in the treatment of Leishmaniasis.
2. **Effects:** Inhibition of conversion to uric acid increases the concentrations of the more soluble hypoxanthine and xanthine, and decreases the concentration of the less soluble uric acid. As a result, there is less likelihood of precipitation of uric acid crystals in joints and tissues.
3. **Pharmacokinetics and clinical use:** Allopurinol is given orally in the management of chronic gout. It is usually withheld for 1–2 weeks after an acute episode of gouty arthritis.
4. **Toxicity:** Allopurinol causes gastrointestinal upset and, rarely, peripheral neuritis and vasculitis.

DRUG LIST

The following drugs are important members of the group discussed in this chapter. Prototypes should be learned in detail; features of the major variants should be known well enough to distinguish the variants from the prototypes and from each other; the other significant agents should be recognized as belonging to a specific subclass.

Subclass	Prototype	Major Variants	Other Significant Agents
Anti-inflammatory drugs Salicylates	Aspirin		Sodium salicylate
Newer nonsteroidals	Ibuprofen	Indomethacin	Naproxen, piroxicam, many others
Slow-acting antirheumatic drugs	Methotrexate	Gold, hydroxychloroquine, penicillamine	
Acetaminophen class	Acetaminophen		Phenacetin
Drugs used in gout Anti-inflammatory drugs	Colchicine		NSAIDs, eg, indomethacin
Uricosurics	Probenecid		Sulfinpyrazone
Xanthine oxidase inhibitors	Allopurinol		

QUESTIONS

DIRECTIONS: Each of the numbered items or incomplete statements in this section is followed by answers or by completions of the sentence. Select the ONE lettered answer or completion that is BEST in each case.

1. Important effects of aspirin include all of the following EXCEPT
   (A) Reduction of fever
   (B) Reduction of prostaglandin synthesis in inflamed tissues
   (C) Respiratory stimulation when taken in toxic dosage
   (D) Reduction of bleeding tendency
   (E) Tinnitus and vertigo

2. Important effects of ibuprofen include all of the following EXCEPT
   (A) Reversal of joint destruction in rheumatoid arthritis
   (B) Reduction of uterine contractions in dysmenorrhea
   (C) Reduction of fever
   (D) Analgesic action in headache
   (E) Reduction of thromboxane synthesis in platelets

3. Drugs that are useful in dysmenorrhea include all of the following EXCEPT
   (A) Colchicine
   (B) Ibuprofen
   (C) Aspirin
   (D) Naproxen
   (E) Piroxicam

4. Drugs that are useful in the treatment of gout include all of the following EXCEPT
   (A) Indomethacin
   (B) Allopurinol
   (C) Colchicine
   (D) Probenecid
   (E) Aspirin

5. Which of the following drug effects is NOT linked with a correct statement about its mechanism of action?
   (A) Allopurinol action in gout: Inhibition of oxidation of hypoxanthine
   (B) Aspirin antiplatelet action: Inhibition of cyclooxygenase
   (C) Hydroxychloroquine antirheumatic action: Interference with T lymphocyte action
   (D) Probenecid uricosuric action: Increased secretion of uric acid by the loop of Henle
   (E) Indomethacin closure of patent ductus arteriosus: Blockade of PGE production in the ductus of the newborn

6. Salicylate intoxication is characterized by all of the following EXCEPT
   (A) Hypothermia
   (B) Hyperventilation
   (C) Metabolic acidosis
   (D) Respiratory alkalosis
   (E) Hypoprothrombinemia

DIRECTIONS: The following section consists of a list of four to twenty-six lettered options followed by several numbered items. For each numbered item, select the ONE option that is most closely associated with it. Each answer may be selected once, more than once, or not at all.
   (A) Aspirin
   (B) Acetaminophen
   (C) Indomethacin
   (D) Hydroxychloroquine
   (E) Colchicine
   (F) Penicillamine
   (G) Phenacetin
   (H) Allopurinol
   (I) Probenecid
   (J) Methotrexate

7. A potent inhibitor of cyclooxygenase; used to accelerate closure of a patent ductus arteriosus
8. A relatively safe antipyretic drug with no anti-inflammatory action
9. A drug that has anti-inflammatory effects only in gout and "Mediterranean fever"
10. An antimalarial agent with a slow anti-inflammatory effect in rheumatoid arthritis
11. A drug that is metabolized to a hepatotoxic product; the antidote is acetylcysteine
12. A slow-acting antirheumatic drug that is cytotoxic and reduces the number of inflammatory cells in rheumatoid joints
13. A drug that is metabolized to a product that inhibits the enzyme that produced it
14. A highly selective inhibitor of microtubule assembly
15. A drug that is metabolized to acetaminophen; it was withdrawn from the US market because of its high incidence of renal damage

ANSWERS

1. Aspirin clearly *increases* bleeding tendency (by its antiplatelet effects). The answer is (**D**).
2. It is not clear that any drug actually reverses the joint damage of rheumatoid arthritis, although it has been claimed that gold salts may do so. The answer is (**A**).
3. Primary dysmenorrhea is caused by excessive production of prostaglandin $F_{2\alpha}$; NSAIDs that inhibit cyclooxygenase are far more effective in relieving symptoms than other analgesics. Colchicine, which is not analgesic and is only anti-inflammatory in gout and "Mediterranean fever," would never be used in this condition. The answer is (**A**).
4. Aspirin should not be used in gout because the drug slows renal secretion of uric acid and raises uric acid blood levels over a large part of the dose range. The answer is (**E**).
5. Probenecid inhibits the reabsorption of uric acid in the proximal tubule. (Both secretion and reabsorption of weak acids occur in the proximal tubule, not the loop of Henle.) The answer is (**D**).
6. Salicylate intoxication is associated with *hyperthermia*, not hypothermia, because the drug causes uncoupling of oxidative phosphorylation, resulting in increased metabolism. The answer is (**A**).
7. The answer is (**C**), indomethacin.
8. The answer is (**B**), acetaminophen.
9. Colchicine has a highly selective effect on leukocytes that are partially responsible for the inflammation associated with urate crystal deposition. The drug's mechanism in the familial disease, Mediterranean fever, is unknown. The answer is (**E**).
10. The answer is (**D**), hydroxychloroquine.
11. Acetaminophen toxicity, a common source of questions on board exams, has been discussed in this chapter and in Chapter 4. Acetaminophen toxicity is more difficult to treat than aspirin toxicity, but acetylcysteine is effective if given early. The answer is (**B**).
12. Methotrexate is cytotoxic (it is an important cancer chemotherapeutic drug) and has become one of the most popular slow-acting antirheumatic drugs. The answer is (**J**).
13. Allopurinol is metabolized to oxipurinol (alloxanthine) by xanthine oxidase; both allopurinol and its metabolite inhibit this enzyme. The answer is (**H**).
14. Colchicine is highly selective in its ability to inhibit microtubule assembly and is a standard agent used in research on these cellular organelles. The answer is (**E**).
15. Phenacetin is a pro-drug of acetaminophen and has been shown in very large epidemiologic studies to cause renal damage in large numbers of patients. The answer is (**G**).

Part VII. Endocrine Drugs

---

36   Hypothalamic & Pituitary Hormones

OBJECTIVES

You should be able to:

- List or describe the major hypothalamic releasing hormones.
- List or describe the major anterior pituitary hormones and their effects.
- List or describe the major posterior pituitary hormones and their effects.
- List or describe the major drugs used as substitutes for the natural hypothalamic and pituitary hormones.

CONCEPTS

The hypothalamus and pituitary gland synthesize several hormones that regulate other glands and tissues throughout the body. One group of hypothalamic hormones (releasing hormones) regulates the release of anterior pituitary hormones. The other hypothalamic hormones (oxytocin and vasopressin) are transported to the posterior pituitary, released from the pituitary into the general circulation, and act directly on distant tissues. The hormones currently recognized as most important (and their targets) are listed in Table 36–1. Except for prolactin-inhibiting hormone (dopamine), all of these endocrine agents are peptides.

Table 36–1. Links between hypothalamic, pituitary, and target organ hormones.

Hypothalamic Hormone	Pituitary Hormone	Target Organ	Target Organ Hormone
Growth hormone-releasing hormone (GHRH)	Growth hormone (GH)	Liver	Somatomedins
Somatostatin			
Thyrotropin-releasing hormone (TRH)	Thyroid-stimulating hormone (TSH)	Thyroid	Thyroxine, triiodothyronine
Corticotropin-releasing hormone (CRH)	Adrenocorticotropin (ACTH)	Adrenal cortex	Glucocorticoids, mineralocorticoids, androgens
Gonadotropin-releasing hormone (GnRH or LHRH)	Follicle-stimulating hormone (FSH)	Gonads	Estrogen, progesterone, testosterone
	Luteinizing hormone (LH)		
Prolactin-releasing hormone (PRH)	Prolactin (PRL)	Lymphocytes	Lymphokines
Prolactin-inhibiting hormone (PIH, dopamine)		Breast	
Oxytocin	None	Smooth muscle, especially uterus	
Vasopressin	None	Renal tubule, smooth muscle	

HYPOTHALAMIC HORMONES

A. Growth Hormone-Releasing Hormone (GHRH): GHRH (also called somatocrinin) has not been precisely characterized. Peptides with GHRH activity have been isolated and synthesized; two of them are available for investigational use. They produce a rapid increase in plasma growth hormone levels and are effective in increasing growth in some patients with short stature. However, most patients with short stature suffer from pituitary insufficiency, not GHRH deficiency. Therefore, the primary use of GHRH preparations is to determine the cause of growth-hormone deficiency.

B. Somatostatin (Somatotropin Release-Inhibiting Hormone, SRIF): Somatostatin has been isolated, sequenced, and synthesized. It is found in the pancreas and other parts of the gastrointestinal system, as well as in the CNS. In addition to inhibiting the release of growth hormone, somatostatin inhibits the release of thyrotropin, glucagon, insulin, and gastrin. Although it can decrease the release of growth hormone in acromegaly, somatostatin is of no clinical value because of its short duration of action. **Octreotide,** a synthetic octapeptide somatostatin analogue with a longer duration of action, has been found useful in the management of acromegaly, carcinoid, gastrinoma, glucagonoma, and other endocrine tumors.

C. Thyrotropin-Releasing Hormone (TRH): TRH is a tripeptide that stimulates release of thyrotropin from the anterior pituitary, possibly through the stimulation of adenylyl cyclase. TRH also increases prolactin production but has no effect on the release of growth hormone or ACTH.

D. Corticotropin-Releasing Hormone (CRH): This 41-amino-acid peptide stimulates secretion of both ACTH and beta-endorphin (a closely related peptide) from the pituitary. This effect is associated with increased cAMP levels in the gland. CRH can be used in the diagnosis of abnormalities of ACTH secretion because ACTH secretion by nonpituitary tumors (eg, of the lung) rarely increases in response to stimulation by CRH, whereas secretion by the pituitary in Cushing's disease consistently increases after CRH stimulation.

E. Gonadotropin-Releasing Hormone (GnRH or LHRH, Gonadorelin): GnRH is a decapeptide; **leuprolide** is a synthetic nonapeptide with similar activity. Several other synthetic peptides with GnRH activity are available. When given in pulsatile doses (resembling physiologic cycling), these agents stimulate gonadotropin release. In contrast, steady dosing causes a marked inhibition of gonadotropin release—in effect, a medical castration. GnRH is used in the diagnosis and treatment (by pulsatile administration) of hypogonadal states. Leuprolide and several analogues (nafarelin, gosarelin, buserelin) are used to suppress gonadotropin secretion (by administration in steady dosage) in patients with prostatic carcinoma or other gonadal steroid-sensitive tumors.

F. Prolactin-Inhibiting Hormone (PIH, Dopamine): Dopamine is the physiologic inhibitor of prolactin release. Because of its peripheral effects and the need for parenteral administration, dopamine is not useful in the control of hyperprolactinemia, but **bromocriptine,** an orally active ergot derivative, is effective in reducing prolactin secretion from the normal gland as well as from pituitary tumors. Bromocriptine may reduce the secretion of other hormones from such tumors; sometimes regression of the tumor may also result.

ANTERIOR PITUITARY HORMONES

A. Growth Hormone (Somatotropin): Growth hormone is a large (191-amino-acid) peptide. In the past it was obtained from the pituitaries of human cadavers. This use was abolished when it was reported that several patients treated with growth hormone from this source developed Creutzfeld-Jakob disease, apparently from slow infectious agents contained in the extracts. Human growth hormone is now available in two forms through recombinant DNA technology: somatrem (somatotropin with an extra methionine) and somatotropin. These products, which are identical in their biologic properties, are useful in the treatment of growth-hormone deficiency in children.

B. Thyroid-Stimulating Hormone (TSH): This peptide stimulates adenylyl cyclase in thyroid cells and increases iodine uptake and production of thyroid hormones. TSH has been used as a diagnostic tool to distinguish primary from secondary hypothyroidism. The hormone is still used occasionally to increase ^{131}I uptake (and tumoricidal effect) in metastatic thyroid carcinoma.

C. Adrenocorticotropin (ACTH): This peptide is formed from a large precursor peptide, proopiomelanocortin. This precursor is also the source of melanocyte-stimulating hormone, beta-endorphin, and met-enkephalin. Although it has been used therapeutically to increase corticosteroid levels, ACTH is now used almost exclusively for diagnostic purposes in patients with abnormal corticosteroid production. **Cosyntropin,** a synthetic analogue consisting of the first 24 amino acids of ACTH, is usually used for this purpose rather than ACTH itself.

D. Follicle-Stimulating Hormone (FSH): FSH is a glycoprotein that stimulates gametogenesis and follicle development in women and spermatogenesis in men. The preparation usually used is urofollitin, a product extracted from the urine of postmenopausal women.

E. Luteinizing Hormone (LH): LH is the major stimulant of gonadal steroid production. In women, LH also regulates follicular development and ovulation. No pure preparation of LH is currently in use. Human chorionic gonadotropin (hCG) has significant LH effect, is synthesized by the placenta, and is available for use (see below).

F. Menotropins (hMG): Menotropins is a preparation of human menopausal gonadotropins that consists of human FSH and LH from postmenopausal urine. The product is often combined with human chorionic gonadotropin (hCG) in the treatment of hypogonadal states in both men and women.

G. Prolactin: Prolactin, a glycoprotein hormone responsible for lactation, is not used in therapy.

POSTERIOR PITUITARY HORMONES

A. Oxytocin: Oxytocin is a nonapeptide synthesized in cell bodies in the paraventricular nuclei of the hypothalamus and transported through the axons of these cells to the posterior pituitary, where the peptide is released into the circulation. Oxytocin is an effective stimulant of uterine contraction and is sometimes used intravenously to induce or reinforce labor. Because it causes contraction of smooth muscle in the myoepithelial cells of the mammary gland, oxytocin also can be used as a nasal spray to stimulate milk "let-down."

B. Vasopressin (Antidiuretic Hormone, ADH): Vasopressin is synthesized in the supraoptic nuclei of the hypothalamus and released from the posterior pituitary. As discussed in Chapter 15, vasopressin acts on V_2 receptors and increases the synthesis or insertion of water channels by a cAMP-dependent mechanism, resulting in an increase in water permeability in the collecting tubules of the kidney. The increased water permeability permits water reabsorption into the hypertonic renal papilla, thus causing the antidiuretic effect. Vasopressin also causes smooth muscle contraction (a V_1 effect). The primary use of vasopressin is in the treatment of pituitary diabetes insipidus.

DRUG LIST

The following drugs are pituitary hormone analogues or agents used for their effects on pituitary-related endocrine function. Many of the natural hormones described in Table 36–1 are also used as drugs.

Drug	Actions	Clinical Use	Comment
Somatrem	Growth hormone	Pituitary deficiency	Protein from recombinant synthesis; has one additional methionine; recombinant somatotropin is also available
Octreotide	Somatostatin analogue	Multiple uses to inhibit glandular secretion	Longer-acting than natural somatostatin
Cosyntropin	ACTH analogue, stimulates adrenal cortex	Corticosteroid substitute; diagnosis; infantile spasms (seizures)	Cosyntropin is a 1–24 amino acid active fragment of ACTH
Leuprolide, goserelin, nafarelin	GnRH analogues	Infertility, cancer	Stimulate gonads if given in pulses; inhibit if given continuously
Urofollitin	FSH-like activity	Infertility	Isolated from human urine
Human chorionic gonadotropin (hCG)	LH-like activity	Infertility	Isolated from human urine
Menotropins	FSH plus LH activity	Infertility	Isolated from human urine
Bromocriptine	Inhibits prolactin release	Stops lactation; inhibits growth of pituitary tumors	An ergot alkaloid with potent dopamine agonist activity
Desmopressin	Antidiuretic hormone analogue	Pituitary diabetes insipidus	A V_2 agonist; longer-acting than ADH

QUESTIONS

DIRECTIONS: Each of the numbered items or incomplete statements in this section is followed by answers or by completions of the sentence. Select the ONE lettered answer or completion that is BEST in each case.

1. All of the following are hormones EXCEPT
   (A) Bromocriptine
   (B) Somatotropin
   (C) Thyrotropin
   (D) Vasopressin
   (E) Somatomedin

2. Drugs useful in the treatment of infertility include all of the following EXCEPT
   (A) Human chorionic gonadotropin
   (B) Bromocriptine
   (C) Gonadotropin-releasing hormone
   (D) Prolactin
   (E) Clomiphene

3. Hormones that increase cAMP in the target organs include
   (A) Vasopressin
   (B) Prolactin
   (C) Luteinizing hormone
   (D) Growth hormone
   (E) Oxytocin

4. Hormones that are synthesized in the hypothalamus include all of the following EXCEPT
   (A) Corticotropin-releasing hormone
   (B) Oxytocin
   (C) Thyrotropin-releasing hormone
   (D) Luteinizing hormone
   (E) Vasopressin

5. Hormones that are useful in the diagnosis of endocrine insufficiency include
   (A) Gonadotropin-releasing hormone
   (B) Thyrotropin-releasing hormone
   (C) Corticotropin-releasing hormone
   (D) Cosyntropin
   (E) All of the above

DIRECTIONS: The following section consists of a list of four to twenty-six lettered options followed by several numbered items. For each numbered item, select the ONE option that is most closely associated with it. Each answer may be selected once, more than once, or not at all.
   (A) Octreotide
   (B) Thyroid-stimulating hormone
   (C) Menotropins
   (D) Leuprolide
   (E) Human chorionic gonadotropin
   (F) Desmopressin
   (G) Cosyntropin
   (H) Bromocriptine
   (I) Somatomedin
   (J) Somatrem

6. A 24-amino-acid peptide with ACTH-like properties
7. A substance derived from the urine of pregnant women; useful for its LH-like activity
8. A substance produced in the liver under the control of growth hormone
9. A recombinant form of growth hormone with one additional amino acid
10. A peptide with GnRH activity but longer duration than the naturally occurring hormone

ANSWERS

1. Bromocriptine, an ergot alkaloid with central dopamine agonist activity, is not produced in the body. The answer is **(A)**.
2. Clomiphene is an ovulation-stimulating partial agonist estrogen (see Chapter 39). Prolactin has inhibitory effects on fertility and is never used in infertility. The answer is **(D)**.
3. Vasopressin acts by increasing cAMP. The other hormones act by other mechanisms. The answer is **(A)**.
4. Luteinizing hormone is synthesized in the anterior pituitary. The answer is **(D)**.
5. All are correct. The answer is **(E)**.
6. Cosyntropin is the form of ACTH usually used. ACTH is now rarely used; cosyntropin is used mainly for diagnostic procedures. The answer is **(G)**.
7. Human chorionic gonadotropin (hCG) is produced by the placenta in pregnant women and has potent LH activity. The answer is **(E)**.
8. The somatomedins are synthesized in the liver under growth hormone control. The answer is **(I)**.
9. Somatrem is recombinant growth hormone with an extra methionine. True somatotropin is also available through recombinant synthesis. The answer is **(J)**.
10. Leuprolide is a longer-acting GnRH analogue. The answer is **(D)**.

Thyroid & Antithyroid Drugs

37

OBJECTIVES

You should be able to:

- List the principal drugs used in the treatment of hypothyroidism.
- List the principal drugs used in the treatment of hyperthyroidism.
- Describe the major toxicities of thyroxine and the antithyroid drugs.

CONCEPTS

The thyroid secretes two types of hormones: iodine-containing amino acids (thyroxine and triiodothyronine) and a peptide (calcitonin). Thyroxine and triiodothyronine have very general effects on growth, development, and metabolism. Calcitonin is important in calcium metabolism and is discussed in Chapter 41.

This chapter describes the drugs used in the treatment of hypo- and hyperthyroidism (Figure 37–1).

THYROID HORMONES

A. Synthesis & Transport of Thyroid Hormones: The thyroid secretes two primary iodine-containing hormones, triiodothyronine (T_3) and thyroxine (T_4). The iodine necessary for the synthesis of these molecules is derived from food or iodine supplements given orally. The uptake of iodine is an active process, and the iodide ion is highly concentrated in the thyroid gland. The tyrosine residues of a protein, thyroglobulin, are iodinated in the gland to form monoiodotyrosine (MIT) or diiodotyrosine (DIT). Thyroxine (T_4) is formed from the combination of two molecules of DIT, while triiodothyronine (T_3) contains one molecule of MIT and one of DIT. Some T_3 is released from the thyroid, but much of the circulating T_3 is formed by the deiodination of T_4 in the tissues. After release from the gland, both T_3 and T_4 are bound to thyroxine-binding globulin, a transport protein in the blood.

Thyroid function is controlled by the pituitary through the release of thyrotropin, and by the availability of iodide. High levels of thyroid hormones inhibit the release of TRH and TSH, providing an effective negative feedback control mechanism. In Graves' disease, lymphocytes release a thyroid-stimulating immunoglobulin (TSI, also called TSH receptor-stimulating antibody, TSH-R Ab[stim]) that causes thyrotoxicosis. Since these lymphocytes are not susceptible to negative feedback, blood concentrations of thyroid hormone may become very high.

Levels of iodide higher than normal inhibit iodination of tyrosine, an effect that is useful in the treatment of thyroid disease. Inadequate iodine intake results in diffuse enlargement of the thyroid (goiter).

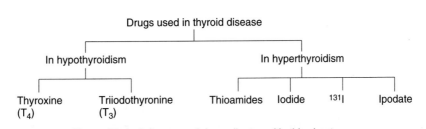

Figure 37–1. Subgroups of drugs discussed in this chapter.

B. Mechanisms of Action of Thyroxine & Triiodothyronine: T_3 appears to be about 10 times more potent than T_4; since T_4 is converted to T_3 in target cells, the liver, and the kidneys, most of the effect of circulating T_4 is probably due to T_3.

Thyroid hormone binds to receptors in the nucleus that control the expression of genes responsible for many metabolic processes. Like many other intracellular hormone receptors, the T_3 receptor exists in two monomeric forms, alpha and beta; they are synthesized in different amounts and different forms ($\alpha 1$, $\alpha 2$, $\beta 1$, or $\beta 2$) in a developmentally specific way. When activated by T_3, the α and β monomers combine to form $\alpha\alpha$, $\beta\beta$, or $\alpha\beta$ dimers. These T_3-activated dimers bind to DNA response elements and control the synthesis of RNA that codes for specific proteins which mediate the actions of thyroid hormones.

The proteins synthesized under T_3 control differ depending upon the tissue involved; these proteins include Na^+/K^+ ATPase, specific contractile proteins in smooth muscle and the heart, enzymes involved in lipid metabolism, important developmental components in the brain, etc. T_3 may also have a separate membrane receptor-mediated effect in some tissues.

1. **Effects of thyroid hormone:** The organ level actions of the thyroid drugs include normal growth and development of nervous, skeletal, and reproductive systems and control of

Table 37–1. Summary of thyroid effects.

System	Thyrotoxicosis	Hypothyroidism
Skin and appendages	Warm, moist skin; sweating; heat intolerance; fine, thin hair; Plummer's nails; pretibial dermopathy (Graves' disease).	Pale, cool, puffy skin; dry and brittle hair; brittle nails.
Eyes, face	Retraction of upper lid with wide stare; periorbital edema; exophthalmos; diplopia (Graves' disease).	Drooping of eyelids; periorbital edema; loss of temporal aspects of eyebrows; puffy, nonpitting facies; large tongue.
Cardiovascular system	Increased peripheral vascular resistance, heart rate, stroke volume, cardiac output, pulse pressure; high-output congestive heart failure; increased inotropic/chronotropic effects; arrhythmias; angina.	Decreased peripheral vascular resistance, heart rate, stroke volume, cardiac output, pulse pressure; low-output congestive heart failure; ECG; bradycardia, prolonged PR interval, flat T wave, low voltage; pericardial effusion.
Respiratory system	Dyspnea; decreased vital capacity.	Pleural effusion; hypoventilation and CO_2 retention.
Gastrointestinal system	Increased appetite; increased frequency of bowel movements; hypoproteinemia.	Decreased appetite; decreased frequency of bowel movements; ascites.
Central nervous system	Nervousness; hyperkinesia; emotional lability.	Lethargy; general slowing of mental processes; neuropathies.
Musculoskeletal system	Weakness and muscle fatigue; increased deep tendon reflexes; hypercalcemia; osteoporosis.	Stiffness and muscle fatigue; decreased deep tendon reflexes; increased alkaline phosphatase, LDH, AST.
Renal system	Mild polyuria; increased renal blood flow; increased glomerular filtration rate.	Impaired water excretion; decreased renal blood flow; decreased glomerular filtration rate.
Hematopoietic system	Increased erythropoiesis; anemia.[1]	Decreased erythropoiesis; anemia.[1]
Reproductive system	Menstrual irregularities; decreased fertility; increased gonadal steroid metabolism.	Hypermenorrhea; infertility; decreased libido; impotency; oligospermia; decreased gonadal steroid metabolism.
Metabolic system	Increased basal metabolic rate; negative nitrogen balance; hyperglycemia; increased free fatty acids; decreased cholesterol and triglycerides; increased hormone degradation; increased requirements for fat- and water-soluble vitamins; increased drug detoxification.	Decreased basal metabolic rate; slight positive nitrogen balance; delayed degradation of insulin, with increased sensitivity; increased cholesterol and triglycerides; decreased hormone degradation; decreased requirements for fat- and water-soluble vitamins; decreased drug detoxification.

[1] The anemia of hyperthyroidism is usually normochromic and caused by increased RBC turnover. The anemia of hypothyroidism may be normochromic, hyperchromic, or hypochromic and may be due to decreased production rate, decreased iron absorption, decreased folic acid absorption, or to autoimmune pernicious anemia.

metabolism of fats, carbohydrates, proteins, and vitamins. The results of excess thyroid activity (thyrotoxicosis) and hypothyroidism (myxedema) are summarized in Table 37–1. A case of thyrotoxicosis is presented in Case 11 (Appendix IV).

2. **Clinical use:**   Thyroid hormone therapy can be accomplished with either thyroxine or triiodothyronine. Synthetic levothyroxine (T_4) is the form of choice for most cases. T_3 is faster-acting but has a shorter half-life and higher cost.
3. **Toxicity:**   Toxicity is that of thyrotoxicosis (Table 37–1).

ANTITHYROID DRUGS

A. **Thioamides:**   Propylthiouracil and methimazole are small sulfur-containing molecules that inhibit thyroid hormone production by several mechanisms. The most important effect is to block iodination of the tyrosine residues of thyroglobulin (Figure 37–2). In addition, these drugs appear to block coupling of DIT and MIT. The thioamides can be used by the oral route and are effective in most patients with uncomplicated hyperthyroidism. Toxic effects include skin rash (common) and severe immune reactions (rare) such as vasculitis, hypoprothrombinemia, and agranulocytosis. These effects are usually reversible.

B. **Iodide Salts & Iodine:**   Iodide salts inhibit organification (iodination of tyrosine) and thyroid hormone release (Figure 37–2); these salts also decrease the size and vascularity of the hyperplastic thyroid gland. These effects of iodide are especially desirable if surgical resection of a hyperactive thyroid is planned. The usual forms of this drug are Lugol's solution (iodine and potassium iodide) and saturated solution of potassium iodide.

C. **Radioactive Iodine:**   Radioactive iodine (^{131}I) is taken up and concentrated in the thyroid gland so avidly that a dose large enough to severely damage the gland can be given without endangering other tissues. Unlike the thioamides and iodide salts, an effective dose of ^{131}I can produce a permanent cure of thyrotoxicosis without surgery.

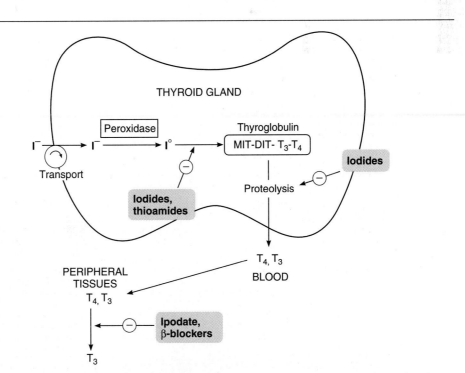

Figure 37–2. Sites of action of some antithyroid drugs. I⁻, iodide ion; I°, elemental iodine. Not shown: radioactive iodine (^{131}I), which destroys the gland through radiation.

D. Iodinated Radiocontrast Media: Certain iodinated radiocontrast media, eg, ipodate, effectively suppress the conversion of T_4 to T_3 in the liver, kidney, and other peripheral tissues (Figure 37–2). Inhibition of hormone release from the thyroid may also play a part. Ipodate has proved to be very useful in rapidly reducing T_3 concentrations in thyrotoxicosis.

E. Other Drugs: Other agents used in the treatment of thyrotoxicosis include the sympatholytic drugs, especially **beta-blockers.** These agents are particularly useful in controlling the tachycardia and other cardiac abnormalities of severe thyrotoxicosis.

DRUG LIST

The following drugs are important members of the group discussed in this chapter. Prototypes should be learned in detail; the other significant agents should be recognized as belonging to a specific subclass.

Subclass	Prototype	Other Significant Agents
Thyroid hormones	Thyroxine (T_4), triiodothyronine (T_3)	
Antithyroid drugs	Propylthiouracil, iodide salts, ^{131}I, ipodate	Methimazole
Miscellaneous	Propranolol	

QUESTIONS

DIRECTIONS: Each of the numbered items or incomplete statements in this section is followed by answers or by completions of the sentence. Select the ONE lettered answer or completion that is BEST in each case.

1. Important drugs used in the treatment of thyrotoxicosis include all of the following EXCEPT
   (A) Propylthiouracil
   (B) Potassium iodide
   (C) Thyroglobulin
   (D) Radioactive iodine
   (E) Methimazole
2. Actions of thyroxine include all of the following EXCEPT
   (A) Stimulation of oxygen consumption
   (B) Acceleration of cardiac rate
   (C) Fine tremor of skeletal muscles
   (D) Decreased glomerular filtration rate
   (E) Increased appetite
3. Effects of iodide salts given in large doses include all of the following EXCEPT
   (A) Decreased size of the thyroid gland
   (B) Decreased vascularity of the thyroid gland
   (C) Decreased hormone release
   (D) Decreased iodination of tyrosine
   (E) Increased ^{131}I uptake
4. Symptoms of hypothyroidism (myxedema) include all of the following EXCEPT
   (A) Slow heart rate
   (B) Dry, puffy skin
   (C) Lethargy, sleepiness
   (D) Increased appetite
   (E) Large tongue and drooping of the eyelids

Items 5–6: A 24-year-old woman is found to have thyrotoxicosis. She appears to be in good health otherwise.

5. It is decided to place her on antithyroid drug therapy. Toxicities that would be considered in this case include all of the following EXCEPT
    (A) Ipodate: Skin rash
    (B) Iodide ion: Acne-like rash
    (C) Methimazole: Agranulocytosis
    (D) Propylthiouracil: Lupus erythematosus-like syndrome
    (E) Radioactive iodine: Radiation damage to the ovaries

6. The patient is lost to follow-up before therapy is begun, but she returns six months later for a prenatal workup. Although 3 months pregnant, she has lost weight, she has a marked tremor, and her resting heart rate is 120/minute. Her thyrotoxicosis is obviously worse and the gland is larger and more vascular. It is decided to correct her thyroid abnormality surgically. Before surgery can be done, however, her gland should be reduced in size and vascularity by administering
    (A) Radioactive iodine
    (B) Propylthiouracil
    (C) Ipodate
    (D) Iodide ion
    (E) Propranolol

DIRECTIONS: The following section consists of a list of four to twenty-six lettered options followed by several numbered items. For each numbered item, select the ONE option that is most closely associated with it. Each answer may be selected once, more than once, or not at all.
    (A) Propylthiouracil
    (B) ^{131}I
    (C) Triiodothyronine
    (D) Ipodate
    (E) Propranolol

7. Produced in the peripheral tissues when thyroxine is administered
8. Useful in "thyroid storm" to control cardiac manifestations
9. Radiocontrast medium that is also useful in thyrotoxicosis
10. Produces a permanent reduction in thyroid activity

ANSWERS

1. Thyroglobulin contains thyroxine in its protein-bound form. This compound would never be used in thyrotoxicosis. Formerly used in hypothyroidism, thyroglobulin is now obsolete. The answer is **(C)**.
2. Thyroid hormone increases glomerular filtration rate. The answer is **(D)**.
3. Iodide has a negative feedback effect on the thyroid. The answer is **(E)**.
4. Appetite decreases in myxedema as the metabolic rate decreases. The answer is **(D)**.
5. The toxicities listed are all possible except radiation damage to the ovaries. Iodine is so avidly taken up by the thyroid that large doses of radioactive iodide can be given without damage to other tissues. The answer is **(E)**.
6. Surgical treatment is often preferred in hyperthyroidism that occurs during pregnancy because this offers minimal risk to the fetus and the fetal thyroid. Before surgical removal, a large, highly vascular thyroid gland should be prepared by administration of iodide ion. This treatment reduces the gland's size and vascularity, and makes surgery much safer. Propylthiouracil may be considered for less severe thyrotoxicosis occurring during pregnancy. The answer is **(D)**.
7. T_4 is converted into T_3 in the periphery. The answer is **(C)**.
8. Beta-blockers are particularly useful in controlling cardiac manifestations of severe thyrotoxicosis ("storm"). The answer is **(E)**.
9. Ipodate is a radiocontrast agent. The answer is **(D)**.
10. Radioactive iodine is the only medical therapy that produces a permanent reduction of thyroid activity. The answer is **(B)**.

38

Corticosteroids & Antagonists

OBJECTIVES

You should be able to:

- Describe the major naturally occurring glucocorticosteroid and its actions.
- List several synthetic glucocorticoids and the differences between these agents and the naturally occurring hormone.
- Describe the actions of the naturally occurring mineralocorticoid and one synthetic agent in this subgroup.
- List the indications for the use of corticosteroids in adrenal disorders and in nonadrenal disorders.
- List or describe the toxic effects of the glucocorticoids when given chronically.

CONCEPTS:

The corticosteroids are those steroid hormones produced by the adrenal cortex. They consist of two primary physiologic and pharmacologic groups: (1) glucocorticoids, which have important effects on intermediary metabolism, catabolism, immune responses, and inflammation; and (2) mineralocorticoids, which regulate sodium and potassium reabsorption in the collecting tubules of the kidney. In addition, some androgenic and estrogenic steroids are also synthesized in the adrenal gland. This chapter reviews the glucocorticoids, mineralocorticoids, and the adrenocorticosteroid antagonists (Figure 38–1).

GLUCOCORTICOIDS

A. Mechanism of Action: Corticosteroids enter the cell and bind to cytosolic receptors that transport the steroid into the nucleus. The steroid-receptor complex alters gene expression by binding to glucocorticoid response elements (GREs) or equivalent mineralocorticoid-specific elements (Figure 38–2). Ligand-bound receptors typically form dimers for optimal binding to the response elements. Tissue-specific responses to steroids are made possible by the presence

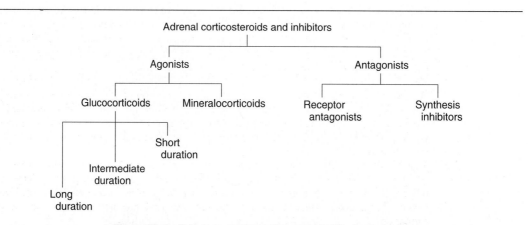

Figure 38–1. Subgroups of drugs discussed in this chapter.

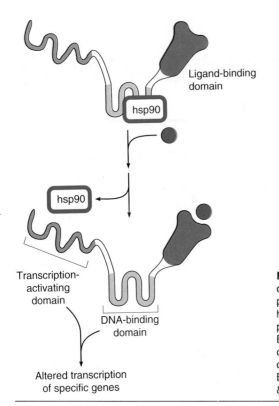

Transcription-
activating
domain

hsp90

DNA-binding
domain

Altered transcription
of specific genes

Figure 38–2. Mechanism of glucocorticoid action. The gluco-corticoid receptor polypeptide is schematically depicted as a protein with three distinct domains. A heat-shock protein, hsp90, binds to the receptor in the absence of hormone and prevents folding into the active conformation of the receptor. Binding of a hormone ligand (filled circle) causes dissociation of the hsp90 stabilizer and permits conversion to the active configuration. (Reproduced, with permission, from Katzung BG [editor]: *Basic & Clinical Pharmacology,* 6th ed. Appleton & Lange, 1995.)

in each tissue of different protein regulators that control the interaction between the hormone-receptor complex and particular response elements.

B. Organ and Tissue Effects:

1. **Metabolic effects:** Glucocorticoids stimulate gluconeogenesis. As a result, blood sugar rises, muscle protein is catabolized, and insulin secretion is stimulated. Both lipolysis and lipogenesis are stimulated, with a net increase of fat deposition in certain areas, eg, face (moon facies) and shoulders and back (buffalo hump).

2. **Catabolic effects:** As noted above, glucocorticoids cause muscle protein catabolism. In addition, lymphoid and connective tissue, fat, and skin undergo wasting under the influence of high concentrations of the corticosteroids. Catabolic effects on bone can lead to osteoporosis. In children, growth is inhibited.

3. **Immunosuppressive effects:** Glucocorticoids inhibit some of the mechanisms involved in cell-mediated immunologic functions, especially those dependent on lymphocytes. These agents are actively lymphotoxic and are important in the treatment of lymphocytic leukemias. The drugs do not interfere with the development of normal acquired immunity but delay rejection reactions in patients with organ transplants.

4. **Anti-inflammatory effects:** Glucocorticoids have a dramatic effect on the distribution and function of leukocytes. These drugs increase neutrophils and decrease lymphocytes, eosinophils, basophils, and monocytes. The migration of leukocytes is also inhibited. The mechanism of these effects probably involves synthesis of inhibitors, which suppress the production of prostaglandins and leukotrienes in the damaged tissue through inhibition of phospholipase (see Chapter 18).

5. **Other effects:** Glucocorticoids such as cortisol are required for normal renal excretion of water loads. The corticosteroids also have effects on the CNS. When given in large doses (especially if given for long periods), these drugs may cause profound behavioral disturbances. Large doses stimulate gastric acid secretion and may decrease resistance to ulcer formation.

Table 38–1. Properties of representative corticosteroids.

Agent	Duration of Action (hours)	Anti-Inflammatory Potency[1]	Salt-Retaining Potency[1]	Topical Activity
Primarily glucocorticoid Cortisol	8–12	1	1	0
Prednisone	12–24	4	0.3	+/–
Triamcinolone	15–24	5	0	+++
Dexamethasone	24–36	30	0	+++++
Primarily mineralocorticoid Aldosterone		0.3	3000	0
Fludrocortisone	8–12	10	125–250	0

[1] Relative to cortisol.

C. **Important Glucocorticoids:** Many glucocorticoids have been developed in an effort to obtain longer duration of action, less mineralocorticoid activity, or better topical activity (Table 38–1).

1. **Cortisol:** The major natural glucocorticoid is cortisol (hydrocortisone), a steroid synthesized in the adrenal cortex from 17-hydroxypregnenolone. The physiologic secretion of cortisol is regulated by ACTH and varies during the day (circadian rhythm), with the peak occurring in the morning and the trough around midnight. In the plasma, cortisol is 95% bound to corticosteroid-binding globulin. Given as a drug, cortisol is well absorbed from the gastrointestinal tract, is cleared by the liver, and has a short duration of action compared to its synthetic congeners (Table 38–1). Although it diffuses poorly across normal skin, cortisol is readily absorbed across inflamed skin and mucous membranes.

   The cortisol molecule also has a small but significant salt-retaining (mineralocorticoid) effect. This is an important cause of hypertension in patients with a corticosteroid-secreting adrenal tumor or a pituitary ACTH-secreting tumor (Cushing's syndrome).

2. **Synthetic glucocorticoids:** The mechanism of action of these agents is identical to that of cortisol. A very large number have been synthesized and are available for use; prednisolone (the active metabolite of prednisone), dexamethasone, and triamcinolone are representative. Their properties (when compared to cortisol) include prolonged half-life and duration of action, reduced salt-retaining effect, and better penetration of lipid barriers for topical activity (Table 38–1). Even greater surface activity can be achieved by adding acetonide or similar groups to the 17-carbon of the steroid ring.

   Special glucocorticoids have been developed for use in asthma and other conditions in which good surface activity on mucous membranes is needed and systemic effects are to be avoided. **Beclomethasone** and **budesonide** readily penetrate the airway mucosa but have very short half-lives after they enter the blood, so that systemic effects and toxicity are greatly reduced.

D. **Clinical Uses:**

1. **Adrenal disorders:** Glucocorticoids are essential to preserve life in patients with severe chronic adrenal cortical insufficiency (Addison's disease). These drugs are also necessary in acute adrenal insufficiency associated with life-threatening shock, infection, or trauma. Glucocorticoids are also used in certain types of congenital adrenal hyperplasia, in which synthesis of abnormal forms of corticosteroids is stimulated by ACTH. Administration of the exogenous normal glucocorticoid suppresses ACTH secretion sufficiently to reduce the synthesis of the abnormal steroids.

2. **Nonadrenal disorders:** Many disorders respond to corticosteroid therapy. Some of these are inflammatory or immunologic in nature, eg, asthma, organ transplant rejection, collagen diseases, etc. Other applications include the treatment of leukemias, neurologic disorders, chemotherapy-induced vomiting, exophthalmos, hypercalcemia, and mountain sickness. The degree of benefit differs considerably in different disorders, however, and the toxicity

of corticosteroids given chronically limits their use. Treatment of one patient with rheumatoid arthritis is described in Case 13 (Appendix IV).

E. Toxicity: Most of the toxic effects of the glucocorticosteroids are predictable from the effects already described. Some are life-threatening and include adrenal suppression (from suppression of ACTH secretion), metabolic effects (growth inhibition, diabetes, muscle wasting, osteoporosis), salt retention, and psychosis. Methods for minimizing these toxicities include local application (eg, aerosols for asthma), alternate day therapy (to reduce pituitary suppression), and tapering the dose soon after achieving a therapeutic response.

MINERALOCORTICOIDS

A. Aldosterone: The major natural mineralocorticoid is aldosterone, which has already been mentioned in connection with hypertension (see Chapter 11) and control of its secretion by angiotensin II (see Chapter 17). Pregnenolone and progesterone are intermediates in the synthesis of this mineralocorticoid. The secretion of aldosterone is regulated by ACTH and by the renin-angiotensin mechanisms and is very important in the regulation of blood volume (see Fig 6–4). Aldosterone has a short half-life and little glucocorticoid activity (Table 38–1). Its mechanism of action is the same as that of the glucocorticoids.

B. Other Mineralocorticoids: Other mineralocorticoids include desoxycorticosterone, the naturally occurring precursor of aldosterone, and **fludrocortisone.** The latter has significant glucocorticoid activity. Because of its long duration of action (Table 38–1), fludrocortisone is favored for replacement therapy after adrenalectomy and in other conditions in which mineralocorticoid therapy is needed.

ADRENOCORTICOSTEROID ANTAGONISTS

A. Receptor Antagonists: **Spironolactone,** an antagonist of aldosterone at its receptor, has been discussed in connection with the diuretics (see Chapter 15). **Mifepristone (RU486)** is an inhibitor at glucocorticoid receptors as well as progesterone receptors (see Chapter 39) and has been used in the treatment of Cushing's syndrome.

B. Synthesis Inhibitors: Several drugs are used in the treatment of adrenal cancer when surgical therapy is impractical or unsuccessful because of metastases. The most important of these drugs are **aminoglutethimide, metyrapone,** and **ketoconazole.** The drugs mitotane (a DDT analogue) and amphenone B also reduce steroid synthesis in the adrenals but are considered too toxic for human use.

Aminoglutethimide is used in the treatment of advanced breast cancer to suppress adrenal secretion of estrogenic steroids. Ketoconazole (an antifungal drug) inhibits the P450 enzymes necessary for the synthesis of all steroids and has been studied in a number of conditions in which reduced steroid levels are desirable, eg, prostate cancer and breast cancer. Metyrapone inhibits the normal synthesis of cortisol but not that of cortisol precursors; the drug can be used in diagnostic tests of adrenal function. A normal response to a test dose of metyrapone (increased levels of cortisol precursors) is evidence that the adrenal cortex is functioning.

DRUG LIST

The following drugs are important members of the group discussed in this chapter. Prototypes should be learned in detail; features of the major variants should be known well enough to distinguish the variants from prototypes and from each other; the other significant agents should be recognized as belonging to a specific subclass.

Subclass	Prototype	Major Variants	Other Significant Agents
Agonists			
Glucocorticoids	Cortisol (hydrocortisone)	Dexamethasone, triamcinolone, beclomethasone	Triamcinolone acetonide
Mineralocorticoids	Aldosterone	Fludrocortisone	
Antagonists			
Receptor antagonists	Spironolactone	Mifepristone	
Synthesis inhibitors	Aminoglutethimide, metyrapone	Ketoconazole	

QUESTIONS

DIRECTIONS: Each of the numbered items or incomplete statements in this section is followed by answers or by completions of the sentence. Select the ONE lettered answer or completion that is BEST in each case.

1. Effects of the glucocorticoids include all of the following EXCEPT
    (A) Reduction in circulating lymphocytes
    (B) Increased skin protein synthesis
    (C) Altered fat deposition
    (D) Inhibition of leukotriene synthesis
    (E) Increased blood glucose
2. Toxic effects of the corticosteroids include all of the following EXCEPT
    (A) Hypoglycemia
    (B) Osteoporosis
    (C) Growth inhibition
    (D) Salt retention
    (E) Psychosis

Items 3–4: A 54-year-old man with miliary tuberculosis has developed signs of severe acute adrenal insufficiency.
3. This patient will probably have all of the following manifestations EXCEPT
    (A) Moon face
    (B) Reduced ability to excrete a water load
    (C) Reduced ability to combat infection
    (D) Hypoglycemia if food is withheld
    (E) Reduced blood volume
4. The patient should be treated immediately. Which of the following combinations is most rational?
    (A) Triamcinolone and dexamethasone
    (B) Aldosterone and fludrocortisone
    (C) Fludrocortisone and metyrapone
    (D) Cortisol and fludrocortisone
    (E) Dexamethasone and metyrapone

DIRECTIONS: The following section consists of a list of four to twenty-six lettered options followed by several numbered items. For each numbered item, select the ONE option that is most closely associated with it. Each answer may be selected once, more than once, or not at all.
    (A) Cortisol
    (B) Triamcinolone acetonide
    (C) Aldosterone
    (D) Fludrocortisone
    (E) Spironolactone

    (F) Prednisolone
    (G) Aminoglutethimide
    (H) Metyrapone
    (I) Ketoconazole
    (J) Beclomethasone

5. Naturally occurring mineralocorticoid
6. Corticosteroid with high salt-retaining potency, some glucocorticoid effect, and long duration of action
7. Glucocorticoid with very low mineralocorticoid activity and very high topical activity
8. Endogenous substance that causes salt retention and buffalo hump in patients with Cushing's syndrome
9. Active metabolite of a synthetic glucocorticoid; has an intermediate duration of action and low topical activity
10. Antifungal agent that inhibits P450 enzymes required for steroid synthesis
11. A drug used by aerosol in the treatment of asthma

ANSWERS

1. Glucocorticoids stimulate protein breakdown (except in the liver). The answer is **(B)**.
2. Corticosteroids may induce hyperglycemia of sufficient magnitude to require insulin therapy. The answer is **(A)**.
3. Moon face is a manifestation of hypercortisolism, not adrenal insufficiency. The answer is **(A)**.
4. A rational combination of drugs should include agents with complementary effects, ie, a glucocorticoid and a mineralocorticoid. The combination with these characteristics is cortisol and fludrocortisone. (Note that while fludrocortisone may have sufficient glucocorticoid activity for a patient with mild disease, a patient in severe acute adrenal insufficiency needs a full glucocorticoid such as cortisol.) The answer is **(D)**.
5. The answer is **(C)**, aldosterone.
6. Fludrocortisone has a much longer duration of action than the naturally occurring mineralocorticoids and has some glucocorticoid activity (Table 38–1). The answer is **(D)**.
7. The answer is **(B)**, triamcinolone acetonide.
8. Cortisol causes buffalo hump. It also has sufficient salt-retaining activity to cause hypertension. Prednisolone would have the same effects (it has some salt-retaining action), but this drug is not present in Cushing's syndrome. The answer is **(A)**.
9. Prednisolone is the active metabolite of prednisone. The answer is **(F)**.
10. Ketoconazole is an antifungal agent that inhibits P450 enzymes in the adrenal gland (and elsewhere). The answer is **(I)**.
11. Beclomethasone has good ability to reduce inflammation in the airways when adminstered by aerosol. The answer is **(J)**.

Gonadal Hormones & Inhibitors

OBJECTIVES

You should be able to:

- Describe the hormonal changes that occur during the menstrual cycle.
- List the benefits and hazards of oral contraceptives.
- Describe the status of pharmacologic contraception in the male.

- List the benefits and hazards of postmenopausal estrogen therapy.
- Describe the use of sex hormones and their antagonists in the treatment of cancer in women and men.
- List or describe the toxic effects of anabolic steroids used to build muscle mass.

CONCEPTS

The gonadal hormones include the steroids of the ovary (estrogens and progestins) and testis (chiefly testosterone) and a few other hormones (eg, peptides) of lesser importance. Sex steroids are also synthesized in the adrenal cortex. Because of their importance in oral contraceptive agents, many synthetic estrogens and progestins have been produced. In the course of development, several partial agonist analogues of the natural hormones have been discovered. Testosterone, partial agonist androgens, and androgen antagonists are of similar importance. This group is outlined in Figure 39–1.

OVARIAN HORMONES

The ovary is the primary source of sex hormones in women during the child-bearing years, ie, between puberty and menopause. When properly regulated by FSH and LH from the pituitary, each menstrual cycle consists of the following events: a follicle in the ovary matures, secretes increasing amounts of estrogen, releases an ovum, and is transformed into a progesterone-secreting corpus luteum. If the ovum is not fertilized and implanted, the corpus luteum degenerates; the uterine endometrium (which has proliferated under the stimulation of estrogen and progesterone) is shed as part of the menstrual flow, and the cycle repeats. The mechanism of action of both estrogen and progesterone involves entry into cells, binding to cytosolic receptors that transport the hormones into the nucleus, and there causing modulation of gene expression.

A. Estrogens: The major ovarian estrogen in women is estradiol. Other estrogens include estrone and estriol, which are produced in other tissues. Almost all of the estrogen in the blood is bound to a sex hormone-binding globulin (SHBG). Estradiol is active by the oral route as replacement therapy but has low bioavailability because of hepatic metabolism. Therefore, semisynthetic derivatives (especially ethinyl estradiol) or other estrogens are usually used (see Drug List).

   1. Effects: Estrogen is essential for normal female sexual development. It is responsible for the growth of the genital structures (vagina, uterus, and uterine tubes) during childhood and for the appearance of secondary sexual characteristics and the growth spurt associated with puberty. Estrogen has many metabolic effects: It modifies serum protein levels, reduces bone resorption, and enhances nutrient absorption in the gastrointestinal tract. It enhances the coagulability of blood and increases plasma triglyceride levels while reducing LDL cholesterol. Estrogen is also an effective feedback suppressant of pituitary FSH (Figure 39–2).

   2. Clinical use: An important therapeutic use of estrogens is in the treatment of hypogonadism in girls (Table 39–1). Another use is in the management of postmenopausal changes

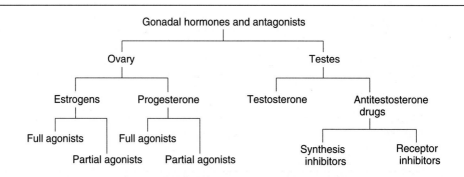

Figure 39–1. Subgroups of drugs discussed in this chapter.

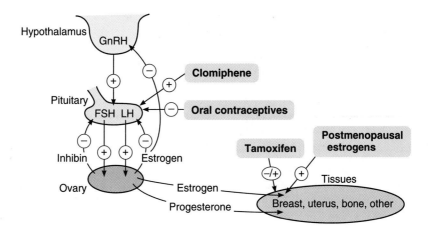

Figure 39–2. Sites of action of several ovarian hormones and their analogues. Clomiphene, a partial agonist, is mainly an antagonist at pituitary estrogen receptors; this prevents negative feedback and increases the output of the pituitary gonadotropic hormones. Tamoxifen is mainly an antagonist at estrogen receptors in the breast but apparently acts as an agonist in bone. Contraceptives reduce FSH and LH output from the pituitary by activating feedback receptors.

in women. Although the hormone is very effective in reducing or preventing the effects of estrogen deprivation after menopause (especially genital changes and osteoporosis), estrogen toxicities are such that routine use in postmenopausal women is still controversial. The estrogens are very important as a component of oral contraceptives. A special use of brief, high-dose therapy is as a "morning-after" contraceptive, ie, to prevent conception as a result of intercourse the night before. Estrogens are sometimes used in the palliative treatment of carcinoma of the prostate.

3. **Toxicity:** The primary toxicity of the estrogens relates to their stimulatory effects on vaginal, uterine, and breast tissue. Moderate doses may cause breast tenderness, endome-

Table 39–1. Representative applications for the gonadal hormones and hormone antagonists.

Clinical Application	Drugs
Hypogonadism in girls, women	Conjugated equine estrogens, ethinyl estradiol
Postmenopausal estrogen replacement	Conjugated equine estrogens, ethinyl estradiol
Intractable dysmenorrhea or uterine bleeding	Ethinyl estradiol, oral contraceptive
"Morning after" contraception	Diethylstilbestrol; quadruple dose of oral contraceptive
Oral contraception	Estrogen: ethinyl estradiol or mestranol; Progestin: norethindrone or norgestrel
Implanted or depot injection contraception	Norgestrel (implant); medroxyprogesterone (IM depot injection)
Infertility	Clomiphene; hMG and hCG; GnRH analogues (pulsatile administration); bromocriptine
Breast cancer	Tamoxifen
Abortifacient	Mifepristone (RU 486) and prostaglandin; methotrexate and prostaglandin
Endometriosis	Danazol; androgen (rare)
Hypogonadism in boys, men; replacement therapy	Testosterone enanthate or cypionate; methyltestosterone; fluoxymesterone
Anabolic protein synthesis	Oxandrolone, stanozolol
Prostate hypertrophy (benign)	Finasteride
Prostate carcinoma	Flutamide, cyproterone; diethylstilbestrol

trial hyperplasia, and breakthrough bleeding. Months-long treatment of pregnant women with diethylstilbestrol (DES), a practice long-since abandoned, may have caused vaginal adenocarcinoma in their daughters. Estrogen use is also associated with an increased incidence of gallbladder disease.

Toxicity of long-term treatment is discussed below (see Oral Contraceptives).

B. Progestins: Progesterone is the major progestin in humans. It is synthesized in the ovary, testis, and adrenal. It is rapidly metabolized in the liver and therefore has a very low bioavailability and a short half-life. Synthetic agents are used for replacement therapy and in oral and implantable contraceptives.

1. **Effects:** Progestins cause development of secretory tissue in the breast and maturation of the uterine endometrium. They have much less effect than the estrogens on plasma proteins but significantly affect carbohydrate metabolism and stimulate the deposition of fat.

2. **Clinical use:** The major therapeutic use of the progestins is as a component of oral or implantable contraceptives. The progestins are occasionally used to produce long-lasting ovarian suppression, eg, in endometriosis. They are of no value in threatened abortion, an indication promoted in the past.

3. **Toxicity:** The toxicity of progestins is rather low. However, they may increase the blood pressure and decrease high-density plasma lipoproteins (HDL).

C. Oral & Implantable Contraceptives: Three different types of oral contraceptives for women are in use in the USA: combination estrogen-progestin tablets that are taken in constant dosage throughout the menstrual cycle (monophasic preparations); combination preparations (biphasic and triphasic) in which the progestin dosage rises during the month (to mimic the natural cycle); and progestin-only preparations. Two parenteral progestin preparations are used: norgestrel implants, which prevent conception for up to 5 years; and medroxyprogesterone acetate depot injections that provide contraceptive action for approximately 3 months.

1. **Mechanism of action:** The combination oral contraceptives have several actions, including inhibition of ovulation (the primary action) and effects on the uterine tubes and endometrium that decrease the likelihood of fertilization and implantation. Oral progestin-only agents do not always inhibit ovulation and may act through the other mechanisms listed. However, implantable and injected progestin-only contraceptives appear to act mainly through inhibition of ovulation.

2. **Toxicity:** Toxicity is an extremely important consideration in the use of contraceptives because they are commonly used over the course of many years.

   a. **Thromboembolism:** The major toxic effects of the oral contraceptives relate to their actions on blood coagulation. There is a well-documented increase in the risk of thromboembolic phenomena (myocardial infarction, stroke, pulmonary embolism) in older women, in smokers, and in women with a family history of such mishaps. However, the risk incurred by the use of these drugs is usually less than the risk engendered by pregnancy.

   b. **Carcinogenesis:** Numerous studies have evaluated the effect of oral contraceptives on the incidence of cancer. Convincing evidence indicates that these agents *reduce* the incidence of endometrial and ovarian carcinoma. Cervical carcinoma incidence is probably unchanged. Evidence regarding the effects on breast cancer is still confusing. A few studies indicate that women who took the pill for many years after it first became available (ie, in high-dose formulations) may have an increased incidence of breast carcinoma. Most studies show no increase.

   c. **Other toxicities:** The other toxicities of the oral contraceptives are much less hazardous and include nausea, breast tenderness, headache, skin pigmentation, acne, and hirsutism. All adverse effects appear to be considerably reduced by the use of preparations containing lower doses of estrogen.

D. Partial Agonist Estrogens & Progestins; Miscellaneous Hormones:

1. **Tamoxifen:** Tamoxifen is an extremely important nonsteroidal partial agonist estrogen that has been used successfully in the treatment of hormone-sensitive breast cancer. In this tissue, tamoxifen's antagonist properties dominate so that endogenous estrogen is prevented from activating receptors in the tumor (Figure 39–2). Major trials are now under way to determine whether tamoxifen can *prevent* breast cancer in women who are at very high risk.

The drug has a low incidence of toxicity and appears to have more agonist than antagonist action on bone, so that it actually prevents osteoporosis in women taking the drug for breast cancer.

2. **Clomiphene:**   Clomiphene is a nonsteroidal partial agonist estrogen that is used in anovulatory women who wish to become pregnant. Clomiphene blocks estrogen receptors in the pituitary, reducing negative feedback and increasing FSH and LH output. The increase in gonadotropins stimulates ovulation.

3. **Mifepristone (RU486):**   Mifepristone is an orally active steroid antagonist of progesterone and glucocorticoids. The drug binds to the cytosolic steroid receptors for these hormones and alters expression of the appropriate genes. Its major use thus far (restricted to a few European countries) has been as an abortifacient. When given in a single oral dose followed by administration of a prostaglandin E or F analogue, a very high percentage of complete abortion is achieved with a low incidence of serious toxicity. This drug also appears to have applications in the treatment of several malignancies.

4. **Danazol:**   Danazol is a partial agonist that binds to progestin, androgen, and glucocorticoid receptors. The drug is used in the treatment of endometriosis and fibrocystic disease of the breast. Danazol may act through suppression of ovarian steroid synthesis.

5. **Relaxin:**   An ovarian *peptide* hormone, relaxin causes relaxation of the pelvic ligaments and softening of the cervix. It may play a physiologic role in parturition but has no documented clinical applications at present.

ANDROGENS

Testosterone and related androgens are produced in the testis, the adrenal, and, to a small extent, in the ovary. Testosterone is synthesized from progesterone and dehydroepiandrosterone. In the plasma, testosterone is partly bound to sex hormone-binding globulin (SHBG), a transport protein. The hormone is converted in several organs (eg, prostate) to **dihydrotestosterone,** which is the active hormone in those tissues. Because of rapid hepatic metabolism, testosterone given by mouth has little effect. It may be given parenterally, or orally active variants may be used (see Table 39–1 and the Drug List).

Many androgens have been synthesized in an effort to increase the anabolic effect (see Effects, below) without increasing androgenic action. **Oxandrolone** and **stanozolol** are examples of drugs that, in laboratory testing, have an increased ratio of anabolic to androgenic action. However, none of these agents are devoid of androgenic effect in clinical use.

A. **Mechanism of Action:**   Like other steroid hormones, androgens enter cells and bind to cytosolic receptors. The hormone-receptor complex enters the nucleus and modulates the expression of certain genes.

B. **Effects:**   Testosterone is necessary for the normal development of the male fetus and infant and is responsible for the major changes in the male at puberty (growth of penis, larynx, and skeleton; development of facial, pubic, and axillary hair; darkening of skin; enlargement of muscle mass). Testosterone causes masculinization of the female.

The major effect of androgenic hormones—other than the development and maintenance of normal male characteristics—is an anabolic action that involves increased muscle size and strength and increased red blood cell production. Excretion of urea nitrogen is reduced ("positive nitrogen balance"). As noted above, the ratio of androgenic to anabolic potency varies somewhat among the synthetic compounds available, but all retain considerable androgenic effect. Therefore, the use of these hormones by athletes to increase muscle strength is attended by the hazards of unwanted androgenic effects.

C. **Clinical Use:**   The clinical uses of the androgens include replacement therapy in hypogonadism, stimulation of red blood cell production in certain anemias, and, rarely, the suppression of estrogen secretion or function in women with severe endometriosis (Table 39–1). The anabolic effects have been exploited illicitly by athletes, especially weight lifters, to increase muscle bulk and strength. The availability of recombinant erythropoietin and other marrow growth factors has rendered obsolete the use of androgens in anemias and agranulocytosis.

D. Toxicity: The toxicity of the androgens is largely a result of their masculinizing effects. In addition, they have caused cholestatic jaundice, elevation of liver enzyme levels, and in a few cases hepatocellular carcinoma. Excessive use by athletes and muscle builders is sometimes associated with behavioral changes including unpredictable rage and hostility. Development of dependence and a withdrawal syndrome have been reported.

ANTIANDROGENS

Reduction of androgen effects is an important mode of therapy for both benign and malignant prostate disease. Drugs are available that act at several different sites in the androgen pathway (Figure 39–3).

A. GnRH Analogues: Reduction of trophic hormones, especially LH, reduces the production of testosterone. This can be effectively accomplished with long-acting depot preparations of **leuprolide** or similar agonist GnRH analogues. These analogues are used in prostatic carcinoma. GnRH antagonists are investigational at present.

B. Inhibitors of Steroid Synthesis: **Ketoconazole,** an antifungal agent, inhibits steroid synthesis. The drug has been used to suppress adrenal steroid synthesis in patients with steroid-dependent metastatic tumors. Spironolactone may have a similar but smaller effect.

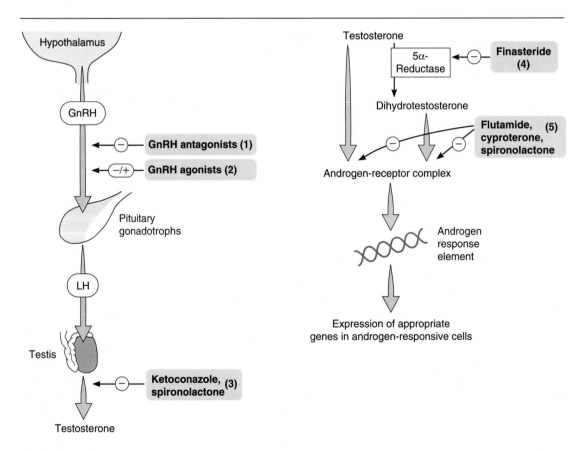

Figure 39–3. Control of androgen secretion and activity and some sites of action of antiandrogens. (1), competitive inhibition of GnRH receptors; (2), stimulation (+) or inhibition(-) by GnRH analogues; (3), inhibition of testosterone synthesis by ketoconazole or spironolactone; (4), inhibition of dihydrotestosterone production by finasteride; (5) inhibition of androgen binding at its receptor by flutamide and other drugs. (Modified and reproduced, with permission, from Katzung BG [editor]: *Basic & Clinical Pharmacology,* 6th ed. Appleton & Lange, 1995.)

C. 5α-Reductase Inhibitors: Testosterone is converted to dihydrotestosterone by the enzyme 5α-reductase. This enzyme can be inhibited by **finasteride,** a heterocyclic steroid. Finasteride has not proved valuable in prostatic carcinoma but may be useful in benign prostatic hypertrophy.

D. Receptor Inhibitors: **Cyproterone** and its acetate derivative are steroidal competitive inhibitors of androgens at the testosterone receptor. Cyproterone also has progestational activity that provides negative feedback to the pituitary. **Flutamide** is a nonsteroidal androgen antagonist with the same action. These drugs have been used to decrease the action of endogenous hormone in prostate carcinoma.

CONTRACEPTION IN THE MALE

Gossypol is a cottonseed oil derivative that was serendipitously discovered to reduce spermatogenesis. It reduces fertility in most males by destroying seminiferous cells. However, gossypol is not nearly as reliable as the oral contraceptives used by women. It causes hypokalemia, and the weakness associated with this side effect may limit its use. Androgenic and estrogenic hormones also reduce spermatogenesis, primarily by suppressing pituitary LH and FSH production. However, the low efficacy of these agents and their other hormonal effects prevent serious consideration of their use as contraceptives.

DRUG LIST

The following drugs are important members of the group discussed in this chapter. Prototypes should be learned in detail; features of the major variants should be known well enough to distinguish the variants from prototypes and from each other; the other significant agents should be recognized as belonging to a specific subclass.

Subclass	Prototype	Major Variants	Other Significant Agents
Estrogens Natural	Estradiol	Conjugated equine estrogens	Estrone, estriol
Synthetic	Ethinyl estradiol	Mestranol	Diethylstilbestrol
Estrogen partial agonists	Tamoxifen, clomiphene		
Progestins Natural	Progesterone		
Synthetic	Norgestrel, medroxyprogesterone		Norethindrone
Partial agonist	Danazol		
Antiprogestin	Mifepristone (RU 486)		
Androgens Natural	Testosterone		
Synthetic	Methyltestosterone	Fluoxymesterone	
Anabolic steroid	Oxandrolone		Stanozolol
Antiandrogens Synthesis inhibitor	Finasteride		
Receptor antagonist	Flutamide	Cyproterone	

QUESTIONS

DIRECTIONS: Each of the numbered items or incomplete statements in this section is followed by answers or by completions of the statement. Select the ONE lettered answer or completion that is BEST in each case.

1. All of the following agents are useful in oral or implantable contraceptives EXCEPT
   (A) Ethinyl estradiol
   (B) Mestranol
   (C) Clomiphene
   (D) Norethindrone
   (E) Norgestrel

2. All of the following are recognized effects of oral contraceptives EXCEPT
   (A) Increased risk of myocardial infarction
   (B) Nausea
   (C) Edema
   (D) Increased risk of endometrial cancer
   (E) Decreased risk of ovarian cancer

3. All of the following are recognized effects of natural androgens or androgenic steroids EXCEPT
   (A) Growth of facial hair
   (B) Increased muscle bulk
   (C) Increased milk production in nursing women
   (D) Induction of a growth spurt in pubertal boys
   (E) Cholestatic jaundice and elevation of SGOT levels in the blood

4. A 50-year-old woman with a positive mammogram undergoes lumpectomy, and a small carcinoma is removed. After this procedure she will probably receive
   (A) Flutamide
   (B) Ketoconazole
   (C) Danazol
   (D) Leuprolide
   (E) Tamoxifen

5. A 60-year-old man is found to have a prostate lump and an elevated PSA (prostate-specific antigen) blood test. MRI examination suggests several enlarged lymph nodes in the lower abdomen and x-ray reveals 2 radiolucent lesions in the bony pelvis. This patient might benefit from any of the following EXCEPT
   (A) Leuprolide
   (B) Flutamide
   (C) Mifepristone
   (D) Cyproterone
   (E) Ketoconazole

6. A young woman complains of severe abdominal pain at the time of menstruation. Careful evaluation indicates the presence of significant endometrial deposits on the pelvic peritoneum. The most appropriate therapy for this patient would be
   (A) Flutamide
   (B) Danazol
   (C) Mestranol
   (D) Estradiol
   (E) Norgestrel

DIRECTIONS: The following section consists of a list of four to twenty-six lettered options followed by several numbered items. For each numbered item, select the ONE option that is most closely associated with it. Each answer may be selected once, more than once, or not at all.
   (A) Cyproterone
   (B) Clomiphene
   (C) Tamoxifen
   (D) Mestranol
   (E) Norgestrel
   (F) Finasteride
   (G) Flutamide
   (H) Danazol
   (I) Leuprolide
   (J) Goserelin
   (K) Ketoconazole

7. A partial agonist estrogen that stimulates ovulation
8. A synthetic estrogen that is useful in oral contraceptives of the combined type
9. A synthetic progestin used in both combination and progestin-only contraceptives
10. A steroid drug that competes with testosterone for its receptor
11. A competitive partial agonist estrogen that is an antagonist in advanced breast cancer tissue but an agonist in bone
12. An antifungal drug that inhibits P450 enzymes required for steroid hormone synthesis
13. A nonsteroidal androgen receptor antagonist used in management of metastatic prostatic carcinoma
14. An inhibitor of 5α-reductase in the prostate

ANSWERS

1. Clomiphene, an antiestrogen, would be of no value in an oral contraceptive. The answer is **(C)**.
2. The oral contraceptives are associated with a decreased risk of both endometrial and ovarian cancer. The answer is **(D)**.
3. Androgens, like estrogens, reduce the pituitary release of prolactin and suppress lactation. The answer is **(C)**.
4. Tamoxifen has proved useful in adjunctive therapy of breast cancer after apparently complete removal; the drug decreases the rate of recurrence of cancer. The answer is **(E)**.
5. Most antiandrogenic drugs are potentially useful in this androgen-dependent type of tumor. Mifepristone (RU 486) has effects at glucocorticoid and progestin receptors, but not at androgen receptors. The answer is **(C)**.
6. In endometriosis, a partial agonist at progesterone and testosterone receptors is useful. Danazol reduces progesterone effects on the ectopic endometrial tissue, while causing feedback inhibition of gonadotropin output from the pituitary. The answer is **(B)**.
7. Clomiphene apparently reduces the feedback inhibition by estrogens of the hypothalamus and pituitary, resulting in an increased production of gonadotropins. The answer is **(B)**.
8. The answer is **(D)**, mestranol.
9. The answer is **(E)**, norgestrel.
10. The answer is **(A)**, cyproterone.
11. Tamoxifen, a competitive partial agonist estrogen, is useful in the treatment of estrogen-dependent breast carcinoma and appears to reduce osteoporosis. The answer is **(C)**.
12. Ketoconazole inhibits P450 enzymes preferentially in fungi, but in high doses it has been shown to have similar effects on mammalian enzymes. The answer is **(K)**.
13. Flutamide is a nonsteroid with strong affinity for the cytosolic androgen receptor. The answer is **(G)**.
14. Finasteride is an effective inhibitor of the enzyme that converts testosterone to dihydrotestosterone. The answer is **(F)**.

40

Pancreatic Hormones & Antidiabetic Agents

OBJECTIVES

You should be able to:

- List the sources of insulin in clinical use.
- List the types of insulin preparations with different durations of action.
- Describe the effects of insulin on the liver, on muscle, and on adipose tissue.
- Describe the major hazards of insulin therapy.
- Describe the mechanisms of action of the two major classes of oral hypoglycemic agents.
- Describe the clinical uses of glucagon.

CONCEPTS:

The Islets of Langerhans (the endocrine pancreas) contain at least four different types of endocrine cells, including **A** (alpha, glucagon-producing), **B** (beta, insulin-producing), **D** (delta, somatostatin-producing), and **F** (PP, pancreatic polypeptide-producing). Of these, the B (insulin-producing) cells are the most numerous.

The most common pancreatic disease requiring pharmacologic therapy is diabetes mellitus, a deficiency of insulin production or effect. Diabetes is treated with several formulations of insulin (all administered parenterally at present) and with two different types of oral hypoglycemic agents (Figure 40–1).

INSULIN

A. **Physiology:** Insulin is synthesized as a prohormone, **proinsulin,** an 86-amino-acid single-chain polypeptide. Cleavage of proinsulin and cross-linking result in the two-chain 51-peptide insulin molecule and a 31-amino-acid residual **C-peptide.** C-peptide is of clinical interest because it can be measured by immunoassay independently of insulin. Neither proinsulin nor C-peptide appear to have any physiologic actions.

B. **Effects:** Insulin has extremely important effects in almost every tissue of the body. Its actions on the liver, muscle, and adipose tissue are set forth in Table 40–1. The insulin receptor, a transmembrane tyrosine kinase, phosphorylates itself and a variety of intracellular proteins

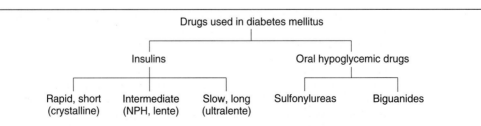

Figure 40–1. Subgroups of drugs discussed in this chapter.

Table 40–1. Endocrine effects of insulin.[1]

Category of Effect	Result
Effects on liver Reversal of catabolic features of insulin deficiency	Inhibits glycogenolysis; inhibits conversion of fatty acids and amino acids to keto acids; inhibits conversion of amino acids to glucose
Anabolic action	Promotes glucose storage as glycogen; (induces glucokinase and glycogen synthase; inhibits phosphorylase); increases triglyceride synthesis and very-low-density lipoprotein formation
Effects on muscle Increased protein synthesis	Increases amino acid transport; increases ribosomal protein synthesis
Increased glycogen synthesis	Increases glucose transport; induces glycogen synthase and inhibits phosphorylase
Effect on adipose tissue Increased triglyceride storage	Induces and activates lipoprotein lipase to hydrolyze triglycerides from ipoproteins; increases glucose transport into the cell to provide glycerol phosphate and permit esterification of fatty acids supplied by lipoprotein transport; inhibits intracellular lipase

[1] Modified and reproduced, with permission, from Katzung BG (editor): *Basic & Clinical Pharmacology,* 6th ed. Appleton & Lange, 1995.

when activated by the hormone. The major target organs for insulin action include the following:

1. **Liver:** Insulin increases the storage of glucose as glycogen in the liver. This involves the insertion of additional **GLUT 2** glucose transport molecules in cell walls, increased synthesis of the enzymes pyruvate kinase, phosphofructokinase, and glucokinase, and the suppression of several other enzymes. Insulin also decreases protein catabolism.

2. **Muscle:** Insulin stimulates glycogen synthesis and protein synthesis. Glucose transport into muscle cells is facilitated by insertion of additional **GLUT 4** transport molecules into cell walls.

3. **Adipose tissue:** Insulin facilitates triglyceride storage by activating plasma lipoprotein lipase, by increasing glucose transport into cells via GLUT 4 transporters, and by reducing intracellular lipolysis.

C. **Types of Insulin Available:** Animal insulin preparations are available from two species (pork, beef). Human insulin is manufactured by bacterial recombinant DNA technology or by chemical modification of pork insulin. The insulin molecule has a half-life of only a few minutes in the circulation, so many preparations for use in diabetes are formulated to release the hormone slowly into the circulation.

The forms available provide three rates of onset and durations of effect: rapid and short-acting, intermediate-acting, and slow and long-acting (Table 40–2). All insulin preparations contain zinc; it is the ratio of zinc (and other substances) to insulin that determines the rate of release of active hormone from the site of administration, and the duration of action.

1. **Rapid- and short-acting:** Crystalline zinc (regular) insulin can be used intravenously in emergencies, or administered subcutaneously in ordinary maintenance regimens, alone or mixed with intermediate- or long-acting preparations. Semilente zinc suspension (prompt), a similar preparation, was available for several years, but is no longer manufactured in the USA.

2. **Intermediate-acting:** These preparations include isophane insulin suspension (NPH insulin) and lente zinc suspension. Both preparations are given by subcutaneous injection; they are not suitable for intravenous use.

3. **Slow onset and long-acting:** Ultralente is the major long-acting preparation. It is often given in the morning to provide maintenance or basal levels for 24 hours. This basal insulin level may be supplemented with individual injections of regular insulin during the day to meet the requirements of carbohydrate intake. Protamine zinc insulin, another long-acting preparation, is no longer available in the USA.

The time course of effect of these preparations is shown in Figure 40–2.

Table 40–2. Insulin: Types and activity.

Pharmacokinetic Type	Species Type	Activity (hours)	
		Peak	Duration
Rapid-acting			
Insulin injection USP (regular, crystalline zinc)	Beef, pork, or human	½–3	5–7
Insulin zinc suspension USP (prompt, semilente)[1]	Beef, pork, or mixture; or human	1–4	12–16
Intermediate-acting			
Isophane insulin suspension USP (NPH insulin)	Beef, pork, or mixture; or human	8–12	18–24
Insulin zinc suspension USP (lente)	Beef, pork, or mixture; or human	8–12	18–24
Long-acting			
Protamine zinc insulin suspension USP (PZI)[1]	Beef, pork, or mixture	8–16	24–36
Insulin zinc suspension extended USP (ultralente)	Beef or human	8–16	24–36

[1] Semilente and PZI insulins are no longer available in the USA.

D. Hazards of Insulin Use: Diabetic patients who use insulin are subject to two types of complications; hypoglycemia, from excessive insulin effect; and immunologic toxic effects, from the development of antibodies. Hypoglycemia is a very dangerous hazard, because brain damage may result. Prompt administration of glucose (sugar or candy by mouth, glucose by vein) or of glucagon (by intramuscular injection or by nasal spray) is essential.

The most common and important form of insulin-induced immunologic complication is the formation of insulin antibodies, which results in resistance to the action of the drug. Of the forms available, bovine insulin is the most antigenic, human the least, and pork insulin intermediate. Lipodystrophy, a change in fatty tissue at the site of injection, was relatively common in the past. Use of more purified, less antigenic forms of insulin has almost eliminated this complication.

ORAL HYPOGLYCEMIC AGENTS

Two groups of drugs are used for the oral treatment of diabetes: the sulfonylureas and the biguanides. Some members of these groups are listed in Table 40–3.

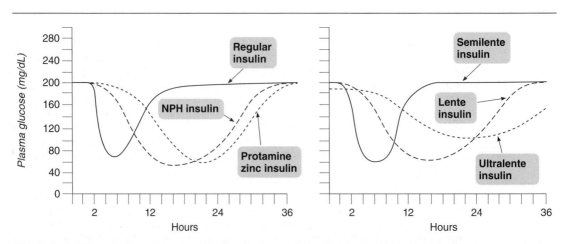

Figure 40–2. Extent and duration of action of various types of insulin (in a fasting diabetic). The durations of action shown are typical of average therapeutic doses; duration increases when dosage is increased. (Reproduced, with permission, from Katzung BG [editor]: *Basic & Clinical Pharmacology,* 6th ed. Appleton & Lange, 1995.)

Table 40–3. Representative oral antidiabetic drugs.

Drug	Dose (grams/day)	Duration of Action (hours)
Sulfonylureas Tolbutamide	0.5–2	6–12
Chlorpropamide	0.1–0.5	up to 60
Glyburide	0.00125–0.02	10–24
Glipizide	0.005–0.02	10–24
Biguanides Phenformin	0.025–0.15	4–6
Metformin	1–3	10–12

A. Sulfonylureas:

1. **Mechanism and effects:** The primary action of the sulfonylureas is to stimulate the release of endogenous insulin. These drugs close potassium channels in the beta cell membrane: channel closure depolarizes the cell and depolarization triggers insulin release. The sulfonylureas are inactive in patients with insulin-dependent diabetes and in adult diabetics who lack functioning islet cells. In addition, it has been proposed that these drugs may reduce glucagon release, and that they may increase the number of functional insulin receptors in peripheral tissues. The "second-generation" sulfonylureas (glyburide, glipizide) are considerably more potent than the older agents (tolbutamide, chlorpropamide, others).

2. **Toxicities:** Adverse effects are relatively uncommon with the sulfonylureas: hypoglycemia due to overdosage, rash (occasionally), and sulfa allergy are all possible. Chlorpropamide has a long duration of action, and liver or kidney disease may greatly increase the blood levels of the drug. Because of their great potency, hypoglycemia is somewhat more common with glyburide and glipizide.

B. Biguanides: The biguanides act by an unknown mechanism. They are effective in some patients who lack functional islet cells. Mechanisms that have been proposed include stimulation of glycolysis in peripheral tissues, reduced hepatic gluconeogenesis, reduction of glucose absorption from the gastrointestinal tract, and reduction of plasma glucagon levels. Several biguanides are in use overseas. In the USA, the use of phenformin was associated with an apparent increase in the incidence of lactic acidosis and no evidence of long-term benefit. The drug was withdrawn from the regular market but has been used in special cases. Metformin, a newer biguanide, is in clinical trials.

TREATMENT OF DIABETES MELLITUS

Diabetes is diagnosed on the basis of more than one fasting blood sugar determination in excess of 140 mg/dL. Two major forms of the disease have been identified: **insulin-dependent diabetes mellitus (IDDM, type I)** and **non-insulin-dependent (NIDDM, type II).** The clinical history and course of these two forms differ considerably, but treatment in both cases requires careful attention to diet and blood sugar levels.

Insulin-dependent diabetes (often called juvenile-onset diabetes) usually has its onset during childhood and results from destruction of the B cells in the pancreatic islets. IDDM is associated with a much higher incidence of ketoacidosis than NIDDM. Non-insulin-dependent diabetes usually has its onset in adulthood and is frequently associated with obesity and insulin resistance rather than insulin deficiency.

A. Insulin-Dependent Diabetes: Therapy of insulin-dependent diabetes involves dietary instruction, parenteral insulin (often a mixture of shorter- and longer-acting forms that mimic physiologic variations in insulin secretion and maintain a stable blood sugar during the day and night), and careful attention by the patient to things that change insulin requirements: exercise, infections, other forms of stress, and deviations from the regular diet. Recent large clinical studies indicate that close control of blood sugar—by frequent blood sugar testing and insulin injections—will reduce the incidence of vascular complications, including renal and retinal damage. The risk of hypoglycemic reactions is increased in close control regimens, but not enough to obviate the benefits of better control. A case of diabetes is presented in Case 10 (Appendix IV).

B. **Non-Insulin-Dependent Diabetes:** Therapy of non-insulin-dependent diabetes starts with attempts to eliminate obesity and to lower blood glucose by dietary means. If this regimen is unsuccessful, oral hypoglycemic agents are begun. A sulfonylurea agent is given to maximum effect or to the onset of side effects. Insulin is used only if both diet and oral hypoglycemic drugs are unsuccessful in controlling the blood sugar.

GLUCAGON

A. **Chemistry, Mechanism, & Effects:** Glucagon is the product of the A cells of the endocrine pancreas. Like insulin, glucagon is a peptide; but unlike insulin, glucagon acts on G protein-coupled receptors. Activation of glucagon receptors, which are located in heart, smooth muscle, and liver, results in activation of adenylyl cyclase and increases intracellular cAMP. The effect is to stimulate heart rate and the force of contraction, to increase hepatic glycogenolysis and gluconeogenesis, and to relax smooth muscle. The smooth muscle effect is particularly marked in the gut.

B. **Clinical Uses:** Glucagon is used to treat severe hypoglycemia in diabetics, but its hyperglycemic action requires intact hepatic glycogen stores. The drug is given intramuscularly or intravenously. A nasal spray for self-administration is in clinical trials. Glucagon is also valuable for x-ray studies of the bowel or abdomen when temporary reduction of motility is necessary for optimal visualization. In the management of severe beta-blocker overdose, glucagon may be the most effective method for stimulating the depressed heart, since it increases cardiac cAMP without requiring access to beta receptors.

QUESTIONS

DIRECTIONS: Each of the numbered items or incomplete statements in this section is followed by answers or by completions of the statement. Select the ONE lettered answer or completion that is BEST in each case.

Items 1–2: A 13-year-old boy, reported to have had a viral infection 3 months earlier, is brought to the hospital complaining of dizziness. He has a recent history of weight loss, polyuria, and polydipsia. Laboratory findings include severe hyperglycemia, ketoacidosis, and a blood pH of 7.15.

1. In order to achieve rapid control of the severe ketoacidosis in this diabetic boy, the appropriate antidiabetic agent to use is
(A) Crystalline zinc insulin
(B) Isophane (NPH) insulin
(C) Protamine zinc or ultralente insulin
(D) Tolbutamide
(E) Glyburide

2. Possible complications of insulin therapy in this patient include
(A) Dilutional hyponatremia
(B) Hypoglycemia
(C) Pancreatitis
(D) Increased bleeding tendency
(E) All of the above

3. A 24-year-old woman with IDDM wishes to try close control of her diabetes to improve her long-term prognosis. Which of the following regimens is most appropriate?
(A) Morning injections of mixed lente and ultralente insulins
(B) Evening injections of mixed regular and lente insulins
(C) Morning and evening injections of regular insulin, supplemented by small amounts of lente insulin at mealtimes

    (D) Morning injections of ultralente insulin, supplemented by small amounts of regular insulin at mealtimes

    (E) Morning injection of semilente insulin and evening injection of lente insulin

4. All of the following act by the same mechanism EXCEPT

    (A) Tolbutamide

    (B) Tolazamide

    (C) Chlorpropamide

    (D) Glipizide

    (E) Phenformin

5. Effects of insulin include all of the following EXCEPT

    (A) Increased glucose transport into cells

    (B) Induction of lipoprotein lipase

    (C) Decreased gluconeogenesis

    (D) Stimulation of glycogenolysis

    (E) Decreased conversion of amino acids into glucose

DIRECTIONS: The following section consists of a list of four to twenty-six lettered options followed by several numbered items. For each numbered item, select the ONE option that is most closely associated with it. Each answer may be selected once, more than once, or not at all.

    (A) Human NPH (isophane) insulin (bacterial origin)

    (B) Porcine regular crystalline zinc insulin

    (C) Bovine ultralente insulin

    (D) Porcine lente insulin

    (E) Glyburide

    (F) Phenformin

    (G) Tolbutamide

6. Longest-acting insulin preparation

7. Most antigenic insulin preparation

8. Less potent agent whose primary action is to release endogenous insulin

9. Oral agent that is not dependent on functioning pancreatic islet cells but is associated with increased incidence of lactic acidosis in some studies

10. Most potent oral hypoglycemic agent

ANSWERS

1. Oral antidiabetic agents are inappropriate in this patient because he clearly has insulin-dependent diabetes (suggested by his age, history, and ketoacidosis). He needs the most rapidly acting insulin preparation that can be given intravenously (Table 40–2). The answer is **(A)**.

2. Because of potential brain damage, the most important complication of insulin therapy is hypoglycemia. The other choices are not common effects of insulin. The answer is **(B)**.

3. Insulin regimens for close control usually take the form of establishing a basal level of insulin with a small amount of a long-acting preparation (ultralente) and supplementing the insulin levels, when called for by food intake, with short-acting insulin (crystalline). Less tight control may be achieved with two injections of intermediate-acting insulin per day. Because intake of glucose is mainly during the day, long-acting insulins are usually given in the morning, not at night. The answer is **(D)**.

4. Phenformin is a biguanide oral antidiabetic agent; the others are all sulfonylureas (Table 40–3). The answer is **(E)**.

5. Insulin stimulates the storage of glucose as glycogen (Table 40–1). The answer is **(D)**.

6. The longest-acting insulin is ultralente. The answer is **(C)**.

7. Porcine insulin differs from the human hormone by only one amino acid. Bovine insulin differs from human by three amino acids and is therefore the most antigenic. The answer is **(C)**.

8. The sulfonylureas are inactive in patients without functioning B cells, ie, these drugs cause the release of endogenous insulin. In contrast, the biguanides lower blood sugar in some patients with IDDM. Tolbutamide is much less potent than glipizide. The answer is **(G)**.

9. The answer is **(F)**, phenformin, a biguanide.

10. The most potent oral hypoglycemic drugs are the second-generation sulfonylureas. The answer is glyburide, **(E)**.

41

Drugs That Affect Bone Mineral Homeostasis

OBJECTIVES

You should be able to:

- List the agents useful in hypercalcemia.
- List the major and minor hormonal regulators of bone mineral homeostasis.
- Describe the major effects of parathyroid hormone on the intestine, the kidney, and bone.
- Describe the major effects of the vitamin D derivatives on the intestine, the kidney, and bone.
- Describe the therapeutic and toxic effects of bisphosphonates.
- Describe the therapeutic and toxic effects of fluoride ion.

CONCEPTS

Calcium and phosphorus are the two major elements of bone. They are also important in the metabolism of other cells in the body, and bone therefore functions as a storage reservoir. The two hormones of primary importance in the regulation of bone mineral homeostasis are parathyroid hormone (PTH) and vitamin D. Less important regulators include calcitonin, glucocorticoids, and estrogens. Exogenous agents of importance in the treatment of bone mineral disorders include the bisphosphonates and fluoride (Figure 41–1).

ENDOGENOUS SUBSTANCES

A. Parathyroid Hormone: Parathyroid hormone (PTH) is an 84-amino-acid peptide. The peptide acts on membrane G protein-coupled receptors to increase cAMP in cells. Increasing cAMP regulates calcium and phosphorus flux across cell membranes in bone and in the renal tubule. At high doses, the hormone increases blood calcium and decreases phosphorus by increasing net bone resorption. At low doses (physiologic levels), the agent may actually increase net bone formation (Table 41–1). A 34-amino-acid agent similar to PTH is under study for the treatment of osteoporosis.

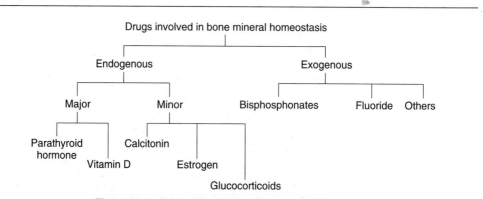

Figure 41–1. Subgroups of drugs discussed in this chapter.

Table 41–1. Actions of PTH and vitamin D on gut, bone, and kidney.[1]

	PTH	Vitamin D
Intestine	Increased calcium and phosphate absorption (by increased 1,25(OH)$_2$D production)	Increased calcium and phosphate absorption (by 1,25(OH)$_2$D)
Kidney	Decreased calcium excretion, increased phosphate excretion	Calcium and phosphate excretion may be decreased by 25(OH)D and 1,25(OH)$_2$D
Bone	Calcium and phosphate resorption increased by high doses. Low doses may increase bone formation	Increased calcium and phosphate resorption by 1,25(OH)$_2$D. Bone formation may be increased by 24,25(OH)$_2$D
Net effect on serum levels	Serum calcium increased, serum phosphate decreased	Serum calcium and phosphate both increased

[1] Reproduced, with permission, from Katzung BG (editor): *Basic & Clinical Pharmacology,* 6th ed. Appleton & Lange, 1995.

B. Vitamin D: Vitamin D, a derivative of 7-dehydrocholesterol, is formed in the skin under the influence of ultraviolet light. Vitamin D is also found in some foods and is commonly used as a food supplement in milk. Several forms of the hormone occur (calcitriol, calciferol, and secalciferol), differing primarily in the number of hydroxyl groups on the molecule (Table 41–2). Some vitamin D is stored in adipose tissue; the rest is cleared by the liver.

Calcitriol is the best studied of the active vitamin D metabolites, and specific receptors for this molecule have been identified. The actions of vitamin D include increased intestinal calcium and phosphorus absorption, decreased renal excretion of these substances, and a net increase in blood levels of both (Figure 41–2, Table 41–1). Bone formation may be increased by one of the isomers of the hormone (secalcifediol, 24,25-dihydroxyvitamin D).

C. Calcitonin: Calcitonin, a peptide hormone secreted by the thyroid gland, decreases bone resorption and serum calcium and phosphate (Figure 41–2). Bone formation is not impaired initially, but ultimately it is reduced. Therefore, calcitonin is not useful in treating conditions in which bone mass is reduced, eg, osteoporosis. The hormone has been used in conditions in which an acute reduction of serum calcium is needed, eg, Paget's disease and hypercalcemia. No disease involving a primary abnormality of calcitonin secretion has been recognized. Although human calcitonin is available, salmon calcitonin is most often selected for clinical use because of its longer half-life and greater potency.

D. Estrogens: The estrogens can prevent or delay bone loss in postmenopausal women. There is no evidence that estrogens stimulate the replacement of bone already lost. Their action may involve the inhibition of parathyroid hormone-stimulated bone resorption. Because of estrogen's proven efficacy in slowing the progression of osteoporosis, many experts strongly recommend these drugs for general use (unless contraindicated) in postmenopausal women.

Table 41–2. Vitamin D and its clinically available metabolites and analogues.[1]

Chemical Name	Abbreviation	Generic Name
Vitamin D$_3$	D$_3$	Cholecalciferol
Vitamin D$_2$	D$_2$	Ergocalciferol
25-Hydroxyvitamin D$_3$	25(OH)D$_3$	Calciferol
1,25-Dihydroxyvitamin D$_3$	1,25(OH)$_2$D$_3$	Calcitriol
24,25-Dihydroxyvitamin D$_3$	24,25(OH)$_2$D$_3$	Secalcifediol
Dihydrotachysterol	DHT	Dihydrotachysterol

[1] Reproduced, with permission, from Katzung BG (editor): *Basic & Clinical Pharmacology,* 6th ed. Appleton & Lange, 1995.

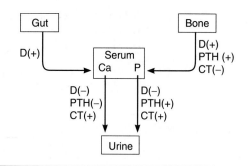

Figure 41–2. Some effects of vitamin D (*D*), parathyroid hormone (*PTH*), and calcitonin (*CT*) on calcium and phosphorus metabolism. Vitamin D increases absorption of calcium from both gut and bone, while PTH increases reabsorption from bone. Both D and PTH reduce urinary excretion of calcium. (Reproduced, with permission, from Katzung BG [editor]: *Basic & Clinical Pharmacology*, 6th ed. Appleton & Lange, 1995.)

E. Glucocorticoids: The glucocorticoids have several effects already referred to (eg, protein catabolism, see Chapter 38) that inhibit bone mineral maintenance. As a result, chronic systemic use of these drugs may be associated with osteoporosis. However, these hormones are useful in the intermediate-term treatment of hypercalcemia.

EXOGENOUS AGENTS

A. Bisphosphonates: The bisphosphonates (eg, etidronate, pamidronate) are short-chain organic polyphosphate compounds that reduce both the resorption and the formation of bone by an action on the basic hydroxyapatite crystal structure. Recent studies suggest that chronic bisphosphonate therapy may halt the progress of postmenopausal osteoporosis and possibly reverse it.

B. Fluoride: Appropriate concentrations of fluoride ion in drinking water (0.5–1 ppm) or as a dentifrice additive have a well-documented ability to reduce dental caries. Chronic exposure to the ion, especially in high concentrations, may increase new bone synthesis. It is not clear, however, whether this new bone is normal in strength.

C. Other Drugs With Effects on Calcium and Bone: Plicamycin (mithramycin) is an antibiotic used to reduce serum calcium and bone resorption in Paget's disease and hypercalcemia. The thiazide diuretics (see Chapter 15) reduce the excretion of calcium by the kidney and have been used to decrease kidney stone formation. The loop diuretics are often used (with saline infusion) to reduce serum calcium in acute hypercalcemia.

QUESTIONS

DIRECTIONS: Each of the numbered items or incomplete statements in this section is followed by answers or by completions of the statement. Select the ONE lettered answer or completion that is BEST in each case.

1. All of the following are useful in the therapy of hypercalcemia EXCEPT
   (A) Calcitonin
   (B) Glucocorticoids
   (C) Thiazides
   (D) Mithramycin
   (E) Parenteral infusion of phosphate
2. Characteristics of vitamin D include which of the following?
   (A) A prohormone produced in the liver
   (B) Active metabolites decrease serum calcium
   (C) Active metabolites increase serum phosphorus
   (D) Active metabolites increase cellular cAMP
   (E) All of the above

3. Which of the following conditions is an indication for the use of calcitonin?
   (A) Osteoporosis
   (B) Paget's disease
   (C) Rickets
   (D) Intestinal osteodystrophy
   (E) Hypoparathyroidism

DIRECTIONS: The following section consists of a list of four to twenty-six lettered options followed by several numbered items. For each numbered item, select the ONE option that is most closely associated with it. Each answer may be selected once, more than once, or not at all.

   (A) Parathyroid hormone
   (B) Vitamin D
   (C) Calcitonin
   (D) Estrogen
   (E) Fluoride
   (F) Pamidronate
   (G) Prednisone
   (H) Furosemide

4. A hormone secreted by the human thyroid; the more commonly used preparation is obtained from salmon
5. An inorganic ion that appears to facilitate new bone formation, especially if ingested in high concentrations
6. Causes decreased renal calcium excretion and increased plasma phosphorus
7. A diuretic used to rapidly lower serum calcium
8. A drug that causes osteoporosis through inhibition of protein synthesis
9. A synthetic phosphate derivative that shows promise in halting or reversing loss of bone density in osteoporosis

ANSWERS

1. Thiazides increase calcium reabsorption from the urine (see Chapter 15) and are never used in patients with hypercalcemia. The answer is **(C)**.
2. Vitamin D is a prohormone whose metabolites increase serum phosphorus. They also increase serum calcium (Table 41–1). The active metabolites are produced in the skin, not the liver. Parathyroid hormone, not vitamin D, acts via cAMP. The answer is **(C)**.
3. Calcitonin is often used in Paget's disease to control hypercalcemia. The answer is **(B)**.
4. The answer is **(C)**, calcitonin.
5. The answer is **(E)**, fluoride.
6. The answer is **(B)**, vitamin D (Table 41–1).
7. Furosemide is used—with saline infusion to prevent hemoconcentration—to reduce serum calcium in the emergency management of hypercalcemia. The answer is **(H)**.
8. Systemic glucocorticoids, eg, prednisone, cause significant osteoporosis when used chronically. The answer is **(G)**.
9. The bisphosphonates are simple synthetic phosphate derivatives that appear to slow osteoporosis significantly. The answer is **(F)**.

Part VIII. Chemotherapeutic Drugs

42   Principles of Antimicrobial Drug Action

OBJECTIVES

You should be able to:

- Describe four different mechanisms of action of antimicrobial drugs.
- List the major antimicrobial drug groups and identify the mechanism of action of each group.
- List four different mechanisms by which microorganisms become resistant to drugs.

Learn the definitions that follow.

Table 42–1. Definitions.

Term	Definition
Selective toxicity	The principle that chemotherapeutic drugs should be more toxic to infecting microbial organisms than to host cells
Bacteriostatic	A drug that inhibits the growth of microorganisms
Bactericidal	A drug that causes the death of microorganisms
Resistance	Decreased susceptibility of microorganisms to drug action; includes chromosomal resistance (spontaneous mutation) and extrachromosomal resistance (plasmid-mediated)
Cross-resistance	Resistance of microorganisms to drugs of similar chemical structure or similar mechanism of action

CONCEPTS

GENERAL PRINCIPLES

A. Selective Toxicity: Ideally, an antimicrobial drug should be much more toxic to the microorganism causing infection than to host cells. This is a requirement for effective and safe chemotherapy of infections caused by invading organisms.

Selective toxicity may result from (1) accumulation of a drug to higher levels in a microorganism than in human cells; (2) a specific action of a drug on cellular structures or biochemical processes that are unique to the microorganism; or (3) actions of a drug on biochemical processes that are more critical to the parasite than to host cells.

B. Bacteriostatic & Bactericidal Actions: The effects of antimicrobial drugs on bacteria can lead to an inhibition of growth (ie, a bacteriostatic effect) that will be reversible upon removal of the drug unless host defense mechanisms have eradicated the organism. Examples of antimicrobial drugs that are usually bacteriostatic include erythromycin, the tetracyclines, and the sulfonamides.

Drugs that act to kill bacteria (ie, bactericidal drugs) are less dependent on defense mechanisms for their therapeutic effects. Beta-lactam antibiotics and the aminoglycosides are usually bactericidal.

C. **Resistance:** Resistance to antimicrobial drugs may result from both genetic and nongenetic mechanisms. Most resistant organisms emerge through chromosomal or extrachromosomal genetic changes followed by selection processes. **Chromosomal resistance** involves spontaneous mutation at a genetic locus that controls susceptibility to specific drugs. **Extrachromosomal resistance** involves **plasmids (R factors)** that carry genes for resistance to one or more drugs. These plasmids can be transferred between organisms by transduction, transformation, translocation, or, most importantly, bacterial conjugation. **Transposons** may carry genes for resistance from plasmids to chromosomes. **Cross-resistance** can occur between antimicrobial drugs, especially if they are chemically related and have similar mechanisms of action.

MECHANISMS OF ACTION

A. **Inhibition of Bacterial Cell Wall Synthesis:** Bacterial cell walls contain complex macromolecules (mucopeptides and peptidoglycans) that are formed via biosynthetic pathways which are absent from mammalian cells. The widely used beta-lactam antibiotics (**penicillins** and **cephalosporins**) bind to specific proteins (**penicillin-binding proteins, PBPs**) that are located in the bacterial cytoplasmic membrane. Binding to PBPs results in inhibition of transpeptidase activities that are required for the cross-linking of the linear peptidoglycan chains, the final step in cell wall synthesis. Inhibition of these enzymes by beta-lactam antibiotics results in decreased cell wall synthesis. These antibiotics also activate autolytic enzymes that are destructive to the cell wall. In susceptible organisms, these actions are bactericidal.

Other antibiotics, including cycloserine and vancomycin, can also interfere with bacterial cell wall synthesis by inhibiting the synthesis of precursors of murein (peptidoglycan) or by preventing the formation of linear peptidoglycan chains.

B. **Inhibition of Protein Synthesis:** The mechanisms of protein synthesis in microorganisms are not identical to those of mammalian cells. Many of the commonly used antimicrobial drugs selectively inhibit bacterial protein synthesis. **Tetracyclines** bind to the 30S ribosomal subunit and block the attachment of aminoacyl-tRNA. **Aminoglycoside** antibiotics also interact with the 30S ribosomal subunit but with different receptors, and this binding blocks the formation of the 70S initiation complex.

The 50S subunit of bacterial ribosomes contains specific receptors for **erythromycin** and **clindamycin.** Both of these drugs can inhibit the formation of the initiation complex and interfere with translocation reactions. **Chloramphenicol** binds to the 50S ribosomal subunit and inhibits peptidyl transferase activity.

Tetracyclines and chloramphenicol are not totally selective in their actions, since they can also inhibit protein synthesis in certain mammalian cells.

C. **Inhibition of Nucleic Acid Synthesis:** Several drugs act at this level. The **quinolones** and **fluoroquinolones** block nucleic acid synthesis by inhibiting DNA gyrase (topoisomerase II), the enzyme that converts supercoiled DNA to the relaxed DNA form. **Rifampin** is an inhibitor of DNA-dependent RNA polymerase.

Nucleic acid synthesis is dependent on folic acid, which acts as a coenzyme in many biosynthetic reactions. Humans obtain folate in the diet, but many microorganisms must synthesize this substance. **Sulfonamides** inhibit bacterial folate synthesis at the level of dihydropteroate synthase by acting as antimetabolites of the endogenous substrate PABA. Similarly, **trimethoprim** is an antimetabolite of folic acid that selectively inhibits dihydrofolate reductases of bacteria and protozoa.

D. **Disruption of Cell Membrane Permeability:** Although the cell membranes of microorganisms function similarly to those of mammalian cells, their chemical composition is distinctive. This difference permits the selectively toxic action of certain antimicrobial drugs. The **polymyxins** disrupt the selective permeability of bacterial cell membranes by insertion into the lipid bilayer and formation of artificial pores. The **polyene antimicrobials** (eg, amphotericin B) bind to membrane components that are present only in microbial cells, eg, ergosterol. The **imidazole** antifungal agents (eg, ketoconazole) act as selective inhibitors of enzymes involved in the synthesis of sterols that are essential components of fungal membranes.

A summary of the mechanisms of action of commonly used antimicrobial agents is set forth in Table 42–2.

Table 42–2. Summary of the mechanisms of action of antimicrobial drugs.

Drug Groups	Mechanism(s) of Action
Penicillins, cephalosporins	Inhibition of the final step (transpeptidation) in bacterial cell wall synthesis and activation of autolytic enzymes
Aminoglycosides	Inhibition of bacterial protein synthesis by blocking formation of the initiation complex; binds to 30S
Chloramphenicol	Inhibition of bacterial protein synthesis by blocking peptidyl transferase; binds to 50S
Macrolides, lincosamides	Inhibition of bacterial protein synthesis by blocking translocase reactions and formation of the initiation complex; binds to 50S
Tetracyclines	Inhibition of bacterial protein synthesis by blocking attachment of aminoacyl-tRNA; binds to 30S
Sulfonamides, trimethoprim	Inhibition of folic acid synthesis in bacteria and other microorganisms
Quinolones, fluoroquinolones	Inhibition of bacterial DNA gyrase
Polyenes, imidazoles	Disruption of fungal cell membrane permeability

MECHANISMS OF RESISTANCE

A. Production of Drug-Inactivating Enzymes: This common mechanism causes resistance to many beta-lactam antibiotics. The synthesis of hydrolytic **beta-lactamase** enzymes **(penicillinases)** that are specific for certain penicillin structures is characteristic of staphylococci and many gram-negative bacteria. A recent therapeutic strategy to counter such resistance has been administration of a penicillin antibiotic in the "protective custody" of an inhibitor (eg, clavulanic acid, sulbactam, tazobactam) of the penicillinases. Beta-lactamase enzymes that hydrolyze cephalosporins can cause resistance to this class of drugs.

Plasmid-mediated resistance to aminoglycosides is caused by the formation of inactivating enzymes **(group transferases)** that catalyze the transfer of acetyl groups and other moieties to the drug molecules.

B. Changes in Receptor Structure: Molecules that act as targets, or receptors, for antimicrobial drugs may undergo changes in molecular structure, rendering them less susceptible to the toxic actions of the drugs. Methylation of a macromolecule that forms part of the erythromycin receptor on the 50S ribosomal subunit is enough to interfere with drug binding and thus lead to resistance. In the same way, apparently minor structural changes in the receptors for aminoglycosides are responsible for marked changes in drug susceptibility of microorganisms.

The structure of target enzymes may also change, leading to a decrease in the inhibitory effects of antimicrobial drugs. This mechanism has been reported for dihydrofolate reductase in organisms resistant to trimethoprim, and for DNA gyrase in organisms resistant to fluoroquinolones. Differences in penicillin binding proteins may also be responsible for the limited susceptibility of many bacteria to the beta-lactam group of drugs.

C. Changes in Drug Permeation & Transport: The antimicrobial action of many drugs depends on their ability to penetrate the cell membranes of an organism and reach effective intracellular concentrations. Aminoglycosides are polar compounds that require oxygen-dependent membrane transport for intracellular accumulation; thus, strict anaerobes are resistant to their effects. Tetracycline resistance is a result of decreased intracellular concentrations of such drugs. This may be because of a decrease in microbial membrane permeability, an increase in the activity of mechanisms involved in extrusion of tetracyclines, or a combination of both.

D. Development of Alternative Metabolic Pathways: Of the antibacterial agents, sulfonamides best illustrate the mechanisms of alternative metabolic pathways. Resistant bacterial strains may produce levels of PABA high enough to overcome the inhibition of dihydropteroate synthase by a sulfonamide. Certain bacteria are able to utilize preformed folic acid from their environment and thus bypass the inhibitory actions of the sulfonamides.

QUESTIONS

DIRECTIONS: Each of the numbered items or incomplete statements in this section is followed by answers or by completions of the statement. Select the ONE lettered answer or completion that is BEST in each case.

1. Which of the following is NOT an action of the beta-lactam antibiotics?
   (A) Inhibition of the cross-linking of peptidoglycan chains
   (B) Binding to specific proteins in the cytoplasmic membrane
   (C) Activation of autolytic enzymes
   (D) Inhibition of peptidyl transferase
   (E) Bactericidal against most susceptible organisms

2. All of the following statements about bacterial resistance to antimicrobial drugs are accurate EXCEPT
   (A) Transposons can transfer resistance factors from plasmids to bacterial chromosomes
   (B) Spontaneous mutation is a frequent cause of clinical resistance during antimicrobial drug therapy in a given patient
   (C) Plasmid-mediated resistance is an example of extrachromosomal resistance
   (D) R factors are plasmids that carry genes for drug resistance
   (E) Bacterial conjugation is an important factor in the spread of plasmid-mediated drug resistance

3. The main reason that sulfonamides have a selective action as antimicrobial drugs is
   (A) Sterol synthesis is essential to microbial but not mammalian cells
   (B) Bacterial cells do not contain dihydrofolate reductase
   (C) The drug sensitivities of dihydrofolate reductases of microbial and mammalian cells are different
   (D) Mammalian cells lack dihydropteroate synthase
   (E) Bacterial ribosomes have a different structure from those of mammalian cells

4. All of the following antimicrobial agents are inhibitors of bacterial protein synthesis EXCEPT
   (A) Erythromycin
   (B) Tetracycline
   (C) Vancomycin
   (D) Streptomycin
   (E) Chloramphenicol

5. The formation of drug-inactivating enzymes is a mechanism of bacterial resistance to all of the following drugs EXCEPT
   (A) Gentamicin
   (B) Fluoroquinolones
   (C) Cefazolin
   (D) Penicillin G
   (E) Chloramphenicol

6. Which ONE of the following drugs acts *directly* to alter fungal cell membrane permeability?
   (A) Polymyxin
   (B) Streptomycin
   (C) Amphotericin B
   (D) Ampicillin
   (E) Tetracycline

7. The selective toxicity of vancomycin as an antibiotic is
   (A) Due to selective accumulation of the drug by bacterial cells
   (B) Because it acts on a biochemical pathway unique to bacteria
   (C) Due to its bioactivation by bacteria
   (D) Because it acts on bacterial folic acid synthesis
   (E) Due to its rapid metabolism in human but not bacterial cells

DIRECTIONS: The following section consists of a list of four to twenty-six lettered options followed by several numbered items. For each numbered item, select the ONE option that is most closely associated with it. Each answer may be selected once, more than once, or not at all.
   (A) Norfloxacin
   (B) Rifampin

      (C) Erythromycin
      (D) Ampicillin
      (E) Penicillin G
      (F) Tobramycin
      (G) Nafcillin
      (H) Polymyxin B

8. This drug is acetylated by group transferase enzymes that are transferred as a plasmid-mediated form of resistance

9. Treatment of bacterial infections with this agent as the sole drug often fails because the spontaneous mutation rate is high and can occur with a frequency of 10^{-5} to 10^{-7}

10. Resistance to this beta-lactam antibiotic, particularly in staphylococci, does not involve the production of beta-lactamases; bacteria resistant to this drug usually exhibit multiple drug resistance

11. This drug acts like a detergent on the lipid membranes of gram-negative bacilli; it is rarely used systemically due to its toxic potential

12. This drug interferes with bacterial nucleic acid synthesis; it is an inhibitor of DNA-dependent RNA polymerases

ANSWERS

1. The beta-lactams (penicillins, cephalosporins) bind to specific membrane proteins, inhibit transpeptidases involved in bacterial cell wall synthesis, and activate autolytic enzymes that attack cell walls. They do not interfere with protein synthesis. The answer is **(D)**.

2. Spontaneous mutation usually occurs with a frequency of 10^{-12} to 10^{-8}. It is not a frequent cause of emergence of clinical resistance during a course of antimicrobial drug therapy. The answer is **(B)**.

3. Mammalian cells do not utilize PABA to synthesize folic acid because they lack dihydropteroate synthase. The answer is **(D)**.

4. Vancomycin is a glycopeptide antibiotic that inhibits the synthesis of bacterial cell walls by binding to precursor subunits. The answer is **(C)**.

5. Resistance to quinolones and fluoroquinolones appears to be due to changes in the drug sensitivity of DNA gyrases and decreased intracellular accumulation of such drugs. The answer is **(B)**.

6. The polyenes (eg, amphotericin) and the polymyxin drugs both disrupt cell membrane permeability in microorganisms. The polyenes have selective actions on fungal cell membranes; the polymyxins have selective actions on bacterial cell membranes. The answer is **(C)**.

7. Vancomycin is an inhibitor of bacterial cell wall synthesis, a process unique to these microorganisms. The answer is **(B)**.

8. Resistance to most of the drugs listed may be plasmid-mediated, but production of specific transferase enzyme activities is the mechanism of resistance to aminoglycosides and to chloramphenicol (not listed). The answer is **(F)**.

9. This is an important exception to the general rule mentioned in answer to question 2. Chromosomal mutants resistant to rifampin occur with a high frequency, and treatment often fails if the drug is used as the sole agent for bacterial infections. The answer is **(B)**.

10. Nafcillin and methicillin (not listed) are members of a subgroup of penicillins resistant to the action of penicillinases. Nafcillin is commonly used for the treatment of known or suspected staphylococcal infections. However, certain strains of this organism are resistant to nafcillin and other members of the subgroup, and to many other antibacterial agents including erythromycin, tetracyclines, and sulfonamides. This is an example of multiple drug resistance. Infections due to methicillin-resistant staphylococcus aureus (MRSA) strains usually require treatment with vancomycin. The answer is **(G)**.

11. The polymyxins disrupt bacterial cell membrane function, acting like cationic detergents. The answer is **(H)**.

12. Only a few antibacterial agents exert selective actions on bacterial nucleic acid synthesis or functions. Quinolones and fluoroquinolones inhibit DNA gyrases. Rifampin is an inhibitor of DNA dependent RNA polymerase. The answer is **(B)**.

Penicillins & Cephalosporins

43

OBJECTIVES

You should be able to:

- Describe the mechanism of antibacterial action of beta-lactam antibiotics.
- Describe the mechanisms underlying the resistance of bacteria to beta-lactam antibiotics.
- Identify the important drugs in each subclass of penicillins and describe their antibacterial activity and clinical uses.
- Identify the three subclasses of cephalosporins and describe their antibacterial activities and clinical uses.
- List the major adverse effects of the penicillins and the cephalosporins.
- Identify the important features of aztreonam and imipenem.

Learn the definitions that follow.

Table 43–1. Definitions.

Term	Definition
Beta-lactam antibiotics	Drugs with structures containing a beta-lactam ring; includes the penicillins and cephalosporins. This ring must be intact for antimicrobial action
Penicillin-binding proteins, PBPs	Bacterial cytoplasmic membrane proteins that act as the initial receptors for penicillins and other beta-lactam antibiotics
Transpeptidases	Bacterial enzymes involved in the cross-linking of linear peptidoglycan chains, the final step in cell wall synthesis
Beta-lactamases	Bacterial enzymes (penicillinases, cephalosporinases) that hydrolyze the beta-lactam ring of certain penicillins and cephalosporins
Peptidoglycan, murein	Polymeric chains of polysaccharides and polypeptides that are cross-linked to form the bacterial cell wall

CONCEPTS

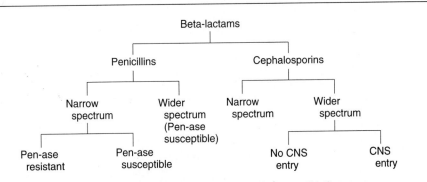

Figure 43–1. Subdivisions of the beta-lactam antibiotics.

PENICILLINS

A. Classification: All penicillins are derivatives of 6-aminopenicillanic acid and contain a beta-lactam ring structure that is essential for antibacterial activity. Penicillin subclasses have additional chemical substituents that confer differences in antimicrobial activity, susceptibility to acid and enzymic hydrolysis, and biodisposition.

B. Pharmacokinetics: Penicillins vary in acid stability and therefore in their oral bioavailability. They are polar compounds and are not metabolized extensively. They are excreted unchanged in the urine via glomerular filtration and tubular secretion, the latter process being inhibited by probenecid. Ampicillin and nafcillin are excreted partly in the bile. The plasma half-lives of most penicillins vary from 0.5 to 1 hour. Procaine and benzathine forms of penicillin G are administered intramuscularly and have long plasma half-lives because the active drug is released very slowly into the bloodstream. Most penicillins cross the blood-brain barrier only when the meninges are inflamed.

C. Mechanism of Action: Beta-lactam antibiotics are bactericidal drugs. They act to inhibit cell wall synthesis by the following steps (see Figure 43–2): (1) binding of the drug to specific receptors (penicillin- binding proteins, **PBPs**) located in the bacterial cytoplasmic membrane; (2) inhibition of **transpeptidase** enzymes that act to cross-link linear peptidoglycan chains that

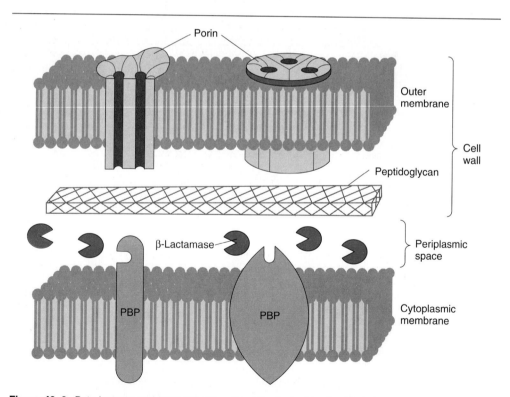

Figure 43–2. Beta-lactams and bacterial cell wall synthesis. In this simplified diagram of the bacterial cell envelope, the outer membrane is present only in gram-negative organisms. It is penetrated by proteins (porins) that are permeable to hydrophilic substances such as beta-lactam antibiotics. The peptidoglycan chains (mureins) are cross-linked by transpeptidases located in the cytoplasmic membrane, closely associated with penicillin-binding proteins (PBPs). Beta-lactam antibiotics bind to PBPs and inhibit transpeptidation, the final step in cell wall synthesis. They also activate autolytic enzymes that cause lesions in the cell wall. Beta-lactamases, which inactivate beta-lactam antibiotics, may be present in the periplasmic space or on the outer surface of the cytoplasmic membrane. (Reproduced, with permission, from Katzung BG [editor]: *Basic & Clinical Pharmacology,* 6th ed. Appleton & Lange, 1995.)

form part of the cell wall; (3) activation of autolytic enzymes that cause lesions in the bacterial cell wall.

Enzymatic hydrolysis of the beta-lactam ring of penicillins leads to inactivation of the drug. The formation of **beta-lactamases (penicillinases)** is a major mechanism of bacterial resistance to this class of drugs. Inhibitors of these enzymes (eg, clavulanic acid, sulbactam, tazobactam) are sometimes used in combination with penicillins to prevent their inactivation. Other resistance mechanisms include decreases in membrane permeability to penicillins and changes in membrane PBPs.

D. Clinical Use:

1. **Narrow spectrum, penicillinase-susceptible agents: Penicillin G** is the prototype of a subclass of penicillins that have a limited spectrum of antibacterial activity and are susceptible to beta-lactamases. Clinical uses include therapy of infections caused by common streptococci, pneumococci, gonococci (some strains are resistant), meningococci, gram-positive bacilli, and spirochetes. Most strains of *Staphylococcus aureus* are resistant. Activity against enterococci is enhanced by aminoglycoside antibiotics. Penicillin V is an oral drug used mainly in common streptococcal infections.

2. **Very narrow spectrum, penicillinase-resistant drugs:**   This subclass of penicillins includes **methicillin (the prototype), nafcillin,** and **oxacillin.** Their sole use is in the treatment of known or suspected staphylococcal infections. Methicillin-resistant staphylococci (MRSA) are resistant to other members of this subgroup and may be resistant to multiple antimicrobial drugs.

3. **Wider spectrum, penicillinase-susceptible drugs:**

    a. **Ampicillin and amoxicillin:**   These drugs comprise a penicillin subgroup that has a wider spectrum of antibacterial activity than penicillin G but remains susceptible to penicillinases. Their clinical uses include indications similar to penicillin G as well as infections due to *Escherichia coli, Proteus mirabilis,* and *Haemophilus influenzae,* although resistant strains occur. When used in combination with inhibitors of penicillinases (clavulanic acid, etc) their antibacterial activity is enhanced.

    b. **Carbenicillin and ticarcillin:**   These drugs have activity against several gram-negative rods, including *Pseudomonas* spp. Most drugs in this subgroup have synergistic actions when used with aminoglycosides against such organisms. Carbenicillin and ticarcillin are susceptible to penicillinases and are sometimes used in combination with penicillinase inhibitors to enhance their activity.

E. Toxicity:

1. **Allergy:**   Allergic reactions include urticaria, severe pruritus, fever, joint swelling, hemolytic anemia, nephritis, and anaphylaxis. About 10–15% of persons with a past history of penicillin reaction have an allergic response when given a penicillin again. Methicillin causes nephritis more often than do other penicillins. Antigenic determinants include degradation products of penicillins, such as penicilloic acid. Complete **cross-allergenicity** between different penicillins should be assumed. Ampicillin frequently causes maculopapular skin rash that may not be an allergic reaction.

2. **Gastrointestinal disturbances:**   Nausea and diarrhea may occur with oral penicillins, especially with ampicillin. Gastrointestinal upsets may be caused by direct irritation, or by overgrowth of gram-positive organisms or yeasts.

3. **Cation toxicity:**   Toxic effects from Na^+ or K^+ may occur when high doses of certain penicillin salts are used in patients with cardiovascular or renal disease.

CEPHALOSPORINS

A. Classification: The cephalosporins are derivatives of 7-aminocephalosporanic acid and contain the beta-lactam ring structure. Many members of this group are in clinical use. They are classified on the basis of their antibacterial activity, but are designated first-, second-, or third-generation drugs according to the time of their introduction into clinical use.

B. Pharmacokinetics: Several cephalosporins are available for oral use, but most are administered parenterally. Cephalosporins with side-chains may undergo hepatic metabolism, but the major elimination mechanism for drugs in this class is renal excretion via active tubular secretion. Cefoperazone and ceftriaxone are excreted mainly in the bile. Most first- and second-generation cephalosporins do not enter the cerebrospinal fluid even when the meninges are inflamed.

C. Mechanism of Action: Cephalosporins bind to PBPs on bacterial cell membranes to inhibit bacterial cell wall synthesis by mechanisms similar to those of the penicillins. Cephalosporins are bactericidal against susceptible organisms.

Structural differences from penicillins render cephalosporins less susceptible to penicillinases produced by staphylococci, but many bacteria are resistant through the production of other beta-lactamases that can inactivate cephalosporins. Resistance can also result from decreases in membrane permeability to cephalosporins and by changes in PBPs. Methicillin-resistant staphylococci are also resistant to most cephalosporins.

D. Clinical Use:

1. **First-generation drugs: Na cephalothin** and **cefazolin** are examples of this subgroup. They are active against gram-positive cocci, including staphylococci and common streptococci. Many strains of *E coli* and *K pneumoniae* are also sensitive. Clinical uses include treatment of infections caused by these organisms and surgical prophylaxis in selected cases. These drugs have minimal activity against gram-negative cocci, enterococci, and most other gram-negative rods.

2. **Second-generation drugs:** Drugs in this subgroup usually have less activity against gram-positive organisms than the first-generation drugs, but have an extended gram-negative coverage. Marked differences in activity occur among the drugs in this subgroup. Examples of clinical uses include infections caused by *Bacteroides fragilis* (**cefotetan, cefoxitin**) and *H influenzae* (**cefuroxime, cefaclor**).

3. **Third-generation drugs:** Characteristic features of third-generation drugs (eg, **cefoperazone, cefotaxime**) include increased activity against resistant gram-negative organisms and ability to penetrate the blood-brain barrier (except cefoperazone and cefixime). Most are active against *Enterobacter* spp, *Providencia* spp, *Serratia marcescens,* and beta-lactamase-producing strains of *H influenzae* and *Neisseria* spp. Individual drugs also have activity against *Pseudomonas* spp (**ceftazidime**) and *B fragilis* (**ceftizoxime**). Drugs in this subclass should usually be reserved for treatment of serious infections, eg, those in debilitated, immunocompromised patients. **Ceftriaxone,** currently the drug of choice in gonorrhea, is an exception.

E. Toxicity:

1. **Allergy:** Cephalosporin use is associated with a range of allergic reactions from skin rashes to anaphylactic shock. These reactions occur less frequently with cephalosporins than with penicillins. Complete cross-hypersensitivity between different cephalosporins should be assumed.

   Cross-reactivity between penicillins and cephalosporins is not complete (10%) so penicillin-allergic patients are sometimes treated successfully with a cephalosporin. However, patients with a history of anaphylaxis to penicillins should not be treated with a cephalosporin.

2. **Other adverse effects:** Cephalosporins may cause pain at intramuscular injection sites and phlebitis after intravenous administration. They may increase the nephrotoxicity of aminoglycosides when the two are administered together. Drugs containing a methylthiotetrazole group (cefoperazone, cefotetan, moxalactam) cause hypoprothrombinemia and may cause disulfiram-like reactions with ethanol. Moxalactam also decreases platelet function and may cause severe bleeding.

OTHER BETA-LACTAM DRUGS

A. Aztreonam: Aztreonam is a monobactam that is resistant to beta-lactamases produced by certain gram-negative rods, including *Klebsiella* spp, *Pseudomonas* spp and *Serratia* spp. The drug has no activity against gram-positive bacteria or anaerobes. It is an inhibitor of cell wall synthesis, preferentially binding to PBP3, and is synergistic with aminoglycosides. Aztreonam is administered intravenously and is eliminated via renal tubular secretion. Half-life is prolonged in renal failure. Adverse effects include gastrointestinal upset with possible superinfection, vertigo and headache, and rare hepatotoxicity. Though skin rash may occur, there is no cross-allergenicity with penicillins.

B. Imipenem: Imipenem is a carbapenem (chemically different from penicillins, but retaining the beta-lactam ring structure) with low susceptibility to beta-lactamases. The drug has wide activity against gram-positive cocci, gram-negative rods, and anaerobes. It is administered parenterally, and is especially useful for infections caused by organisms resistant to other antibiotics. Imipenem is rapidly inactivated by renal dihydropeptidase I and is always administered in combination with cilastatin, an inhibitor of this enzyme. Combination with cilastatin increases the plasma half-life of imipenem and inhibits the formation of a potentially nephrotoxic metabolite. Adverse effects of imipenem-cilastatin include gastrointestinal distress and skin rash, and CNS toxicity (confusion, encephalopathy, seizures) at very high plasma levels. There is partial cross-allergenicity with the penicillins.

DRUG LIST

The following drugs are important members of the group discussed in this chapter. Prototypes should be learned in detail; features of the major variants should be known well enough to distinguish the variants from prototypes and from each other.

Subclass	Prototype	Major Variants
Penicillins Limited spectrum	Penicillin G	Penicillin V
Beta-lactamase-resistant	Methicillin	Nafcillin, oxacillin, cloxacillin
Wider spectrum	Ampicillin, carbenicillin	Amoxicillin, ticarcillin
Cephalosporins First-generation	Na cephalothin	Cefazolin, cephradine, cephapirin
Second-generation	Cefamandole	Cefaclor, cefotetan, cefoxitin
Third-generation	Cefoperazone	Cefotaxime, ceftazidime, ceftriaxone
Carbapenem	Imipenem	
Monobactam	Aztreonam	
Beta-lactamase inhibitors[1]	Clavulanic acid	Sulbactam, tazobactam

[1] Negligible antimicrobial activity when given alone

QUESTIONS

DIRECTIONS: Each of the numbered items or incomplete statements in this section is followed by answers or by completions of the statement. Select the ONE lettered answer or completion that is BEST in each case.

1.   All of the following statements about the biodisposition of penicillins and cephalosporins are accurate EXCEPT
  (A) Oral bioavailability of such drugs depends on their stability in gastric acid
  (B) Cephalosporins are more likely to cross the blood-brain barrier than most penicillins
  (C) The half-life of penicillin is prolonged if it is administered as the procaine salt
  (D) Penicillins are polar compounds and are not metabolized extensively by liver enzymes
  (E) Nafcillin and cefoperazone are eliminated mainly via biliary secretion

2.   The mechanism of antibacterial action of cephalosporins involves
  (A) Inhibition of the synthesis of precursors of peptidoglycans
  (B) Interference with the synthesis of ergosterol
  (C) Inhibition of transpeptidase enzymes
  (D) Inhibition of beta-lactamases
  (E) Binding to cytoplasmic receptor proteins

3. Which of the following drugs is LEAST likely to be effective in the treatment of an infection caused by *S aureus*?
   (A) Amoxicillin
   (B) Nafcillin
   (C) Cefazolin
   (D) Oxacillin
   (E) Erythromycin

4. All of the following statements about the beta-lactam antibiotics are accurate EXCEPT
   (A) Penicillin G is the drug of choice for syphilis
   (B) Cefoxitin and cefotetan are effective in the treatment of peritonitis and diverticulitis because they have activity against anaerobes including *B fragilis*
   (C) Resistance of staphylococci to methicillin is an example of multiple drug resistance
   (D) Skin rashes occur more commonly with penicillin G than with ampicillin
   (E) Bleeding episodes following moxalactam are partly due to interference with platelet function

5. Which of the following drugs is most likely to interfere with vitamin K availability, leading to hypoprothrombinemia and possible bleeding disorders?
   (A) Cefoperazone
   (B) Procaine penicillin G
   (C) Imipenem
   (D) Cefazolin
   (E) Nafcillin

6. An elderly, debilitated patient has a fever believed to be due to an infection. He has extensive skin lesions, scrapings of which reveal the presence of large numbers of gram-positive cocci. The most appropriate drug to use for treatment of this patient is
   (A) Amoxicillin
   (B) Aztreonam
   (C) Moxalactam
   (D) Nafcillin
   (E) Penicillin G

7. A patient recently treated for leukemia is admitted to hospital with malaise, chills and high fever. Gram stain of blood reveals the presence of gram-negative bacilli. The initial diagnosis is bacteremia, and parenteral antibiotics are indicated. The records of the patient reveal that she had a severe urticarial rash, hypotension, and respiratory difficulty following oral penicillin V about 7 months ago. The most appropriate drug to administer is
   (A) Ampicillin plus sulbactam
   (B) Aztreonam
   (C) Ticarcillin plus clavulanic acid
   (D) Cefazolin
   (E) Imipenem plus cilastatin

8. The drug of choice for treatment of meningococcal meningitis in an adult patient with no drug allergies is
   (A) Penicillin G
   (B) Methicillin
   (C) Sulbactam
   (D) Cefazolin
   (E) Ticarcillin

9. All of the following statements about imipenem are accurate EXCEPT
   (A) It has a wide spectrum of antibacterial action
   (B) Its renal elimination is not inhibited by probenecid
   (C) There is partial cross-allergenicity between imipenem and penicillins
   (D) Dosage reductions are unnecessary in renal impairment because the drug is metabolized
   (E) It is not active against methicillin-resistant staphylococci

DIRECTIONS: The following section consists of a list of four to twenty-six lettered options followed by several numbered items. For each numbered item, select the ONE option that is most closely associated with it. Each answer may be selected once, more than once, or not at all.
   (A) Ceftriaxone
   (B) Penicillin V

    (C) Dicloxacillin
    (D) Ticarcillin
    (E) Imipenem
    (F) Ampicillin
    (G) Penicillin G
    (H) Cefaclor
    (I) Aztreonam
    (J) Sulbactam

10. This drug is often effective in the treatment of infections caused by *Pseudomonas aeruginosa* but is susceptible to penicillinases produced by certain strains of this organism

11. This drug has minimal activity against gram-negative rods and is susceptible to penicillinases. Its clinical uses are restricted to the treatment of infections caused by streptococci and oral pathogens. This drug is stable in gastric acid

12. A second-generation cephalosporin commonly used to treat sinusitis and otitis media

13. To prevent the rapid inactivation of this drug, it must be administered in combination with cilastatin, an inhibitor of renal dihydropeptidase

14. The spectrum of activity of this antibiotic includes penicillinase-producing *S aureus* and many gram-negative bacteria including meningococci, *E coli*, *Haemophilus influenzae,* and *Klebsiella* spp. Most pseudomonal strains are resistant. The drug is effective in the empiric treatment of suspected bacterial meningitis in children

ANSWERS

1. Penicillins enter the CSF when the meninges are inflamed and are effective in the treatment of meningitis caused by susceptible bacteria. In contrast, most first- and second-generation cephalosporins do not cross the blood-brain barrier. The answer is **(B)**.

2. The cephalosporins act at the transpeptidation stage to inhibit peptidoglycan cross-linking and have no actions on the synthesis of precursor molecules. The answer is **(C)**.

3. It is important to recall that ampicillin and amoxicillin are susceptible to penicillinases. These drugs are unlikely to be effective in infections caused by staphylococci unless they are administered in combination with inhibitors of beta-lactamases. The answer is **(A)**.

4. While all penicillins may cause skin rashes, they occur most commonly with ampicillin. The answer is **(D)**.

5. Hypoprothrombinemia is associated with the use of third-generation cephalosporins that contain a methylthiotetrazole group. This effect can be prevented by administration of vitamin K. The answer is **(A)**.

6. Bacterial lesions of the skin are often caused by staphylococci or streptococci, and may lead to systemic infections; they should be treated promptly. Virtually all strains of *S aureus* are penicillinase-producing, so amoxicillin and penicillin G would not be effective. Aztreonam is only active against gram-negative bacilli, and third-generation cephalosporins (eg, moxalactam) have limited activity against gram-positive organisms. In addition, moxalactam carries the risk of bleeding disorders in elderly, debilitated patients. Nafcillin is resistant to penicillinases and has activity against most strains of *S aureus* and common streptococci. The answer is **(D)**.

7. The drugs listed all have activity against some gram-negative bacilli. All penicillins should be avoided in patients with a history of allergic reactions to any individual penicillin drug. Cephalosporins should also be avoided in patients who have had anaphylaxis or other severe hypersensitivity reactions following use of a penicillin. There is no cross-reactivity between the penicillins and aztreonam. The answer is **(B)**.

8. In the adult patient, penicillin G remains the drug of choice for the treatment of meningitis due to meningococci or pneumococci. However, penicillin G does not provide coverage for gram-negative bacilli in the presumptive management of suspected bacterial meningitis. The answer is **(A)**.

9. Severe CNS toxicity, including seizures, will occur if the dose of imipenem is not reduced in patients with renal impairment. The answer is **(D)**.

10. Ticarcillin is a member of the penicillin subgroup that has activity against selected gram-negative rods including *Pseudomonas aeruginosa*. However, its activity against penicillinase-producing strains of such organisms is greatly enhanced if the drug is administered in combination with clavulanic acid. The answer is **(D)**.

11. Penicillin V is equivalent to penicillin G in terms of its activity against streptococci. Unlike penicillin G, penicillin V is stable in gastric acid and is effective by mouth. The answer is **(B)**.
12. Cefaclor is the only second-generation cephalosporin listed. The answer is **(H)**.
13. Imipenem is resistant to beta-lactamases and has a wide antibacterial activity. The antibiotic is rapidly inactivated by renal dihydropeptidases, and cilastatin must be used in combination with it to prolong its effects. The answer is **(E)**.
14. The antibacterial spectrum and clinical use described is that of the third-generation cephalosporin, ceftriaxone. The answer is **(A)**.

Chloramphenicol & Tetracyclines

OBJECTIVES

You should be able to:

- Describe the mechanisms of action of chloramphenicol and tetracyclines.
- Describe the mechanisms responsible for clinical bacterial resistance to these drugs.
- List the major clinical uses of these drugs.
- Describe the pharmacokinetic features of these agents that are most relevant to their clinical use.
- List the main toxic effects of chloramphenicol and tetracyclines.

CONCEPTS

Chloramphenicol and the tetracyclines constitute the first **broad spectrum** antibiotics discovered. Because they were thought to have very low toxicities, they were overused, and many bacterial species became resistant. These drugs are now used for more selected targets.

CHLORAMPHENICOL

A. Classification & Pharmacokinetics: Chloramphenicol has a simple and distinctive structure, and no other antimicrobials have been discovered in this chemical class. Effective orally as well as parenterally, it is distributed throughout all tissues and readily crosses the placental and blood-brain barriers. The drug undergoes enterohepatic cycling, and a small fraction of the dose is excreted in the urine unchanged. Most of the drug is inactivated by a hepatic glucuronosyltransferase.

B. Mechanism of Action: Chloramphenicol has a wide spectrum of antimicrobial activity (ie, it is a broad-spectrum drug) and is usually bacteriostatic. It binds to the 50S ribosomal subunit of bacteria and inhibits peptidyl transferase (Figure 44–1). This ribosomal enzyme is responsible for peptide bond formation, and thus protein synthesis is inhibited in the presence of chloramphenicol. Though selectively toxic to bacteria, chloramphenicol can also inhibit mitochondrial protein synthesis in mammalian cells. Resistance to chloramphenicol, which is plasmid-mediated, occurs through the formation of inactivating acetyltransferases.

C. Clinical Use: Because of its toxicity, chloramphenicol is reserved for severe infections caused by *Salmonella* and *Haemophilus* spp and for the treatment of pneumococcal and meningococcal meningitis in penicillin-sensitive persons. Note that some *H influenzae* strains

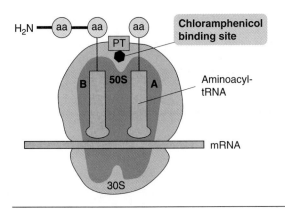

Figure 44–1. Chloramphenicol inhibits peptide bond formation. The binding site for chloramphenicol is on the larger ribosomal subunit (50S) of bacteria, adjacent to peptidyl transferase (PT), the ribosomal enzyme that catalyzes peptide bond formation. Drug binding interferes with the action of this enzyme, preventing the transfer of amino acids (aa) from aminoacyl-tRNA to the growing peptide chain.

are resistant to chloramphenicol; therefore ceftriaxone or another third-generation cephalosporin is usually preferred. Chloramphenicol is sometimes used for rickettsial diseases and for infections caused by anaerobes such as *Bacteroides fragilis*. Chloramphenicol is commonly used as a topical antimicrobial agent because of its broad spectrum of activity.

D. Toxicity:

1. **Gastrointestinal disturbances:** These may occur from direct irritation and from superinfections, especially candidiasis.
2. **Bone marrow:** Inhibition of red-cell maturation leads to a decrease in RBCs. This action is dose-dependent and reversible.
3. **Aplastic anemia:** This is a rare (approximately 1 case in 25,000–40,000 patients treated) idiosyncratic reaction. It is usually irreversible and may be fatal.
4. **Gray baby syndrome:** This syndrome occurs in infants and is characterized by cyanosis and cardiovascular collapse. Neonates, especially premature neonates, are deficient in hepatic glucuronosyltransferase, the enzyme required for chloramphenicol elimination. These infants are therefore very sensitive to doses of the drug that would be tolerated in older infants.
5. **Drug interactions:** Chloramphenicol inhibits the metabolism of several drugs, including phenytoin, coumarins, and tolbutamide.

TETRACYCLINES

A. Classification: Drugs in this class are structural congeners that have a broad range of antimicrobial activity and only minor differences in their activities against specific organisms. **Tetracycline** is representative of older members of the group; **doxycycline** and **minocycline** are newer agents.

B. Pharmacokinetics: Oral absorption is variable, especially for the older drugs, and may be impaired by foods and multivalent cations (calcium, iron, aluminum). These drugs have a wide tissue distribution and enter mammalian cells. They cross the placental barrier, but CNS penetration is limited. All of the tetracyclines undergo enterohepatic cycling. Doxycycline is excreted mainly in feces; the other drugs are eliminated primarily in the urine. The half-lives of doxycycline and minocycline are longer than those of other tetracyclines.

C. Mechanism of Action: Tetracyclines are bacteriostatic inhibitors of protein synthesis. They are accumulated intracellularly via energy-dependent transport systems present in bacterial membranes. As shown in Figure 44–2, the binding site for tetracyclines is present on the smaller bacterial ribosomal subunit (30S). The bulky structure of the drug interferes with binding of **aminoacyl-tRNA** to the A site on the ribosomal complex. This blocking action prevents alignment of the aminoacyl-tRNA anticodons with mRNA, and peptide bond synthesis is inhibited. The selective toxicity of tetracyclines occurs mainly because mammalian cells lack the membrane transporting systems that lead to drug accumulation.

Plasmid-mediated resistance to tetracyclines is widespread. Tetracycline-resistant organisms

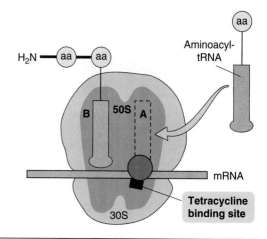

Figure 44–2. Tetracyclines inhibit binding of aminoacyl-tRNA. The interaction of tetracycline with components of the smaller ribosomal subunit (30S) blocks the binding of aminoacyl-tRNA to the A-site on the ribosomal complex, and protein synthesis is inhibited. Compare with Figure 44–1 (aa, amino acid).

show decreased intracellular accumulation of the drugs. The probable mechanisms are decreased activity of the uptake systems and development of mechanisms for active extrusion of tetracyclines out of the organism.

D. Clinical Use:
1. **Primary uses:** Tetracyclines are the drugs of first choice in the treatment of infections caused by *Mycoplasma pneumoniae* (in adults), chlamydiae, rickettsiae, and vibrios.
2. **Secondary uses:** Tetracyclines are alternative drugs in the treatment of syphilis and gonorrhea (a tetracycline or other agent may be required for accompanying chlamydial infections even if penicillin is used). Tetracyclines are also used in the treatment of respiratory infections caused by susceptible organisms, in the prophylactic treatment of chronic bronchitis, the management of leptospirosis, and the treatment of acne.
3. **Selective uses:** Specific tetracyclines are used in the treatment of bacterial enteritis and Lyme disease (doxycycline), and the meningococcal carrier state (minocycline). Demeclocycline inhibits the renal actions of ADH and is used in the management of patients with ADH-secreting tumors (Chapter 15).

E. Toxicity:
1. **Gastrointestinal disturbances:** Effects on the gastrointestinal system range from mild nausea and diarrhea to severe, possibly life-threatening colitis. Disturbances in the normal flora lead to candidiasis (oral and vaginal) and, more rarely, bacterial superinfections due to *S aureus* or *Clostridium difficile.*
2. **Bony structures and teeth:** Fetal exposure to tetracyclines may lead to tooth enamel dysplasia and irregularities in bone growth. Treatment of younger children may cause enamel dysplasia and crown deformations when permanent teeth appear.
3. **Hepatic toxicity:** High doses of tetracyclines, especially in pregnant patients or in patients with preexisting hepatic disease, may impair liver function and lead to hepatic necrosis.
4. **Renal toxicity:** One form of renal tubular acidosis, Fanconi syndrome, has been attributed to use of outdated tetracyclines. Though not directly nephrotoxic, tetracyclines may exacerbate preexisting renal dysfunction.
5. **Photosensitivity:** Tetracyclines, especially demeclocycline, may cause enhanced skin sensitivity to ultraviolet light.
6. **Vestibular toxicity:** Dose-dependent, reversible dizziness and vertigo have been noted with minocycline.

DRUG LIST

The following drugs are important members of the groups discussed in this chapter. Prototypes should be learned in detail; features of the major variants should be known well enough to distinguish the variants from the prototypes and from each other; the other significant agents should be recognized as belonging to a specific subclass.

Subclass	Prototype	Major Variants	Other Significant Agents
Chloramphenicol	Chloramphenicol		
Tetracyclines	Tetracycline	Demeclocycline	Doxycycline, minocycline

QUESTIONS

DIRECTIONS: Each of the numbered items or incomplete statements in this section is followed by answers or by completions of the statement. Select the ONE lettered answer or completion that is BEST in each case.

1. All of the following statements about chloramphenicol are accurate EXCEPT
   (A) The drug is completely absorbed following oral administration
   (B) When it is given to neonates, their limited hepatic glucuronosyltransferase activity may result in cyanosis
   (C) Chloramphenicol is usually bacteriostatic
   (D) Clinical resistance occurs through changes in the structure of bacterial peptidyl transferase
   (E) The dose of chloramphenicol should be reduced in hepatic failure

2. Chloramphenicol is likely to be effective in all of the following EXCEPT
   (A) Salmonellosis
   (B) Chlamydial infections of the eye
   (C) Pneumococcal meningitis in a penicillin-allergic person
   (D) Initial therapy of meningitis suspected to be caused by *H influenzae*
   (E) Brain abscess caused by anaerobes

3. The mechanism of antibacterial action of tetracyclines involves
   (A) Inhibition of the conversion of lanosterol to ergosterol
   (B) Inhibition of DNA-dependent RNA polymerase
   (C) Blockade of binding of aminoacyl-tRNA to bacterial ribosomes
   (D) Selective inhibition of ribosomal peptidyl transferases
   (E) Inhibition of translocase activity

4. Appropriate statements about the clinical uses of tetracyclines include all of the following EXCEPT
   (A) The tetracyclines are drugs of choice in the treatment of rickettsial infections
   (B) Doxycycline is an effective prophylactic drug for traveler's diarrhea
   (C) The tetracyclines should not be used for the therapy of respiratory infections caused by *Mycoplasma pneumoniae*
   (D) The efficacy of tetracyclines may be decreased in patients taking antacids
   (E) At full doses for 7 days, a tetracycline will usually be effective in gonorrhea and also control co-existing chlamydial infections

5. All of the following statements about tetracyclines are accurate EXCEPT
   (A) They cross the placental barrier and are excreted in the milk of nursing mothers
   (B) Suppression of normal flora by tetracyclines may lead to superinfections from resistant bacteria or yeast
   (C) Tetracyclines are chelating agents that bind to calcium in developing bone and teeth
   (D) They have minimal activity against most strains of *Pseudomonas* spp
   (E) Clinical resistance is due to formation of enzymes that inactivate tetracyclines

6. A 2-year-old child is brought to the hospital after ingesting pills that a parent had used for bacterial dysentery when traveling outside the United States. The physician is informed that the child had been vomiting for over 24 hours, and has had diarrhea with green stools. He is now lethargic with an ashen color. Other signs and symptoms include hypothermia, hypotension, and abdominal distension. The drug most likely to be the cause of this problem is

(A) Doxycycline
(B) Chloramphenicol
(C) Ampicillin
(D) Trimethoprim-sulfamethoxazole
(E) Minocycline

7. Which ONE of the following drugs is most likely to be effective in the treatment of both Rocky Mountain Spotted fever and meningococcal meningitis?
(A) Tetracycline HCl
(B) Penicillin G
(C) Ceftriaxone
(D) Chloramphenicol
(E) Doxycycline

8. A 24-year-old woman has primary syphilis. She has a history of penicillin hypersensitivity, so tetracycline will be used to treat the infection. All of the following statements about the proposed drug management of this patient are accurate EXCEPT
(A) She should be told that she has to take the drug for 15 days
(B) She should avoid taking supplementary iron tablets at the same time as she takes the drug
(C) She may experience anorexia and gastrointestinal distress
(D) She should eat plenty of yogurt to prevent vaginal candidiasis
(E) She should call her physician if she develops severe diarrhea

DIRECTIONS: The following section consists of a list of four to twenty-six lettered options followed by several numbered items. For each numbered item, select the ONE option that is most closely associated with it. Each answer may be selected once, more than once, or not at all.

(A) Doxycycline
(B) Minocycline
(C) Chloramphenicol
(D) Erythromycin
(E) Demeclocycline
(F) Aztreonam
(G) Tetracycline HCl
(H) Cyclosporine

9. The appearance of markedly vacuolated, nucleated red cells in the marrow, anemia, and reticulocytopenia are characteristic dose-dependent side effects of this drug

10. Decreased renal function has little effect on the rate of elimination of this tetracycline. It has a longer plasma half-life than other drugs in its class

11. Loss of balance, dizziness, nausea, and tinnitus may occur in up to 70% of patients receiving this drug for meningococcal prophylaxis

12. In addition to its antibacterial actions, this drug has ADH-inhibiting effects. It has caused abnormal reddening of the skin when patients were exposed to sunlight

13. This is the preferred tetracycline for management of acute respiratory infections in patients with chronic bronchitis, and it also has greater activity against anaerobes than other drugs in its class

14. This drug is traditionally regarded as the preferred agent for treatment of typhoid fever

ANSWERS

1. Clinical resistance to chloramphenicol involves the plasmid-mediated formation of acetyltransferases that inactivate the drug. Although it is usually bacteriostatic, the drug may be bactericidal to some strains of pneumococci and meningococci. The answer is **(D)**.

2. Chloramphenicol penetrates into the aqueous humor and, because of its wide spectrum of activity, is used topically in the treatment of eye infections. However, it is not effective in chlamydial infections. All of the other indications are reasonable, although chloramphenicol may not be the drug of first choice. The answer is **(B)**.

3. Tetracyclines inhibit bacterial protein synthesis by interfering with the binding of aminoacyl-tRNA molecules to bacterial ribosomes. Peptidyl transferase is inhibited by chloramphenicol. The answer is **(C)**.

4. Tetracyclines are highly effective in the treatment of respiratory infections due to *Mycoplasma pneumoniae* and may be the drugs of choice in adult patients. However, tetracyclines are not usually regarded as appropriate drugs to treat such infections in children or in pregnant women. The answer is **(C)**.

5. Decreased intracellular accumulation of tetracyclines is the major mechanism involved in the development of resistance to this class of drugs. The development of inactivating transferase enzymes is the mechanism of resistance to chloramphenicol. The answer is **(E)**.

6. Although the gray baby syndrome is most common in neonates, it has occurred with over-dosage of chloramphenicol in older children and adults, especially those with hepatic dysfunction. The answer is **(B)**.

7. Beta-lactam antibiotics are not effective in rickettsial infections, and many strains of *N meningitides* are resistant to the tetracyclines. The answer is **(D)**.

8. The ingestion of foods containing multivalent cations (yogurt contains calcium and magnesium) can interfere with gastrointestinal absorption of tetracyclines and impair their clinical efficacy. The answer is **(D)**.

9. Reversible, dose-dependent bone marrow dysfunction occurs with chloramphenicol, due to maturation arrest. Serum iron concentration increases and blood levels of phenylalanine decrease. These actions are unrelated to the rare occurrence of aplastic anemia. The answer is **(C)**.

10. Doxycycline is excreted almost entirely in the feces, mainly via biliary secretion. This is the only tetracycline that does not require major dosage adjustments in patients with renal impairment. The answer is **(A)**.

11. Among the adverse effects of tetracyclines, vestibular toxicity is unique to minocycline. The answer is **(B)**.

12. Photosensitivity reactions can occur with any tetracycline but appear to be more common with demeclocycline. The answer is **(E)**.

13. Doxycycline offers a number of pharmacologic advantages over conventional tetracyclines. It has good bioavailability, effective tissue penetration, and a long half-life. Doxycycline is also more effective against pathogens associated with acute exacerbations of chronic bronchitis (pneumococci, *H influenzae, M catarrhalis*) and has better activity against most anaerobes than other tetracyclines. The answer is **(A)**.

14. Chloramphenicol is an effective drug in typhoid fever. However, because of this drug's toxicity and minimal efficacy in eliminating the carrier state, many specialists in the USA prefer other antimicrobial drugs to treat acute typhoid fever. These may include ampicillin/amoxicillin, trimethoprim-sulfamethoxazole, a third-generation cephalosporin, or a fluoroquinolone. The answer is **(C)**.

Aminoglycosides & Polymyxins

45

OBJECTIVES

You should be able to:

- Describe the mechanism of action of aminoglycoside antibiotics and the mechanism by which bacterial resistance to this class of drugs occurs.
- List the major clinical applications of aminoglycosides and describe their main toxic effects.
- Describe the pharmacokinetics of this drug class, with special reference to the importance of renal clearance and its relationship to toxicity.
- Describe the mechanism of action, clinical uses, and major toxic effects of polymyxins.

CONCEPTS

The aminoglycosides and polymyxins are very different in their structures and mechanisms of action, but they share activity against gram-negative bacteria.

AMINOGLYCOSIDES

A. Classification: The drugs in this class are structurally related amino sugars attached by glycosidic linkages. The main differences among the individual drugs lie in their activities against specific organisms, particularly gram-negative rods.

B. Pharmacokinetics: Aminoglycosides are polar compounds and must be given parenterally for systemic effect; they are not absorbed after oral administration. They have limited tissue penetration and no significant metabolism by the host. Glomerular filtration is the major mode of excretion, and plasma levels of these drugs are greatly affected by changes in renal function. Each member of the group has a particular range of optimal plasma levels below which the drug has limited antibacterial activity and above which it causes toxic effects. This range of drug concentrations defines the therapeutic window (Figure 3–6). Monitoring of plasma levels of aminoglycosides is an important requirement for safe and effective dosage selection and adjustment.

C. Mechanism of Action: Aminoglycosides are bactericidal inhibitors of protein synthesis. Their penetration through the bacterial cell envelope is partly via oxygen-dependent, active transport, and they have little activity against strict anaerobes. Inside the cell, streptomycin (the best-studied aminoglycoside) binds to the 30S ribosomal subunit and interferes with protein synthesis in three ways: (1) block of the initiation complex, which prevents its transition to a chain-elongating functional ribosomal complex; (2) misreading of the code on the mRNA template, which causes miscoding of amino acids in the peptide; and (3) disruption of polysomes into nonfunctional monosomes (Figure 45–1). Other aminoglycosides have a similar but not identical mechanism of action.

D. Mechanism of Resistance: Resistance to aminoglycosides involves the plasmid-mediated formation of inactivating enzymes. These enzymes are **group transferases** that catalyze the acetylation of amine functions and the transfer of phosphoryl or adenylyl groups to the oxygen atoms of hydroxyl groups on the aminoglycoside. Individual aminoglycosides have varying susceptibilities to such enzymes. Currently, **amikacin** and **netilmicin** are susceptible to only a few such enzymes, and these drugs are often active against more strains of organisms than are other aminoglycosides.

E. Clinical Uses:

1. **Primary uses:** Three aminoglycosides (gentamicin, tobramycin, amikacin) are important drugs for the treatment of serious infections caused by aerobic gram-negative bacteria, including *E coli* and *Enterobacter, Klebsiella, Proteus, Pseudomonas*, and *Serratia* spp (Table 45–1). Drug choice depends on susceptibility patterns. Antibacterial synergy may occur when aminoglycosides are used in combination with beta-lactam antibiotics. Examples include their combined use in the treatment of serious pseudomonal and enterococcal infections.

2. **Other indications:**
   a. **Streptomycin:** Streptomycin is used in the treatment of tuberculosis, plague, and tularemia. Because of the risk of ototoxicity, streptomycin should not be used when other drugs will serve.
   b. **Neomycin:** Due to its toxic potential, neomycin is only used topically or locally, eg, in the gastrointestinal tract.
   c. **Netilmicin:** A relatively new drug, netilmicin is usually reserved for organisms resistant to the other aminoglycosides.
   d. **Spectinomycin:** The sole use of spectinomycin, an aminocyclitol related to the aminoglycosides, is in the treatment of gonorrhea.

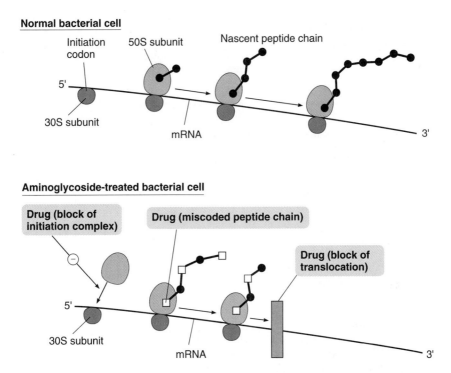

Figure 45–1. Putative mechanisms of action of the aminoglycosides. Normal protein synthesis is shown in the top panel. At least three different aminoglycoside effects have been described as shown in the bottom panel: block of formation of the initiation complex; miscoding of amino acids in the emerging peptide chain due to misreading of the mRNA; and block of translocation on mRNA. Block of movement of the ribosome may occur after the formation of a single initiation complex, resulting in an mRNA chain with only a single ribosome on it, a so-called monosome.

F. **Toxicity:**
   1. **Ototoxicity:**   Auditory or vestibular damage (or both) can occur with any aminoglycoside and may be irreversible. Ototoxicity risk is proportionate to the plasma levels, and thus is especially high if dosage is not appropriately modified in a patient with renal dysfunction. Ototoxicity may be increased by the use of loop diuretics.
   2. **Nephrotoxicity:**   Renal toxicity usually takes the form of acute tubular necrosis. This adverse effect, which is often reversible, is more common in elderly patients and in those receiving cephalosporin antibiotics.
   3. **Neuromuscular blockade:**   Though rare, a curare-like block can occur at high doses of aminoglycosides and may result in respiratory paralysis. Neuromuscular blockade from an aminoglycoside is usually reversible by treatment with calcium and neostigmine, but ventilatory support may be required.
   4. **Skin reactions:**   Allergic skin reactions may occur in patients, and contact dermatitis may occur in personnel handling the drug. Of the aminoglycosides, neomycin is the most likely to cause this adverse effect.

Table 45–1. Clinical applications of the aminoglycosides.

Drug	Application
Gentamicin, amikacin, tobramycin, netilmicin	Serious infections with aerobic gram-negative bacteria, including *E coli* and *Enterobacter, Klebsiella, Proteus, Pseudomonas,* and *Serratia* spp
Streptomycin	Tuberculosis; rare: plague, brucellosis, tularemia, infective endocarditis
Neomycin, kanamycin	Bowel sterilization, skin infections
Spectinomycin	Gonorrhea

POLYMYXINS

A. **Chemistry & Mechanism:** The polymyxins are fatty acid-containing basic polypeptides that are bactericidal against gram-negative bacteria. These drugs interact with a specific **lipopolysaccharide** component of the outer cell membrane that is also a binding site for calcium. Membrane lipid structure is distorted, with an increase in permeability to polar molecules, resulting in marked changes in cell metabolism.

B. **Clinical Uses & Toxicities:** Because of toxicity, the clinical applications of the polymyxins are limited to topical therapy of resistant gram-negative infections, including those caused by *Enterobacter* and *Pseudomonas* spp. These drugs are occasionally administered into infected cavities, eg, the joints and the pleural and peritoneal cavities.

Adverse effects include neurotoxicity (paresthesias, dizziness, ataxia) and acute renal tubular necrosis (hematuria, proteinuria, nitrogen retention).

DRUG LIST

The following drugs are important members of the group discussed in this chapter. Prototypes should be learned in detail; features of the major variants should be known well enough to distinguish the variants from the prototypes and from each other; the other significant agents should be recognized as belonging to a specific subclass.

Subclass	Prototype	Major Variants	Other Significant Agents
Aminoglycosides Systemic	Gentamicin	Tobramycin	Amikacin, netilmicin, streptomycin
Local	Neomycin		Gentamicin, kanamycin
Aminocyclitols	Spectinomycin		
Polymyxins	Polymyxin B	Colistin (polymyxin E)	

QUESTIONS

DIRECTIONS: Each of the numbered items or incomplete statements in this section is followed by answers or by completions of the statement. Select the ONE lettered answer or completion that is BEST in each case.

1. All of the following statements about the mechanism of action of aminoglycosides are accurate EXCEPT
   (A) They induce misreading of the code on the mRNA template
   (B) They prevent polysome formation
   (C) They bind to the 50S ribosomal subunit and inhibit peptidyl transferase
   (D) They block the formation of the initiation complex
   (E) They are bactericidal

2. All of the following statements about the clinical uses of the aminoglycosides are accurate EXCEPT
   (A) Due to their polar nature they are not absorbed following oral administration
   (B) Aminoglycosides are often used in combination with cephalosporins in the empiric treatment of life-threatening bacterial infections
   (C) Amikacin is more likely to be effective than streptomycin in the treatment of a hospital-acquired infection caused by *Serratia marcescens*
   (D) The primary indication for spectinomycin is the treatment of hospital-acquired gram-negative infections in the immunocompromised patient
   (E) Gentamicin is used with ampicillin for synergistic effects in the treatment of enterococcal endocarditis

3. All of the following statements about the toxic effects of aminoglycosides are accurate EXCEPT
   (A) When used in combination, cephalosporins potentiate the nephrotoxicity of aminoglycosides
   (B) Muscle paralysis due to high concentrations of aminoglycosides is usually reversible by infusion of calcium gluconate

    (C)   Loop diuretics increase the rate of renal elimination of aminoglycosides and decrease the likelihood of toxic effects

    (D)   Headache and vertigo in the upright position are early signs of aminoglycoside neurotoxicity

    (E)   Oral administration of neomycin may lead to intestinal malabsorption and superinfection

4. A 70-kg patient with creatinine clearance of greater than 90 mL/min has a gram-negative infection. Amikacin is administered intramuscularly at a dose of 5 mg/kg every 8 hours, and the patient begins to respond. After 2 days, creatinine clearance declines to 30 mL/min. Assuming that there is no information available about amikacin plasma levels, what would be a reasonable approach to management of the patient at this point?

    (A)   Decrease daily dose to a total of 100 mg

    (B)   Decrease the dosage to 120 mg every 8 hrs

    (C)   Maintain the patient on the present dosage and test auditory function

    (D)   Administer 5 mg/kg every 12 hrs

    (E)   Discontinue amikacin and switch to gentamicin

5. All of the following statements about polymyxins are accurate EXCEPT

    (A)   They are bactericidal for many gram-negative rods including *Pseudomonas* spp

    (B)   Polymyxin activity against gram-positive bacteria is minimal

    (C)   They are effective against intracellular pathogens since they effectively penetrate mammalian cell membranes

    (D)   Paresthesias and incoordination are potential toxic effects of polymyxins

    (E)   Polymyxin-induced injury to renal tubules results in hematuria and proteinuria

6. An adult patient (weight 70 kg) has bacteremia suspected to be due to a gram-negative rod. Tobramycin is to be administered, and the loading dose must be calculated based on a required plasma level of 3 mg/L. Assume the patient has normal renal function. Pharmacokinetic parameters of tobramycin in this patient are: Vd = 20L; $t_{1/2}$ = 3 hr; CL = 80 mL/min. What loading dose should be given?

    (A)   80 mg

    (B)   60 mg

    (C)   24 mg

    (D)   15 mg

    (E)   9 mg

7. Which of the following statements about bacterial resistance to aminoglycosides is MOST accurate?

    (A)   Resistance is due to the production of peptidyltransferases

    (B)   Bacteria resistant to aminoglycosides have characteristic alterations in the pathway of folic acid synthesis

    (C)   Emergence of resistance during the course of drug treatment is common

    (D)   Clinical resistance mainly occurs through plasmid-mediated formation of group transferase enzymes

    (E)   Staphylococci resistant to methicillin (MRSA) are usually sensitive to aminoglycosides

8. Bubonic plague sometimes reaches epidemic proportions in the developing countries of the world. The most helpful drug in such epidemics is

    (A)   Neomycin

    (B)   Spectinomycin

    (C)   Chloramphenicol

    (D)   Polymyxin B

    (E)   Streptomycin

DIRECTIONS: The following section consists of a list of four to twenty-six lettered options followed by several numbered items. For each numbered item, select the ONE option that is most closely associated with it. Each answer may be selected once, more than once, or not at all.

    (A)   Tobramycin

    (B)   Polymyxin B

    (C)   Neomycin

    (D)   Vancomycin

    (E)   Streptomycin

    (F)   Ticarcillin

    (G)   Spectinomycin

    (H)   Amikacin

9. The systemic use of this drug has been largely abandoned due to its toxicity. It is used topically and for its local effects in the gastrointestinal tract

10. This drug is used in the treatment of tularemia. When administered in combination with other agents in tuberculosis, this drug delays the emergence of resistant mycobacteria

11. This drug is active against some gentamicin-resistant gram-negative bacilli because its metabolic inactivation by bacterial enzymes is sterically hindered

12. This drug has a spectrum of activity and properties similar to those of gentamicin, except that the drug in question shows poor activity in combination with penicillin against enterococci.

13. Synergistic actions occur when this drug is used in combination with gentamicin in the treatment of infections due to *Pseudomonas aeruginosa*

14. This drug is commonly used as a component of antibacterial ointments or creams for topical application; its antibacterial action does not involve inhibition of protein synthesis

ANSWERS

1. Bacterial protein synthesis is inhibited by aminoglycosides through their binding to specific components of the 30S ribosomal subunit. The answer is **(C)**.

2. Spectinomycin's only clinical use is the treatment of gonorrhea, as an alternative drug in cases of resistance, or patient allergy. The answer is **(D)**.

3. Aminoglycosides are excreted via glomerular filtration, and their rate of elimination is not directly affected by ethacrynic acid or furosemide. However, the loop diuretics are potentially ototoxic and may worsen hearing loss when used with aminoglycosides. The answer is **(C)**.

4. Monitoring plasma drug levels is important when aminoglycosides are used. In this case, the patient seems to be improving, so a decrease of the amikacin dose in proportion to decreased creatinine clearance is most appropriate. Since creatinine clearance is only one-third of the starting value, a dose reduction should be made to one-third of that given initially. The answer is **(B)**.

5. Polymyxins are cationic basic polypeptides that do not readily penetrate mammalian cell membranes. These drugs have limited activity against intracellular pathogens. The answer is **(C)**.

6. The loading dose of any drug may be calculated by multiplying the desired plasma concentration (mg/L) by the volume of distribution (L). The answer is **(B)**.

7. Clinical resistance to aminoglycosides results from their metabolic inactivation. The emergence of resistance during drug treatment is rare. Aminoglycosides are not active against staphylococci resistant to methicillin. The answer is **(D)**.

8. The treatment of choice in bubonic plague is a combination of streptomycin with tetracycline (not listed), but streptomycin alone is often effective. The answer is **(E)**.

9. When used parenterally, neomycin causes renal damage and ototoxicity. It is used topically and for local actions, including gastrointestinal tract infections, sterilization prior to bowel surgery, and to reduce ammonia intoxication in hepatic coma. The answer is **(C)**.

10. Streptomycin is not commonly used to treat infections caused by gram-negative rods, since many organisms are resistant. The drug does have special clinical uses, including the treatment of plague, tularemia, and tuberculosis. The answer is **(E)**.

11. Due to its chemical structure, amikacin is less susceptible than gentamicin to the actions of group transferase enzymes produced by resistant gram-negative organisms. The answer is **(H)**.

12. Tobramycin is almost identical to gentamicin in its properties. However, it is much less active than either gentamicin or streptomycin when used in combination with a penicillin in the treatment of enterococcal endocarditis. The answer is **(A)**.

13. The antipseudomonal action of ticarcillin is enhanced when used in combination with gentamicin. This is a good example of antibacterial drug synergy at the clinical level. The answer is **(F)**.

14. Gentamicin (not listed), neomycin, and polymyxin B are all used as topical antibacterial agents. The polymyxins exert their antibacterial actions by the disruption of membrane lipid structure. The answer is **(B)**.

Antimycobacterial Drugs

46

OBJECTIVES

You should be able to:

- Describe the special problems of chemotherapy for mycobacterial infections.
- Describe the pharmacodynamic and pharmacokinetic properties of the first-line drugs used in tuberculosis (isoniazid, ethambutol, pyrazinamide, and rifampin).
- Identify the second-line drugs used in tuberculosis and describe their limitations.
- Identify the drugs used in leprosy and in atypical mycobacterial disease and describe their major toxic effects.

CONCEPTS

The chemotherapy of infections caused by *M tuberculosis, M leprae,* and *M avium-intracellulare* is complicated by numerous factors, including (1) limited information about the mechanisms of antimycobacterial drug actions; (2) the development of resistance; (3) the intracellular location of mycobacteria; and (4) the chronic nature of mycobacterial disease, which accentuates drug toxicities.

Chemotherapy of mycobacterial infections almost always involves the use of **drug combinations** to delay the emergence of resistance and to enhance antimycobacterial efficacy. The major drugs used in tuberculosis are isoniazid (INH), rifampin, ethambutol, pyrazinamide, and streptomycin. The main drug for leprosy is dapsone, and it is commonly given with either rifampin or clofazimine. Suppression of *M avium-intracellulare* in the immunocompromised patient also requires multidrug treatment. The subgroups of drugs used in these conditions are shown in Figure 46–1.

DRUGS FOR TUBERCULOSIS

A. Isoniazid:

1. **Mechanisms:** Isoniazid (INH) is a structural congener of pyridoxine. Its mechanism of action involves inhibition of enzymes required for the synthesis of mycolic acids and mycobacterial cell walls. Resistance can emerge rapidly if the drug is used alone. In some cases resistance may be associated with deletion of a gene (*kat*G) that codes for catalase and peroxidase enzymes in the mycobacterium.

2. **Pharmacokinetics:** INH is well absorbed orally and penetrates cells to act on intracellular mycobacteria. The liver metabolism of INH is by acetylation and is under genetic control. Patients may be fast (half-life 1 to 1.5 hours) or slow (half-life 3 hours) inactivators of the drug. The proportion of fast acetylators is higher among people of Asian origin (including Native Americans) than those of European or African origin.

3. **Clinical use:** INH is the single most important drug used in tuberculosis, and it is a component of most drug combination regimens. In the prophylaxis of skin test converters, and in close contacts of patients with active disease, INH is given as the sole drug.

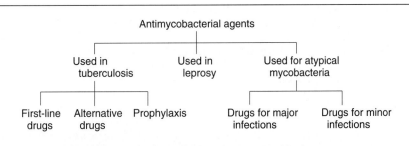

Figure 46–1. Subgroups of drugs discussed in this chapter.

4. **Toxicity and interactions:** Neurotoxic effects are common and include peripheral neuritis, restlessness, muscle twitching, and insomnia. These effects can be alleviated (without blocking the antibacterial effects) by administration of pyridoxine. INH is hepatotoxic and may cause abnormal liver function tests, jaundice, and hepatitis (rare in children). INH may inhibit the hepatic metabolism of drugs, eg, phenytoin. Hemolysis has occurred in patients with glucose-6-phosphate dehydrogenase deficiency.

B. Rifampin:

1. **Mechanisms:** Rifampin, a derivative of rifamycin, is bactericidal to *M tuberculosis*. The drug inhibits DNA-dependent RNA polymerase in *M tuberculosis* and many other microorganisms. Resistance (via changes in drug sensitivity of the polymerase) emerges rapidly if the drug is used alone.

2. **Pharmacokinetics:** When given orally, rifampin is well absorbed and is distributed to most body tissues, including the CNS. The drug undergoes enterohepatic cycling and is partially metabolized in the liver. Both free drug and metabolites (which are orange-colored) are eliminated mainly in the feces.

3. **Clinical uses:** In tuberculosis, rifampin is always used in combination with other drugs. When used with dapsone in leprosy, rifampin delays the emergence of resistance if given monthly. Rifampin is used as the sole drug in the treatment of the meningococcal carrier state.

4. **Toxicity and interactions:** Rifampin commonly causes light chain proteinuria and may impair antibody responses. Occasional side effects include skin rashes, thrombocytopenia, nephritis, and liver dysfunction. If given less than twice weekly, rifampin may cause a flu-like syndrome and anemia. Rifampin strongly induces liver drug-metabolizing enzymes and enhances the elimination rate of many drugs including contraceptive steroids, ketoconazole, methadone, and warfarin.

C. Ethambutol:

1. **Mechanisms:** Ethambutol acts on mycobacteria by unknown mechanisms, and resistance occurs rapidly if the drug is used alone.

2. **Pharmacokinetics:** The drug is well-absorbed orally and distributes to most tissues including the CNS. A large fraction of drug is eliminated unchanged in the urine. Dose reduction is necessary in renal failure.

3. **Clinical use:** The only use of ethambutol is in tuberculosis, and it is always given in combination with other drugs.

4. **Toxicity:** The most common adverse effects are dose-dependent visual disturbances, including decreased visual acuity, optic neuritis, and possible retinal damage (with prolonged use at high doses). Most of these effects regress on drug discontinuance. Other neurotoxic effects include headache, confusion, and peripheral neuritis.

D. Pyrazinamide:

1. **Mechanisms:** The mechanism of pyrazinamide's action is not known; however, its bacteriostatic action appears to require metabolic conversion via pyrazinamidases present in *M tuberculosis*. Resistant mycobacterial strains lack these enzymes, and resistance develops rapidly if the drug is used alone. There is minimal cross-resistance with other antimycobacterial drugs.

2. **Pharmacokinetics:** Pyrazinamide is well absorbed orally and penetrates most body tissues including the CNS. The drug is partly metabolized to pyrazinoic acid, and both parent molecule and metabolite are excreted in the urine. The plasma half-life of pyrazinamide is increased in hepatic or renal failure.

3. **Clinical use:** The combined use of pyrazinamide with other antitubercular drugs is an important factor in the success of "short-course" (6 month) treatment regimens.

4. **Toxicity:** Approximately 40% of patients develop nongouty polyarthralgia. Hyperuricemia occurs commonly, but is usually asymptomatic. Other adverse effects include myalgia, gastrointestinal irritation, maculopapular rash, hepatic dysfunction, porphyria, and photosensitivity reactions.

E. Streptomycin: This aminoglycoside is now used more frequently than hitherto, because of the growing prevalence of drug-resistant strains of *M tuberculosis*. Streptomycin is used principally in drug combinations for the treatment of life-threatening tuberculous disease, including meningitis, miliary dissemination, and severe organ tuberculosis. The pharmacodynamic and pharmacokinetic properties of streptomycin are similar to those of other aminoglycosides (see Chapter 45).

F. Alternative Drugs: The second-line antimycobacterial drugs are used in cases that are resistant to the first-line agents; they are considered second-line drugs because they are no more effective, and their toxicities are often more serious than those of the major drugs. **Ethionamide** is a congener of INH, but cross-resistance does not occur. The major disadvantage of ethionamide is that intense gastrointestinal irritation and adverse neurologic effects occur at doses needed for effective plasma levels. **Aminosalicylic acid (PAS)** is now rarely used because of its toxicity: gastrointestinal irritation, peptic ulceration, hypersensitivity reactions, and effects on kidney, liver, and thyroid function. Other drugs occasionally used include the antibiotics **capreomycin, cycloserine,** and **viomycin.**

DRUGS FOR LEPROSY

A. Sulfones: **Dapsone** (diaminodiphenylsulfone) remains the most active drug against *M leprae.* The mechanism of action of sulfones may involve inhibition of folic acid synthesis. Resistance may develop, especially if low doses are given. Dapsone can be given orally, penetrates tissues well, undergoes enterohepatic cycling, and is eliminated in the urine partly as acetylated metabolites. Common adverse effects include gastrointestinal irritation, fever, skin rashes, and methemoglobinemia. Hemolysis may occur, especially in patients with glucose-6-phosphate dehydrogenase deficiency. **Acedapsone** is a repository form that provides inhibitory plasma concentrations for several months. In addition to its use in leprosy, dapsone is an alternative drug for the treatment of *Pneumocystis carinii* pneumonia in AIDS patients.

B. Other Agents: Alternative drugs for leprosy include rifampin (see above), **clofazimine,** and **amithiozone.** Clofazimine is given in cases of dapsone resistance or intolerance. The drug causes gastrointestinal irritation and marked skin discoloration. Amithiozone is also an alternative to dapsone, but emergence of resistance, together with gastrointestinal and hepatotoxic effects, limit its use.

DRUGS FOR ATYPICAL MYCOBACTERIAL INFECTIONS

Infections due to atypical mycobacteria (eg, *M marinum, M avium-intracellulare, M ulcerans*), though sometimes asymptomatic, may be treated with the described antimycobacterial drugs (eg, ethambutol, rifampin) or with other antibiotics (eg, erythromycin, amikacin). Attempts to suppress *M avium-intracellulare* infections in AIDS patients have included treatment with antituberculosis drugs, the newer macrolides (azithromycin, clarithromycin), fluoroquinolones (eg, ofloxacin), clofazimine, and rifabutin, a congener of rifampin.

DRUG LIST

The following drugs are important members of the group discussed in this chapter. Prototypes should be learned in detail; other significant agents should be recognized as belonging to a specific subclass.

Subclass	Prototype	Other Significant Agents
Drugs for tuberculosis Pyridines	Isoniazid	Ethionamide, pyrazinamide
Rifamycins	Rifampin	
Diamines	Ethambutol	
Aminoglycosides	Streptomycin	
Others		Aminosalicylic acid, capreomycin, cycloserine, viomycin
Drugs for leprosy Sulfones	Dapsone	Acedapsone
Phenazines	Clofazimine	
Thiosemicarbazones	Amithiozone	

QUESTIONS

DIRECTIONS: Each of the numbered items or incomplete statements in this section is followed by answers or by completions of the statement. Select the ONE lettered answer or completion that is BEST in each case.

1. The primary reason for the use of drug combinations in the treatment of tuberculosis is to
   - **(A)** Prolong the plasma half-life of each drug
   - **(B)** Lower the incidence of adverse effects
   - **(C)** Enhance activity against metabolically inactive mycobacteria
   - **(D)** Delay emergence of resistance
   - **(E)** Prevent other bacterial infections

2. All of the following statements concerning isoniazid (INH) are accurate EXCEPT
   - **(A)** Some patients on INH have experienced flushing, palpitations, sweating, and dyspnea after ingestion of tyramine-containing foods
   - **(B)** Native Americans may require higher maintenance doses of INH than other persons in the USA
   - **(C)** Daily consumption of ethanol increases the risk of hepatotoxicity due to INH
   - **(D)** Peripheral neuritis may occur during treatment with INH
   - **(E)** Use of INH by a patient taking warfarin may result in decreased anticoagulant effect

3. All of the following statements concerning rifampin are accurate EXCEPT
   - **(A)** Rifampin may decrease the efficacy of oral contraceptives
   - **(B)** Most of the toxic effects of rifampin result from inhibition of human DNA-dependent RNA polymerase
   - **(C)** Mutant organisms resistant to rifampin occur at a frequency of 1 in 10^7 or greater
   - **(D)** Hepatitis occurs less frequently with rifampin than with INH
   - **(E)** Rifampin has low in vitro activity against *M avium-intracellulare*

4. All of the following statements concerning pyrazinamide are accurate EXCEPT
   - **(A)** It is effective orally and penetrates into cerebrospinal fluid
   - **(B)** It decreases the plasma half-life of warfarin
   - **(C)** Hepatic dysfunction occurs in 1–5% of patients treated with pyrazinamide
   - **(D)** Mycobacteria resistant to INH are usually sensitive to pyrazinamide
   - **(E)** Arthralgia and myalgia are common side effects of the drug

5. A 10-year-old boy has uncomplicated pulmonary tuberculosis. After initial hospitalization, he is now being treated at home with isoniazid, rifampin, and ethambutol. All of the following statements about this case are accurate EXCEPT
   - **(A)** Care-givers should not worry about orange-colored tears if he cries
   - **(B)** Periodic tests of liver function should be considered
   - **(C)** Pyridoxine should be administered in an amount equivalent to the dose of INH
   - **(D)** His mother (who takes care of him) should receive INH prophylaxis, but this is inadvisable for his younger siblings
   - **(E)** The boy may develop symptoms similar to those of influenza

6. All of the following statements concerning drugs used in leprosy are accurate EXCEPT
   - **(A)** The mechanism of action of dapsone probably involves inhibition of folic acid synthesis
   - **(B)** Single intramuscular injections of acedapsone maintain inhibitory levels of dapsone in tissues for up to 3 months
   - **(C)** Monthly doses of rifampin delay the emergence of resistance to dapsone
   - **(D)** Clofazimine should not be given to patients who are intolerant to dapsone or who fail to improve during treatment with dapsone
   - **(E)** Clofazimine may cause skin discoloration

DIRECTIONS: The following section consists of a list of four to twenty-six lettered options followed by several numbered items. For each numbered item, select the ONE option that is most closely associated with it. Each answer may be selected once, more than once, or not at all.
   - **(A)** Isoniazid
   - **(B)** Ethionamide
   - **(C)** Dapsone
   - **(D)** Rifabutin
   - **(E)** PAS

    (F) Pyrazinamide
    (G) Clofazimine
    (H) Rifampin
    (I) Ethambutol
    (J) Streptomycin

7. This drug eliminates a majority of meningococci from carriers, but highly resistant strains may be selected out during treatment

8. Patients taking this drug might be advised to test their vision by reading the small print in the newspaper from time to time

9. A chemical congener of isoniazid, this second-line antitubercular drug is poorly tolerated because it causes intense gastric irritation and neurologic symptoms

10. Hemolysis is a common side effect of this drug, especially in patents with G6PD deficiency. Methemoglobinemia also occurs quite commonly

11. Of the drugs listed, this agent is the most likely to cause loss of equilibrium and auditory damage

12. Patients in methadone maintenance programs may experience symptoms of yawning, piloerection, lacrimation, anxiety, and muscle jerking when they take this drug

ANSWERS

1. While it is sometimes possible to achieve synergistic effects against mycobacteria with drug combinations, the primary reason for their use is to delay the emergence of resistance. The answer is **(D)**.

2. Isoniazid inhibits hepatic cytochrome P450 and increases plasma levels of several drugs including benzodiazepines, phenytoin, and warfarin. Note that INH can also inhibit monoamine oxidase type A. The answer is **(E)**.

3. Rifampin inhibits RNA synthesis in bacteria and chlamydia, but human RNA polymerases are not sensitive to its actions. The answer is **(B)**.

4. Hepatic dysfunction may occur during treatment with pyrazinamide, but the drug is not an inducer of liver drug-metabolizing enzymes. It does not increase the rate of metabolism of other drugs (compare with rifampin). The answer is **(B)**.

5. Hepatic dysfunction due to INH is rare in persons under age 20. However, periodic tests of liver function may be advisable in younger patients who are also receiving rifampin, especially if higher doses of these drugs are used. Prophylaxis with INH is advisable for all household members and very close contacts of patients with active tuberculosis, *especially* children. A flu-like syndrome has occurred following intermittent high dose administration of rifampin. The answer is **(D)**.

6. Clofazimine is not related chemically to dapsone, and there is little cross-resistance. The drug is used in sulfone-resistant leprosy and for patients who are unable to tolerate dapsone. The answer is **(D)**.

7. Resistance emerges rapidly when rifampin is used as a single agent in the treatment of bacterial infections. When used to treat the meningococcal carrier state, up to 10% of treated carriers may harbor rifampin-resistant organisms. The answer is **(H)**.

8. Decreased visual acuity, optic neuritis, and possible retinal damage are characteristic adverse effects of ethambutol. Ocular toxicity is dose-dependent and is usually reversible when ethambutol is discontinued. Periodic testing of visual acuity is advisable during treatment. The answer is **(I)**.

9. Ethionamide and pyrazinamide are both related chemically to INH. Ethionamide has a metallic taste and causes severe nausea, vomiting, and diarrhea, unless taken with food to minimize gastric irritation. The drug is a second-line agent in the treatment of tuberculosis. The answer is **(B)**.

10. Hematologic abnormalities are common with dapsone and may include methemoglobinemia, hemolysis, leukopenia, and thrombocytopenia. Note also that isoniazid may precipitate acute hemolysis in patients with glucose-6-phosphate dehydrogenase deficiency. The answer is **(C)**.

11. Ototoxicity is characteristic of the aminoglycoside antibiotics. While disturbances of equilibrium may occur with overdosage of PAS, the drug does not cause hearing loss. Note that viomycin (not listed) is even more toxic to the 8th nerve than streptomycin. The answer is **(J)**.

12. The chronic use of rifampin causes the induction of hepatic microsomal drug-metabolizing enzymes. A number of drug interactions have been attributed to this effect of rifampin. The symptoms described are characteristic of the opioid withdrawal syndrome, and result from an increase in the rate of methadone metabolism. The answer is **(H)**.

47

Sulfonamides & Trimethoprim

OBJECTIVES

You should be able to:

- Describe the mechanisms of action of sulfonamides and trimethoprim on bacterial folic acid synthesis.
- Describe the mechanisms of resistance to sulfonamides and trimethoprim.
- List the major clinical uses of sulfonamides and trimethoprim, singly and in combination.
- Indicate the major pharmacokinetic features of sulfonamides and trimethoprim.
- Describe the toxic effects of sulfonamides and trimethoprim.

Learn the definitions that follow.

Table 47–1. Definitions.

Term	Definition
Antimetabolite	A drug that through chemical similarity is able to interfere with the role of an endogenous compound in cellular metabolism. The term includes antibacterial agents that inhibit bacterial folic acid metabolism
Sequential blockade	The combined action of two drugs that act at sequential steps in a pathway of bacterial metabolism

CONCEPTS

A. Classification & Pharmacokinetics:

1. Sulfonamides: The sulfonamides are weakly acidic compounds that have a common chemical nucleus resembling p-aminobenzoic acid **(PABA).** Members of this group differ mainly in their pharmacokinetic properties and clinical uses (see Figure 47–1). Pharmacokinetic features include modest tissue penetration, hepatic metabolism, and excretion of both intact drug and acetylated metabolites in the urine. Solubility may be decreased in acidic urine, resulting in precipitation of the drug or its metabolites. Because of the solubility limitation, a combination of three separate sulfonamides **(triple sulfas)** has been used to reduce the likelihood that any one drug will precipitate. The sulfonamides may be classified as

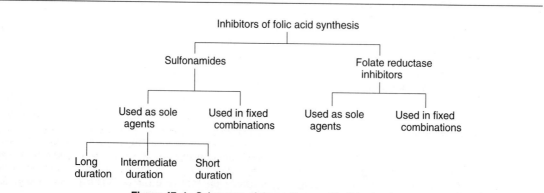

Figure 47–1. Subgroups of drugs discussed in this chapter.

short-acting (eg, sulfisoxazole), intermediate-acting (eg, sulfamethoxazole), and long-acting (eg, sulfadoxine). Sulfonamides bind to plasma proteins at sites shared by bilirubin and by other drugs.

2. **Trimethoprim:** This drug is structurally similar to folic acid. It is a weak base and is trapped in acidic environments, reaching high concentrations in prostatic and vaginal fluids. (The trapping of a congener, pyrimethamine, is illustrated in Figure 1–1). A large fraction of trimethoprim is excreted unchanged in the urine. The half-life of this drug is similar to that of sulfamethoxazole (10–12 hr).

B. Mechanisms of Action:
  1. **Sulfonamides:** The sulfa drugs are bacteriostatic inhibitors of folic acid synthesis. As antimetabolites of PABA, they are competitive inhibitors of dihydropteroate synthase (Figure 47–2). They can also act as substrates for this enzyme, resulting in the synthesis of nonfunctional forms of folic acid. The selective toxicity of sulfonamides results from the inability of mammalian cells to synthesize folic acid; they must use preformed folic acid that is present in the diet.
  2. **Trimethoprim:** Trimethoprim is a selective inhibitor of bacterial dihydrofolate reductase that prevents the formation of the active tetrahydro form of folic acid (Figure 47–2). Bacterial dihydrofolate reductase is 4–5 orders of magnitude more sensitive than the mammalian enzyme to inhibition by trimethoprim.
  3. **Trimethoprim and sulfamethoxazole:** When the two drugs are used in combination, antimicrobial synergy results from the **sequential blockade** of folate synthesis (Figure 47–2). The drug combination is bactericidal against susceptible organisms.

C. Resistance: Bacterial resistance to sulfonamides is common and may be plasmid-mediated. It may result from decreased intracellular accumulation of the drug, increased production of PABA by bacteria, or a change in the sensitivity of dihydropteroate synthase to the sulfonamides. Clinical resistance to trimethoprim results from the production of dihydrofolate reductase that has a reduced affinity for the drug.

D. Clinical Use:
  1. **Sulfonamides:** The sulfonamides are active against a wide range of gram-positive and gram-negative organisms, chlamydia, and *Nocardia* spp. Specific members of the sulfonamide group are used by the following routes for the conditions indicated:
     a. **Simple urinary tract infections:** Oral (eg, triple sulfas, sulfisoxazole).
     b. **Ocular infections:** Topical (eg, sulfacetamide).
     c. **Burn infections:** Topical (eg, mafenide, silver sulfadiazine).
     d. **Ulcerative colitis:** Oral (eg, sulfasalazine).
  2. **Trimethoprim and sulfamethoxazole (TMP-SMZ):** This important combination medication is currently accepted treatment for complicated urinary tract infections, and for respi-

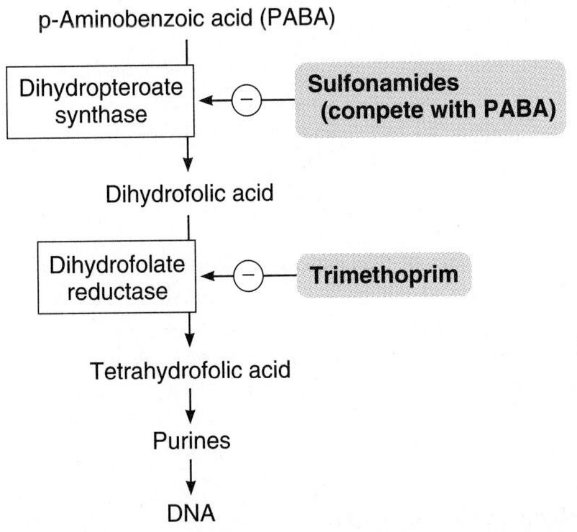

Figure 47–2. Inhibitory effects of sulfonamides and trimethoprim on folic acid synthesis. Inhibition of two successive steps in the formation of tetrahydrofolic acid constitutes sequential blockade and results in antibacterial synergy. (Modified and reproduced, with permission, from Katzung BG [editor]: *Basic & Clinical Pharmacology,* 6th ed. Appleton & Lange, 1995.)

ratory, ear, and sinus infections due to *H influenzae* and *Moraxella catarrhalis.* In the immunocompromised patient, TMP-SMZ is used for infections due to *Aeromonas hydrophila* and in *Pneumocystis carinii* pneumonia. TMP-SMZ is also active against *Shigella, Salmonella,* and *Serratia* spp. Trimethoprim has been used as the sole drug for some community-acquired urinary tract infections.

E. Toxicity of Sulfonamides:
1. **Hypersensitivity:** Allergic reactions, including skin rashes and fever, occur commonly. Cross-allergenicity between the individual drugs, including other sulfonamide families (diuretics, oral hypoglycemics, etc.), should be assumed. Though rare, exfoliative dermatitis, polyarteritis nodosa, and Stevens-Johnson syndrome have also occurred.
2. **Gastrointestinal:** Nausea, vomiting, and diarrhea occur commonly. Mild hepatic dysfunction can occur, but hepatitis is uncommon.
3. **Hematotoxicity:** Though rare, sulfonamides can cause granulocytopenia, thrombocytopenia, and aplastic anemia. Acute hemolysis may occur in persons with glucose-6-phosphate dehydrogenase deficiency.
4. **Nephrotoxicity:** Sulfonamides may precipitate in the urine at acidic pH, causing crystalluria and hematuria.
5. **Drug interactions:** Competition with warfarin and methotrexate for plasma protein binding transiently increases the plasma levels of these drugs. Sulfonamides can displace bilirubin from plasma proteins, with the risk of kernicterus in the neonate.

F. Toxicity of Trimethoprim: Trimethoprim may cause the predictable adverse effects of an antifolate drug including megaloblastic anemia, leukopenia, and granulocytopenia. These effects are usually ameliorated by supplementary folinic acid. The combination of trimethoprim-sulfamethoxazole may cause any of the adverse effects associated with the sulfonamides. AIDS patients given TMP-SMZ have a high incidence of adverse effects, including fever, rashes, leukopenia, and diarrhea.

DRUG LIST

The following drugs are important members of the group discussed in this chapter. Prototypes should be learned in detail; features of the major variants should be known well enough to distinguish the variants from the prototypes and from each other; the other significant agents should be recognized as belonging to a specific subclass.

Subclass	Prototype	Major Variants	Other Significant Agents

Sulfonamides
  Oral agents
	Sulfisoxazole	Triple sulfas,
		  sulfamethoxazole
			Sulfadiazine

Local agents, agents
  for special applications
		Sulfacetamide,
		  sulfasalazine, mafenide,
		  sulfadiazine	

Combination	Trimethoprim- sulfamethoxazole		Pyrimethamine-sulfadoxine
Folate reductase inhibitors	Trimethoprim		Pyrimethamine

QUESTIONS

DIRECTIONS: Each of the numbered items or incomplete statements in this section is followed by answers or by completions of the statement. Select the ONE lettered answer or completion that is BEST in each case.

1. All of the following statements about sulfonamides are accurate EXCEPT
   (A) They inhibit bacterial dihydrofolate reductase
   (B) Dysfunction of the basal ganglia may occur in the newborn if sulfonamides are administered late in pregnancy
   (C) Cross-allergenicity may occur with thiazides

      (D)   Crystalluria is most likely to occur at low urinary pH

      (E)   They are antimetabolites of PABA

2. All of the following statements about the clinical use of sulfonamides are accurate EXCEPT

      (A)   Resistant bacterial strains may have a decreased intracellular accumulation of sulfonamides

      (B)   Sulfonamides have activity against *C trachomatis* and can be used topically for the treatment of chlamydial infections of the eye

      (C)   The sulfonamides are effective in Rocky Mountain Spotted Fever in patients allergic to tetracyclines

      (D)   The use of a sulfonamide as the sole antibacterial agent is unlikely to be effective in the treatment of chronic prostatitis in an elderly patient

      (E)   Some strains of bacteria become resistant by an increased production of PABA

3. All of the following adverse effects may occur with sulfonamide therapy EXCEPT

      (A)   Neurologic effects including headache, dizziness, and lethargy

      (B)   Hematuria

      (C)   Fanconi aminoaciduria syndrome

      (D)   Kernicterus in the newborn

      (E)   Urticaria

4. All of the following statements about the combination of trimethoprim plus sulfamethoxazole are accurate EXCEPT

      (A)   This combination is effective in the treatment of pneumonia due to *Pneumocystis carinii*

      (B)   The drugs produce a sequential blockade of folic acid synthesis

      (C)   Fever and pancytopenia occur frequently when these drugs are used in AIDS patients

      (D)   The combination is appropriate for the treatment of streptococcal pharyngitis

      (E)   The combination is effective in the management of acute exacerbations of chronic bronchitis

Items 5–6:   A 27-year-old African-American man with a history of recurrent, mild urinary tract infections presents with prostatitis. He also has type II diabetes, which he manages by diet and weight control, and with an oral hypoglycemic drug. Trimethoprim-sulfamethoxazole is prescribed.

5. All of the following statements about this case are accurate EXCEPT

      (A)   TMP-SMZ is often effective in bacterial prostatitis

      (B)   The dose of the oral hypoglycemic drug should be increased because he has an infection

      (C)   He should be informed about the possibility of an acute hemolytic reaction due to the drug

      (D)   It is probably advisable that he take supplementary folinic acid

      (E)   He should maintain high fluid intake

6. In this case, the physician should also be concerned if the patient is taking any of the following medications EXCEPT

      (A)   Methotrexate

      (B)   Phenytoin

      (C)   Warfarin

      (D)   Diazepam

      (E)   Thiazides

7. In addition to its use in *Pneumocystis* pneumonia, the combination of trimethoprim and sulfamethoxazole is also effective against which ONE of the following opportunistic infections in the AIDS patient?

      (A)   Disseminated herpes simplex

      (B)   Cryptococcal meningitis

      (C)   Toxoplasmosis

      (D)   Oral candidiasis

      (E)   Tuberculosis

DIRECTIONS: The following section consists of a list of four to twenty-six lettered options followed by several numbered items. For each numbered item, select the ONE option that is most closely associated with it. Each answer may be selected once, more than once, or not at all.

      (A)   Trimethoprim

      (B)   Sulfinpyrazone

      (C)   Sulfamethoxazole

      (D)   Methenamine

      (E)   Sulfasalazine

      (F) Sulfadiazine
      (G) Sulindac
      (H) Mafenide
      (I) Sulfisoxazole
      (J) Trimethaphan

8. Used orally in ulcerative colitis, this agent has both antibacterial and anti-inflammatory actions

9. This drug is rarely used for treatment of urinary tract infections, but it is the preferred agent for nocardiosis

10. This sulfonamide is only available for topical use; when applied to burns, it is effective in controlling colonization of bacteria including *Pseudomonas* spp

11. Supplementary folinic acid may prevent hematotoxicity in folate-deficient persons who use this drug; it is a weak base and achieves tissue levels similar to those in plasma

12. This drug is frequently active against amoxicillin-resistant strains of *H influenzae*; in combination with erythromycin, this drug is used to treat otitis media caused by such strains

ANSWERS

1. Know the specific enzymes in bacterial folic acid synthesis that are inhibited by sulfonamides and trimethoprim: sulfonamides inhibit dihydropteroate synthase; dihydrofolate reductase is inhibited by trimethoprim. The answer is **(A)**.

2. Sulfonamides have minimal therapeutic actions in rickettsial infections. Chloramphenicol may be used for Rocky Mountain Spotted fever in patients with established allergy or other contraindication to tetracyclines. The answer is **(C)**.

3. Renal dysfunction including crystalluria, hematuria, nephrosis, and allergic nephritis occurs with sulfonamides. However, the Fanconi syndrome, characterized by low back pain, aminoaciduria, polydipsia, and polyuria, is associated with the use of out-dated tetracyclines. The answer is **(C)**.

4. The combination of trimethoprim and sulfamethoxazole is often effective in respiratory infections due to susceptible *S pneumoniae* and *H influenzae*. However, in streptococcal pharyngitis the organisms are not eradicated. The answer is **(D)**.

5. Sulfonamides can displace sulfonylurea hypoglycemics from binding sites on plasma proteins. This elevates the free concentration of the sulfonylurea in the blood, which leads to an increase in hypoglycemic action. Thus the dose of the drug should *not* be increased. The answer is **(B)**.

6. Sulfonamides can also displace anticoagulants, phenytoin, and methotrexate from plasma protein binding sites, increasing their pharmacologic (and toxic) actions. Hyponatremia may occur following use of trimethoprim with diuretics. The answer is **(D)**.

7. Trimethoprim-sulfamethoxazole is not effective in the treatment of infections due to viruses, fungi, or mycobacterial species. However, the drug combination is active against specific protozoans including *Toxoplasma* spp. The answer is **(C)**.

8. Sulfasalazine is converted by intestinal microflora to yield sulfapyridine, which is antibacterial, and 5-aminosalicylate, which has anti-inflammatory activity. The answer is **(E)**.

9. Sulfadiazine is not recommended for the treatment of urinary tract infections because high doses are required, and alkalinization of the urine is necessary. It is the preferred drug in nocardiosis. In combination with pyrimethamine (an effective dihydrofolate reductase inhibitor in protozoa), sulfadiazine is also effective in toxoplasmosis. The answer is **(F)**.

10. Mafenide (sulfamylon) is the only sulfonamide listed that is used *solely* as a topical agent. Mafenide and silver sulfadiazine are used prophylactically as topical agents in burns to prevent bacterial colonization. Topical application of mafenide is painful and may lead to fungal superinfections. The answer is **(H)**.

11. Trimethoprim is a weak base with high lipid-solubility at blood pH. It penetrates membrane barriers more effectively than sulfonamides. Because prostatic and vaginal fluid pH is usually more acid than blood pH, levels of the drug in these organs are similar to—and often higher than—those in plasma. (The opposite is true of sulfonamides, which are weak acids.) Leukopenia and thrombocytopenia may occur in folate deficiency when the drug is used alone or in combination with sulfamethoxazole. The answer is **(A)**.

12. Sulfisoxazole is very soluble in the urine and is commonly used for the treatment of acute, uncomplicated urinary tract infections. The drug is also active against some common causative agents of otitis media, including *H influenzae* and pneumococci. For the treatment of otitis media, sulfisoxazole is usually given in a fixed-ratio combination with erythromycin. The answer is **(I)**.

Antifungal Agents

48

OBJECTIVES

You should be able to:

- Describe the mechanisms of action of the major drugs used for fungal infections.
- Describe the clinical uses and pharmacokinetics of amphotericin B, flucytosine, fluconazole, griseofulvin, and ketoconazole.
- Indicate the major toxic effects of the antifungal drugs listed above.
- Identify the main topical antifungal agents.

CONCEPTS

DRUGS FOR SYSTEMIC FUNGAL INFECTIONS

Several different drug groups are available for the treatment of fungal infections (Figure 48–1). These drugs act by a variety of mechanisms as described below.

A. Amphotericin B:
1. **Classification and pharmacokinetics:** Amphotericin B is a polyene antibiotic related to nystatin. Amphotericin is poorly absorbed from the gastrointestinal tract, is usually administered intravenously, and is widely distributed to body tissues, except the CNS. The drug undergoes slow renal elimination, largely in unchanged form. In renal dysfunction, the dose must be reduced.
2. **Mechanism of action:** The fungicidal action of amphotericin B is due to changes it produces in the permeability and transport properties of fungal membranes. Polyenes bind to **ergosterol,** a sterol specific to fungal cell membranes, and cause the formation of artificial pores (Figure 48–2). Resistance can occur via a decreased level of, or structural change in, membrane ergosterol.
3. **Clinical uses:** Amphotericin B is the most important of the drugs available for the treatment of systemic mycoses. It is active against *Aspergillus, Blastomyces, Coccidioides, Cryptococcus, Histoplasma,* and *Mucor* spp and *Candida albicans.* In systemic infections, the drug is usually given by slow intravenous infusion. In fungal meningitis, intrathecal administration is required.
4. **Toxicity:** Adverse effects are extensive and commonly include fever, chills, vomiting, and headache. Electrolyte imbalance (especially hypokalemia), a shock-like fall in blood pressure, and neurologic symptoms may also occur. Amphotericin B decreases glomerular filtration rate and changes renal tubular function. The nephrotoxic effects of the drug are dose-limiting. Dose reduction (with lowered toxicity) may be possible in some fungal infections if rifampin or a tetracycline is used concomitantly. A liposomal preparation of amphotericin B may have reduced toxic effects.

B. Flucytosine (5-fluorocytosine, 5-FC):
1. **Classification and pharmacokinetics:** 5-FC is a pyrimidine antimetabolite related to the anticancer drug 5-fluorouracil (5-FU). 5-FC is effective orally and is distributed to most body tissues, including the CNS. The drug is eliminated intact in the urine, and the dose must be reduced in patients with renal impairment.
2. **Mechanism of action:** The drug is accumulated in fungal cells by the action of a membrane permease and converted by cytosine deaminase to 5-FU, an inhibitor of thymidylate synthase (Figure 48–2). Selective toxicity occurs because mammalian cells have low levels of permease and deaminase. Resistance can occur rapidly and involves decreased activity

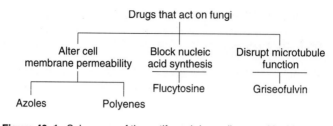

Figure 48–1. Subgroups of the antifungal drugs discussed in this chapter.

of the fungal permeases or deaminases. When 5-FC is given with amphotericin B, emergence of resistance is decreased and synergistic antifungal effects may occur.

3. **Clinical uses:** The antifungal spectrum of 5-FC is narrow; its clinical use is limited to the treatment, in combination with amphotericin B, of infections due to *Cryptococcus* spp and *C albicans*.

4. **Toxicity:** Prolonged high plasma levels of flucytosine cause reversible bone marrow depression, alopecia, and liver dysfunction. The hematotoxic effects can be reduced by administration of uracil.

C. Azole Antifungal Agents:

1. **Classification and pharmacokinetics:** The azoles used for systemic mycoses include **ketoconazole, fluconazole,** and **itraconazole.** These drugs have good oral bioavailability (normal gastric acidity is required) and are distributed to most body tissues. With the exception of fluconazole, drug levels achieved in the CNS are low. Liver metabolism is responsible for the elimination of ketoconazole and itraconazole.

Fluconazole is a new azole that is more reliably absorbed via the oral route than ketoconazole. The drug is distributed widely and readily enters the CNS. Fluconazole is eliminated by the kidneys, largely in unchanged form.

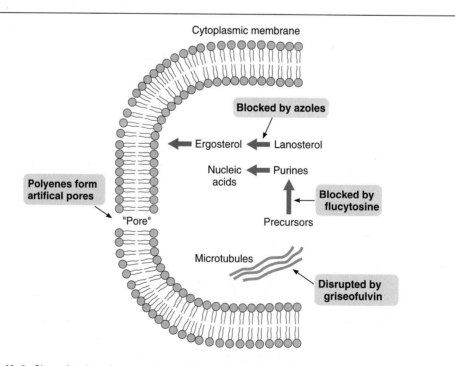

Figure 48–2. Sites of action of some antifungal drugs. The cell cytoplasmic membrane shown is that of a typical fungus. Because ergosterol is not a component of mammalian membranes, significant selective toxicity is achieved with the azole drugs.

2. **Mechanism of action:** The azoles interfere with fungal cell membrane permeability by inhibiting the synthesis of ergosterol. These drugs act at the step of 14α-demethylation of lanosterol, which is catalyzed by a cytochrome P450 isozyme. Development of resistance is rare.

3. **Clinical uses:**

   a. **Ketoconazole:** This drug is active in systemic infections caused by certain *Blastomyces, Coccidioides,* and *Histoplasma* spp and *C albicans.* In chronic mucocutaneous candidiasis, ketoconazole is usually the drug of choice. Oral ketoconazole is also effective against dermatophytes.

   b. **Fluconazole:** Fluconazole has a wide spectrum of antifungal activity, but in systemic mycoses it is usually an alternative agent to amphotericin B. Fluconazole is the drug of choice in esophageal and oropharyngeal candidiasis and is also used to suppress cryptococcal meningitis in immunodeficient patients.

   c. **Itraconazole:** The most common use of itraconazole is as an alternative agent in the treatment of infections caused by *Aspergillus, Coccidioides, Cryptococcus,* and *Histoplasma* spp. However, it is the drug of choice in subcutaneous chromoblastomycosis.

   d. **Miconazole and clotrimazole:** Miconazole and clotrimazole, more commonly used topically for fungal infections of the skin and mucous membranes, have also been used intravenously for systemic mycoses. While effective in some infections, they appear to be more toxic than ketoconazole or fluconazole when used systemically.

4. **Toxicity:** Adverse effects of the azoles include vomiting, diarrhea, rash, and sometimes hepatotoxicity (especially in patients with preexisting liver dysfunction). Ketoconazole (and probably most azoles) inhibits hepatic cytochrome P450 isozymes and may increase the plasma levels of other drugs including anticoagulants, oral hypoglycemics, and phenytoin. Inhibition of P450 also decreases the synthesis of adrenal steroids and androgens, and appears to be responsible for the cardiotoxicity of astemizole and terfenadine when these antihistaminic drugs are given concomitantly with ketoconazole (see Chapter 16).

A SYSTEMIC DRUG FOR SUPERFICIAL FUNGAL INFECTIONS: GRISEOFULVIN

A. **Pharmacokinetics:** Oral absorption of griseofulvin depends on the physical state of the drug (ultramicrosize formulations, which have finer crystals or particles, are more effectively absorbed), and is aided by high-fat foods. The drug is distributed to the stratum corneum where it binds to keratin. Biliary excretion is responsible for its elimination.

B. **Mechanism of Action:** Griseofulvin interferes with microtubule function (Figure 48–2) and may also inhibit the synthesis and polymerization of nucleic acids. Sensitive fungi take up the drug by an energy-dependent mechanism, and resistance can occur via decrease in this transport.

C. **Clinical Uses:** The antifungal activity of griseofulvin is restricted to dermatophytes including *Epidermophyton, Microsporum,* and *Trichophyton* spp. The drug is indicated for severe dermatophytoses of the skin, hair, and nails.

D. **Toxicity:** Adverse effects include headaches, mental confusion, gastrointestinal irritation, photosensitivity, and changes in liver function. A drug interaction may enhance coumarin metabolism, resulting in decreased anticoagulant effect. Griseofulvin is teratogenic and carcinogenic in animals.

TOPICAL DRUGS FOR SUPERFICIAL INFECTIONS

A number of antifungal drugs are used topically for superficial infections caused by *C albicans* and dermatophytes. **Nystatin** is a polyene antibiotic (related to amphotericin) that disrupts fungal membranes by binding to ergosterol. Nystatin is commonly used topically to suppress local *Candida* infections and has been used orally to eradicate gastrointestinal fungi in patients with impaired defense mechanisms. Other topical antifungal agents include the azole compounds **miconazole** and **clotrimazole** and the nonazoles **haloprogin, tolnaftate,** and **undecylenic acid.**

DRUG LIST

The following drugs are important members of the group discussed in this chapter. Prototypes should be learned in detail; the other significant agents should be recognized as belonging to a specific subclass.

Subclass	Prototype	Other Significant Agents
Drugs for systemic mycoses	Amphotericin B	Flucytosine, fluconazole, itraconazole, ketoconazole
Drugs for superficial infections Oral	Griseofulvin	Ketoconazole
Topical	Nystatin	Miconazole, clotrimazole, tolnaftate

QUESTIONS

DIRECTIONS: Each of the numbered items or incomplete statements in this section is followed by answers or by completions of the statement. Select the ONE lettered answer or completion that is BEST in each case.

1. Each of the following statements about the mechanisms of action of antifungal drugs and resistance are accurate EXCEPT
   (A) Flucytosine is deaminated and converted to a metabolite that inhibits fungal thymidylate synthase
   (B) Polyene antifungals inhibit the synthesis of ergosterol
   (C) Fungal resistance to amphotericin B is rare
   (D) Ketoconazole inhibits a fungal cytochrome P450 isozyme
   (E) Dermatophytes resistant to griseofulvin do not accumulate the drug
2. Each of the following statements about ketoconazole is accurate EXCEPT
   (A) It is effective in disseminated blastomycosis
   (B) It can be used orally in dermatophytosis
   (C) Its oral absorption may be impaired by antacids
   (D) It inhibits the synthesis of cortisol
   (E) It is effective in the treatment of fungal meningitis
3. Each of the following statements about the adverse effects of individual antifungal agents is accurate EXCEPT
   (A) Severe hypotension occurs with rapid intravenous administration of amphotericin B
   (B) Headache, lethargy, and mental confusion are adverse effects of griseofulvin
   (C) Flucytosine inhibits androgen synthesis and may cause gynecomastia
   (D) Ketoconazole is not recommended during pregnancy because it has teratogenic potential
   (E) A major problem with using nystatin for oral candidiasis is that it has an extremely unpleasant taste
4. Each of the following statements about griseofulvin is accurate EXCEPT
   (A) It disrupts microtubule function in some fungi that cause superficial mycoses
   (B) Its oral absorption may be increased by consumption of fatty foods
   (C) It may reduce the efficacy of some oral contraceptives
   (D) It is effective topically against many dermatophytes
   (E) In animal studies the drug is teratogenic and carcinogenic
5. A New York resident is transferred by his employer to Stockton, California, for 6 months. On his return he complains of periodic mild respiratory problems, which are thought by his physician to be due to a fungal infection of the lungs, contracted during his stay in the San Joaquin Valley. This patient should be treated immediately with
   (A) Amphotericin B
   (B) Griseofulvin
   (C) Ketoconazole
   (D) Itraconazole
   (E) None of the above drugs
6. Each of the following drugs is likely to be effective in the treatment of infections due to *C albicans* EXCEPT
   (A) Nystatin
   (B) Griseofulvin
   (C) Clotrimazole

    (D) Ketoconazole
    (E) Amphotericin B

DIRECTIONS: The following section consists of a list of four to twenty-six lettered options followed by several numbered items. For each numbered item, select the ONE option that is most closely associated with it. Each answer may be selected once, more than once, or not at all.

    (A) Flucytosine
    (B) Nystatin
    (C) Amphotericin B
    (D) Ketoconazole
    (E) Itraconazole
    (F) Griseofulvin
    (G) Fluconazole
    (H) Clotrimazole

  7. With chronic use, this drug causes hypochromic normocytic anemia, as well as renal dysfunction leading to the urinary loss of K^+ and Mg^{2+}. When used to treat fungal meningitis, the drug must be administered via intrathecal infusion

  8. After oral administration of this antimetabolite, the cerebrospinal fluid levels achieved are almost as high as plasma levels. Resistance may emerge during the treatment of systemic mycoses if the drug is used as the sole antifungal agent

  9. The oral absorption of this drug is impaired by antacids and by histamine H_2 receptor-blocking agents. Cardiac arrhythmias have occurred during concomitant administration of terfenadine

10. This drug is used as an oral agent in esophageal candidiasis; more than 90% of a dose is eliminated in the urine as unchanged drug

11. The symptoms of the "shake and bake" syndrome caused by this drug may be diminished by aspirin

ANSWERS

  1. The *synthesis* of ergosterol is decreased by azole antifungal drugs through their inhibition of cytochrome P450-mediated demethylation of lanosterol. Polyene antifungals *bind* to ergosterol to form artificial pores in the cell membrane. The answer is **(B).**

  2. The level of ketoconazole achievable in the cerebrospinal fluid in fungal meningitis is approximately 1% of the plasma concentration. Therefore, the drug has limited effectiveness in such infections. The answer is **(E).**

  3. Adverse effects of prolonged treatment with flucytosine include reversible bone marrow depression, alopecia, and gastrointestinal distress. While hormonal changes may occur, gynecomastia has not been reported with flucytosine, although it is a known adverse effect of treatment with ketoconazole. The answer is **(C).**

  4. Topical application of griseofulvin has minimal antifungal effects; the drug must be given orally. The answer is **(D).**

  5. A travel history can be important in the diagnosis of fungal disease. If this patient has a fungal infection of the lungs, it is likely to be due to *C immitis,* which is endemic in dry regions of the western United States. Pulmonary symptoms of coccidioidomycosis are usually self-limited, and drug therapy is not commonly required. However, in progressive or disseminated forms of the disease, amphotericin B is the recommended therapy. Additional diagnostic information is needed. The answer is **(E).**

  6. Griseofulvin has no activity against *Candida* species and is not effective in the treatment of superficial infections caused by such organisms. The answer is **(B).**

  7. The characteristics described should permit identification of amphotericin B. The answer is **(C).**

  8. Flucytosine is converted to the antimetabolite 5-fluorouracil, which causes inhibition of thymidylate synthase. Flucytosine is usually used in combination with amphotericin B. The answer is **(A).**

  9. An acidic environment is required for the dissolution of ketoconazole. Cardiotoxicity has occurred when ketoconazole was combined with terfenadine or with astemizole, possibly due to the ability of ketoconazole to inhibit hepatic drug-metabolizing enzymes. The answer is **(D).**

10. The pharmacokinetic properties of fluconazole are different from those of other azoles used in systemic fungal infections. For example, effective cerebrospinal fluid levels are achievable after its oral administration, and it is not eliminated by hepatic metabolism. The answer is (G).

11. Chills, fever, headache, and gastrointestinal disturbances occur commonly during the intravenous administration of amphotericin B. Most of these adverse effects may be decreased by a temporary reduction in dose, or by the administration of nonsteroidal anti-inflammatory agents or antihistaminic drugs. The answer is (C).

49 Antiviral Chemotherapy & Prophylaxis

OBJECTIVES

You should be able to:

- Identify the main steps in viral replication.
- Describe the mechanisms of action of the major antiviral drugs.
- Describe the clinical uses of the major antiviral drugs.
- List the toxic effects of the systemic antiviral drugs.
- Describe the actions of methisazone and rifampin.
- List the newer drugs used in immunosuppressed patients.

CONCEPTS

A. **Classification of Antiviral Drugs:** The antiviral drugs are conveniently classified on the basis of their target in the viral replication process (Figure 49–1).

1. **Adsorption and penetration of the virus:** The first steps in viral replication involve adsorption to the host cell membrane, penetration into the cell via endocytosis, and viral particle uncoating. Drugs that act at this stage include the **immune gamma globulins,** which contain specific antibodies to viral antigens and can block cell penetration (Figure 49–1). The process of fusion of the viral particle with the endosomal membrane requires low pH. **Amantadine** and **rimantadine** inhibit this step, partly because they are basic and raise the endosomal pH. At low concentrations, amantadine also binds to a specific protein in the surface coat of the influenza virus to prevent fusion. The investigational drug **disoxaril** binds to and stabilizes the surface coat of some viruses and prevents uncoating, so that the viral genome is not released into the infected cell.

2. **Early protein synthesis:** Certain biguanide drugs inhibit viral RNA polymerases and thus interfere with the synthesis of nonstructural proteins and enzymes. Resistance to these compounds occurs rapidly, however, and no clinically useful drugs act at this stage in viral replication (Figure 49–1).

3. **Nucleic acid synthesis:** Many useful antiviral drugs act as antimetabolites because they are structurally similar to purine or pyrimidine bases. As shown in Figure 49–2, drugs such as **zidovudine (AZT)** undergo phosphorylation by host cell kinases to form nucleotide analogues that may inhibit viral DNA polymerases or act as substrates for viral enzymes (or both), resulting in their incorporation into viral nucleic acids. Selective toxicity may result, because viral DNA polymerases are more sensitive to inhibition by these antimetabolites than are mammalian polymerases.

   Acyclovir is more selectively toxic than the drugs that require phosphorylation only by host cell enzymes. This increased selectivity is partly a result of acyclovir's initial phosphorylation by a *viral* thymidine kinase that is absent in uninfected cells (Figure 49–2, top).

   The **interferons** exert multiple actions that affect viral RNA and DNA synthesis. Interferons induce the formation of enzymes, including a protein kinase that phosphorylates a

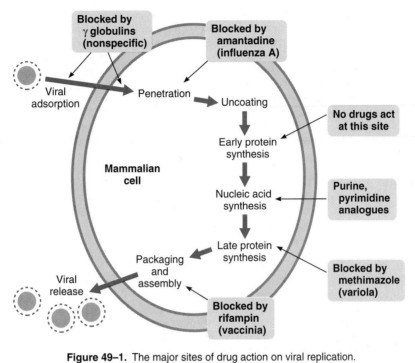

Figure 49–1. The major sites of drug action on viral replication.

factor which blocks peptide chain initiation, a phosphodiesterase that degrades terminal nucleotides of tRNA, and enzymes that activate RNase.

4. **Late protein synthesis and viral assembly:** Few clinically useful drugs act at the later stages of viral replication (Figure 49–1). **Methisazone,** however, effectively interferes with synthesis of a late structural protein in variola (smallpox), resulting in blockade of particle assembly. **Rifampin** blocks a step in the formation of the viral envelope of pox viruses, preventing the assembly of enveloped mature particles.

B. **Clinical Uses & Toxicity:**

1. **Acyclovir (acycloguanosine):** Acyclovir is active against herpes simplex virus, Epstein-Barr virus, and varicella-zoster. Some resistant strains of herpes (TK⁻ strains) lack thymidine kinase, the enzyme involved in the initial bioactivation of acyclovir (Figure 49–2).

Clinical uses of acyclovir include treatment of mucocutaneous and genital herpes lesions,

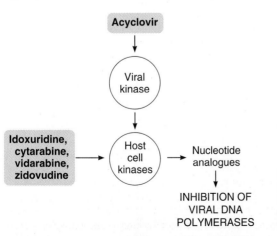

Figure 49–2. Antiviral actions of purine and pyrimidine analogues. Acyclovir (top) is metabolized first by viral kinase to an intermediate. This intermediate and the drugs shown on the left are then metabolized by host cell kinases to nucleotide analogues that inhibit viral replication.

and prophylaxis in AIDS and in other immunocompromised patients (eg, those undergoing organ transplantation). Acyclovir can be administered by the topical, oral, and intravenous routes. Renal excretion is the major route of elimination of acyclovir, and dosage should be reduced in patients with renal impairment. Toxic effects with parenteral administration include delirium, tremor, seizures, hypotension, and nephrotoxicity. Acyclovir has no significant toxicity on the bone marrow.

2. **Amantadine:** Amantadine is active against influenza A and rubella viruses. The drug is prophylactic (not curative) in influenza, but modifies symptoms if given early. Drug-resistant influenza A virus mutants can emerge and infect contacts of patients in treatment.

   Amantadine is orally active and is eliminated unchanged in the urine at a rate proportionate to creatinine clearance; dosage modification is required in renal insufficiency. Toxic effects include dizziness, ataxia, and slurred speech. **Rimantadine** is equally effective, has a longer half-life, and requires no dosage adjustment in renal failure.

3. **Foscarnet:** This drug is a phosphonoformate derivative that does not require phosphorylation for antiviral activity; foscarnet is not an antimetabolite. It is given intravenously in cytomegalovirus (CMV) infections (including CMV retinitis) and has activity against ganciclovir-resistant strains of this virus (Table 49–1). Foscarnet inhibits herpes DNA polymerase in acyclovir-resistant strains that are thymidine kinase-deficient and may suppress such resistant herpetic infections in patients with AIDS. Adverse effects include nephrotoxicity and disturbances in electrolyte balance (especially calcium and magnesium). Foscarnet increases the severity of anemia in zidovudine-treated patients.

4. **Ganciclovir:** Ganciclovir, a guanine derivative, is an antimetabolite that is phosphorylated by cellular kinases to form a nucleotide that inhibits DNA polymerases of cytomegalovirus (CMV). The drug is used intravenously in immunocompromised patients (eg, those with AIDS and those undergoing cancer chemotherapy or organ transplantation). Resistant strains of CMV can emerge during prolonged treatment. Systemic toxic effects include leukopenia, thrombocytopenia, mucositis, hepatic dysfunction, and seizures. The drug may cause severe neutropenia when used with other myelosuppressive agents.

5. **Interferons:** Interferons are glycoproteins produced in human leukocytes (IFN-α), fibroblasts (IFN-β), and immune cells (IFN-γ), and are now manufactured by recombinant DNA technology. Clinical uses include the prevention of herpes zoster virus dissemination in cancer patients, suppression of viremia with hepatitis B virus, and cancer chemotherapy. Toxic effects include gastrointestinal irritation, fatigue, anemia, myalgia, mental confusion, and cardiovascular dysfunction.

6. **Ribavirin:** This drug inhibits the replication of both RNA and DNA viruses by interfering with guanidine monophosphate formation and subsequent nucleic acid synthesis. Ribavirin is used in aerosol form for respiratory syncytial virus infections, and may shorten the symptoms of influenza A and B infections.

7. **Vidarabine:** The purine nucleoside analogue vidarabine is used in severe herpes simplex virus diseases, including encephalitis, keratitis, and neonatal herpes, but has no effect on genital lesions. Vidarabine also prevents the dissemination of varicella-zoster virus in immunocompromised patients. The drug is available for topical use, but can be used intravenously in serious infections. Systemic toxic effects include gastrointestinal irritation, paresthesias, tremor, convulsions, and hepatic dysfunction.

8. **Zidovudine (ZDV):** Formerly called azidothymidine (AZT), zidovudine is an antimetabolite that is phosphorylated and inhibits DNA polymerase (reverse transcriptase) of

Table 49–1. Major clinical uses of antiviral drugs.

Virus	Drug of Choice	Alternative Drugs
Cytomegalovirus	Ganciclovir	Foscarnet
Hepatitis B, C	Interferon α-2b	
Herpes simplex	Acyclovir	Foscarnet, vidarabine
HIV	Zidovudine	Didanosine
Influenza A	Amantadine	Rimantadine
Respiratory syncytial virus	Ribavirin	
Varicella-zoster	Acyclovir	Foscarnet

the human immunodeficiency retrovirus. The viral enzyme is more susceptible to inhibition than are mammalian DNA polymerases. Zidovudine is active orally and is eliminated by both hepatic metabolism and renal excretion. The drug temporarily reduces mortality and morbidity in patients with AIDS and AIDS-related complex. In asymptomatic HIV-positive individuals, zidovudine slows the rate of progression to AIDS. Toxic effects include bone marrow suppression (which may require transfusions), granulocytopenia, thrombocytopenia, headaches, myalgia, agitation, and insomnia.

9. **Newer drugs:** Newer drugs with activity against zidovudine-resistant strains of HIV include **dideoxyinosine (DDI, didanosine)** and **dideoxycytidine (DDC).** DDI is not hematotoxic and may be active against HIV strains resistant to zidovudine. A recent strategy in the treatment of patients with AIDS is to institute treatment with zidovudine and to replace the drug with didanosine after 6 months. DDI may cause dose-dependent peripheral neuropathy and pancreatitis. Dideoxycytidine has been used with zidovudine in AIDS patients with advanced HIV infection. Though not markedly hematotoxic, DDC may cause severe peripheral neuropathy and gastrointestinal adverse effects including nausea, diarrhea, and gastric and esophageal ulceration.

10. **Topical antiviral drugs:** Several antiviral agents with marked systemic toxicity (bone marrow, hepatic, renal) are used mainly as topical drugs for herpes simplex eye infections, including corneal keratitis. These drugs include three antimetabolites: **idoxuridine, cytarabine,** and **trifluorothymidine.**

DRUG LIST

The following drugs are important members of the group discussed in this chapter. Prototypes should be learned in detail; features of the other significant agents should be known well enough to distinguish them from the prototypes and from each other.

Subclass	Prototype	Other Significant Agents
Purine and pyrimidine analogues Topical	Idoxuridine	Trifluorothymidine, cytarabine
Systemic	Acyclovir	Dideoxyinosine, ganciclovir, ribavirin, vidarabine, zidovudine
Phosphonacetic acid derivatives	Foscarnet	
Tricyclic symmetric amines	Amantadine	Rimantadine
Proteins	Immune globulin, interferon	

QUESTIONS

DIRECTIONS: Each of the numbered items or incomplete statements in this section is followed by answers or by completions of the statement. Select the ONE lettered answer or completion that is BEST in each case.

1. Each of the following statements about the antiviral drugs that act on nucleic acid synthesis is accurate EXCEPT
   (A) The initial step in activation of vidarabine is its phosphorylation by viral thymidine kinase
   (B) The reverse transcriptase of HIV is 30–50 times more sensitive to inhibition by zidovudine than host cell DNA polymerases
   (C) Acyclovir is an antimetabolite related to guanosine
   (D) Increased activity of host cell phosphodiesterases that degrade tRNA is one of the antiviral actions of interferons
   (E) Foscarnet is not an antimetabolite
2. This drug has activity against herpes simplex virus type 1 and is used only topically. Systemic administration results in bone marrow depression, hepatic dysfunction, and nephrotoxicity.
   (A) Ganciclovir
   (B) Acyclovir
   (C) Amantadine

    (D) Vidarabine

    (E) Idoxuridine

3. Each of the following statements about antiviral agents is accurate EXCEPT

    (A) Interferons may prevent dissemination of herpes zoster in cancer patients and reduce CMV shedding after renal transplantation

    (B) The oral absorption of acyclovir is slow and incomplete, but this process is not affected by foods

    (C) Dosage modification of amantadine is required in renal insufficiency

    (D) Peripheral neuropathy is the major dose-limiting toxic effect of ganciclovir

    (E) Topical use of vidarabine requires caution during pregnancy because systemic absorption occurs, and the drug is potentially mutagenic and teratogenic

4. Each of the following statements about the antiviral drugs used in patients with AIDS is accurate EXCEPT

    (A) Treatment with acyclovir does not prevent transmission of herpes during sexual intercourse

    (B) Dideoxycytidine has activity against certain HIV strains resistant to zidovudine

    (C) The development of neutropenia and thrombocytopenia in asymptomatic HIV-positive AIDS patients is not related to treatment with zidovudine

    (D) Acute treatment with ganciclovir halts the progression of CMV retinitis

    (E) Zidovudine dosage should be reduced in patients with cirrhosis or uremia

5. Which ONE of the following drugs is active against the human immunodeficiency virus and, when used in AIDS, causes peripheral neuropathies and pancreatitis?

    (A) Amantadine

    (B) Didanosine

    (C) Ganciclovir

    (D) Interferon alpha

    (E) Zidovudine

Items 6–7: A 27-year-old nursing mother is diagnosed as suffering from herpes simplex genitalis. She has a prior history of this viral infection. Previously, she responded to a drug used topically. Apart from her current problem, she is in good health.

6. Which of the following drugs is most likely to be prescribed at this time?

    (A) Amantadine

    (B) Acyclovir

    (C) Foscarnet

    (D) Rifampin

    (E) Trifluridine

7. All of the following statements about the drug management of herpes simplex genitalis in this patient are accurate EXCEPT

    (A) Topical administration of the antiviral drug will provide minimal clinical benefit

    (B) Oral use of the antiviral drug will reduce pain and shorten the duration of disease manifestations

    (C) It is probably advisable to terminate use of the antiviral drug if she becomes pregnant

    (D) Prompt intravenous treatment with the antiviral drug will prevent recurrent disease

    (E) She should not breast-feed the infant while taking the antiviral drug

DIRECTIONS: The following section consists of a list of four to twenty-six lettered options followed by several numbered items. For each numbered item, select the ONE option that is most closely associated with it. Each answer may be selected once, more than once, or not at all.

    (A) Interferon alpha-2b

    (B) Acyclovir

    (C) Ribavirin

    (D) Cytarabine

    (E) Rimantadine

    (F) Zidovudine

    (G) Ganciclovir

    (H) Vidarabine

    (I) Didanosine

    (J) Foscarnet

8. This drug is used occasionally as a topical agent in herpes simplex ocular infections, and may also be administered systemically for its antineoplastic effects
9. The antiviral actions of this drug include inhibition of both RNA and DNA synthesis. The drug is used for the treatment of severe respiratory syncytial virus infections in neonates
10. At the initiation of therapy with this drug, most patients experience a flu-like syndrome. Clinical uses of the drug include the treatment of Kaposi's sarcoma, hairy-cell leukemias, and genital warts
11. Over 90% of this drug is excreted in the urine in intact form. Because its urinary solubility is low, patients should be well hydrated to prevent nephrotoxicity
12. This drug is active against resistant herpes strains that are thymidine kinase-deficient

ANSWERS

1. Initial phosphorylation by viral thymidine kinase is a distinctive feature of the activation of acyclovir. Vidarabine and other antiviral agents that act as antimetabolites are activated exclusively by host cell kinases. The answer is **(A)**.
2. Due to its systemic toxicity, idoxuridine is used solely as a topical agent for the treatment of herpes ocular infections. When applied to the cornea, the drug does not penetrate the deep stroma and is not significantly absorbed into the blood stream. The answer is **(E)**.
3. The adverse effects of ganciclovir are similar to those caused by radiation therapy. The major dose-limiting adverse effects—myelosuppression, gastrointestinal distress, and mucositis—occur commonly. The toxic effects of ganciclovir are enhanced by concomitant administration of other drugs that suppress bone marrow. The answer is **(D)**.
4. The incidence and severity of zidovudine's hematotoxicity in AIDS patients is related to the dose and the severity of the disease when treatment is begun. Anemia, neutropenia, and thrombocytopenia may occur in the asymptomatic patient at relatively low doses of zidovudine. The answer is **(C)**.
5. Didanosine causes dose-dependent peripheral neuropathy and pancreatic dysfunction. The risk of pancreatitis is greatest in patients with a history of alcoholism and in those with advanced HIV infection. The answer is **(B)**.
6. Three of the drugs listed (acyclovir, foscarnet, trifluridine) are active against strains of herpes simplex virus. Foscarnet is not used in genital infections (HSV-2) because clinical efficacy has not been established and the drug causes many toxic effects. Trifluridine is used only for herpes keratoconjunctivitis (HSV-1) and only topically. The answer is **(B)**.
7. First episodes of genital HSV usually respond to the topical use of acyclovir, but oral or parenteral administration is necessary to treat recurrent disease. Acyclovir treatment, by any mode of administration, does not eradicate latent herpes and will not prevent recurrence of the disease. Note that the drug is secreted in breast milk and, while there are no reports of human teratogenicity, acyclovir is a potential mutagen. The answer is **(D)**.
8. Herpes simplex infections of the eye that are resistant to idoxuridine may respond to cytarabine. A CCS anticancer drug, cytarabine is used intravenously in acute leukemias and can cause dose-dependent neuritis, peripheral neuropathy, and depression of bone marrow. The answer is **(D)**.
9. The antiviral actions of ribavirin include inhibition of RNA polymerases, inhibition of DNA and RNA synthesis, and interference with viral coating. Ribavirin is used by aerosol inhalation for respiratory syncytial virus infections in premature infants and children with cardiopulmonary disease. The answer is **(C)**.
10. Headache, fever, chills, and muscle aches are common side effects of treatment with interferons. Patients are advised to take acetaminophen, since aspirin aggravates gastrointestinal irritation and may promote bleeding. Interferons may also cause neurotoxicity, cardiovascular dysfunction, and bone marrow depression. The answer is **(A)**.
11. Acyclovir is eliminated in the urine via filtration and by active tubular secretion, which is inhibited by probenecid. Nephrotoxic effects, including hematuria and crystalluria, are enhanced in patients who are dehydrated or who have pre-existing renal dysfunction. The answer is **(B)**.
12. Foscarnet is active against cytomegalovirus and certain TK⁻ (thymidine kinase-deficient) strains of herpes resistant to acyclovir. The answer is **(J)**.

50 Miscellaneous Antimicrobial Agents & Urinary Antiseptics

OBJECTIVES

You should be able to:

- Describe the mechanisms of antibacterial action of clindamycin, erythromycin, fluoroquinolones, and vancomycin.
- Describe the clinical uses, significant features of biodisposition, and main toxic effects of clindamycin, erythromycin, vancomycin, and the fluoroquinolones.
- Identify the clinical uses of metronidazole and bacitracin.
- Identify the drugs commonly used as urinary antiseptics, and describe their toxic effects.

CONCEPTS

The drugs discussed in this chapter comprise two major groups: drugs suitable for systemic use (further divided into cell wall inhibitors, protein synthesis inhibitors, and nucleic acid synthesis inhibitors) and drugs used as urinary tract antiseptics, see Figure 50–1.

CELL WALL INHIBITORS

A. Vancomycin: Vancomycin is an important drug used for serious infections caused by drug-resistant gram-positive organisms, including beta-lactamase-producing staphylococci and *C difficile*. Vancomycin is a bactericidal inhibitor of the synthesis of cell wall mucopeptides, and resistance is rare. The drug is not absorbed from the gastrointestinal tract but may be given orally for bacterial enterocolitis. When given parenterally, vancomycin penetrates most tissues and is eliminated unchanged in the urine. Dose modification is necessary in patients with renal impairment. Toxic effects following parenteral use include chills, fever, phlebitis, ototoxicity, and nephrotoxicity. Rapid intravenous infusion may cause diffuse flushing ("red man" syndrome).

B. Bacitracin: Bacitracin is a polypeptide that interferes with a late stage in cell wall synthesis in gram-positive organisms. Because of marked nephrotoxicity, the drug is limited to topical use.

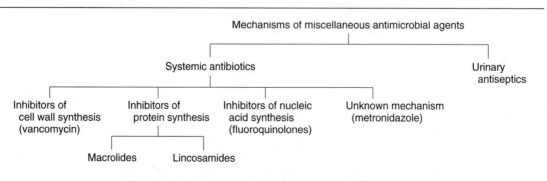

Figure 50–1. Subgroups of the drugs discussed in this chapter.

PROTEIN SYNTHESIS INHIBITORS

A. Macrolides:

1. **Classification and pharmacokinetics:** The macrolide antibiotics (**erythromycin, azithromycin** and **clarithromycin**) are large cyclic lactone-ring structures with attached sugars. The drugs have good oral bioavailability, but azithromycin absorption is impeded by food. Macrolides distribute to most body tissues, but azithromycin is unique in that the tissue levels achieved are considerably higher (10–100 fold) than those in the plasma. The elimination of erythromycin (via biliary excretion) and clarithromycin (via hepatic metabolism and urinary excretion of intact drug) is fairly rapid (half-life 2–5 hr). Azithromycin is eliminated slowly (half-life 2–4 days), mainly as unchanged drug in the urine.

2. **Mechanism of action:** The macrolides are inhibitors of bacterial protein synthesis and can be either bactericidal or bacteriostatic against susceptible microorganisms. Erythromycin binds to a 23S rRNA component of the 50S ribosomal subunit to prevent formation of the initiation complex and block ribosomal translocation.

    Resistance can result from plasmid-mediated formation of enzymes that methylate this receptor, preventing drug binding. Another type of resistance is found among coliforms, in which a transmissible plasmid occurs that specifies an esterase that hydrolyzes the lactone ring of erythromycin. Cross-resistance occurs among macrolide drugs.

3. **Clinical uses:** Erythromycin is effective in the treatment of infections caused by *Mycoplasma pneumoniae, Corynebacterium spp, C trachomatis, Legionella pneumophila, Ureaplasma urealyticum,* and *Bordetella pertussis.* The drug is also active against gram-positive cocci including beta-lactamase-producing staphylococci, but not methicillin-resistant strains. Azithromycin has a similar spectrum of activity, but is more active against *H influenza, M catarrhalis,* and *Neisseria* spp. A single dose of azithromycin is usually effective in the treatment of urethritis or cervicitis due to *C trachomatis.* Clarithromycin is also similar to erythromycin in its antibacterial spectrum, except that it has activity against *M avium-intracellulare* and *Helicobacter pylori.*

4. **Toxicity:** Adverse effects are minor and include gastrointestinal irritation, skin rashes, and eosinophilia. A hypersensitivity-based acute cholestatic hepatitis may occur with erythromycin estolate, but is rare in children. Erythromycin inhibits hepatic cytochrome P450 and can increase the plasma levels of anticoagulants, carbamazepine, digoxin, theophylline, astemizole, and terfenadine. Cardiac arrhythmias have occurred when erythromycin was administered with astemizole or terfenadine. Such drug interactions have yet to be documented with the newer macrolides, but caution is advised.

B. Fluoroquinolones:

1. **Classification and pharmacokinetics:** Fluoroquinolones are structurally related to the older quinolone antibiotic, nalidixic acid. The prototypical fluoroquinolone is **norfloxacin;** others in the group include **ciprofloxacin, ofloxacin,** and **temafloxacin.** All of the drugs are well absorbed after oral administration and penetrate most body tissues with the exception of the CNS. Elimination is partly by metabolism but mainly through the kidneys via active tubular secretion (which can be blocked by probenecid).

2. **Mechanism of action:** The fluoroquinolones are inhibitors of bacterial topoisomerase II (DNA gyrase). They block the relaxation of supercoiled DNA that is required for normal transcription and duplication. Fluoroquinolones are usually bactericidal against susceptible organisms. Resistance occurs during treatment with a frequency of about 1 in 10^9 organisms, especially in staphylococci, *Pseudomonas,* and *Serratia* spp, and is due to an altered drug sensitivity of DNA gyrase, or to decreased intracellular accumulation of the drug.

3. **Clinical uses:** The fluoroquinolones are effective in the treatment of infections of the urinary, gastrointestinal, and respiratory tracts caused by gram-negative organisms including gonococci, *E coli, Klebsiella pneumoniae, Campylobacter jejuni,* and *Enterobacter, Salmonella,* and *Shigella* spp. These drugs have also been used to treat the meningococcal carrier state and in the prophylaxis of neutropenic patients.

4. **Toxicity:** Gastrointestinal distress occurs commonly, and the fluoroquinolones may cause skin rashes, headache, dizziness, insomnia, tendonitis, and abnormal liver function. Superinfections due to *C albicans* and streptococci have occurred. The fluoroquinolones are not recommended for use in children or in pregnancy because animal studies have shown that

these drugs cause cartilage erosion. Ciprofloxacin increases the plasma levels of theophylline and other methylxanthines.

C. Lincosamides: **Lincomycin** and **clindamycin** have few clinical uses. They inhibit bacterial protein synthesis via a mechanism similar to that of erythromycin, and are usually bacteriostatic. The clinical uses of clindamycin are limited to gram-positive cocci and anaerobes such as *Bacteroides* spp.

Good tissue penetration occurs after oral absorption. The lincosamides are eliminated partly by metabolism and partly by biliary and renal excretion. The toxicity of clindamycin includes marked gastrointestinal irritation, skin rashes, neutropenia, hepatic dysfunction, and possible superinfections such as *C difficile* pseudomembranous colitis.

METRONIDAZOLE

An antiprotozoal agent, metronidazole is also active against *Gardnerella vaginalis* and anaerobes such as *Bacteroides* and *Clostridium* spp. The bactericidal actions of metronidazole probably result from the formation of toxic metabolites in the bacterial cell. The drug is effective orally and penetrates most tissues, including abscesses and the CNS. Toxic effects include gastrointestinal irritation, headache, vestibular dysfunction, and disulfiram-like reactions with ethanol. Metronidazole is teratogenic in some animals.

URINARY ANTISEPTICS

Urinary antiseptics are oral drugs that are rapidly excreted and act in the urine to suppress bacteriuria. The drugs lack systemic antibacterial effects but may be toxic. Urinary antiseptics are often administered with acidifying agents, because bacterial growth in urine is inhibited at low pH.

A. Nitrofurantoin: This drug is active against many urinary tract pathogens (but not *Proteus* or *Pseudomonas* spp), and resistance emerges slowly. The drug is active orally and is excreted in the urine via filtration and secretion; toxic levels may occur in the blood of patients with renal dysfunction. Adverse effects of nitrofurantoin include gastrointestinal irritation, skin rashes, neuropathies, and hemolysis in patients with glucose-6-phosphate dehydrogenase deficiency.

B. Nalidixic Acid: This quinolone acts against many gram-negative organisms (but not *Proteus* or *Pseudomonas* spp) by mechanisms that may involve acidification or inhibition of DNA gyrase. Resistance emerges rapidly. The drug is active orally and is excreted in the urine partly unchanged and partly as the inactive glucuronide. Toxic effects include gastrointestinal irritation, glycosuria, skin rashes, photosensitization, visual disturbances, and CNS stimulation.

C. Methenamine: Methenamine mandelate and methenamine hippurate combine acidification with the release of the antibacterial compound formaldehyde at pH levels below 5.5. These drugs are not usually active against *Proteus* spp because these organisms alkalinize the urine. Insoluble complexes form between formaldehyde and sulfonamides, and the drugs should not be used together.

D. Cycloserine: Cycloserine inhibits the incorporation of D-alanine into cell wall mucopeptides. The drug is active against coliforms, mycobacteria, and *Proteus* spp. The clinical use of cycloserine is limited by serious toxicity, including headache, tremor, vertigo, convulsions, and psychotic reactions.

E. Other Urinary Antibiotics: Many systemically active antimicrobial agents are effective in the treatment of urinary tract infections; these agents include penicillins, cephalosporins, fluoroquinolones, sulfonamides, trimethoprim-sulfamethoxazole, and aminoglycosides.

DRUG LIST

The following drugs are important members of the group discussed in this chapter. Prototypes should be learned in detail; features of the major variants should be known well enough to distinguish the variants from the prototypes and from each other.

Subclass	Prototype	Major Variants
Macrolides	Erythromycin	Azithromycin, clarithromycin
Fluoroquinolones	Norfloxacin	Ciprofloxacin, ofloxacin, temafloxacin
Lincosamides	Lincomycin	Clindamycin
Glycopeptides	Vancomycin	
Nitroimidazoles	Metronidazole	
Urinary tract antiseptics Nitrofurans	Nitrofurantoin	
Quinolones	Nalidixic acid	Cinoxacin
Methenamine salts	Methenamine mandelate	Methenamine hippurate
Cycloserine	Cycloserine	

QUESTIONS

DIRECTIONS: Each of the numbered items or incomplete statements in this section is followed by answers or by completions of the statement. Select the ONE lettered answer or completion that is BEST in each case.

1. Each of the following statements about the macrolide antibiotics is accurate EXCEPT
   (A) Children rarely develop cholestatic hepatitis with erythromycin estolate
   (B) Azithromycin is rapidly and highly concentrated in polymorphonuclear leukocytes
   (C) Resistance to erythromycin can occur through methylation of its receptor on 23S rRNA
   (D) Erythromycin is the drug of choice for the treatment of *Mycoplasma pneumoniae* infections in the pregnant patient
   (E) Clarithromycin is active against methicillin-resistant staphylococci

2. Each of the following statements about the fluoroquinolones is accurate EXCEPT
   (A) Antacids containing multivalent cations may decrease the oral bioavailability of fluoroquinolones
   (B) Resistance to fluoroquinolones may involve changes in DNA gyrase
   (C) Streptococcal superinfections have occurred during treatment with fluoroquinolones
   (D) A fluoroquinolone would be appropriate for an uncomplicated urinary tract infection in a 10-year-old girl
   (E) Modification of fluoroquinolone dosage is required in renal insufficiency

3. All of the following statements about the lincosamides are accurate EXCEPT
   (A) Lincomycin and clindamycin are bacteriostatic inhibitors of protein synthesis
   (B) They are active versus *S aureus* and common streptococci
   (C) Lincomycin is effective in the treatment of infections caused by *B fragilis*
   (D) They are excreted mainly in the bile
   (E) Clindamycin use may lead to pseudomembranous colitis

4. Each of the following statements about vancomycin is accurate EXCEPT
   (A) Vancomycin inhibits the synthesis of bacterial cell wall precursor molecules
   (B) The dosage of vancomycin must be increased in patients on hemodialysis
   (C) Rapid infusion of vancomycin may cause the "red man" syndrome
   (D) Toxic effects will occur if vancomycin dosage is not decreased in renal impairment
   (E) Vancomycin may be used for severe infections caused by resistant *S aureus*

5. Each of the following statements about metronidazole is accurate EXCEPT
   (A) Metronidazole is a useful alternative drug for infections caused by pneumococci in patients allergic to penicillins
   (B) The drug is effective orally and penetrates into the CNS

(C) Peripheral neuropathies have occurred during the use of metronidazole

(D) Caution is advised during pregnancy because metronidazole has teratogenic effects in some animals

(E) It is effective in the treatment of pseudomembranous colitis due to *C difficile*

Items 6–7: A 31-year-old man has gonorrhea that is to be treated with ceftriaxone. He has no drug allergies, but he recalls that a few years ago while in Africa he had acute hemolysis following use of an antimalarial drug. The physician is concerned that the patient has an accompanying urethritis due to *C trachomatis*, although no culture or enzyme tests have been conducted.

6. Which ONE of the following agents will eradicate nongonococcal urethritis due to *C trachomatis* in a single dose?

(A) Erythromycin

(B) Ciprofloxacin

(C) Azithromycin

(D) Tetracycline

(E) Nitrofurantoin

7. If the nongonococcal urethritis in this patient happened to be caused by a *Mycoplasma* or by *Ureaplasma urealyticum,* which ONE of the following agents would be the drug of choice for treatment of this organism?

(A) Erythromycin

(B) Ciprofloxacin

(C) Sulfisoxazole

(D) Clarithromycin

(E) Trimethoprim-sulfamethoxazole

8. A 24-year-old woman has returned from a vacation abroad suffering from traveler's diarrhea. Her problem has not responded to antidiarrheal drugs and, since gram-negative bacilli have been recovered from the feces, an antibiotic is prescribed. Which ONE of the following drugs is most likely to be effective in the treatment of this patient?

(A) Erythromycin

(B) Norfloxacin

(C) Metronidazole

(D) Nitrofurantoin

(E) Vancomycin

DIRECTIONS: The following section consists of a list of four to twenty-six lettered options followed by several numbered items. For each numbered item, select the ONE option that is most closely associated with it. Each answer may be selected once, more than once, or not at all.

(A) Methenamine

(B) Erythromycin

(C) Nalidixic acid

(D) Vancomycin

(E) Azithromycin

(F) Nitrofurantoin

(G) Ciprofloxacin

(H) Metronidazole

(I) Clarithromycin

(J) Cycloserine

9. This drug has activity against gram-negative bacteria in urinary tract infections, but resistance may develop during the course of treatment. There is cross-resistance with cinoxacin. The drug has no useful systemic antibacterial effects

10. A urinary antiseptic, this drug is not effective in the treatment of urinary tract infections caused by *Proteus* spp. The agent releases formaldehyde, which may form an insoluble complex with sulfonamides

11. Symptoms of CNS excitation, including seizures, have occurred in asthmatic patients taking theophylline when they are administered this inhibitor of bacterial protein synthesis

12. This inhibitor of cell wall synthesis may be used in endocarditis caused by viridans streptococci in patients allergic to penicillins. In combination with an aminoglycoside, the drug is also effective in enterococcal endocarditis, but ototoxicity may occur

13. Neuropathies are more likely to occur with this urinary antiseptic when it is used in patients with renal dysfunction. The drug may cause acute hemolysis in patients with G6PD deficiency

14. Flushing, headache, nausea, and vomiting are likely effects if patients ingest alcoholic beverages while taking this drug

ANSWERS

1. The macrolides are effective against common streptococci and penicillinase-producing staphylococci. However, most methicillin-resistant staphylococci are resistant to erythromycin, azithromycin, and clarithromycin. For infections caused by such organisms, vancomycin is the drug of choice. The answer is **(E)**.

2. The fluoroquinolones should not be used to treat uncomplicated first-time urinary tract infections. In this child, the infection is almost certainly due to *E coli* that are sensitive to many other drugs. In addition, because of possible effects on cartilage, fluoroquinolones are not recommended for use in children. The answer is **(D)**.

3. The antibacterial activity of lincomycin is essentially restricted to gram-positive cocci, including penicillinase-producing staphylococci. The drug has minimal activity against anaerobes. However, clindamycin is active against *B fragilis* and, though not the drug of choice, continues to be used for infections caused by strains of this organism. The answer is **(C)**.

4. The dosage of some dialyzable drugs may have to be increased in patients on hemodialysis. Vancomycin is not dialyzable and, since patients on hemodialysis ordinarily have minimal renal function, dosage must be *lowered* in such patients to avoid auditory and renal damage. The answer is **(B)**.

5. In addition to its use as an antiprotozoal agent, metronidazole is also active against anaerobic cocci and bacilli. The drug has minimal activity against aerobes, because anoxic or hypoxic conditions are necessary for the formation of cytotoxic metabolites. The answer is **(A)**.

6. Urinary tract infections due to *C trachomatis* are likely to respond to all of the drugs listed except nitrofurantoin. However, azithromycin is effective following a single dose, presumably due to its extensive tissue accumulation and prolonged half-life. The answer is **(C)**.

7. In nongonococcal urethritis, *C trachomatis* is the causative organism in only 50% of cases. Erythromycin is the drug of choice when *Mycoplasma* or *Ureaplasma urealyticum* are implicated. Doxycycline (not listed) is also effective in nongonococcal urethritis. Avoid sulfonamides (which are also active against chlamydia) in patients who have experienced acute hemolysis from drugs that act as oxidizing agents. The answer is **(A)**.

8. The fluoroquinolones are very effective in diarrhea caused by bacterial pathogens including *E coli,* and *Shigella* and *Salmonella* spp. None of the other drugs listed have significant activity against these organisms. Doxycycline (not listed) would also be effective. The answer is **(B)**.

9. Nalidixic acid, a quinolone, is structurally related to cinoxacin. Both drugs are used in the treatment of urinary tract infections, and cross-resistance may occur. Quinolone derivatives may lower seizure threshold in susceptible individuals. The answer is **(C)**.

10. Methenamine is a urinary antiseptic with antibacterial actions that are mainly due to release of formaldehyde at acidic pH. Sulfonamides may form complexes with formaldehyde, resulting in mutual antagonism. The answer is **(A)**.

11. Erythromycin inhibits the metabolism of methylxanthines, including theophylline and caffeine. The resulting increase in the plasma level of theophylline causes CNS stimulation. Fluoroquinolone antibiotics (which act by a different mechanism) may cause a similar drug interaction. The answer is **(B)**.

12. In addition to its important clinical use in staphylococcal infections, vancomycin is effective in bacterial endocarditis. Vancomycin causes ototoxicity that may be irreversible; this occurs more frequently when it is administered with other ototoxic drugs. The answer is **(D)**.

13. Acute hemolytic reactions in G6PD deficiency occur with drugs that are oxidizing agents, including antimalarials, nalidixic acid, sulfonamides, and the nitrofurans. Severe polyneuropathies, with both motor and sensory nerve degeneration, may occur with nitrofurantoin. These reactions are more likely to occur in patients with renal dysfunction. The answer is **(F)**.

14. Metronidazole may cause disulfiram-like reactions when ethanol is ingested. The answer is **(H)**.

51

Disinfectants & Antiseptics

OBJECTIVES

You should be able to:

- Identify the compounds used as antiseptics and disinfectants.
- Describe the advantages and disadvantages of the most commonly used antiseptics and disinfectants.

Learn the definitions that follow.

Table 51–1. Definitions.

Term	Definition
Antiseptic	An agent used to inhibit bacterial growth in vitro and in vivo
Disinfectant	An agent used to kill microorganisms in an inanimate environment
Sterilization	Procedures that kill microorganisms on instruments and dressings; methods include autoclaving, dry heat, and exposure to ethylene oxide
Chlorine demand	The amount of chlorine bound to organic matter in water and thus unavailable for antimicrobial activity

CONCEPTS

Although the terms are often used interchangeably, **disinfectant** should be used to refer to a compound that is used to kill microorganisms in an inanimate environment, whereas **antiseptic** denotes a compound that is used to inhibit bacterial growth in vitro and when in contact with the surfaces of living tissues. Disinfectants and antiseptics do not have selective toxicity, and their clinical use is confined to inanimate objects and topical application (with the exception of urinary antiseptics; see Chapter 50). Most antiseptics delay wound healing.

A. Alcohols, Aldehydes & Acids: **Ethanol** (70%) and **isopropanol** (70–90%) are effective skin antiseptics, since they denature microbial proteins. **Formaldehyde,** which also denatures proteins, is too irritating for topical use but is a disinfectant for instruments. **Acetic acid** (1%) is used in surgical dressings and has activity against gram-negative bacteria, including *Pseudomonas* spp, when used as a urinary irrigant and in the external ear. **Salicylic acid** and **undecylenic acid** are useful antidermatophytes.

B. Halogens: **Iodine tincture** is an effective antiseptic for intact skin and is commonly used in preparing the skin before taking blood samples, though it can cause dermatitis. Iodine complexed with povidone **(povidone-iodine)** is widely used, particularly as a preoperative skin antiseptic, but solutions can become contaminated with aerobic gram-negative bacteria.

    Hypochlorous acid, formed when chlorine dissolves in water, is antimicrobial. This is the basis for the use of chlorine and halazone in water purification. Organic matter binds chlorine, thus preventing antimicrobial actions. In a given water sample, this process is referred to as the **"chlorine demand,"** since the chlorine-binding capacity of the organic material must be exceeded before bacterial killing is accomplished. Many preparations of chlorine for water purification do not eradicate all bacteria or *Entamoeba* cysts.

C. Oxidizing Agents: **Hydrogen peroxide** exerts short-lived antimicrobial action through the release of molecular oxygen. The agent is used as a mouthwash, for cleansing wounds, and for disinfection of contact lenses. Potassium permanganate is an effective bactericidal agent, but has the disadvantage of causing persistent brown stains on skin and clothing.

D. Heavy Metals: **Mercuric ions** precipitate proteins and inactivate sulfhydryl groups of enzymes. These agents are toxic if ingested but may be used as skin antiseptics. Organic mercurials such as **nitromersol** and **thimerosal** are more effective and less toxic than inorganic salts. **Merbromin** is a very weak antiseptic and has the additional disadvantage of staining tissues a brilliant red color. **Silver** is a protein precipitant and inhibitor of microbial metabolism, but it can be irritating to tissues. Its uses as the nitrate salt include the prevention of neonatal gonococcal ophthalmia and the treatment of burns. **Silver sulfadiazine** (a sulfonamide) is also used to decrease bacterial colonization in burns.

E. Chlorinated Phenols: Phenol, the first antiseptic agent, is irritating to tissues and is now used only as a disinfectant of inanimate objects. Chlorinated phenolic compounds are less irritating. **Hexachlorophene** is widely used in surgical scrub routines and in deodorant soaps. If used routinely, the drug forms antibacterial deposits on the skin, decreasing the population of resident bacteria. Hexachlorophene has also been used to protect against staphylococcal infections in neonates, but repeated use on the skin in infants can lead to absorption of the drug, resulting in CNS white matter degeneration. Antiseptic soaps may also contain other chlorinated phenols such as **triclocarban** and **chlorhexidine.** While chlorhexidine is not very effective against strains of *Pseudomonas* or *Serratia,* it is commonly used in hospital scrub routines to cleanse skin sites. All antiseptic soaps may cause allergies or photosensitization.

    Lindane (gamma benzene hexachloride) is used to treat infestations with mites or lice, and it is also an agricultural insecticide. The agent can be absorbed through the skin; if excessive amounts are applied, toxic effects, including blood dyscrasias and convulsions, may occur.

F. Cationic Surfactants: **Benzalkonium chloride** and **cetylpyridinium chloride** are used as antiseptics on skin and as disinfectants of surgical instruments. The antimicrobial action of these agents is antagonized by soaps. A serious disadvantage of their use is that certain gramnegative bacteria (eg, *Pseudomonas* spp) may not be eradicated. **Nitrofurazone** is an antimicrobial agent often used on skin lesions. Although it does not impair wound healing, the drug can cause allergic reactions.

DRUG LIST

The following drugs are important members of the group discussed in this chapter. Prototypes should be learned in detail; features of the major variants should be known well enough to distinguish the variants from prototypes and from each other.

Subclass	Prototype	Major Variants
Alcohols, aldehydes, and acids	Ethanol, formaldehyde, acetic acid	Isopropanol, glutaraldehyde, salicylic acid
Halogens	Iodine, chlorine	Povidone-iodide, halazone
Heavy metals	Silver nitrate, mercury bichloride	Silver sulfadiazine, nitromersol, thimerosal
Chlorinated phenols	Hexachlorophene	Triclocarban, chlorhexidine
Cationic surfactants	Benzalkonium chloride	Cetylpyridinium chloride

QUESTIONS

DIRECTIONS: Each of the numbered items or incomplete statements in this section is followed by answers or by completions of the statement. Select the ONE lettered answer or completion that is BEST in each case.

1. All of the following statements about antiseptics and disinfectants are accurate EXCEPT
   (A) Chlorhexidine disrupts bacterial cell membranes, especially those of gram-positive organisms
   (B) Mercuric ions precipitate microbial proteins
   (C) Dilute (0.25%) acetic acid is particularly active against aerobic gram-negative bacteria
   (D) Benzalkonium chloride will effectively eradicate *Pseudomonas* and other gram-negative bacteria when applied to the skin

2. All of the following statements about antiseptics and disinfectants are accurate EXCEPT
   (A) Most soaps are anionic surfactants that form strongly alkaline solutions in water
   (B) Triclocarban is an effective topical antiseptic that acts to promote wound healing
   (C) Ninety percent isopropanol is an effective skin antiseptic
   (D) Though too irritating for use on tissues, formaldehyde is widely employed as a disinfectant for instruments

3. All of the following statements about heavy metal antiseptics are accurate EXCEPT
   (A) By binding to sulfhydryl groups, these antiseptics are selective inhibitors of bacterial enzymes and exhibit selective toxicity
   (B) Silver sulfadiazine is applied topically and prevents bacterial colonization of burns
   (C) Organic mercurials are less toxic than inorganic mercury salts
   (D) Merbromin is a weak antiseptic agent that can stain tissues

4. All of the following statements about halogens used as antiseptics or disinfectants are accurate EXCEPT
   (A) Chlorine has antibacterial activity because it forms hypochlorous acid when it dissolves in an aqueous solution
   (B) "Chlorine demand" refers to the utilization of chlorine for metabolic processes in microorganisms
   (C) Bacteria can often survive after treatment of water samples with chlorine preparations
   (D) Povidone-iodine is an effective antibacterial agent that kills vegetative forms and clostridial spores

5. Which ONE of the following compounds is used topically to treat scabies and pediculosis?
   (A) Hexachlorophene
   (B) Nitrofurazone
   (C) Lindane
   (D) Silver sulfadiazine

DIRECTIONS: The following section consists of a list of four to twenty-six lettered options followed by several numbered items. For each numbered item, select the ONE lettered option that is most closely associated with it. Each answer may be selected once, more than once, or not at all.
   (A) Hexachlorophene
   (B) Silver nitrate
   (C) Halazone
   (D) Formaldehyde
   (E) Chlorhexidine
   (F) Salicylic acid
   (G) Lindane
   (H) Potassium permanganate
   (I) Undecylenic acid
   (J) Cetylpyridinium chloride

6. This compound is used in tablet form to purify drinking water. If a large quantity of organic material is present, cysts of *Entamoeba histolytica* may not be eradicated

7. This agent can reduce infection of burns and decrease the mortality rate in burn cases. The drug is irritating to tissues and can be reduced by bacterial enzymes to form a compound that causes methemoglobinemia

8. Daily use of this substituted phenol results in a bacteriostatic deposit on the skin. The compound may be absorbed and has caused neurotoxic effects in neonates when used as an antistaphylococcal agent

9. This agent is commonly incorporated into soaps used for skin antisepsis and surgical scrub procedures. The compound has minimal activity against *Pseudomonas* and *Serratia* spp

10. The antimicrobial actions of this antiseptic are antagonized by soaps

ANSWERS

1. Cationic surfactants cannot be employed safely as skin antiseptics because they form a film under which microorganisms can survive. Infections due to *Pseudomonas* spp and other gram-negative organisms occur. The answer is (**D**).

2. No antiseptic in current use is able to promote wound healing, and most agents do the opposite. In general, cleansing of abrasions and superficial wounds with soap and water is just as effective and less damaging than the application of topical antiseptics. The answer is (**B**).

3. Heavy metal antiseptics inhibit sulfhydryl-containing enzymes in all organisms and are not selectively toxic in bacteria. Most of the toxic actions of mercury and lead in humans occur through interaction with sulfhydryl groups on enzymes. The answer is (**A**).

4. "Chlorine demand" refers to the chlorine concentration required for bactericidal action in a water sample. Water samples with a high content of organic materials "demand" higher levels of chlorine for purification. The answer is (**B**).

5. Of the four agents listed, only lindane is an effective scabicide and pediculicide. There is some concern about the systemic absorption of topically applied lindane, which may cause neurotoxicity. Accidental ingestion in children has caused seizures. The answer is (**C**).

6. The addition of 4–8 mg of halazone per liter will sterilize most water samples in about 30 minutes, but will not kill cysts of *Entamoeba histolytica*. The answer is (**C**).

7. Silver nitrate destroys many microorganisms upon contact and is used to prevent neonatal gonococcal ophthalmia and to reduce infections in burns. Reduction of nitrate to nitrite by microorganisms may cause methemoglobinemia. The answer is (**B**).

8. Repeated bathing of newborns with hexachlorophene to prevent staphylococcal colonization may permit systemic absorption, which leads to neurotoxic effects (eg, spongiform degeneration of white matter). The answer is (**A**).

9. Chlorhexidine is a bisdiguanide that disrupts bacterial cytoplasmic membranes, especially of gram-positive organisms. The agent is less effective against *Pseudomonas* and *Serratia* spp. Hospital uses include hand-washing, wound cleansing, and preparation of skin sites for operative procedures. The answer is (**E**).

10. Cationic surfactant agents, including benzalkonium and cetylpyridinium salts, are antagonized by anionic agents and are thus incompatible with soaps. The answer is (**J**).

Clinical Use of Antimicrobials

52

OBJECTIVES

You should be able to:

- List the steps that should be taken prior to the initiation of empiric antimicrobial therapy.
- Describe the importance of susceptibility testing and analyses of serum drug levels or bactericidal titers in antimicrobial chemotherapy.
- Identify the antimicrobial drugs that require major modifications of dosage when renal or hepatic function change, or when dialysis is used.
- Describe the valid reasons for use of antimicrobial drugs in combination and the probable mechanisms involved in drug synergy.
- Describe the principles underlying valid antimicrobial chemoprophylaxis and give examples of surgical and nonsurgical prophylaxis.

Learn the definitions that follow.

Table 52–1. Definitions.

Term	Definition
Empiric (presumptive) antimicrobial therapy	Initiation of drug treatment prior to identification of a specific pathogen
Susceptibility testing	Laboratory methods to determine the sensitivity of the isolated pathogen to antimicrobial drugs
Minimum inhibitory concentration (MIC)	An estimate of the drug sensitivity of pathogens for comparison with anticipated levels in blood or tissues
Antimicrobial prophylaxis	The use of antimicrobial drugs to decrease the risk of infection
Combination antimicrobial drug therapy	The use of two or more drugs together to increase efficacy more than can be accomplished with the use of a single agent

CONCEPTS

A. Guidelines for Antimicrobial Therapy: **Empiric antimicrobial therapy** is antimicrobial therapy that is begun before a specific pathogen has been identified and is based on the presumption of an infection that requires immediate drug treatment. Prior to initiation of such therapy, accepted practice involves making a clinical diagnosis of microbial infection, obtaining specimens for laboratory analyses, making a microbiologic diagnosis, deciding whether treatment should precede the results of laboratory tests, and, finally, selecting the optimal drug or drugs. A variety of publications provide annually updated lists of antimicrobial drugs of choice for specific pathogens. Such lists can provide a useful guide to empiric therapy based on presumptive microbiologic diagnosis. Table 52–2 sets forth the current drugs of choice and alternative agents for common pathogens.

Table 52–2. Examples of empiric antimicrobial therapy based on microbiologic etiology.

Pathogen	Drug(s) of First Choice	Alternative Drug(s)
Gram-positive cocci *Pneumococcus*	Penicillin G, ampicillin	Erythromycin, cephalosporin
Streptococcus (common)	Penicillin G	Erythromycin, cephalosporin
Staphylococcus (penicillinase-producing)	Penicillinase-resistant penicillin	Cephalosporin, vancomycin, macrolide
Staphylococcus (methicillin-resistant)	Vancomycin	TMP-SMZ
Enterococcus	Penicillin G plus gentamicin	Vancomycin plus gentamicin
Gram-negative cocci *Gonococcus*	Ceftriaxone	Penicillin G, ampicillin, spectinomycin
Meningococcus	Penicillin G, ampicillin	Cefotaxime, cefuroxime, chloramphenicol
Gram-negative rods *E coli, Proteus, Klebsiella*	Aminoglycosides, third-generation cephalosporin	TMP-SMZ, fluoroquinolone, extended spectrum penicillin
Shigella	Fluoroquinolone	TMP-SMZ, ampicillin
Enterobacter, Citrobacter, Serratia	Imipenem, fluoroquinolone	TMP-SMZ, extended spectrum penicillin
Hemophilus spp	Cefuroxime or third-generation cephalosporin	TMP-SMZ, ampicillin, chloramphenicol
Pseudomonas aeruginosa	Aminoglycoside plus extended spectrum penicillin	Ceftazidime, aztreonam, imipenem
Bacteroides fragilis	Metronidazole, clindamycin	Imipenem, chloramphenicol, ampicillin/sulbactam
Miscellaneous *Mycoplasma pneumoniae*	Erythromycin, tetracycline	Fluoroquinolone
Treponema pallidum	Penicillin G	Erythromycin, tetracycline

B. **Principles of Antimicrobial Therapy:**   Antimicrobial therapy in established infections is guided by the following principles:
   1. **Susceptibility testing:**   The results of susceptibility testing establish the drug sensitivity of the organism. These results usually predict the **minimum inhibitory concentrations (MICs)** of a drug for comparison with anticipated blood or tissue levels. The two most common methods of susceptibility testing are disk diffusion (Kirby-Bauer) and broth dilution. For some bacteria (eg, gonococci, enterococci, *H influenzae*), a direct test for beta-lactamase can be substituted, since susceptibility patterns are identical for all strains except for the production of beta-lactamase.
   2. **Drug concentration in blood:**   The measurement of drug concentration in the blood may be appropriate when using agents with a low therapeutic index (eg, aminoglycosides, vancomycin) and when investigating poor clinical response to a drug treatment regimen.
   3. **Serum bactericidal titers:**   In certain infections in which host defenses may contribute minimally to cure, the estimation of serum bactericidal titers can confirm the appropriateness of choice of drug and dosage. Serial dilutions of serum are incubated with standardized quantities of the pathogen isolated from the patient, and killing at a dilution of 1:8 is generally considered satisfactory.
   4. **Route of administration:**   Parenteral therapy is preferred in most cases of serious microbial infections. Chloramphenicol, the fluoroquinolones, and trimethoprim-sulfamethoxazole (TMP-SMZ) may be effective orally.
   5. **Monitoring of therapeutic response:**   Therapeutic responses to drug therapy should be monitored clinically and microbiologically to detect the development of resistance or superinfections. The duration of drug therapy required depends on the pathogen (eg, longer courses of therapy are required for infections due to fungi or mycobacteria), the site of infection (eg, endocarditis and osteomyelitis require longer duration of treatment) and the immunocompetence of the patient.

C. **Clinical Failure of Antimicrobial Therapy:**   Inadequate clinical or microbiologic response to antimicrobial therapy can result from multiple causes, including laboratory testing errors; problems with the drug (eg, incorrect choice, poor tissue penetration, inadequate dose); the patient (poor host defenses, undrained abscesses); or the pathogen (resistance, superinfection).

D. **Factors Influencing Antimicrobial Drug Use:**
   1. **Drug elimination mechanisms:**   Changes in hepatic and renal function, and the use of dialysis, can influence the pharmacokinetics of antimicrobials and may necessitate dosage modifications. The major mechanisms of elimination of commonly used antimicrobial drugs are shown in Table 52–3. In anuria (creatinine clearance <5 mL/min), the elimination half-life of drugs that are eliminated by the kidney is markedly increased, usually necessitating major reductions in drug dosage. Erythromycin, clindamycin, chloramphenicol, rifampin, and ketoconazole are notable exceptions, requiring no change in dosage in renal failure. Reductions in dosage may also be required for drugs that undergo hepatic elimination, especially in patients with biliary dysfunction or cirrhosis. Dialysis, especially hemodialysis, may markedly decrease the plasma levels of many antimicrobials; supplementary doses of such drugs may be required to reestablish effective plasma levels following these procedures. Drugs that are not removed from the blood by hemodialysis include amphotericin B, cefonicid, cefoperazone, ceftriaxone, erythromycin, nafcillin, tetracyclines, and vancomycin.

Table 52–3. Elimination of commonly used antimicrobial agents.

Mode of Elimination	Drugs or Drug Groups
Renal	Acyclovir, aminoglycosides, amphotericin B, most cephalosporins, imipenem, most penicillins, sulfonamides, tetracyclines (except doxycycline), TMP-SMZ, vancomycin
Hepatic	Amphotericin B, ampicillin, cefoperazone, chloramphenicol, clindamycin, erythromycin, isoniazid, ketoconazole, nafcillin, rifampin
Hemodialysis	Acyclovir (and most antiviral agents), aminoglycosides, cephalosporins (not cefonicid, cefoperazone, ceftriaxone), penicillins (not nafcillin), sulfonamides

2. **Pregnancy and the newborn:** Antimicrobial therapy during pregnancy and the neonatal period requires special consideration. Tetracyclines cause tooth enamel dysplasia and inhibition of bone growth. Sulfonamides, by displacing bilirubin from serum albumin, may cause kernicterus in the neonate. Chloramphenicol may cause the gray baby syndrome. Other drugs that should be used with extreme caution during pregnancy include most antiviral and antifungal agents. The fluoroquinolones are not recommended for use in pregnancy or in children because of effects on growing cartilage.

3. **Drug interactions:** Interactions sometimes occur between antimicrobials and other drugs (see also Chapter 62). Interactions include enhanced nephrotoxicity or ototoxicity when aminoglycosides are given with loop diuretics, vancomycin, or cisplatin. Several drug interactions with sulfonamides are based on competition for plasma protein binding; these include excessive hypoglycemia with sulfonylureas and increased hypoprothrombinemia with warfarin. Disulfiram-like reactions to ethanol occur with metronidazole and with several newer cephalosporins (see Chapter 43). Erythromycin inhibits the hepatic metabolism of a number of drugs, including phenytoin, terfenadine, theophylline, and warfarin. Rifampin, a strong inducer of hepatic drug-metabolizing enzymes, decreases the effects of digoxin, ketoconazole, oral contraceptives, propranolol, quinidine, and warfarin.

E. **Antimicrobial Drug Combinations:** Therapy with multiple antimicrobials may be indicated in the following clinical situations:

1. **Emergency situations:** In severe infections (eg, sepsis, meningitis), combinations of antimicrobial drugs are used empirically to suppress all of the most likely pathogens.

2. **To delay resistance:** The combined use of drugs is valid in situations where the rapid emergence of resistance impairs the chances for cure. For this reason, combined drug therapy is especially important in the treatment of tuberculosis.

3. **Mixed infections:** Multiple organisms may be involved in some infections. For example, peritoneal infections may be caused by several pathogens (eg, anaerobes and coliforms); a combination of drugs may be required to achieve coverage. Skin infections are often due to mixed bacterial, fungal, or viral pathogens.

4. **To achieve synergistic effects:** The use of a drug combination against a specific pathogen may result in an effect that is greater than that achieved with a single drug. Examples include the use of penicillins with gentamicin in enterococcal endocarditis, the use of a beta-lactam drug plus an aminoglycoside in *Pseudomonas aeruginosa* infections, and the combined use of amphotericin B and flucytosine in cryptococcal meningitis.

   In terms of bactericidal actions, the outcome of the combined use of two antimicrobials may be indifference, synergism, potentiation, or antagonism (see Chapter 62). Such actions are more readily demonstrated in vitro than at the clinical level. Some mechanisms that may account for synergism follow.

   a. **Sequential blockade:** The combined use of drugs may cause inhibition of two or more steps in a metabolic pathway. For example, trimethoprim and sulfamethoxazole (TMP-SMZ) block different steps in the formation of tetrahydrofolic acid.

   b. **Blockade of drug-inactivating enzymes:** Clavulanic acid, sulbactam, and tazobactam inhibit penicillinases and are often combined with penicillinase-sensitive beta-lactam drugs.

   c. **Enhanced drug uptake:** Increased permeability to aminoglycosides after exposure of certain bacteria to cell wall-inhibiting antimicrobials (eg, beta-lactams) is thought to underlie synergistic effects.

F. **Antimicrobial Chemoprophylaxis:** The general principles of antimicrobial chemoprophylaxis can be summarized as follows: (1) Prophylaxis should always be directed towards a *specific pathogen*, (2) *no resistance* should develop during the period of drug use, (3) prophylactic drug use should be of *limited duration*, (4) conventional *therapeutic doses* should be employed, and (5) prophylaxis should be employed only in situations of documented *drug efficacy*.

Examples of clinical situations in which nonsurgical antimicrobial prophylaxis is highly effective are given in Table 52–4. These include contacts in cases of meningococcal infections, gonorrhea, syphilis, and tuberculosis, as well as prophylaxis against streptococcal infections in patients with rheumatic fever. Though somewhat less effective, antimicrobial prophylaxis is also commonly used for animal or human bite wounds, influenza A, recurrent otitis media, and chronic bronchitis. Severely leukopenic patients are often given prophylactic antibiotics.

Table 52–4. Examples of nonsurgical antimicrobial prophylaxis with established efficacy.

Disease Prevented	Subjects for Prophylaxis	Drug(s)	Comments
Group A streptococcal infection	Prior rheumatic fever or rheumatic heart disease	Penicillin G, sulfadiazine	Does not prevent endocarditis
Meningococcal infection	Close contacts of index case	Rifampin, minocycline	
Gonorrhea	1. Contacts of index case 2. Newborn	1. As for active gonorrhea 2. Silver nitrate	
Syphilis	Contacts of index case	Benzathine penicillin G	
Urinary tract infections	History of recurrent UTI	TMP-SMZ	Alternatively, treat each episode
Pneumocystis carinii pneumonia	Immunosuppressed	TMP-SMZ	Aerosolized pentamidine is an alternative

Prophylaxis against postsurgical infections should be limited to procedures that are associated with infection in more than 5% of cases under optimal conditions. Prophylaxis should embody the principles listed above, with drug selection based on the most likely infecting organism, and treatment initiated just prior to surgery and continued for no more than 24–48 hours. Ideally, the agent should be nontoxic and not essential for treatment of severe microbial infections. Situations in which surgical prophylaxis is of benefit (or commonly used) include gastrointestinal procedures, vaginal hysterectomy, cesarean section, joint replacement, open fracture surgery, and dental procedures in patients with valvular disease or prostheses.

QUESTIONS

DIRECTIONS: Each of the numbered items or incomplete statements in this section is followed by answers or by completions of the statement. Select the ONE lettered answer or completion that is BEST in each case.

Items 1–3: A hospitalized AIDS patient is receiving zidovudine, but no antimicrobial prophylaxis. He develops sepsis with fever, suspected to be caused by a gram-negative bacillus. Treatment will include antibiotics, and the drugs under consideration include aminoglycosides, cephalosporins, fluoroquinolones, and imipenem.

1. Antimicrobial treatment of this severely immune-depressed patient should not be initiated before
   (A) The pathogen has been identified by the microbiology laboratory
   (B) The results of a gram stain are available
   (C) Specimens have been taken for laboratory tests and examinations
   (D) Antipyretic drugs have been given to reduce body temperature
   (E) The results of antibacterial drug susceptibility tests are available

2. If an aminoglycoside is used systemically in the treatment of this patient, monitoring of serum drug level is important because
   (A) If administered orally, the drug is unstable in gastric acid
   (B) The drug's antibacterial action will be antagonized by cephalosporins
   (C) The aminoglycosides have a narrow therapeutic window
   (D) The aminoglycoside will not readily penetrate into the cerebrospinal fluid
   (E) The aminoglycosides are hematotoxic

3. A combination of drugs might be given to this patient to provide coverage of multiple organisms or to obtain a synergistic action. Examples of antimicrobial drug synergism established at the clinical level include all of the following EXCEPT
   (A) Penicillin and vancomycin in enterococcal infections
   (B) Amphotericin B and flucytosine in cryptococcal meningitis
   (C) Carbenicillin and gentamicin in pseudomonal infections
   (D) Penicillin and tetracycline in bacterial meningitis
   (E) Trimethoprim and sulfamethoxazole in coliform infections

Items 4–5: A 27-year-old pregnant patient with a past history of pyelonephritis has developed a severe upper respiratory tract infection that appears to be due to a bacterial pathogen. The woman is hospitalized and an antibacterial agent is to be selected for treatment.

4. Assuming that the physician is concerned about the effects of renal impairment on drug dosage in this patient, which one of the following drugs is LEAST likely to require dosage reduction, even if creatinine clearance is less than 10 mL/min?

   (A) Trimethoprim-sulfamethoxazole
   (B) Clindamycin
   (C) Cefazolin
   (D) Ampicillin
   (E) Tetracycline

5. Because of their possible teratogenic or toxic effects in this pregnant patient, all of the following drugs should be avoided (or used with extreme caution) EXCEPT

   (A) Sulfadiazine
   (B) Metronidazole
   (C) Ciprofloxacin
   (D) Tetracycline
   (E) Erythromycin

6. A common drug interaction that occurs with the use of antimicrobial drugs, particularly drugs that have a wide antibacterial spectrum of activity, is

   (A) Antabuse-like reactions when ethanol is ingested
   (B) Increased ototoxicity if administered to a patient on furosemide
   (C) Enhancement of the anticoagulant effects of warfarin
   (D) Increased adverse effects if acetaminophen is administered as an antipyretic
   (E) Hypertension with ingestion of red wine and cheese

7. Antimicrobial prophylaxis is of established benefit in all of the following situations EXCEPT

   (A) Contacts of the index case in gonorrhea
   (B) Traveler's diarrhea
   (C) Contacts of the index case in mycoplasmal pneumonia
   (D) Recurrent urinary tract infection
   (E) Tuberculin convertors

8. Established mechanisms of antimicrobial drug synergy include all of the following EXCEPT

   (A) Drugs A and B block successive steps in a bacterial metabolic pathway
   (B) Drug A promotes the accumulation of drug B within the bacterium
   (C) Drug A induces enzymes that convert drug B to a more polar form
   (D) Drug A inhibits an enzyme that inactivates drug B

Items 9–10: A 48-year-old patient is scheduled for a vaginal hysterectomy. An antimicrobial drug will be used for prophylaxis against postoperative infection. It is proposed that cefazolin, a first-generation cephalosporin, be given intravenously at the normal therapeutic dose immediately prior to surgery and continued until the patient is released from the hospital.

9. The proposed drug management of this patient follows all of the established principles of surgical antimicrobial practice EXCEPT

   (A) Without prophylaxis, the infection rate following this procedure exceeds 5% under optimal conditions
   (B) The drug is to be administered immediately prior to surgery
   (C) Probable pathogens do not become rapidly resistant to this drug
   (D) Nosocomial (hospital-acquired) infection will be prevented by treatment throughout the period of hospitalization
   (E) Prophylaxis has documented efficacy in this type of surgical procedure

10. If the above patient had been scheduled for elective colonic surgery, optimal prophylaxis against infection would be achieved by mechanical bowel preparation and the use of

    (A) Intravenous cefotetan
    (B) Oral ampicillin
    (C) Oral neomycin and erythromycin
    (D) Intravenous third-generation cephalosporin
    (E) Oral fluoroquinolone

11. Antimicrobial drugs known to affect the metabolism of other pharmacological agents or endogenous compounds include all of the following EXCEPT

(A) Chloramphenicol
(B) Ampicillin
(C) Erythromycin
(D) Rifampin
(E) Ketoconazole

12. Antimicrobial drugs that require supplementation of dosage following hemodialysis include all of the following EXCEPT
(A) Vancomycin
(B) Cefazolin
(C) Ampicillin
(D) Ganciclovir
(E) Gentamicin

ANSWERS

1. To delay therapy until laboratory results are available is inappropriate in serious bacterial infections, but specimens for possible laboratory identification must be obtained before drugs are administered. The answer is **(C)**.

2. Monitoring plasma aminoglycoside levels is important because these drugs have a low therapeutic index; toxicity occurs when plasma levels are only 2–3 times higher than those needed for antibacterial action. Decreases in renal function may elevate the plasma levels of aminoglycosides to toxic levels within a few hours. The answer is **(C)**.

3. Combinations of antimicrobial drugs are not always synergistic. In the treatment of bacterial meningitis, two drugs may *not* be better than one. For example, the combination of penicillin and a tetracycline cures fewer patients with pneumococcal meningitis than the same dose of penicillin used alone. The answer is **(D)**.

4. Antimicrobial drugs that are eliminated via hepatic metabolism or biliary excretion include erythromycin, cefoperazone, clindamycin, doxycycline, isoniazid, ketoconazole, and nafcillin. The answer is **(B)**.

5. Several groups of antimicrobial drugs are relatively safe in pregnancy, including penicillins, cephalosporins, the macrolides, and the lincosamides. The answer is **(E)**.

6. Disturbance of the gut microbial flora often leads to decreased availability of vitamin K, with enhancement of the anticoagulant effects of coumarins. The answer is **(C)**. Can you name the drugs in the other drug interactions listed?

7. Tetracycline has been administered to subjects exposed to mycoplasmal pneumonia, but the effectiveness of such treatment has not been documented. The answer is **(C)**.

8. Increased activity of enzymes that make drugs more polar is likely to inactivate an antimicrobial drug and will not lead to increased antibacterial activity. Specific examples of mechanisms that *do* result in synergy include **(A)** the combination of trimethoprim and sulfamethoxazole; **(B)** the combination of a penicillin and an aminoglycoside; **(D)** the combination of clavulanic acid and amoxicillin. The answer is **(C)**.

9. With few exceptions, the postoperative use of prophylactic antibiotics should not be continued beyond 24 hours. Following routine surgical procedures, the risk of superinfection (from disturbances in microbial flora) *increases* in a hospitalized patient if prophylaxis is prolonged; there is also more likelihood of drug toxicity. The answer is **(D)**.

10. The second-generation cephalosporin, cefotetan, is more active than cefazolin against bowel anaerobes such as *B fragilis,* and is sometimes used for prophylaxis in "dirty" surgical procedures. However, for elective bowel surgery most authorities favor the oral use of neomycin together with a poorly absorbed formulation of erythromycin. In cases of bowel perforation, the use of cefoxitin (or cefotetan) is more appropriate. The answer is **(C)**.

11. Chloramphenicol, ketoconazole, and erythromycin can inhibit the hepatic metabolism of various drugs. Rifampin is an inducer of liver microsomal drug-metabolizing enzymes. The answer is **(B)**.

12. Vancomycin is not removed from the blood during hemodialysis, and no change in dosage is required. The answer is **(A)**.

53

Basic Principles of Antiparasitic Chemotherapy

OBJECTIVES

You should be able to:

- Describe the mechanisms of drugs whose targets are enzymes unique to parasites, ie, not found in host cells.
- Describe the mechanisms of drugs whose targets are enzymes indispensable to parasites but not to their hosts.
- Describe the mechanisms of drugs whose targets are biochemical functions common to host and parasite cells.

Learn the definitions that follow.

Table 53–1. Definitions.

Term	Definition
Glycosome	A membrane-bounded intracellular organelle in trypanosomes that contains glycolytic enzymes
Hydrogenosome	A membrane-bounded intracellular organelle in certain anaerobic protozoans that contains hydrogenase
Salvage enzymes	Nucleoside phosphotransferases involved in the salvage of purines and pyrimidines in protozoans
Suicide substrate	A chemical that forms a stable complex with an enzyme leading to its irreversible inhibition; suicide compounds are chemically related to natural enzyme substrates
Sequential blockade	The term describes the actions of two or more drugs that act at sequential steps in a metabolic pathway of a microorganism

CONCEPTS

Rational approaches to antiparasite chemotherapy utilize the principle of **selective toxicity,** which exploits biochemical and physiologic differences between parasite and host cells. Many antiparasitic agents target enzymes that are unique to, or indispensable to, parasites; other drugs affect cellular functions common to both host and parasite cells (Table 53–2).

A. Mechanisms Involving Enzymes Unique to Parasites: These enzymes are not found in the host's cells.

  1. **Dihydropteroate synthase:** Sporozoans (*Plasmodium, Toxoplasma,* and *Eimeria* spp) lack the ability to utilize exogenous folate and therefore possess enzymes for its synthesis; these enzymes can be inhibited by drugs. **Sulfonamides,** which are antimetabolites of PABA, inhibit dihydropteroate synthase. **Sequential blockade** can be achieved with a sulfonamide and an inhibitor of dihydrofolate reductase (eg, pyrimethamine); such drug combinations are effective in malaria and toxoplasmosis.

  2. **Pyruvate-ferredoxin oxidoreductase:** Certain anaerobic protozoans (*Trichomonas, Entamoeba*) lack mitochondria and possess a pyruvate-ferredoxin oxidoreductase of low redox potential that generates acetyl-CoA via electron transport. In trichomonal flagellates, this enzyme is coupled to a hydrogenase located in hydrogenosomes. Under anaerobic conditions, electron transport results in formation of hydrogen. The system also transfers elec-

Table 53–2. Identified targets and mechanisms of action of some antiparasitic drugs.

Mechanism	Parasites	Examples of Drugs
Act on enzymes specific to parasites		
Dihydropteroate synthase	Sporozoa	Sulfonamides, sulfones
Pyruvate-ferredoxin oxidoreductase	Anaerobic protozoa	Nitroimidazoles
Nucleoside phosphoreductase	Flagellated protozoa	Allopurinol riboside
Trypanothione reductase	Kinetoplastida	Nifurtimox, melarsoprol
Act on enzymes indispensable to parasites		
Purine phosphoribosyl transferase	Protozoa	Allopurinol
Ornithine decarboxylase	Protozoa	α-Difluoromethylornithine
Glycolytic enzymes	Kinetoplastida	Glycerol plus salicylhydroxamic acid and suramin
Act on functions common to both host and parasites[1]		
Thiamine transporter	Coccidia	Amprolium
Mitochondrial electron transporter	Coccidia	4-Hydroxyquinolines
Microtubules	Helminths	Benzimidazoles
Neurotransmission, muscle contraction	Helminths and ectoparasites	Levamisole, piperazines, avermectins, milbemycins

[1] Differences in the structures of regulatory macromolecules among parasites and host cells and differences in drug access may account for the selective toxicities of drugs in this subgroup.

trons from pyruvate to the nitro groups of nitroimidazoles (eg, **metronidazole**), forming cytotoxic products that inhibit growth by binding to the parasite's proteins and DNA.

3. **Nucleoside phosphotransferases:** Protozoan parasites depend critically on purine salvage pathways because these organisms are unable to synthesize purine nucleotides de novo. In *Leishmania,* purine nucleoside phosphotransferase (a **salvage enzyme** that transfers phosphate groups to the 5′ position of purine nucleosides) also phosphorylates purine nucleoside analogues such as **allopurinol riboside, formycin B,** and **thiopurinol riboside.** The triphosphate derivatives of these drugs may be incorporated into nucleic acids or may inhibit enzymes in purine metabolism. Toxicity is low because mammalian cells lack this salvage enzyme.

Trichomonads need to salvage pyrimidines (as well as purines), since these organisms lack dihydrofolate reductase and thymidylate synthase. Conversion of exogenous thymidine to thymidine 5′-phosphate can only be carried out in these parasites by the action of a thymidine phosphotransferase. This enzyme can be selectively inhibited by antimetabolites (eg, **guanosine**).

4. **Trypanothione reductase:** In the protozoans known as kinetoplastidans, glutathione exists largely in the form of trypanothione, a unique conjugate with spermidine. Trypanothione, via the action of a specific trypanothione reductase, plays a central role in maintaining the reduced state of intracellular thiols and is essential for the survival of such parasites. **Nifurtimox** and certain trivalent arsenicals used as antitrypanosomal agents inhibit trypanothione reductase.

B. **Mechanisms Involving Enzymes Indispensable to Parasites:** These enzymes are present in the host as well as the parasite, but they are essential only to the parasite or they differ in their substrate specificities.

1. **Purine phosphoribosyl transferases:** Hypoxanthine-guanine phosphoribosyltransferase (HGPRTase) is a key enzyme in purine synthesis in many parasites, including *Leishmania, Schistosoma,* and *Trypanosoma* spp. **Allopurinol** is a good substrate for this enzyme in certain parasites (but not for the mammalian enzyme); the drug is metabolized to the ribotide, which is incorporated after phosphorylation into RNA forms that interfere with normal growth. Purine salvage in *Giardia* depends critically on adenine phosphoribosyltransferase and guanine phosphoribosyltransferase. Unlike mammalian forms of these enzymes, the parasitic enzymes do not utilize hypoxanthine, xanthine, or adenine as substrates and are thus amenable to inhibition by a designed inhibitor.

2. **Ornithine decarboxylase:** This enzyme controls the formation of the polyamine, putrescine, and appears to be more critical for the growth of certain parasites than for the growth of mammalian cells. **Alpha-difluoromethylornithine (DFMO)** is a **suicide substrate** of ornithine decarboxylase and has antiparasitic activity against *Trypanosoma, Plasmodium,* and *Giardia* spp. In *T brucei,* DFMO transforms the organism into a nondividing form that can be eliminated by the host immune system.

3. **Glycolytic enzymes:** The bloodstream form of the African trypanosome *T brucei* is entirely dependent on glycolysis for generation of ATP. The enzymes involved are arranged in close proximity to each other in glycosomes. Glycerol-3-phosphate oxidase is a key enzyme that can be inhibited by **salicylhydroxamic acid (SHAM),** bringing the parasite into an anaerobic state. The addition of glycerol inhibits the reversed glycerol kinase reaction, stops glycolysis, and results in the death of the parasite. Biogenesis of glycosomes may also be a target for antiparasitic drugs. Suramin, a very large, polar molecule, binds to glycolytic enzymes, and may prevent the incorporation of the enzymes into the glycosome.

C. **Mechanisms Involving Biochemical Functions Common to Host & Parasite:** Several processes that occur in both parasites and hosts are nevertheless more susceptible to inhibition in the parasite.

1. **Thiamine transporter:** Carbohydrate metabolism is the primary energy source in coccidia. Inhibition of the cellular transport of thiamine by the structurally similar agent **amprolium** leads to a deficiency of this cofactor in coccidia.

2. **Mitochondrial electron transporter:** **4-Hydroxyquinoline** drugs with anticoccidial effects interact with components of the respiratory chain that are specific to *Eimeria* spp and inhibit electron transport in the mitochondria of these organisms. Mitochondrial respiration in other parasites and in mammals is not inhibited by these drugs.

3. **Microtubules:** The microtubules of the cytoskeleton and mitotic spindle consist of tubulin polymers. These tubulins are heterogeneous among species. Structural features of alpha-tubulins in helminths may account for the selective toxicity of benzimidazole drugs (eg, **mebendazole**). These agents bind to microtubules in helminths to block transport processes.

4. **Neurotransmission and muscle contraction:** The antiparasitic effect of nicotinic agonist drugs (eg, **levamisole, pyrantel pamoate**) in nematodes is caused by stimulation of neuromuscular transmission, which leads to muscle contraction. **Piperazine** acts as a GABA receptor agonist in nematodes, causing flaccid paralysis; facilitation of the actions of GABA appears to underlie the actions of **milbemycins** and **avermectins.** These natural products do not cross the blood-brain barrier in mammalian hosts and are relatively nontoxic. **Praziquantel,** an antischistosomal and antitapeworm agent, stimulates Ca^{2+} entry into muscles of these parasites and causes unphysiologic contraction.

QUESTIONS

DIRECTIONS: Each of the numbered items or incomplete statements in this section is followed by answers or by completions of the statement. Select the ONE lettered answer or completion that is BEST in each case.

1. Certain anaerobic protozoan parasites lack mitochondria and generate energy-rich compounds, such as acetyl-CoA, by means of enzymes present in organelles called hydrogenosomes. An important enzyme involved in this process is
   (A) Cytochrome P450
   (B) Glycerol-3-phosphate oxidase
   (C) Pyruvate-ferredoxin oxidoreductase
   (D) Hypoxanthine-guanine phosphoribosyltransferase
   (E) Thymidylate synthase

2. Which of the following compounds is a good substrate for hypoxanthine-guanine phosphoribosyltransferase in trypanosomes (but not mammals) and is eventually converted into metabolites that are incorporated into RNA?
   (A) Alpha-difluoromethylornithine
   (B) Salicylhydroxamic acid

    (C) Allopurinol

    (D) Mebendazole

    (E) Glycerol

3. One chemotherapeutic strategy used to eradicate the bloodstream form of African trypanosomes is based on the absolute dependence of the organism on

    (A) Mitochondrial respiration

    (B) Cytochrome-dependent electron transfer

    (C) Lactate dehydrogenase

    (D) Glycolysis

    (E) Dihydropteroate synthesis

4. Which of the following drugs enhances GABA actions on the neuromuscular junctions of nematodes and arthropods?

    (A) Pyrantel pamoate

    (B) Ivermectin

    (C) Picrotoxin

    (D) Glutamic acid

    (E) Thiamine

5. Which of the following drugs is an antimetabolite that inhibits a trypanosomal enzyme that synthesizes putrescine?

    (A) Alpha-fluorodeoxyuridine

    (B) Metronidazole

    (C) Thiopurinol riboside

    (D) Alpha-difluoromethylornithine

    (E) Polymyxin

6. All of the following statements about the mechanisms of action of antiparasitic drugs are accurate EXCEPT

    (A) 4-Hydroxyquinolines inhibit phospholipase C

    (B) Metronidazole is activated in the parasite to a cytotoxic product

    (C) Salicylhydroxamic acid is an inhibitor of glycerol-3-phosphate oxidase

    (D) Mebendazole binds to tubulins to alter the transport functions of microtubules

7. Enzymes unique to parasites include all of the following EXCEPT

    (A) Trypanothione reductase

    (B) Dihydropteridine pyrophosphokinase

    (C) Hypoxanthine-guanine phosphoribosyltransferase

    (D) Purine nucleoside phosphotransferase

8. All of the following statements about specific antiparasitic drugs are accurate EXCEPT

    (A) Sulfadoxine is an inhibitor of dihydropteroate synthase in the malarial parasite

    (B) Allopurinol riboside is a potent inhibitor of mitochondrial electron transfer

    (C) Amprolium is an inhibitor of thiamine transport in *Eimeria* spp

    (D) Suramin binds to glycolytic enzymes and prevents their incorporation into glycosomes

ANSWERS

1. In *T vaginalis,* conversion of pyruvate to acetyl-CoA takes place via the actions of pyruvate-ferredoxin oxidoreductase. The answer is **(C).**

2. Allopurinol is a good substrate for HGPRTase in trypanosomes but not mammals. Recall that allopurinol is also an inhibitor of xanthine oxidase and is used in gout and cancer chemotherapy. The answer is **(C).**

3. Glycolytic enzyme inhibitors (such as SHAM) that inhibit glycerol-3-phosphate oxidase may be selectively toxic to African trypanosomes. The answer is **(D).**

4. Several antiparasitic drugs enhance GABA neurotransmission in nematodes and arthropods and cause muscle paralysis. These drugs include piperazine, milbemycins, and avermectins (eg, ivermectin). The answer is **(B).**

5. DFMO is a suicide inhibitor of ornithine decarboxylase. Although it also inhibits mammalian ornithine decarboxylase, DMFO is less toxic to the host because of more rapid turnover and replacement of the irreversibly inhibited enzyme in the host than in parasites. The answer is **(D).**

6. The anticoccidial 4-aminoquinolines inhibit mitochondrial respiration in *Eimeria* spp, probably through interaction with a component between NADH oxidase and cytochrome b in the electron transport chain. The answer is **(A)**.
7. HGPRTase, an enzyme involved in purine salvage, is present in both parasites and mammals. The answer is **(C)**.
8. *Leishmania* species possess the unique salvage enzyme, purine nucleoside phosphotransferase. This enzyme phosphorylates allopurinol riboside to form the corresponding nucleotide, which interferes with purine and nucleic acid metabolism. The answer is **(B)**.

54 Antiprotozoal Drugs

OBJECTIVES

You should be able to:

- List the major groups of antiprotozoal drugs.
- Describe the pharmacodynamic and pharmacokinetic properties of the major antimalarial drugs (chloroquine, quinine, primaquine, and the antifolate agents).
- Describe the pharmacodynamic and pharmacokinetic properties of the major amebicides (diloxanide, emetine, iodoquinol, and metronidazole). List other clinical applications of metronidazole.
- Identify the major trypanosomicidal drugs and list their toxic effects.

CONCEPTS

DRUGS FOR MALARIA

Malaria parasites have a complex life cycle that permits drug action at several points. *Plasmodium* species that infect humans (*P falciparum, P malariae, P ovale, P vivax*) are spread by the female *Anopheles* mosquito and, after inoculation into the human host, undergo a primary developmental stage in the liver (primary tissue phase). They then enter the blood and parasitize erythrocytes (erythrocytic phase). *P falciparum* and *P malariae* have only one cycle of liver cell invasion; thereafter, multiplication is confined to erythrocytes. The other species have a dormant hepatic stage (in which they become **hypnozoites**) that is responsible for recurrent infections and relapses after apparent recovery of the host from the initial infection.

Primary tissue **schizonticides** (eg, primaquine) kill schizonts in the liver soon after infection, whereas blood schizonticides (eg, chloroquine, quinine) kill these parasitic forms only in the erythrocyte. Antimalarial drugs may exert multiple actions. Primaquine is **gametocidal,** since it kills gametes in the blood; the drug also destroys the secondary exoerythrocytic (liver) schizonts that cause the relapsing fevers of malaria. **Sporonticides** (proguanil, pyrimethamine) prevent sporogony and multiplication in the mosquito (Table 54–1).

A. **Chloroquine:**
   1. **Classification and pharmacokinetics:** Chloroquine is a 4-aminoquinoline derivative. The drug is rapidly absorbed when given orally, is widely distributed to tissues, and has an extremely large volume of distribution. Chloroquine is excreted largely unchanged in the urine.
   2. **Mechanism of action:** Chloroquine forms a complex with hemin that has deleterious effects on cellular membranes. Chloroquine is a weak base and may buffer intracellular pH,

Table 54–1. Drugs used in malaria.

Drug	Acute Attacks	Eradication of Liver Stages	Prophylaxis
Chloroquine	Yes	No	Yes, except in regions where *P falciparum* is resistant
Quinine, mefloquine	Yes, in resistant *P falciparum*	No	Yes, mefloquine is used in regions with chloroquine-resistant *P falciparum*
Primaquine	No	Yes, *(P vivax, P ovale)*	Yes, but only if exposed to *P vivax* or *P ovale*
Antifols	Yes, but only in resistant *P falciparum*	No	Not usually advised

thereby inhibiting cellular invasion by parasitic organisms. The selective toxicity of the drug is due to an energy-dependent carrier mechanism in parasitized cells. Chloroquine-resistant parasites are able to expel the drug via a membrane P-glycoprotein pump.

3. **Clinical use:** Chloroquine is used for acute attacks of malaria and as a chemosuppressant, except in regions where *P falciparum* is resistant. The drug is solely a blood schizonticide and will not eradicate secondary tissue schizonts. Chloroquine is also used in amebic liver disease and in autoimmune disorders.

4. **Toxicity:** At low doses, chloroquine causes gastrointestinal irritation, skin rash, and headaches. High doses may cause severe skin lesions, peripheral neuropathies, myocardial depression, retinal damage, auditory impairment, and toxic psychosis. Chloroquine may also precipitate porphyria attacks.

B. Quinine & Mefloquine:

1. **Classification and pharmacokinetics:** Quinine is the principal alkaloid derived from the bark of the cinchona tree. Quinine is rapidly absorbed orally and is metabolized before renal excretion. Intravenous administration of quinine is possible in severe infections.

   Mefloquine is a synthetic 4-quinoline derivative chemically related to quinine. Because of local irritation, mefloquine can only be given orally, although it is subject to variable absorption. Mefloquine binds to plasma and tissue proteins and has a long plasma half-life (>6 days).

2. **Mechanism of action:** Quinine complexes with double-stranded DNA to prevent strand separation, resulting in block of DNA replication and transcription to RNA. The mechanism of action of mefloquine is unknown but does not appear to involve binding to DNA. Quinine and mefloquine are blood schizonticides and have no effect on liver stages of the malaria parasite.

3. **Clinical use:** The main use of these drugs is in *P falciparum* infections resistant to chloroquine. To delay emergence of resistance, the drugs should not be used routinely for prophylaxis.

4. **Toxicity:** Quinine commonly causes **cinchonism,** whose symptoms include gastrointestinal distress, headache, vertigo, blurred vision, and tinnitus. Severe overdose results in disturbances in cardiac conduction that resemble quinidine toxicity. Hematotoxic effects occur, including hemolysis in glucose-6-phosphate dehydrogenase-deficient patients. **Blackwater fever** (intravascular hemolysis) is a rare and sometimes fatal complication in quinine-sensitized persons.

   Mefloquine is less toxic than quinine; its adverse effects include gastrointestinal distress, skin rash, headache, and dizziness. At high doses, mefloquine may cause neurologic symptoms and seizures.

C. Primaquine:

1. **Classification and pharmacokinetics:** Primaquine is a synthetic 8-aminoquinoline. Absorption is complete after oral administration and is followed by extensive metabolism.

2. **Mechanism of action:** The drug forms quinoline-quinone metabolites, which are electron-transferring redox compounds that act as cellular oxidants. The drug is a tissue schizonticide and also limits malaria transmission by acting as a gametocide.

3. **Clinical use:** Primaquine is not effective in acute attacks but is used to eradicate liver stages of *P vivax* and *P ovale*. The drug should be used in conjunction with a blood schizonticide.

4. **Toxicity:** Primaquine is usually well tolerated but may cause gastrointestinal distress, pruritus, headaches, and methemoglobinemia. More serious toxicity involves hemolysis in glucose-6-phosphate dehydrogenase-deficient patients; this is thought to be a result of the formation of redox intermediates.

D. Antifolate Drugs:

1. **Classification and pharmacokinetics:** This group includes pyrimethamine, proguanil, sulfadoxine, and dapsone. All of these drugs are absorbed orally and are excreted in the urine, partly in unchanged form. Proguanil has a shorter half-life (12–16 hr) than other drugs in this subclass (half-life >100 hr).

2. **Mechanisms of action:** Sulfonamides act as antimetabolites of PABA and block folic acid synthesis in certain protozoans by inhibiting dihydropteroate synthase. Proguanil (chloroguanide) is bioactivated to cycloguanil. Pyrimethamine and cycloguanil are selective inhibitors of protozoan dihydrofolate reductases, preventing formation of tetrahydrofolate. The combination of pyrimethamine with sulfadoxine has synergistic antimalarial effects through the **sequential blockade** of two steps in folic acid synthesis.

3. **Clinical use:** The antifols are blood schizonticides that act mainly against *P falciparum*. Pyrimethamine with sulfadoxine in fixed combination (Fansidar) is used in the treatment of chloroquine-resistant forms of this species, although the onset of activity is slow. Many strains of *P falciparum* are now resistant to antifols, and the drugs are not commonly used for prophylaxis due to their toxic potential. However, pyrimethamine with sulfadiazine is the treatment of choice in toxoplasmosis.

4. **Toxicity:** The toxic effects of sulfonamides include skin rashes, gastrointestinal distress, hemolysis, kidney damage, and drug interactions caused by competition for plasma protein binding sites. Pyrimethamine may cause folic acid deficiency when used in high doses.

DRUGS FOR AMEBIASIS

Tissue amebicides (**chloroquine, emetines, metronidazole**) act on organisms in the bowel wall and the liver; luminal amebicides (**diloxanide furoate, iodoquinol, paromomycin**) act only in the lumen of the bowel. The choice of a drug depends on the form of amebiasis. For asymptomatic disease, diloxanide furoate is the choice. For mild-to-severe intestinal infection, metronidazole is used with diloxanide furoate or iodoquinol. The latter regimen, plus chloroquine, is recommended in amebic liver abscess (see Table 54–2). The mechanisms of amebicidal action of most drugs in this subclass are unknown.

A. Diloxanide Furoate: This drug is commonly used as the sole agent for the treatment of asymptomatic amebiasis, and is also useful in mild intestinal disease when used with other drugs. Diloxanide furoate is converted in the gut to the diloxanide free-base form, which is the active amebicide. Toxic effects are mild and are usually restricted to gastrointestinal symptoms.

B. Emetines: Emetine and dehydroemetine inhibit protein synthesis by blocking ribosomal movement along messenger RNA. These alkaloids are used as back-up drugs for treatment of

Table 54–2. Drugs used in the treatment of amebiasis.[1]

Disease Form	Drug(s) of Choice	Alternative Drug(s)
Asymptomatic intestinal	Diloxanide furoate	Iodoquinol, paromomycin
Mild-to-severe intestinal	Metronidazole plus diloxanide or iodoquinol	Diloxanide (plus doxycycline), chloroquine, paromomycin
Hepatic abscess	Metronidazole plus diloxanide, followed by chloroquine	Emetines, followed by chloroquine plus diloxanide

[1] Adapted, with permission, from Katzung BG (editor): *Basic & Clinical Pharmacology*, 6th ed. Appleton & Lange, 1995.

severe intestinal or hepatic amebiasis in hospitalized patients. Emetines are given parenterally, are widely distributed to tissues, and are excreted slowly by the kidney. The drugs may cause severe toxicity, including gastrointestinal distress, muscle weakness, and cardiovascular dysfunction (arrhythmias and congestive heart failure).

C. Iodoquinol: Iodoquinol is a halogenated hydroxyquinoline with an unknown mechanism of action. The drug is an orally active luminal amebicide used as an alternative drug for mild-to-severe intestinal infections. Adverse gastrointestinal effects are common but usually mild. Systemic absorption after high doses may lead to thyroid enlargement and neurotoxic effects, including peripheral neuropathy and visual dysfunction.

D. Metronidazole:
   1. **Pharmacokinetics:** Metronidazole is effective orally and distributed widely to tissues. Elimination of the drug requires hepatic metabolism.
   2. **Mechanism of action:** Metronidazole undergoes a reductive bioactivation of its nitro group by ferredoxin (present in anaerobic parasites) to form reactive cytotoxic products.
   3. **Clinical use:** Metronidazole is the drug of choice in severe intestinal wall disease and in hepatic abscess and other extraintestinal amebic disease. Metronidazole is commonly used with a luminal amebicide. Other important clinical uses of metronidazole include treatment of trichomoniasis, giardiasis, and infections caused by *Gardnerella vaginalis* and anaerobic bacteria *(B fragilis, C difficile)*.
   4. **Toxicity:** Adverse effects include gastrointestinal irritation, headache, and discoloration of urine. More serious toxicity includes leukopenia, dizziness, and ataxia. Drug interactions with metronidazole include a disulfiram-like reaction with ethanol and potentiation of coumarin anticoagulant effects. Because of its teratogenicity in animals, the drug should be avoided in pregnant women and in nursing mothers.

E. Paromomycin: This drug is an aminoglycoside antibiotic used as a second-line luminal amebicide. Adverse gastrointestinal effects are common, and systemic absorption may lead to headaches, dizziness, rashes, and arthralgia. Tetracyclines (eg, doxycycline) are sometimes used with a luminal amebicide in mild intestinal disease.

DRUGS FOR TRYPANOSOMIASIS

A. Pentamidine:
   1. **Classification and pharmacokinetics:** Pentamidine is an aromatic diamidine. For systemic effect, the drug is administered parenterally. Pentamidine is strongly bound to tissues, has a long half-life (2–4 weeks), and is excreted unchanged in the urine. The drug may be used as an aerosol for prophylaxis of *Pneumocystis carinii* pneumonia.
   2. **Mechanism of action:** The mechanism of action is unknown, but may involve inhibition of glycolysis or interference with nucleic acid metabolism of trypanosomes. Preferential accumulation of the drug by the parasite may account for its selective toxicity.
   3. **Clinical use:** Pentamidine is commonly used in the hemolymphatic stages of disease caused by *Trypanosoma gambiense* and *T rhodesiense*. Because it does not cross the blood-brain barrier, pentamidine is not used in later stages of trypanosomiasis. Other clinical uses include the prophylaxis and therapy of *Pneumocystis carinii* infections (eg, AIDS patients) and treatment of the kala azar form of leishmaniasis (Table 54–3).
   4. **Toxicity:** Adverse effects following parenteral use include respiratory stimulation followed by depression, hypotension due to peripheral vasodilation, nephrotoxicity, and pancreatic beta cell dysfunction. Systemic toxicity in AIDS patients is reduced by aerosol inhalation.

B. Other Trypanosomicidal Agents:
   1. **Melarsoprol (Mel B):** This drug is an organic arsenical that inhibits enzyme sulfhydryl groups. Because it enters the CNS, melarsoprol is the drug of choice in African sleeping sickness. Melarsoprol is given parenterally because it causes gastrointestinal irritation; it may cause a reactive encephalopathy that can be fatal.
   2. **Nifurtimox:** This drug is a nitrofurazone derivative that inhibits the unique enzyme try-

Table 54–3. Drugs used in the treatment of other protozoal infections.

Drug	Primary Indications
Melarsoprol	Drug of choice in African sleeping sickness (late, CNS stage of trypanosomiasis); also used in mucocutaneous forms of the disease
Nifurtimox	Trypanosomiasis due to *T cruzi*
Pentamidine	Hemolymphatic stage of trypanosomiasis; also used in *Pneumocystis carinii* pneumonia
Pyrimethamine plus sulfadiazine	Drug combination of choice in toxoplasmosis
Sodium stibogluconate	Drug of choice for leishmaniasis (all species)
Suramin	Drug of choice for hemolymphatic stage of trypanosomiasis *(T brucei gambiense, T rhodesiense)*
Trimethoprim-sulfamethoxazole	Drug combination of choice in *Pneumocystis carinii* infections

panothione reductase. Nifurtimox is the drug of choice in American trypanosomiasis and has also been effective in mucocutaneous leishmaniasis. The drug causes severe toxicity, including allergies, gastrointestinal irritation, and CNS effects.

3. **Suramin:** This polyanionic drug has been used for the early stages of African trypanosomiasis (before CNS involvement). Suramin is used parenterally and causes skin rashes, gastrointestinal distress, and neurologic complications.

DRUGS FOR LEISHMANIASIS

Leishmania, parasitic protozoa transmitted by flesh-eating flies, cause various diseases ranging from cutaneous or mucocutaneous lesions to splenic and hepatic enlargement with fever. **Sodium stibogluconate** (pentavalent antimony), the primary drug in all forms of the disease, appears to kill the parasite by inhibition of glycolysis or effects on nucleic acid metabolism. Alternative agents include pentamidine (for visceral leishmaniasis), metronidazole (for cutaneous lesions), and amphotericin B (for mucocutaneous leishmaniasis).

DRUG LIST

See drugs in Tables 54–1, 54–2, and 54–3.

QUESTIONS

DIRECTIONS: Each of the numbered items or incomplete statements in this section is followed by answers or by completions of the statement. Select the ONE lettered answer or completion that is BEST in each case.

1. All of the following statements about antimalarial drugs are accurate EXCEPT
   (A) Chloroquine is a blood schizonticide but does not affect secondary tissue schizonts
   (B) Proguanil is converted to a reactive metabolite that is sporonticidal
   (C) Primaquine acts primarily on exoerythrocytic stages of the malarial life cycle
   (D) Mefloquine destroys secondary exoerythrocytic schizonts
2. Which of the following antimalarial drugs causes a dose-dependent toxic state that includes flushed and sweaty skin, dizziness, nausea, diarrhea, tinnitus, blurred vision, and impaired hearing?
   (A) Amodiaquine
   (B) Primaquine
   (C) Quinine
   (D) Pyrimethamine
3. Plasmodial resistance to chloroquine is due to
   (A) Induction of inactivating enzymes
   (B) Change in receptor structure
   (C) Increase in the activity of DNA repair mechanisms
   (D) Decreased carrier-mediated drug transport

Items 4–6:   A photographer traveled in a jungle region where chloroquine resistant *P falciparum* is endemic. She took a drug for prophylaxis but nevertheless developed a severe attack of *P vivax* malaria.

4.   The drug she took for prophylaxis is probably
     (A)   Mefloquine
     (B)   Chloroquine
     (C)   Primaquine
     (D)   Pyrimethamine

5.   Which of the following drugs should be used for oral treatment of the photographer's acute attack of *P vivax* malaria?
     (A)   Chloroquine
     (B)   Mefloquine
     (C)   Primaquine
     (D)   Pyrimethamine plus dapsone

6.   Which of the following drugs should be given later in order to eradicate schizonts and latent hypnozoites in the patient's liver?
     (A)   Proguanil
     (B)   Chloroquine
     (C)   Quinine
     (D)   Primaquine

7.   All of the following statements about amebicides are accurate EXCEPT
     (A)   Paromomycin is effective in extraintestinal amebiasis
     (B)   Diloxanide furoate is a luminal amebicide
     (C)   Metronidazole has little activity in the gut lumen
     (D)   Systemic use of iodoquinol may cause thyroid enlargement and peripheral neuropathy

Items 8–9:   A male patient presents with lower abdominal discomfort, flatulence, and occasional diarrhea. A diagnosis is made of intestinal amebiasis and *E histolytica* is identified in his diarrheal stools. An oral drug is prescribed and reduces his intestinal symptoms. Later he presents with severe dysentery, right upper quadrant pain, weight loss, fever, and an enlarged liver. Amebic liver abscess is diagnosed.

8.   The drug that he *should* have been given for the initial mild-to-moderate intestinal symptoms is
     (A)   Diloxanide furoate
     (B)   Metronidazole
     (C)   Emetine
     (D)   Tetracycline

9.   The drug regimen most likely to be effective in treating both his intestinal symptoms and the hepatic abscess is
     (A)   Diloxanide plus iodoquinol
     (B)   Paromomycin plus mefloquine
     (C)   Metronidazole plus iodoquinol
     (D)   Chloroquine alone

10.   All of the following statements about antiprotozoal drugs are accurate EXCEPT
     (A)   Nifurtimox is selectively toxic to some protozoans because it inhibits trypanothione reductase
     (B)   Pyrimethamine is synergistic with sulfadoxine against malarial parasites ("sequential blockade")
     (C)   Blackwater fever occurs in patients sensitized to chloroquine
     (D)   Intravenous injection of pentamidine produces a sharp fall in blood pressure that is only partially blocked by atropine

11.   All of the following statements about antiprotozoal drugs are accurate EXCEPT
     (A)   Metronidazole may have a disulfiram-like effect with ethanol
     (B)   Irreversible retinopathy and ototoxicity may occur with long-term use of chloroquine
     (C)   Toxic effects on pancreatic B cells have been associated with pentamidine use
     (D)   Given parenterally, sodium stibogluconate may cause fatal encephalopathy

DIRECTIONS: The following section consists of a list of four to twenty-six lettered options followed by several numbered items. For each numbered item, select the ONE option that is most closely associated with it. Each answer may be selected once, more than once, or not at all.

     (A) Quinine
     (B) Primaquine
     (C) Melarsoprol
     (D) Pentamidine
     (E) Metronidazole
     (F) Nifurtimox
     (G) Sodium stibogluconate
     (H) Diloxanide furoate
     (I) Paromomycin
     (J) Emetine

12. This antimalarial drug may cause acute hemolysis in patients with glucose-6-phosphate dehydrogenase deficiency

13. This agent is used as an alternative drug in severe intestinal or hepatic amebiasis; atrial and ventricular arrhythmias have occurred during its use

14. This drug can clear trypanosomes from the blood and lymph nodes and is active in the late central nervous system stages of African sleeping sickness

15. The clinical uses of this drug include the treatment of amebiasis, trichomoniasis, giardiasis, and infections caused by anaerobic bacteria

ANSWERS

1. Mefloquine has many properties similar to those of quinine. Both drugs are effective blood schizonticides, and both have minimal effects on the secondary exoerythrocytic (liver) schizonts that cause the relapsing fevers of malaria. The answer is **(D)**.

2. These dose-related symptoms are characteristic adverse effects of cinchona alkaloids (quinine, quinidine) and are termed cinchonism. The answer is **(C)**.

3. Resistance occurs through decreases in the activity of a carrier-mediated transport system. The answer is **(D)**.

4. Mefloquine is the preferred drug for prophylaxis in regions of the world with chloroquine-resistant *P falciparum*. Doxycycline is an alternative drug for this indication. The answer is **(A)**.

5. Chloroquine is the drug of choice for the treatment of an acute attack of malaria due to *P vivax* but will not eradicate exoerythrocytic forms of the parasite. Quinine is a possible second-line drug. The answer is **(A)**.

6. Primaquine is the only antimalarial drug that reliably acts on tissue schizonts in liver cells. The answer is **(D)**.

7. Paromomycin is an aminoglycoside antibiotic used as a back-up drug in the treatment of amebiasis. The drug acts only on organisms in the lumen of the bowel because the aminoglycosides are not absorbed when used orally (Chapter 45). The answer is **(A)**.

8. Metronidazole is the drug of choice in nondysenteric amebic colitis. Diloxanide furoate is commonly used as the sole agent in asymptomatic intestinal infection and may also be used as a supplement to treatment with metronidazole. The answer is **(B)**.

9. Metronidazole plus iodoquinol (or diloxanide) is the regimen of choice for the treatment of hepatic abscess due to *E histolytica*. Chloroquine is often used as a follow-up drug. The answer is **(C)**.

10. Massive intravascular hemolysis (blackwater fever) is now a rare complication of the treatment of malaria with quinine. Blackwater fever does not occur in the few patients who may be sensitive to chloroquine. The answer is **(C)**.

11. Sodium stibogluconate is a pentavalent antimonial, the drug of choice in leishmaniasis. The drug is painful on injection, causes gastrointestinal distress, myalgia and arthralgia, but is not neurotoxic. Encephalopathy is associated with use of the trypanosomicidal drug, melarsoprol. The answer is **(D)**.

12. Primaquine is the prototypical drug that induces hemolysis in persons deficient in glucose-6-phosphate dehydrogenase. The answer is **(B)**.

13. Emetine causes severe side effects that include congestive heart failure, hypertension, and cardiac arrhythmias. The answer is **(J)**.

14. In African sleeping sickness, melarsoprol is the drug of choice because it effectively enters the CNS, unlike pentamidine. The answer is **(C)**.

15. Of the drugs listed, only metronidazole has both antiprotozoal activity and clinically useful activity in bacterial infections. The answer is **(E)**.

Antihelmintic Drugs

55

OBJECTIVES

You should be able to:

- Identify the drugs of choice for treatment of common infections caused by nematodes, trematodes, and cestodes.
- Describe the mechanisms of action (if known), important pharmacokinetic features, and the major toxic effects of these drugs.
- Describe the main features of important back-up antihelmintics.

CONCEPTS

Antihelmintic drugs have diverse chemical structures, mechanisms of action, and properties. Most were discovered by empiric screening methods; many act against specific parasites, and few are devoid of significant toxicity to host cells. In addition to the direct toxicity of the drugs, reactions to dead and dying parasites may cause serious toxicity in patients. In the text that follows the drugs are subdivided on the basis of the type of helminth affected (nematodes, trematodes, and cestodes). The drugs of choice and alternative agents for selected important helminthic infections are listed in Table 55–1.

Table 55–1. Major helmintic infections and the drugs used to treat them.

Infecting Organism	Drugs of Choice	Alternative Drugs
Nematodes *Ascaris lumbricoides* (roundworm)	Pyrantel pamoate	Levamisole, mebendazole
Necator americanus, Ancylostoma duodenale (hookworm)	Pyrantel pamoate, mebendazole	Albendazole, levamisole
Trichuris trichiura (whipworm)	Mebendazole	Albendazole, pyrantel pamoate
Strongyloides stercoralis (threadworm)	Thiabendazole	Albendazole, mebendazole
Enterobius vermicularis (pinworm)	Mebendazole, pyrantel pamoate	Albendazole
Larva migrans	Thiabendazole	Albendazole, diethylcarbamazine
Wuchereria bancrofti, Brugia malayi	Diethylcarbamazine	Ivermectin
Onchocerca volvulus	Ivermectin	Diethylcarbamazine plus suramin
Trematodes (flukes) *Schistosoma haematobium*	Praziquantel	Metrifonate
Schistosoma mansoni	Praziquantel	Oxamniquine
Schistosoma japonicum	Praziquantel	None
Paragonimus westermani	Praziquantel	Bithionol
Fasciola hepaticum	Bithionol	Dehydroemetine, praziquantel
Cestodes (tapeworms) *Taenia saginata*	Niclosamide	Praziquantel, mebendazole
Taenia solium	Niclosamide	Praziquantel, mebendazole
Diphyllobothrium latum	Niclosamide	Praziquantel
Cysticercosis	Praziquantel	None
Hydatid disease	Mebendazole	Albendazole

DRUGS THAT ACT AGAINST NEMATODES (ROUNDWORMS)

A. Mebendazole: Mebendazole acts by selectively inhibiting microtubule synthesis in nematodes. It is the drug of choice for pinworm and whipworm infections, for combined infections with ascarids and hookworm, and for treatment of hydatid disease. It is also a back-up drug in certain cestode and trematode infections. Less than 10% of the drug is absorbed systemically after oral use, and this portion is metabolized rapidly. The drug has a high therapeutic index, and its toxic effects are limited to gastrointestinal irritation. Mebendazole is contraindicated in pregnancy because of possible embryotoxicity.

B. Thiabendazole: A structural congener of mebendazole, thiabendazole has a similar action on microtubules. Thiabendazole is the drug of choice to treat threadworm infections and cutaneous and visceral forms of larva migrans. Thiabendazole is rapidly absorbed from the gut and is metabolized by liver enzymes. The drug has anti-inflammatory and immunorestorative actions in the host. Toxic effects include gastrointestinal irritation, headache, dizziness, leukopenia, hematuria, and allergic reactions, including intrahepatic cholestasis. Reactions caused by dying parasites include fever, chills, lymphadenopathy, and skin rash.

C. Diethylcarbamazine: This piperazine derivative has an unknown mechanism of action. Diethylcarbamazine is the drug of choice for filariasis and an alternative drug, when used in combination with suramin, for onchocerciasis. Microfilariae are killed more readily than adult worms. The drug is rapidly absorbed from the gut and is excreted in the urine. Toxic effects include headache, malaise, weakness, and anorexia. Reactions to proteins released by dying filariae include fever, rashes, ocular damage, joint and muscle pain, and lymphangitis. In onchocerciasis, the **Mazzotti reaction** includes most of these symptoms, as well as hypotension, pyrexia, respiratory distress, and prostration.

D. Ivermectin: Ivermectin intensifies GABA-mediated neurotransmission in nematodes and causes immobilization of parasites, facilitating their removal by the reticuloendothelial system. Selective toxicity results because GABA is a neurotransmitter in humans only in the CNS, and ivermectin does not cross the blood-brain barrier. Ivermectin, the drug of choice for onchocerciasis, acts more slowly than diethylcarbamazine and causes fewer systemic and ocular reactions. Other potential uses of ivermectin include treatment of filariasis and strongyloidiasis. Single-dose oral treatment in onchocerciasis results in multiple reactions that include fever, headache, dizziness, rashes, pruritus, tachycardia, hypotension, and pain in joints, muscles, and lymph glands. These symptoms are usually of short duration, and most can be controlled with antihistamines and nonsteroidal anti-inflammatory drugs.

E. Pyrantel Pamoate: Pyrantel pamoate and its congener, **oxantel pamoate,** cause neuromuscular blockade by interaction with nicotinic receptors, and this blockade leads to paralysis of parasites. Pyrantel pamoate is the drug of choice in *Ascaris* infections and is equivalent to mebendazole for hookworm and *Trichostrongylus* infections. Both pyrantel pamoate and oxantel pamoate are poorly absorbed from the gut when given orally. Toxic effects are minor but include gastrointestinal distress, headache, and weakness.

F. Levamisole: Levamisole causes a depolarizing neuromuscular blockade by stimulating nicotinic receptors. This agent is the drug of choice for infections caused by *Angiostrongylus cantonensis* and an alternative agent in *Ascaris* and hookworm diseases. The drug affects host defenses by promoting cell-mediated immune responses, including macrophage and T cell functions. Toxic effects of this oral drug are limited to gastrointestinal irritation. The drug is not labeled for antihelmintic use in the USA.

G. Albendazole: The mechanism of action of albendazole is unclear. The drug blocks glucose uptake in both larval and adult parasites, which leads to decreased formation of ATP and subsequent parasite immobilization. The actions of albendazole may also include inhibition of microtubule assembly, as has been described for the other benzimidazoles, mebendazole and thiabendazole. Albendazole has a wide antihelmintic spectrum and is an important alternative drug for hookworm and pinworm infections and for the treatment of ascariasis, strongyloidiasis, trichuriasis, and hydatid diseases. The drug is effective orally. Toxic effects during short courses of therapy are minimal. Reversible leukopenia, alopecia, and changes in liver enzymes may occur with prolonged use. Long-term animal toxicity studies report bone marrow suppression and fetal toxicity.

DRUGS THAT ACT AGAINST TREMATODES (FLUKES)

A. Praziquantel: Praziquantel increases membrane permeability to calcium, causing marked contraction initially and then paralysis of trematode muscles; this is followed by vacuolization and parasite death. Praziquantel is the drug of choice for schistosomiasis (all species), infections due to *Paragonimus westermani,* and certain tapeworm infections (cysticercosis, *Hymenolepis nana*). The drug is active against immature and adult schistosomal forms. Absorption from the gut is rapid, and the drug is metabolized to inactive products. Common adverse effects include headache, dizziness, malaise, and less frequently, gastrointestinal irritation, skin rash, and fever. Increased rates of abortion with praziquantel therapy preclude its use in pregnancy.

B. Bithionol: This agent is the drug of choice for treatment of fascioliasis (sheep liver fluke), and it is an alternative agent in paragonimiasis. The mechanism of action of the drug is unknown. Bithionol is orally effective and is eliminated in the urine. Common adverse effects include nausea and vomiting, diarrhea and abdominal cramps, dizziness, and headache. Less frequently, pyrexia, tinnitus, proteinuria, and leukopenia may occur.

C. Alternative Agents:
   1. **Metrifonate:** This drug is an organophosphate pro-drug that forms the cholinesterase inhibitor, dichlorvos. The active metabolite acts solely against *Schistosoma haematobium mansoni* (bilharziasis). Toxic effects occur from excess cholinergic stimulation.
   2. **Oxamniquine:** This tetrahydroquinolone derivative is effective solely in *Schistosoma mansoni* infections, acting on male immature forms and adult schistosomal forms. Dizziness is a common adverse effect; headache, gastrointestinal irritation, and pruritus may also occur. Reactions to dying parasites include eosinophilia, urticaria, and pulmonary infiltrates. It is not advisable to use the drug in pregnancy or in patients with past history of seizure disorders.

DRUGS THAT ACT AGAINST CESTODES (TAPEWORMS)

A. Niclosamide: This is the most important drug in the subclass used against cestodes. A salicylamide derivative, the drug may act by uncoupling oxidative phosphorylation or by activating ATPases. Niclosamide is a drug of choice for all tapeworm infections except cysticercosis (for which praziquantel is used) and those caused by *Echinococcus granulosus* (for which mebendazole is used). Scoleces and cestode segments are killed, but ova are not. The drug is minimally absorbed from the gut. Toxic effects are usually mild, but include gastrointestinal distress, headache, rash, and fever. Some of these effects may result from systemic absorption of antigens from disintegrating parasites.

DRUG LIST

See Table 55–1.

QUESTIONS

DIRECTIONS: Each of the numbered items or incomplete statements in this section is followed by answers or by completions of the statement. Select the ONE lettered answer or completion that is BEST in each case.

1. This drug is currently an alternative agent in onchocerciasis; its use is associated with a severe reaction (the Mazzotti reaction) from dying parasites.
    (A) Albendazole
    (B) Pyrantel pamoate
    (C) Diethylcarbamazine
    (D) Mebendazole

2. A patient with a tapeworm infection is to be treated with niclosamide. All of the following statements concerning this case and its treatment are accurate EXCEPT
    (A) Niclosamide is active against *T solium* and *T saginata*
    (B) The drug will kill ova of the parasite
    (C) The patient probably became infected by eating raw or undercooked pork or beef
    (D) Niclosamide is only effective against intestinal worms

3. The mechanism of antiparasitic action of mebendazole and thiabendazole is thought to involve
    (A) Stimulation of acetylcholine receptors at neuromuscular junctions
    (B) Inhibition of dihydrofolate reductase
    (C) Interference with microtubule synthesis and assembly
    (D) Block of thiamine transport

4. All of the following statements about pyrantel pamoate are accurate EXCEPT
    (A) Pyrantel pamoate is effective in roundworm infections
    (B) Pyrantel pamoate blocks nicotinic receptors, leading to muscle paralysis in parasites
    (C) Toxic effects of pyrantel pamoate mainly concern the gastrointestinal tract because little of an oral dose is absorbed
    (D) Pyrantel pamoate is equivalent in efficacy to niclosamide in the treatment of tapeworm infections

5. A student studying medicine at a Caribbean university develops fever, chills, and diarrhea due to *S mansoni* and oxamniquine is prescribed. All of the following statements about the proposed therapy are accurate EXCEPT
    (A) Oxamniquine is likely to be effective in all stages of the disease, including hepatosplenomegaly
    (B) Oxamniquine should not be used if the patient has a history of seizure disorders
    (C) Oxamniquine is effective in other forms of schistosomiasis
    (D) Oxamniquine is contraindicated in pregnancy

6. All of the following statements about ivermectin are accurate EXCEPT
    (A) Ivermectin is the drug of choice in onchocerciasis
    (B) Fever, rash, pruritus, and joint pain may occur during treatment of onchocerciasis with ivermectin
    (C) Ivermectin enhances the actions of GABA in neurotransmission
    (D) Ivermectin commonly causes CNS side effects

7. A young woman with a combined gastrointestinal infection due to *Ascaris* and hookworm is to be treated with mebendazole. All of the following statements about this drug therapy are accurate EXCEPT
    (A) Mebendazole would not be effective if the patient had a combined infection due to hookworm and *Trichuris*
    (B) Mebendazole has a high therapeutic index
    (C) Mebendazole is contraindicated in pregnancy
    (D) Fat-containing foods increase the oral absorption of mebendazole

8. Which ONE of the following is an alternative drug for nematode infections, including those caused by hookworm, pinworm, and roundworm? Long-term use may cause alopecia, changes in liver enzymes, and reversible leukopenia.
    (A) Albendazole
    (B) Oxantel pamoate
    (C) Diethylcarbamazine
    (D) Levamisole

9. All of the following statements about praziquantel are accurate EXCEPT
    (A) Praziquantel is effective in the treatment of trichinosis
    (B) Praziquantel causes muscle paralysis in parasites by increasing membrane permeability to calcium
    (C) Malaise, headache, anorexia, and gastrointestinal distress are less common adverse effects of praziquantel in children than in adults

(D) Praziquantel is the drug of choice for schistosomiasis

10. Which ONE of the following is thought to promote host defense mechanisms by increasing cell-mediated immune responses?
    (A) Praziquantel
    (B) Metrifonate
    (C) Levamisole
    (D) Albendazole

Items 11–12: A patient living in a rural area of the southern United States presents with fever, cough, and eosinophilia. He has had watery stools for some time. The presumptive diagnosis of strongyloidiasis is confirmed by the presence of the ova of *S stercoralis* in the stools.

11. The drug most likely to be effective in strongyloidiasis with possible pneumonitis is
    (A) Praziquantel
    (B) Niclosamide
    (C) Thiabendazole
    (D) Pyrantel pamoate

12. Which ONE of the following adverse effects of the drug is most likely to occur?
    (A) Dizziness and drowsiness
    (B) Skin rash and angioedema
    (C) Cholestatic jaundice
    (D) Peripheral neuropathy

ANSWERS

1. The Mazzotti reaction results from the rapid killing of parasites by diethylcarbamazine. The answer is **(C)**.

2. Niclosamide is the major drug used to treat cestode infections. Scoleces and cestode segments are killed, but ova are not. The answer is **(B)**.

3. Mebendazole and thiabendazole bind to tubulin and cause a selective loss of cytoplasmic microtubules in affected worms. The answer is **(C)**.

4. Pyrantel pamoate is not equivalent to niclosamide in the treatment of infections caused by cestodes. Niclosamide is the drug of choice in most tapeworm infections. The answer is **(D)**.

5. Oxamniquine is an alternative drug for *S mansoni* but is not effective against other *Schistosoma* species. CNS side effects are common, and the drug has caused seizures in susceptible persons. Oxamniquine is teratogenic in animals. The answer is **(C)**.

6. Ivermectin intensifies the actions of GABA in nematodes but not in the brain of the host; it has no CNS side effects. The answer is **(D)**.

7. Mebendazole is the drug of choice to treat combined infections caused by hookworm, pinworm, roundworm, and whipworm. Note that the drug has embryotoxic potential and is relatively contraindicated in pregnancy. The answer is **(A)**.

8. Albendazole has a wide antihelmintic spectrum and is an important back-up drug in the treatment of nematode infections. The answer is **(A)**.

9. The antiparasitic activity of praziquantel is restricted to trematodes (flukes) and does not include whipworm. The response to drug treatment of trichinosis is variable, but mebendazole with corticosteroids may be effective in severe disease. The answer is **(A)**.

10. In the United States, levamisole is currently approved only as an adjunct in the treatment of colon cancer. However, the drug is useful in hookworm infections and is the drug of choice for treatment of *Angiostrongylus cantonensis*. Properties of levamisole include stimulation of macrophage and T cell functions. The answer is **(C)**.

11. The drug of choice to treat threadworm infections is thiabendazole, which is well absorbed orally and penetrates most tissues. Ivermectin and mebendazole are possible back-up drugs. The answer is **(C)**.

12. The most frequent side effects of thiabendazole are dizziness, gastrointestinal disturbances, and drowsiness. The answer is **(A)**.

56

Cancer Chemotherapy

OBJECTIVES

You should be able to:

- Describe the relevance of cell cycle kinetics to the modes of action and clinical uses of anticancer drugs.
- Identify the major subclasses of anticancer drugs, describe the mechanisms of action of the main drugs in each subclass, and describe the mechanisms by which tumor cells develop drug resistance.
- Identify the drugs of choice for the more important neoplastic diseases and describe their pharmacokinetics and their characteristic toxic effects.
- Understand the rationale underlying the strategies of combination drug chemotherapy and rescue therapies.

Learn the definitions that follow.

Table 56–1. Definitions

Term	Definition
Cell cycle-specific (CCS) drug	An anticancer agent that acts selectively on tumor cells when they are traversing the cell cycle and not when they are in the G_0 phase
Cell cycle-nonspecific (CCNS) drug	An anticancer agent that acts on tumor cells when they are traversing the cell cycle and when they are in the resting phase
Log kill hypothesis	A concept used in cancer chemotherapy to denote that anticancer drugs kill a fixed proportion of a tumor cell population, not a fixed number of tumor cells. For example, a 1-log kill will decrease a tumor cell population by one order of magnitude, ie, 90% of the cells will be eradicated
Growth fraction	The proportion of cells in a tumor population that are actively dividing
Rescue therapy	The administration of normal metabolites to counteract the effects of anticancer drugs on normal (non-neoplastic) cells

CONCEPTS

The treatment of cancer requires a variety of different types of drugs, acting on several different targets (Figure 56–1).

CANCER CELL CYCLE KINETICS

A. Cell Cycle Kinetics: Cancer cell population kinetics and the cancer cell cycle are important determinants of the actions and clinical uses of anticancer drugs. Some anticancer drugs act specifically on tumor cells undergoing cycling (cell cycle-specific [CCS] drugs) and others (cell cycle-nonspecific [CCNS] drugs) kill tumor cells in both cycling and resting phases of the cell cycle. CCS drugs may be more active in a specific phase of the cell cycle (Figure 56–2). In general, CCS drugs are particularly effective when a large proportion of the tumor cells are proliferating (ie, when the growth fraction is high).

B. The Log Kill Hypothesis: Cytotoxic drugs act with first-order kinetics, a given dose killing a constant *proportion* of a cell population rather than a constant *number* of cells. The log kill

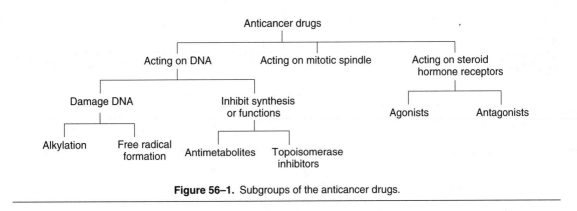

Figure 56–1. Subgroups of the anticancer drugs.

hypothesis describes the magnitude of tumor cell kill by anticancer drugs as a logarithmic function. For example, a 3-log kill dose of an effective drug will reduce a cancer cell population of 10^{12} cells to 10^9 (a total kill of $10^{12} - 10^9$ or 999×10^9 cells); the same dose would reduce a starting population of 10^6 cells to 10^3 cells (a kill of 999×10^3 cells). In both cases the dose reduces the numbers of cells by three orders of magnitude or "3 logs."

C. Resistance to Anticancer Drugs: Drug resistance is a major problem in cancer chemotherapy. In many cases, the resistance mechanisms involve changes in gene expression in neoplastic cells that can result in resistance either to an individual drug or to multiple anticancer drugs.

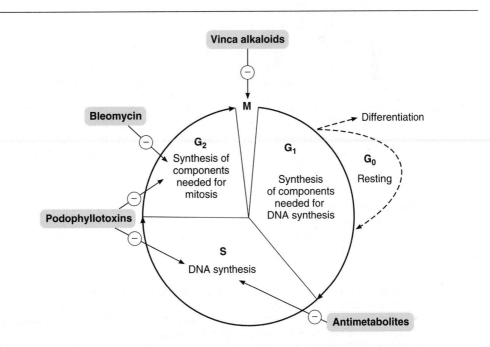

Figure 56–2. Phases of the cell cycle that are susceptible to the actions of cell cycle-specific (CCS) drugs. All cells—normal and neoplastic—must traverse these cell cycle phases before and during cell division. CCS drug actions may not be restricted to a specific phase, but tumor cells are usually most responsive to specific drugs (or drug groups) in the phases indicated. Cell cycle-nonspecific (CCNS) drugs act on tumor cells while they are actively cycling and while they are in the resting phase (G_0). (Adapted, with permission, from Katzung BG [editor]: *Basic & Clinical Pharmacology*, 6th ed. Appleton & Lange, 1995.)

Mechanisms of resistance include:

1. **Increased DNA repair:**   An increased rate of DNA repair in tumor cells is responsible for resistance to several groups of anticancer drugs and is particularly important in the case of most alkylating agents and cisplatin.

2. **Formation of trapping agents:**   Some tumor cells increase their production of thiol trapping agents (eg, glutathione), which interact with anticancer drugs that form reactive electrophilic species. This mechanism of resistance is seen with the alkylating agents, bleomycin, cisplatin, and the anthracyclines.

3. **Changes in target enzymes:**   Changes in the drug sensitivity of a target enzyme, dihydrofolate reductase, and increased synthesis of the enzyme are mechanisms of resistance of tumor cells to methotrexate. Resistance to the *Vinca* alkaloids can involve changes in the structure of their target, the tubulin proteins.

4. **Decreased activation of pro-drugs:**   Resistance to the purine antimetabolites (mercaptopurine, thioguanine) and the pyrimidine antimetabolites (cytarabine, fluorouracil) can result from a decrease in the activity of the tumor cell enzymes needed to convert these prodrugs to their cytotoxic metabolites.

5. **Inactivation of anticancer drugs:**   Increased activity of enzymes capable of inactivating anticancer drugs is a mechanism of tumor cell resistance to most of the purine and pyrimidine antimetabolites.

6. **Decreased drug accumulation:**   This form of multidrug resistance often involves the increased expression of a normal gene (the *MDR1* gene) for a cell surface glycoprotein (P-170 glycoprotein). This transport molecule is involved in the accelerated efflux of many anticancer drugs in resistant cells.

ANTICANCER DRUGS

A. Alkylating Agents:

1. **Chemistry:**   The alkylating agents include nitrogen mustards (**chlorambucil, cyclophosphamide, mechlorethamine),** nitrosureas (**carmustine [BCNU], lomustine [CCNU]**), and alkylsulfonates (**busulfan**). Other drugs that may act in part as alkylating agents include **cisplatin, dacarbazine,** and **procarbazine.**

2. **Mechanisms of action:**   The alkylating agents are CCNS drugs. They form reactive molecular species that alkylate nucleophilic groups on DNA bases, particularly the N7 position of guanine. This leads to cross-linking of bases, abnormal base pairing, or DNA strand breakage. Tumor cell resistance to the drugs occurs through increased DNA repair, decreased drug permeability, or the production of trapping agents such as thiols.

3. **Pharmacokinetics:**   These drugs vary widely in terms of their oral bioavailability, distribution, and elimination. The most distinctive features include: (1) the direct cytotoxicity of mechlorethamine (it does not require conversion to a reactive intermediate); (2) a requirement for hepatic cytochrome P450-mediated biotransformation of cyclophosphamide for antitumor activity; and (3) the high lipophilicity of the nitrosureas, which is important for their use in the treatment of CNS tumors.

4. **Clinical use:**   The alkylating agents are important in combination regimens for the therapy of lymphomas, leukemias, and myelomas (see Table 56–2). For example, mechlorethamine is a component of a multidrug regimen for Hodgkin's disease. Cyclophosphamide is used in ovarian cancers and neuroblastoma, and busulfan is the drug of choice in chronic myelogenous leukemia (CML).

5. **Toxicity:**   Common toxic effects of alkylating agents include bone marrow suppression (leukopenia, thrombocytopenia), gastrointestinal irritation, and changes in gonadal function. The use of cyclophosphamide is associated with a high incidence of alopecia and the occurrence of hemorrhagic cystitis. Busulfan has an atypical toxicity profile, causing adrenal insufficiency, pulmonary fibrosis, and increased skin pigmentation.

B. Antimetabolites:

1. **Chemistry:**   The antimetabolites are structurally similar to endogenous compounds and are antagonists of folic acid (**methotrexate**), purines (**6-mercaptopurine, thioguanine**), or pyrimidines (**5-fluorouracil, cytarabine**).

2. **Mechanisms of action:**   The antimetabolites are CCS drugs. The sites of action of the antimetabolites on DNA synthetic pathways are shown in Figure 56–3.

Table 56–2. Selected examples of effective cancer chemotherapy.[1,2]

Diagnosis	Current Drug Therapy of Choice
Acute lymphocytic leukemia	Induction: vincristine plus prednisone. Maintenance: mercaptopurine, methotrexate, and cyclophosphamide in various combinations
Acute myelogenous leukemia	Induction: Cytarabine plus mitoxantrone or daunorubicin. Maintenance: cytarabine plus etoposide or daunorubicin
Breast carcinoma (early stage)	Cyclophosphamide plus methotrexate and fluorouracil
Burkitt's lymphoma	Cyclophosphamide plus methotrexate and vincristine
Ewing's sarcoma	Cyclophosphamide plus doxorubicin and vincristine
Hodgkin's disease	See text: Examples of combination chemotherapy
Non-Hodgkin's lymphoma	Cyclophosphamide plus doxorubicin, vincristine, and prednisone
Small cell lung carcinoma	Multiple combinations that include cyclophosphamide, cisplatin, doxorubicin, etoposide, and vincristine
Trophoblastic (gestational)	Methotrexate (plus other agents if high risk)
Testicular carcinoma	See text: Examples of combination chemotherapy
Wilms' tumor	Dactinomycin plus vincristine (plus other agents for tumors with unfavorable histology)

[1] Cancers that respond to chemotherapy with prolonged patient survival and some cures.
[2] Modified and reproduced, with permission, from Katzung BG (editor): *Basic & Clinical Pharmacology*, 6th ed. Appleton & Lange, 1995.

a. **Methotrexate:** Methotrexate is an inhibitor of dihydrofolate reductase. This action leads to a decrease in the synthesis of thymidylate, purine nucleotides, and amino acids and thus interferes with nucleic acid and protein metabolism. Tumor cell resistance mechanisms include decreased drug accumulation and changes in the drug sensitivity or activity of dihydrofolate reductase.

b. **Purine antimetabolites:** Mercaptopurine and thioguanine are activated by hypoxanthine-guanine phosphoribosyltransferases (HGPRTase) to toxic nucleotide forms that inhibit several enzymes involved in purine metabolism. Resistant tumor cells have decreased activity of HGPRTase, or they may increase their production of alkaline phosphatases that inactivate the toxic nucleotides.

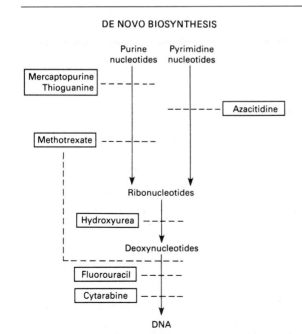

Figure 56–3. Sites of action of antimetabolites on DNA synthetic pathways.

    c. Pyrimidine antimetabolites: Fluorouracil is biotransformed to 5-fluoro-2′-deoxyuridine-5′-monophosphate (5-FdUMP), which inhibits thymidylate synthase and leads to "thymineless death" of cells. Tumor cell resistance mechanisms include decreased metabolism of 5FU, increased thymidylate synthase activity, and reduced drug sensitivity of this enzyme. Cytarabine (cytosine arabinoside, AraC) is activated by kinases to AraCTP, an inhibitor of DNA polymerases. Of all the antimetabolites, cytarabine is the most specific for the S phase of the tumor cell cycle. Resistance to cytarabine can occur through decreased uptake of AraC or a decreased conversion to AraCTP.

  3. Pharmacokinetics: Fluorouracil and the purine antimetabolites are effective after oral administration; the pyrimidine antimetabolites are usually given intravenously. Biodisposition features of particular importance include the dependence of methotrexate on renal function for its elimination and the metabolism of mercaptopurine by xanthine oxidase, which can be inhibited by allopurinol.

  4. Clinical uses: Antimetabolites are used in drug combinations for acute leukemias; cytarabine is an important component in such regimens for the treatment of acute myelogenous leukemia (AML). Methotrexate, alone or combined with other drugs, is effective in choriocarcinoma, and the drug is also used for non-Hodgkin's and cutaneous T cell lymphomas. Fluorouracil is only useful in the treatment of solid tumors and as a topical agent for skin cancers. Some of the uses of the antimetabolites in neoplastic disease are listed in Table 56–2. The antimetabolites also have immunosuppressive actions.

  5. Toxicity: Common adverse effects include bone marrow suppression and toxic effects on the skin and gastrointestinal mucosa (mucositis). Purine antimetabolites may cause dose-dependent hepatic dysfunction. The toxic effects of methotrexate on normal cells may be reduced by administration of folinic acid (leucovorin); this strategy is called **"leucovorin rescue."**

C. Plant Alkaloids:

  1. Chemistry: This subclass includes the *Vinca* alkaloids **(vinblastine, vincristine)**, podophyllotoxins (eg, **etoposide**), and **paclitaxel.** These plant alkaloids are CCS drugs.

  2. Pharmacokinetics: Vinblastine and vincristine have low oral bioavailability and are given parenterally. The major mode of elimination of both drugs is via biliary excretion. Paclitaxel is also given intravenously. Etoposide is absorbed after oral administration and distributes to most body tissues. Elimination of etoposide is mainly via the kidneys, and dose reductions should be made in patients with renal impairment.

  3. Mechanisms of action: Vinblastine and vincristine prevent the assembly of tubulin dimers into microtubules, blocking the assembly of the mitotic spindle. They are therefore called **spindle poisons.** They act primarily in the M phase of the cancer cell cycle. Paclitaxel is also a spindle poison but acts by preventing tubulin *disassembly.* Etoposide increases degradation of DNA, possibly via activation of topoisomerase II, and also inhibits mitochondrial electron transport. The drug is most active in the late S and early G_2 phases of the cell cycle. Resistance to the plant alkaloids may occur from increased efflux of the drugs from tumor cells via the membrane drug-transporter.

  4. Clinical use: Vincristine is a component of the MOPP and COP* regimens used in lymphomas and is also used in Wilms' tumor and choriocarcinoma. Vinblastine is a component of the ABVD* regimen for Hodgkin's disease and the PVB* regimen for testicular carcinoma. Etoposide is used in combination drug regimens for therapy of lung (oat cell), prostate, and testicular carcinoma. Paclitaxel is most useful in ovarian cancer and is also used in advanced breast cancer.

  5. Toxicity: Vinblastine causes gastrointestinal distress, alopecia, and bone marrow suppression. Vincristine does not cause serious myelosuppression, but the drug has neurotoxic actions and may cause areflexia, peripheral neuritis, and paralytic ileus. Etoposide is a gastrointestinal irritant and causes alopecia and bone marrow suppression. Paclitaxel causes neutropenia, thrombocytopenia, and neuropathy.

D. Antibiotics:

  1. Chemistry: This subclass is made up of several structurally dissimilar drugs, including the anthracyclines **(doxorubicin, daunorubicin), bleomycin, dactinomycin, mitomycin, and mithramycin.**

---

* Combination chemotherapy regimens.

2. **Mechanisms of action:**
   a. **Anthracyclines:** These are CCNS drugs that can intercalate between base pairs to block DNA and RNA synthesis, but they also cause membrane disruption and generation of free radicals that lead to cardiotoxicity.
   b. **Bleomycin:** This agent is a mixture of glycopeptides that generate free radicals which bind to DNA and cause strand breaks and inhibit DNA synthesis. These peptides are CCS drugs active in the G_2 phase of the tumor cell cycle.
   c. **Dactinomycin:** This is a CCNS drug that binds to double-stranded DNA and inhibits DNA-dependent RNA synthesis.
   d. **Mitomycin:** This antibiotic is a CCNS drug that is metabolized by liver enzymes to form an alkylating agent that cross-links DNA.
3. **Pharmacokinetics:** Important features include: (1) the metabolism of anthracyclines by liver enzymes to form both active and inactive metabolites that are excreted in the bile; (2) the inactivation of bleomycins by tissue aminopeptidases (but some renal clearance of intact drug also occurs); and (3) the short half-life of dactinomycin, with intact drug excreted in the bile.
4. **Clinical use:** Doxorubicin is a component of the ABVD regimen used in Hodgkin's disease and is used in therapy of myelomas and sarcomas. The main use of daunorubicin is the treatment of acute leukemias. Bleomycin is a component of the ABVD regimen and the PVB regimen for testicular carcinoma. Dactinomycin is used in melanomas and Wilms' tumor. Mitomycin acts against hypoxic tumor cells and is used for cervical carcinoma. Some other chemotherapeutic uses of the antibiotics are indicated in Table 56–2.
5. **Toxicity:**
   a. **Anthracyclines:** These drugs cause bone marrow suppression, gastrointestinal distress and severe alopecia. Their most distinctive adverse effect is cardiotoxicity, which includes initial ECG irregularities with the possibility of arrhythmias and a slowly developing cardiomyopathy and congestive heart failure.
   b. **Bleomycin:** The toxicity profile of this agent is unusual: pulmonary toxicity (pneumonitis, fibrosis) develops slowly and is dose-limiting. Hypersensitivity reactions (chills, fever, anaphylaxis) are common, as are mucocutaneous reactions (alopecia, blister-formation, hyperpigmentation).
   c. **Dactinomycin:** This drug causes bone marrow suppression, skin reactions, and gastrointestinal irritation.
   d. **Mitomycin:** Mitomycin causes severe myelosuppression and can be nephrotoxic. A form of interstitial pneumonia can occur.

E. Hormones & Hormone Antagonists:

1. **Glucocorticoids:** **Prednisone** is the most commonly used glucocorticoid in cancer chemotherapy. The hormone has applications in drug regimens for chronic lymphocytic leukemia, Hodgkin's disease (MOPP regimen), and other lymphomas.
2. **Sex hormones:** The estrogens, progestins, androgens are used in some hormone-dependent cancers to change the hormone balance.
3. **Sex hormone antagonists:** **Tamoxifen,** an estrogen receptor partial agonist, blocks the binding of estrogen to receptors of estrogen-sensitive cancer cells. It is used in therapy of breast cancer and also acts against progestin-resistant endometrial carcinoma. **Flutamide** is an androgen receptor antagonist used in prostatic carcinoma.
4. **Gonadotropin-releasing hormone analogues:** **Leuprolide, goserelin** and **nafarelin** are GnRH agonists. When administered in steady doses, they *inhibit* release of pituitary LH and FSH. These agents are as active as diethylstilbestrol in prostatic carcinoma and cause fewer adverse effects.
5. **Aminoglutethimide:** This drug is an aromatase inhibitor: it blocks the final step in estrogen synthesis. Aminoglutethimide is used in drug regimens for metastatic breast cancer in postmenopausal women.

F. Possible Alkylating Agents:

1. **Procarbazine:** This reactive agent forms hydrogen peroxide, which generates free radicals that cause DNA strand scission. Several of its metabolites are cytotoxic, and one is an MAO inhibitor. The primary use of the drug is as a component of the MOPP regimen for Hodgkin's disease. Procarbazine is myelosuppressive and causes gastrointestinal irritation. The drug may also cause CNS dysfunction, peripheral neuropathy, and skin reactions. Pro-

carbazine inhibits many enzymes, including those involved in hepatic drug metabolism. Disulfiram-like reactions have occurred with ethanol.

2. **Dacarbazine:** This drug is activated by liver enzymes to form methylcarbonium species that act as alkylating agents and interfere with nucleic acid metabolism. Used in Hodgkin's disease (as part of the ABVD regimen), dacarbazine causes marked myelosuppression and gastrointestinal distress.

3. **Cisplatin:** A platinum complex, this CCNS drug binds to DNA, alters its structure, and inhibits nucleic acid synthesis. The drug is used in combination regimens for testicular and lung carcinomas. Cisplatin causes nephrotoxicity and acoustic nerve damage. Renal damage may be reduced by the use of mannitol with adequate hydration. **Carboplatin** is less nephrotoxic than cisplatin and is less likely to cause tinnitus and hearing loss, but carboplatin has significant myelosuppressive actions.

4. **Newer anticancer drugs:**
   a. **Mitoxantrone:** This anthracene compound probably acts via the alkylation of DNA bases. Mitoxantrone is used in combination regimens for refractory acute leukemia. Myelosuppression, gastrointestinal effects, and cardiac arrhythmias are toxic effects of the drug.
   b. **Interferons:** The interferons are endogenous glycoproteins with antineoplastic, immunosuppressive, and antiviral actions. Interferons alpha-2a and alpha-2b (produced by recombinant DNA technology) are effective against a number of neoplasms, including hairy cell leukemia, the early stage of chronic myelogenous leukemia, and T cell lymphomas. Toxic effects of the interferons include myelosuppression and neurologic dysfunction.

STRATEGIES IN CANCER CHEMOTHERAPY

A. **Principles of Combination Therapy:** Chemotherapy with combinations of anticancer drugs usually increases log kill markedly, and, in some cases, synergistic effects are achieved (see section B, below). Combinations are often cytotoxic to a heterogeneous population of cancer cells and may prevent development of resistant clones. Drug combinations using CCS and CCNS drugs may be cytotoxic to dividing and resting cancer cells. The following principles are important for selecting appropriate drugs to use in combination chemotherapy:
(1) Each drug should be active when used alone against the particular cancer.
(2) The drugs should have different mechanisms of action.
(3) Cross-resistance between drugs should be minimal.
(4) The drugs should have different toxic effects.

B. **Examples of Combination Chemotherapy:**
1. **Hodgkin's disease:**
   a. **MOPP regimen:** Mechlorethamine, Oncovin (vincristine), procarbazine, and prednisone. This regimen is effective and was the mainstay of drug treatment of stages III and IV of the disease. It is now being replaced—for initial therapy—by the ABVD regimen.
   b. **ABVD regimen:** Adriamycin (doxorubicin), bleomycin, vinblastine, and dacarbazine. The ABVD regimen is equally effective and appears to be less likely to cause sterility and secondary malignancies (leukemia) than the MOPP regimen. If the neoplasm becomes resistant, the MOPP regimen may be alternated with the ABVD regimen.
2. **Non-Hodgkin's lymphoma:** The COP regimen, which includes cyclophosphamide, Oncovin (vincristine), and prednisone, is commonly used with or without doxorubicin.
3. **Testicular carcinoma:** The PVB regimen, which includes Platinol (cisplatin), vinblastine, and bleomycin, is the standard treatment and is very effective. A more recently introduced regimen, in which cisplatin is replaced by etoposide, appears to be equally effective.
4. **Breast carcinoma:** Postoperative chemotherapy commonly involves use of the CMF regimen (cyclophosphamide, methotrexate, and fluorouracil) with or without tamoxifen.

C. **Additional Strategies in Chemotherapy:**
1. **Pulse therapy:** Intermittent, or pulse, treatment with high doses of an anticancer drug has been used as an alternative to continuous daily therapy. Intensive drug treatment every 3–4 weeks allows for maximum effects on neoplastic cells, with hematologic and immunologic recovery between courses. This type of regimen is used successfully in therapy of acute leukemias, testicular carcinomas, and Wilms' tumor.

2. **Recruitment and synchrony:** The strategy of **recruitment** involves initial use of a CCNS drug to achieve a significant log kill, which results in the recruitment into cell division of resting cells in the G_0 phase of the cell cycle. With subsequent administration of a CCS drug that is active against dividing cells, maximal cell kill may be achieved. A similar approach involves **synchrony,** one example being the use of *Vinca* alkaloids to hold cancer cells in the M phase. Subsequent treatment with another CCS drug, such as the S phase-specific agent, cytarabine, may result in a greater killing effect on the neoplastic cell population.

3. **Rescue therapy:** Toxic effects of anticancer drugs can sometimes be alleviated by rescue strategy. For example, high doses of methotrexate may be given for 36–48 hours and terminated before severe toxicity occurs to cells of the gastrointestinal tract and blood. **Leucovorin** (formyl tetrahydrofolate), which is accumulated more readily by normal than by neoplastic cells, is then administered. This results in rescue of the normal cells, since leucovorin bypasses the dihydrofolate reductase step in folic acid synthesis.

DRUG LIST

The following drugs are important members of the group discussed in this chapter. Prototypes should be learned in detail; features of the major variants should be known well enough to distinguish the variants from the prototypes and from each other; the other significant agents should be recognized as belonging to a specific subclass.

Subclass	Prototype	Major Variants	Other Significant Agents
Alkylating agents Nitrogen mustards	Cyclosphosphamide		Mechlorethamine, chlorambucil
Nitrosureas	Carmustine	Lomustine	Semustine
Alkylsulfonates	Busulfan		
Platinum complex	Cisplatin	Carboplatin	
Triazenes	Dacarbazine		
Hydrazines	Procarbazine		
Antimetabolites Folate analogues	Methotrexate		
Purine analogues	Mercaptopurine		Thioguanine
Pyrimidine analogues	Fluorouracil		Cytarabine
Plant alkaloids *Vinca* alkaloids	Vinblastine	Vincristine	
Podophyllotoxins	Etoposide	Teniposide	
Other	Paclitaxel		Taxotere
Antibiotics Anthracyclines	Doxorubicin	Daunorubicin	
Bleomycins	Bleomycin		
Actinomycins	Dactinomycin		
Mitomycins	Mitomycin		
Hormones Adrenocorticoids	Prednisone	Hydrocortisone	
Androgens	Testosterone	Fluoxymesterone	
Estrogens	Diethylstilbestrol	Ethinyl estradiol	
Progestins	Hydroxyprogesterone	Medroxy-progesterone	
Antiestrogens	Tamoxifen		
Antiandrogens	Flutamide		
Gonadotropin-releasing hormone agonists	Leuprolide	Goserelin	

QUESTIONS

DIRECTIONS: Each of the numbered items or incomplete statements in this section is followed by answers or by completions of the statement. Select the ONE lettered answer or completion that is BEST in each case.

1. This drug is a nitrogen mustard that must be activated by liver enzymes to become an alkylating agent. The drug causes adverse effects that include amenorrhea, bone marrow depression, gastrointestinal distress, and hemorrhagic cystitis.
    (A) Cytarabine
    (B) Cyclophosphamide
    (C) Carmustine
    (D) Methotrexate

2. An antimetabolite used in acute myelogenous leukemia, this drug is phosphorylated to form a nucleotide inhibitor of DNA polymerases. Its major toxic effect is myelosuppression.
    (A) Mechlorethamine
    (B) Vincristine
    (C) Prednisone
    (D) Cytarabine

3. This agent is used to treat testicular carcinoma. Adequate hydration of the patient and the use of an osmotic diuretic decrease the toxicity of the drug.
    (A) Bleomycin
    (B) Cisplatin
    (C) Etoposide
    (D) Vinblastine
    (E) Leuprolide

Items 4–5: A patient with metastatic choriocarcinoma is to be treated with methotrexate (MTX) in a pulse dosage regimen, with the first drug course to continue for no more than 72 hours. Serum creatinine levels will be monitored, and rescue treatment with leucovorin is anticipated. Prior to drug treatment, glucose and bicarbonate will be given over 8–12 hours.

4. During this initial course of drug treatment, it is important to monitor serum MTX levels because
    (A) Resistance to MTX can occur within a few days
    (B) Renal toxicity is likely to occur
    (C) High MTX levels in the blood require additional leucovorin rescue
    (D) MTX levels in the blood are predictive of gastrointestinal mucositis

5. Hydration and alkalinization are important prior to drug treatment in this patient because
    (A) They reduce myelosuppressive side effects
    (B) MTX is a weak acid
    (C) Leucovorin toxicity is increased in a dehydrated patient
    (D) They decrease gastrointestinal distress

6. Concerning mechanisms of action of anticancer drugs, all of the following statements are accurate EXCEPT
    (A) Alkylating agents commonly attack the nucleophilic N7 position in guanine
    (B) Fluorouracil can cause "thymineless death" of cancer cells
    (C) Anthracyclines intercalate with base pairs to block nucleic acid synthesis
    (D) Mercaptopurine is an irreversible inhibitor of HGPRTase

7. Mechanisms of cancer cell resistance to drugs include all of the following EXCEPT
    (A) Increase in DNA repair
    (B) Increase in cytochrome P450
    (C) Increase in production of drug-trapping molecules, eg, glutathione
    (D) Change in properties of a target enzyme
    (E) Decreased activity of activating enzymes

8. Characteristic toxic effects of anticancer drugs include all of the following EXCEPT
    (A) Myelosuppression with vincristine
    (B) Cardiotoxicity with doxorubicin
    (C) Ototoxicity with cisplatin
    (D) Pulmonary dysfunction with procarbazine

Items 9–10: A 23-year-old woman with Hodgkin's disease was treated unsuccessfully with the MOPP regimen; she subsequently underwent a successful course of therapy with the ABVD regimen.

9. Which ONE of the following classes of anticancer drugs used in the treatment of this patient is cell cycle-specific (CCS) and is used in both the MOPP and ABVD regimens?
   (A) Antibiotics
   (B) Alkylating agents
   (C) Plant alkaloids
   (D) Glucocorticoids

10. During the second course of drug treatment (ABVD regimen), this patient experienced chills and fever, developed blisters on the palms of the hands and soles of the feet, and later had symptoms of pulmonary dysfunction. The drug most likely to cause these side effects is
    (A) Mechlorethamine
    (B) Vincristine
    (C) Dacarbazine
    (D) Bleomycin

DIRECTIONS: The following section consists of a list of four to twenty-six lettered options followed by several numbered items. For each numbered item, select the ONE option that is most closely associated with it. Each answer may be selected once, more than once, or not at all.

   (A) Mercaptopurine
   (B) Vincristine
   (C) Procarbazine
   (D) Leuprolide
   (E) Cisplatin
   (F) Busulfan
   (G) Dacarbazine
   (H) Mechlorethamine
   (I) Flutamide
   (J) Doxorubicin
   (K) Etoposide
   (L) Bleomycin
   (M) Methotrexate
   (N) Tamoxifen
   (O) Diethylstilbestrol

11. When used for prostatic carcinoma, this agent decreases the release of gonadotropins from the pituitary gland
12. The plasma levels of this anticancer drug are increased dramatically if it is used concomitantly with allopurinol
13. This alkylating agent is the treatment of choice for palliation of chronic myelogenous leukemia
14. A component of a combination drug regimen for Hodgkin's disease, this drug is thought to be cytotoxic via the generation of free radicals from hydrogen peroxide. Ethanol should be avoided by patients taking this drug
15. This drug is used in combination therapy for testicular carcinoma. It is a cell cycle-specific (CCS) drug that acts mainly in the late S and G_0 phases of the tumor cell cycle

ANSWERS

1. Only two of the drugs listed are alkylating agents. Carmustine (BCNU) is a nitrosourea that decomposes spontaneously in aqueous environments to form reactive products. Cyclophosphamide is a nitrogen mustard pro-drug that is activated by hepatic cytochrome P450 to form reactive metabolites. The answer is **(B)**.
2. Antimetabolites are almost always structurally similar to endogenous molecules. Cytarabine (cytosine arabinoside) undergoes phosphorylation to become an inhibitor of DNA polymerase. The answer is **(D)**.
3. The characteristic nephrotoxicity of cisplatin may be reduced by slow intravenous infusion, the maintenance of good hydration, and the administration of mannitol (to maximize urine flow).

You should recall that cisplatin also has dose-dependent neurotoxic effects. The answer is **(B)**.

4. Resistance to methotrexate does not occur within a few days; a longer time period is required. Serum MTX levels are not predictive of mucositis but are related to potential myelosuppressive toxicity of the drug. Renal toxicity is unlikely to occur in this patient with the proposed protocol. The answer is **(C)**.

5. Nephrotoxicity can be a problem with high doses of methotrexate, but it is less likely to occur than myelosuppression, especially if the patient is well hydrated and the urine is alkalinized. As a weak acid, MTX is more water-soluble at alkaline pH and is thus eliminated more rapidly in the urine. The answer is **(B)**.

6. To exert anticancer activity, mercaptopurine (and thioguanine) must first be activated to nucleotides by HGPRTase. If mercaptopurine were an irreversible inhibitor of this enzyme, this bioactivation process could not occur. The answer is **(D)**.

7. Increases in the activity of cytochrome P450 have not been reported as a mechanism of resistance to anticancer drugs. In fact, one might predict *enhanced* cytotoxic effects of drugs that are activated by this enzyme system, eg, cyclophosphamide. Increased drug inactivation through increased production of alkaline phosphatases is a mechanism of resistance to purine antimetabolites. The answer is **(B)**.

8. Myelosuppression is a common toxic effect of anticancer drugs, particularly alkylating agents, antimetabolites, antibiotics, and plant alkaloids. However, vincristine is an exception! It causes characteristic neurotoxicity and, unlike vinblastine, has little effect on bone marrow. The other toxic effects listed are distinctive for the particular drugs. The answer is **(A)**.

9. The cell cycle-specific drugs used in standard treatment protocols for Hodgkin's disease are bleomycin and the *Vinca* alkaloids. Vinblastine is used in the ABVD regimen, and vincristine (Oncovin) is used in the MOPP regimen. The answer is **(C)**.

10. The toxic profile described in this patient is characteristic of bleomycin used in the ABVD regimen. The answer is **(D)**.

11. Leuprolide is a synthetic peptide that acts like gonadotropin-releasing hormone if given in pulse doses. Administered in steady, continuous doses or as a depot injection, leuprolide *inhibits* the release of pituitary gonadotropins. The answer is **(D)**.

12. Allopurinol, a xanthine oxidase inhibitor, is given to control the hyperuricemia that occurs as a result of large cell kills in the successful drug therapy of malignant diseases. The antimetabolite 6-mercaptopurine is metabolized by xanthine oxidase, and, in the presence of an inhibitor of this enzyme (eg, allopurinol), toxic levels of the drug may be reached rapidly. The answer is **(A)**.

13. Although many anticancer drugs are used for the palliative treatment of chronic myelogenous leukemia, busulfan is the treatment of choice. The drug is also used in polycythemia vera and has been used to ablate the host's bone marrow prior to bone marrow transplantation. The answer is **(F)**.

14. Procarbazine is a highly reactive chemical that generates hydrogen peroxide and toxic free radicals. Adverse effects of the drug include myelosuppression, gastrointestinal distress, disulfiram-like reactions with ethanol, and neurotoxicity. Procarbazine is teratogenic and carcinogenic. Despite these problems, procarbazine is a component of the MOPP anticancer drug regimen used in Hodgkin's disease, the gains presumably outweighing the risks. (Note, however, that ABVD is supplanting the MOPP regimen in most centers.) The answer is **(C)**.

15. Vinblastine is a cell cycle-specific drug used in testicular cancers, but it acts in the M phase of the cell cycle. The answer is **(K)**.

Immunopharmacology

57

OBJECTIVES

You should be able to:

- Describe cellular and serologic immunity.
- Identify the therapeutic similarities and the differences between immunosuppressant and anti-cancer drugs.
- Describe the mechanisms of action, clinical uses, and toxicities of glucocorticoids, cyclosporine, azathioprine, and cyclophosphamide in immunopharmacology.
- Describe the mechanisms of action, clinical uses, and toxicities of antibodies used as immunosuppressants.
- Identify the major cytokines and other immunomodulating agents.
- List the different types of immunologic reactions to drugs.

Learn the definitions that follow.

Table 57–1. Definitions.

Term	Definition
B cells	Lymphoid cells derived from the bone marrow that mediate serologic immunity through the formation of antibodies
T cells	Lymphoid cells derived from the thymus that mediate cellular immunity and can modify serologic immunity. The class includes CD4+ ("helper") cells and CD8+ ("suppressor") cells
Antigen-presenting cells (APCs)	Dendritic and Langerhans cells, macrophages, and B lymphocytes involved in the processing of antigens into cell-surface forms recognizable by lymphoid cells
Clusters of differentiation (CDs)	Specific cell surface constituents (characterized by monoclonal antibodies) identified by number (CD1, CD2, etc)
Major histocompatibility complex (MHC)	Cell surface molecules of antigen-presenting cells that bind antigen fragments for recognition by helper T cells
Cytokines	Polypeptide modulators of cellular functions; include interferons, interleukins, and growth stimulating factors
Lymphokine	A cytokine that is capable of modulating lymphoid cell functions

CONCEPTS

The drugs used to alter immunologic processes comprise a wide variety of chemical and pharmacologic types (Figure 57–1).

IMMUNE MECHANISMS

A. Development of Immunity: The development of specific immunity requires the following steps: (1) antigen recognition and processing; (2) proliferation of lymphoid cells; (3) differentiation of lymphoid cells; and (4) immune effects. The critical initial step (antigen recognition and processing) involves **antigen-presenting cells,** including those derived from macrophages, which change antigens so that they become more recognizable to lymphoid cells. The cell types involved in the immune response can be identified by monoclonal antibodies to specific cell

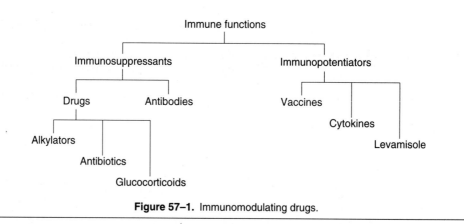

Figure 57–1. Immunomodulating drugs.

surface components designated **clusters of differentiation (CDs),** eg, CD4+, CD8+. Among the most important antigen-presenting cell surface molecules are the **major histocompatibility complex (MHC)** class II antigens (also called Ia antigens).

The **T (thymus) lymphoid cells** recognize and make contact with antigens. The clonal proliferation and differentiation of T cells lead to **cellular immunity** (Figure 57–2). T cells, either by direct cytotoxic effects or by the release of lymphokines (endogenous immunomodulators), mediate delayed hypersensitivity reactions and are important in tissue graft rejection.

The **B (bone marrow) lymphoid cells,** which differentiate into specific antibody-forming cells, are responsible for **serologic immunity.** B cells respond to specific antigens by rapid proliferation, a process controlled by T helper (CD4+) or suppressor (CD8+) cells.

Antibody-antigen interactions lead to precipitation of viruses, phagocytosis of bacteria, or lysis of red cells. Lymphoid cell proliferation may be inhibited by the endogenous eicosanoids

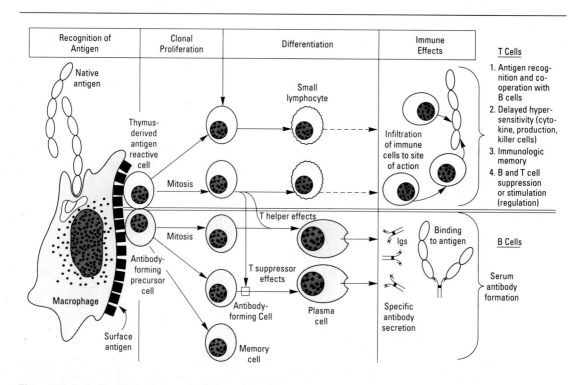

Figure 57–2. A simplified scheme of cellular and humoral immunity. (Reproduced, with permission, from Katzung BG [editor]: *Basic & Clinical Pharmacology,* 6th ed. Appleton & Lange, 1995.)

(eg, prostaglandin E_2) and stimulated by the cytokines (eg, interferons, interleukins, and peptide growth factors).

Natural killer (NK) lymphoid cells are of unknown origin and may also play an important role in immune defense mechanisms, including tumor rejection and viral immunity.

B. Immunocompetence: The techniques used to assess immunologic competence and to measure drug effects on competence include delayed hypersensitivity testing with skin test antigens; assays of serum immunoglobulins, complement and specific antibodies; measurement of antibody response to primary or secondary immunization; absolute circulating lymphocyte count; and others.

C. Sites of Action of Immunosuppressant Agents: Sites of action of immunosuppressive agents are shown in Figure 57–3. Drugs that act at the step of antigen recognition are antibodies and include Rh$_o$(D) immune globulin, lymphocyte immune globulin (antithymocyte globulin, ATG), and a monoclonal antibody, muromonab-CD3. Lymphoid cell proliferation, a primary target of the cytotoxic drugs, is also inhibited by cyclosporine, glucocorticoids, and ATG. The stages of differentiation of B and T cells are inhibited to some extent by cyclosporine, dactinomycin, and lymphocyte immune globulin. Corticosteroids also modify tissue injury from immune responses via their anti-inflammatory properties.

D. Immunosuppression Compared to Cancer Chemotherapy: Since most cytotoxic drugs act on proliferating cells, there is a similarity between immunosuppressant agents and the drugs used in cancer chemotherapy. However, the therapeutic principles involved are not identical. In contrast to growth in most neoplasms, immune cell proliferation is **synchronized.** This permits a greater selective toxicity of anti-immune cytotoxic drugs if they are given at the time of initial antigen exposure. In addition, immunosuppressant drugs are usually given in *low doses, continuously,* whereas anticancer drug therapy often follows *intermittent, high-dose* regimens.

IMMUNOSUPPRESSANT DRUGS

A. Corticosteroids:
1. **Mechanism of action:** Glucocorticoids act at multiple cellular sites, leading to broad effects on inflammatory and immune processes (see Chapter 38). At the biochemical level, their actions on gene expression lead to decreases in the synthesis of prostaglandins, leukotrienes, and lymphokines (eg, interleukins, platelet activating factor). At the cellular

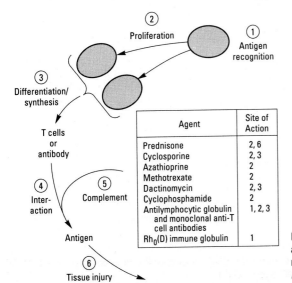

Figure 57–3. The sites of action of immunosuppressive agents on the immune response. (Reproduced, with permission, from Katzung BG [editor]: *Basic & Clinical Pharmacology,* 6th ed. Appleton & Lange, 1995.)

level, the glucocorticoids inhibit the proliferation of T lymphocytes (suppressing cellular immunity), but B cells are less affected. At doses used for immunosuppression, the glucocorticoids are cytotoxic to certain subsets of T cells. Continuous therapy lowers IgG levels by increasing catabolism of this class of immunoglobulins.

2. **Clinical use:** Prednisone is the drug of choice in several autoimmune diseases, including idiopathic thrombocytopenic purpura, autoimmune hemolytic anemia, and acute glomerulonephritis. Corticosteroids are also used in combination with other agents as immunosuppressants in organ transplantation.

3. **Toxicity:** Predictable adverse effects include adrenal suppression, growth inhibition, muscle wasting, osteoporosis, salt retention, diabetogenesis, and possible psychoses (Chapter 38).

B. Cyclosporine:

1. **Mechanism of action:** This peptide antibiotic inhibits early stages of the differentiation of T cells and blocks their activation. Cyclosporine inhibits the synthesis of factors that stimulate the growth of T cells, including interleukins (IL-2, IL-3) and interferons (IFN-γ). The drug binds to a protein (cyclophilin) and the complex inhibits a cytoplasmic phosphatase (calcineurin) that is needed for the activation of a T cell-specific transcription factor. However, cyclosporine does not block the effects of such factors on primed T cells, nor does it block interaction with antigen.

2. **Clinical use:** Cyclosporine can be used orally, but since bioavailability is erratic, serum levels should be monitored. The drug undergoes slow hepatic metabolism and has a long half-life. Cyclosporine is the drug of choice for immunosuppression in organ transplantation and is used in the graft-versus-host syndrome in bone marrow transplants. Cyclosporine has been used in combination with glucocorticoids (and sometimes cytotoxic drugs) but may be equally effective used alone. The drug may also be useful in autoimmune diseases including the early treatment of type I diabetes.

3. **Toxicity:** The most frequent adverse effects are renal dysfunction, hypertension, hirsutism, and neurotoxicity. Cyclosporine may also cause hyperglycemia and hyperlipidemia. Transient liver dysfunction and an increase in viral infections may also occur. One virtue of cyclosporine is its low incidence of bone marrow toxicity. Drugs that stimulate or inhibit liver microsomal drug-metabolizing enzymes may alter the plasma levels of cyclosporine.

C. Azathioprine:

1. **Mechanism of action:** This pro-drug is transformed to the antimetabolite mercaptopurine, which, upon further metabolic conversion, inhibits enzymes involved in purine metabolism. Azathioprine is cytotoxic in the early phase of lymphoid cell proliferation and has a greater effect on the activity of T cells than B cells. The drug has minimal effects on established graft rejections.

2. **Clinical use:** Azathioprine is used in several autoimmune diseases, including lupus erythematosus and severe rheumatoid arthritis. The drug is also used for immunosuppression in renal homografts.

3. **Toxicity:** The major toxic effect is bone marrow suppression, but gastrointestinal irritation, skin rashes, and liver dysfunction also occur. The use of azathioprine is associated with an increased incidence of neoplasms. The active compound, mercaptopurine, is metabolized by xanthine oxidase, and toxic effects may be increased by allopurinol given for hyperuricemia.

D. Cyclophosphamide:

1. **Mechanism of action:** This orally active pro-drug is transformed by liver enzymes to an alkylating agent that is cytotoxic to proliferating lymphoid cells. The drug has a greater effect on B cells than T lymphocytes and will inhibit an established immune response. Other cytotoxic drugs act similarly and are sometimes used as immunosuppressants; these include cytarabine, dactinomycin, methotrexate, and vincristine (see Chapter 56).

2. **Clinical use:** Cyclophosphamide is effective in autoimmune diseases (including hemolytic anemia), antibody-induced red cell aplasia, bone marrow transplants, and possibly other organ transplants. Cyclophosphamide does not prevent the graft-versus-host reaction in bone marrow transplantation.

3. **Toxicity:** Large doses of the drug (usually needed for immunosuppression) cause pancytopenia, gastrointestinal distress, hemorrhagic cystitis, and alopecia. Cyclophosphamide (and other alkylating agents) may cause sterility.

E. **Tacrolimus (FK 506):** This immunosuppressive antibiotic has a mechanism of action similar to that of cyclosporine. The drug may be more effective in liver transplantation than cyclosporine, in terms of graft and patient survival. The toxicity of tacrolimus is similar to that of cyclosporine. **Rapamycin** is a new investigational immunosuppressive antibiotic with structural similarities to tacrolimus but a different mechanism of action.

ANTIBODIES AS IMMUNOSUPPRESSANTS

A. **Lymphocyte Immune Globulin:**
1. **Mechanism of action:** Lymphocyte immune globulin, or antithymocyte globulin (ATG), is usually produced in horses by immunization against human thymus cells. ATG binds to T cells involved in antigen recognition, initiating their destruction by serum complement. ATG selectively blocks cellular immunity rather than antibody formation, which accounts for its clinical use to suppress organ graft rejection.
2. **Clinical use:** ATG is used in combination with cyclosporine or cytotoxic drugs (or both) for bone marrow, heart, and renal transplantations. ATG has induced remissions in patients with aplastic anemia who are not candidates for bone marrow transplantation.
3. **Toxicity:** Since serologic immunity may remain intact, injection of ATG may cause hypersensitivity reactions, including serum sickness and anaphylaxis. Pain and erythema occur at injection sites, and histiocytic lymphoma has been noted as a late complication.

B. **Muromonab-CD3 (OKT-3):**
1. **Mechanism of action:** Muromonab-CD3 is a murine monoclonal antibody to the T3 (CD3) antigen on the surface of human thymocytes and mature T cells. The antibody blocks the killing action of cytotoxic T cells and probably interferes with other T cell functions.
2. **Clinical use:** Muromonab-CD3 is used intravenously to reverse renal allograft rejection crisis.
3. **Toxicity:** First-dose effects include fever, chills, dyspnea, and pulmonary edema. Hypersensitivity reactions may also occur.

C. **$Rh_o(D)$ Immune Globulin (Rh_oGAM):**
1. **Mechanism of action:** Rh_oGAM is a human IgG preparation that contains antibodies against red cell $Rh_o(D)$ antigens. Administration of this antibody to $Rh_o(D)$-negative, D^u-negative mothers at time of antigen exposure (ie, birth of an $Rh_o(D)$-positive, D^u-positive child) blocks the primary immune response to the foreign cells. The mechanism probably involves "feedback immunosuppression."
2. **Clinical use:** $Rh_o(D)$ is used for prevention of Rh hemolytic disease of the newborn. In women treated with $Rh_o(D)$, maternal antibodies to Rh-positive cells are not produced in subsequent pregnancies, and hemolytic disease of the neonate is averted.

IMMUNOMODULATING AGENTS

Agents that act as stimulators of immune responses represent a new area in immunopharmacology, with the potential for important therapeutic uses, including the treatment of immune-deficiency diseases, chronic infectious diseases, and cancer.

A. **Levamisole:** This antiparasitic drug can also act as an immunopotentiator. Levamisole stimulates the maturation and proliferation of T cells in patients with impaired immune function. The drug enhances T cell-mediated immune responses and restores delayed hypersensitivity. One of the actions of levamisole is to promote the oxidation of an endogenous precursor molecule to soluble immune response repressor substance (SIRS). The drug has been used in the treatment of the nephrotic syndrome and adjunctively in cancer chemotherapy. Levamisole may also be useful in rheumatoid arthritis and in the immunodeficiency of Hodgkin's disease.

B. Aldesleukin: This agent is recombinant interleukin-2 (IL-2). IL-2 is an endogenous lymphokine that promotes the proliferation and differentiation of lymphocytes into cytotoxic cells and activates natural killer cells. Aldesleukin is indicated for the adjunctive treatment of renal cell carcinoma. The agent is investigational for possible efficacy in restoring immune function in AIDS and other immunocompromised patients.

C. Other Cytokines:
1. **Filgrastim and sargramostim:** These agents are recombinant forms of human colony stimulating factors G-CSF and GM-CSF (Chapter 32). They are indicated for the acceleration of marrow recovery in patients who are undergoing cytotoxic therapy for cancer.
2. **Interferon gamma-1b:** This interferon is a primary endogenous activator of phagocytosis and appears to act by increasing the synthesis of tumor necrosis factor (TNF). The recombinant form is used to decrease the incidence and severity of infections in patients with chronic granulomatous disease.

D. BCG (Bacille Calmette-Guerin): BCG has been used for immunization against tuberculosis and as an immunostimulant in cancer therapy. BCG activates macrophages and may enhance immune responses in patients with superficial bladder cancer.

E. Thymosin: Thymosin is a protein hormone from the thymus gland that stimulates the maturation of pre-T cells and promotes the formation of T cells from ordinary lymphoid stem cells. Thymosin-containing preparations have been used in DiGeorge syndrome, but their efficacy in other immune deficiency states has not been established.

MECHANISMS OF DRUG ALLERGY

A. Type I (Immediate) Drug Allergy: This form of drug allergy involves **IgE**-mediated reactions to animal and plant stings as well as drugs. Such reactions include anaphylaxis, urticaria, and angioedema. Small drug molecules can act as haptens when linked to carrier proteins, initiating B cell proliferation and formation of IgE antibodies. These antibodies bind to tissue mast cells and blood basophils, which become sensitized. On subsequent exposure, the antigenic drug is bound to antibodies, triggering release of mediators of vascular responses and tissue injury, including histamine, kinins, prostaglandins, and leukotrienes. Drugs that commonly cause type I reactions include penicillins and sulfonamides.

B. Type II Drug Allergy: This involves **IgG** or **IgM** antibodies, which bind to circulating blood cells. On re-exposure to the antigen, complement-dependent cell lysis occurs. Type II reactions include autoimmune syndromes such as hemolytic anemia from methyldopa, systemic lupus erythematosus from hydralazine or procainamide, thrombocytopenic purpura from quinidine, and agranulocytosis from exposure to any of a number of drugs.

C. Type III Drug Allergy: This complex type of reaction involves complement-fixing **IgM** or **IgG** antibodies and possibly **IgE** antibodies. Drug-induced serum sickness and vasculitis are examples of Type III reactions; Stevens-Johnson syndrome (associated with sulfonamide therapy) may also result from type III mechanisms.

D. Type IV Drug Allergy: This cell-mediated reaction can occur from topical application of drugs. It results in contact dermatitis.

E. Modification of Drug Allergies: Drugs that modify allergic responses to other drugs or toxins may act at several steps of the immune mechanism. For example, corticosteroids inhibit lymphoid cell proliferation and reduce tissue injury and edema. However, most drugs that are useful in type I reactions (eg, isoproterenol, theophylline, epinephrine) block mediator release or act as physiologic antagonists of the mediators.

DRUG LIST

The following drugs are important members of the group discussed in this chapter. Prototypes should be learned in detail; features of the major variants should be known well enough to distinguish the variants from prototypes and from each other; the other significant agents should be recognized as belonging to a specific subclass.

Subclass	Prototype	Major Variants	Other Significant Agents
Steroids	Prednisone		
Antibiotics	Cyclosporine	Tacrolimus	Dactinomycin, rapamycin
Antimetabolites	Azathioprine	Mercaptopurine	Cytarabine, methotrexate
Alkylating agents	Cyclophosphamide		Chlorambucil
Antibodies	Lymphocytic immune globulin, muromonab-CD3, Rh$_o$(D) globulin		
Immunostimulators	Filgrastim, interferon-gamma, levamisole, sargramostim		

QUESTIONS

DIRECTIONS: Each of the numbered items or incomplete statements in this section is followed by answers or by completions of the statement. Select the ONE lettered answer or completion that is BEST in each case.

1. Cyclosporine is effective in organ transplantation. Although its precise mechanism of action is unknown, cyclosporine
   (A) Interferes with antigen recognition
   (B) Blocks tissue responses to inflammatory mediators
   (C) Inhibits differentiation of T cells
   (D) Increases catabolism of IgG antibodies
   (E) Stimulates production of NK cells

2. Azathioprine
   (A) Is an inhibitor of dihydrofolate reductase
   (B) Is metabolized to a cytotoxic intermediate by xanthine oxidase
   (C) Blocks both cellular and serologic immune mechanisms
   (D) Is not toxic to bone marrow cells
   (E) Prevents Rh hemolytic disease of the newborn

   Items 3–4: A renal transplant recipient is given a combination of immunosuppressive agents to prevent allograft rejection. During the course of drug therapy, the patient develops fever, vomiting, cutaneous lesions, and lymphadenopathy.

3. The agent most likely to cause these symptoms is
   (A) Cyclophosphamide
   (B) Dactinomycin
   (C) Lymphocytic immune globulin
   (D) Cyclosporine

4. If the patient had developed upper extremity tremor, limb paresthesias, and hallucinations, the most likely causative agent would have been
   (A) Cyclosporine
   (B) Prednisone
   (C) Lymphocytic immune globulin
   (D) Methotrexate

5. This drug is a widely used agent that suppresses cellular immunity, inhibits prostaglandin and leukotriene synthesis, and increases the catabolism of IgG antibodies.

    (A) Mercaptopurine
    (B) Cyclophosphamide
    (C) Prednisone
    (D) Levamisole
    (E) Cyclosporine

6. This agent promotes the proliferation of T cells, stimulates the differentiation of lymphocytes into cytotoxic cells, and activates natural killer cells.
    (A) Aldesleukin
    (B) Cyclosporin
    (C) Levamisole
    (D) Macrophage colony-stimulating factor

7. Functions of T cells include all of the following EXCEPT
    (A) Serologic memory
    (B) Antigen recognition
    (C) Regulation of B cells
    (D) Production of cytokines

8. Actions of lymphocytic immune globulin include all of the following EXCEPT
    (A) Facilitates complement-mediated destruction of T cells
    (B) Stimulates release of cytokines
    (C) Blocks "antigen recognition"
    (D) Causes type III drug allergies

9. All of the following statements about cyclosporine are accurate EXCEPT
    (A) Mannitol diuresis decreases its nephrotoxic effects
    (B) Viral infections can occur during treatment
    (C) It causes severe myelosuppression
    (D) It is used orally, but its bioavailability is variable

Items 10–11: An immunosuppressed patient was treated for a bacterial infection with a parenteral penicillin. Within a few minutes of the penicillin injection, he developed severe bronchoconstriction, laryngeal edema, and hypotension. Due to the rapid administration of epinephrine, the patient survived. Unfortunately, a year later he was treated with an antipsychotic drug and developed agranulocytosis.

10. The type of drug reaction that was caused by the penicillin is
    (A) A type II drug allergy
    (B) An autoimmune syndrome
    (C) A cell-mediated reaction
    (D) Mediated by IgE

11. The type of drug reaction that was caused by the antipsychotic drug is
    (A) A type III drug reaction
    (B) Mediated by IgG or IgM antibodies
    (C) A type IV drug reaction
    (D) The Stevens-Johnson syndrome

12. Which of the following is NOT a cytokine?
    (A) Muromonab-CD3
    (B) Interferon alpha
    (C) Interleukin-2
    (D) Tumor necrosis factor
    (E) Granulocyte colony-stimulating factor

ANSWERS

1. Cyclosporine inhibits early stages in the differentiation of T cells and blocks their activation. The drug inhibits the synthesis of factors that stimulate T cell growth. The answer is **(C)**.

2. Azathioprine blocks both cellular and serologic immunity. The answer is **(C)**.

3. Lymphocytic immune globulin is produced mainly through the immunization of large animals. As a mixture of foreign proteins, the agent may cause a wide range of hypersensitivity reactions, including skin reactions, serum sickness, and even anaphylaxis. The symptoms described are typical of serum sickness. The answer is **(C)**.

4. Neurotoxic effects associated with the use of cyclosporine include limb paresthesias (incidence 50%), distal tremor (incidence 25%), hallucinations, and seizures. The answer is (A).

5. The corticosteroid prednisone is used extensively as an immunosuppressant in autoimmune diseases and organ transplantation. Glucocorticoids have multiple actions, including those described. The answer is (C).

6. Aldesleukin activates natural killer cells (NK cells) and lymphokine-activated killer cells (LAK cells). Investigational use of aldesleukin in AIDS patients is based on the fact that lymphocytes from such individuals produce significantly less IL-2 than from healthy controls. The answer is (A).

7. Serologic immunity consists of antibodies produced by B cells after their differentiation into specific clones of antibody-forming cells. T cells are responsible for cellular immunity. The answer is (A).

8. Lymphocytic immune globulin increases T cell destruction and blocks cellular immunity. Since serologic immunity remains intact, the injection of lymphocyte immune globulin may cause hypersensitivity reactions. The agent does not stimulate the release of cytokines. The answer is (B).

9. Cyclosporine is relatively free of bone marrow-suppressive effects. The answer is (C).

10. The patient experienced an anaphylactic response to the penicillin. This is a type I (immediate) drug reaction, mediated by IgE antibodies. The answer is (D).

11. Autoimmune syndromes that can be drug-induced include agranulocytosis and systemic lupus erythematosus. They are type II reactions involving IgM and IgG antibodies that bind to circulating blood cells. The patient was probably treated with clozapine for his psychosis (see clozapine toxicity, Chapter 28). The answer is (B).

12. Cytokines are immunoregulatory proteins synthesized by lymphoreticular and other cells. They usually exert their effects via interaction with cell surface receptors. This class of endogenous compounds includes interferons, interleukins, colony-stimulating factors, and tumor necrosis factors. Muromonab-CD3 is a murine monoclonal *antibody* directed against a surface component of human lymphocytes and mature T cells. The answer is (A).

Part IX. Toxicology

Introduction to Toxicology   58

OBJECTIVES

You should be able to:

- List four major air pollutants and their clinical effects.
- List the major toxicities of benzene, chlorinated hydrocarbon insecticides, and the organophosphate insecticides.
- List two important herbicides and their major toxicities.
- Describe the source of dioxin exposure and the source of PCB exposure.

Learn the definitions that follow.

Table 58–1. Definitions.	
Term	**Definition**
Toxicology	The area of pharmacology that deals with the adverse effects of chemicals on biologic systems
Occupational toxicology	The area that deals with the toxic effects of chemicals found in the workplace; regulated by the Occupational Safety & Health Agency (OSHA)
Environmental toxicology	The area that deals with the effects of agents found in the environment (air, water, etc); regulated by the Environmental Protection Agency (EPA)
Ecotoxicology	The area that deals with the untoward effects of agents found in the environment on whole populations, as opposed to single individuals
Risk	The expected frequency of occurrence of a particular toxic effect in response to a particular agent
Threshold Limit Value (TLV)	Denotes the amount of exposure to a given agent that is deemed safe for a stated time period. It is higher for shorter periods than for longer periods
Generally recognized as safe (GRAS)	An official list of substances that through testing or experience do not appear to have significant toxicity
Bioaccumulation	The increasing concentration of a substance in the environment as the result of environmental persistence and physical properties (eg, lipid solubility) that permits it to accumulate in the tissues of organisms
Biomagnification	The further concentration of chemicals within organisms that feed on other organisms and thereby concentrate the chemicals found in the tissues of the prey species

CONCEPTS

Chemicals in the environment (including home, workplace, atmosphere, etc) may constitute important health hazards. Some of these chemical groups are indicated in Figure 58–1.

AIR POLLUTANTS

A. Classification & Prototypes: The major air pollutants in industrialized countries include carbon monoxide (which accounts for about 50% of the total amount of air pollutants), sulfur oxides (18%), hydrocarbons (12%), particulate matter (eg, smoke particles, 10%), and nitrogen oxides (6%). Ambient air pollution appears to be a contributing factor in bronchitis, obstructive pulmonary disease, and lung cancer.

B. Carbon Monoxide: CO is an odorless, colorless gas that competes avidly with oxygen for hemoglobin. The affinity of CO for hemoglobin is more than 200-fold greater than that of oxygen. The threshold limit value (TLV) of CO for an 8 hour workday is 25 parts per million (PPM); in heavy traffic, the concentration of CO may exceed 100 PPM.

   1. Effects: Carbon monoxide causes tissue hypoxia. Headache is one of the first symptoms, followed by confusion, loss of visual acuity, tachycardia, syncope, coma, convulsions, and

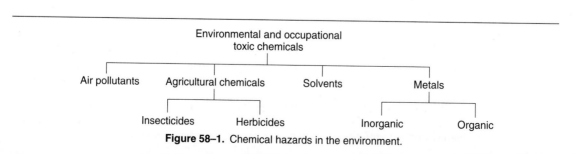

Figure 58–1. Chemical hazards in the environment.

death. Collapse and syncope occur when approximately 40% of hemoglobin has been converted to carboxyhemoglobin. These adverse effects may be aggravated by high ambient temperature and high altitude.

2. **Treatment:** Removal of the source of carbon monoxide, and breathing pure oxygen comprise the major treatment. Hyperbaric oxygen accelerates the clearance of carbon monoxide.

C. **Sulfur Dioxide:** SO_2 is a colorless, irritating gas formed from the combustion of fossil fuels.
1. **Effects:** SO_2 forms sulfurous acid on contact with moist mucous membranes; this acid is responsible for most of the pathologic effects. Conjunctival and bronchial irritation (especially in asthmatics) are the primary signs of exposure. Five to ten PPM in the air is enough to cause severe bronchospasm. Severe exposure may lead to delayed pulmonary edema.
2. **Treatment:** Removal from exposure and relief of irritation and inflammation comprise the major treatment.

D. **Nitrogen Oxides:** Nitrogen dioxide (NO_2), a brownish irritant gas, is the primary member of this group. It is formed in fires and in silage on farms.
1. **Effects:** NO_2 causes deep lung irritation and pulmonary edema. Farm workers exposed to high concentrations of the gas within enclosed silos may die of acute pulmonary edema very rapidly. Irritation of the eyes, nose, and throat is also common.
2. **Treatment:** No specific treatment is available; measures to reduce inflammation and pulmonary edema are important.

E. **Ozone:** O_3 is a bluish, irritant gas produced in air and water purification devices and in electrical fields.
1. **Effects:** Exposure to 0.01–0.1 PPM may cause irritation and dryness of the mucous membranes. Pulmonary function may be impaired at higher concentrations. Chronic exposure leads to bronchitis, bronchiolitis, fibrosis, and emphysema.
2. **Treatment:** No specific treatment is available. Measures that reduce inflammation and pulmonary edema are emphasized.

F. **Hydrocarbons:** Solvents used in industry and to clean clothing are the major sources of hydrocarbon exposure. Examples include the aliphatic hydrocarbons (eg, carbon tetrachloride and trichloroethylene) and aromatic compounds (eg, benzene and toluene).
1. **Effects:** The hydrocarbons are potent CNS depressants. The acute effects of excessive exposure are nausea, vertigo, locomotor disturbance, headache, and coma. Benzene, a bone marrow suppressant, may cause aplastic anemia, thrombocytopenia, or leukopenia.
2. **Treatment:** Removal from exposure is the only direct treatment available. Serious CNS depression must be treated with support of vital signs (Chapter 60).

INSECTICIDES

A. **Classification & Prototypes:** The three major classes of insecticides are the chlorinated hydrocarbons (DDT and its analogues), acetylcholinesterase inhibitors (carbaryl, malathion, etc), and the botanical agents (nicotine, rotenone, pyrethrum alkaloids).

B. **Chlorinated Hydrocarbons:** DDT and its analogues are long-persistence chemicals that accumulate in body fat and thus are subject to both bioaccumulation and biomagnification. These hydrocarbons are banned in many countries.
1. **Effects:** Chlorinated hydrocarbons block physiologic inactivation in the sodium channels of nerve membranes and cause uncontrolled firing of action potentials. This is probably the mode of insecticidal action. In mammals, the same effect may occur with very high doses. Chronic exposure to lower concentrations leads to impaired egg survival in birds and may result in increased tumorigenesis in mammals.
2. **Treatment:** No specific treatment is available for toxicity caused by chlorinated hydrocarbons. Their extremely long half-lives in the environment (years) resulted in their removal from the market to prevent more severe environmental toxicity.

C. Cholinesterase Inhibitors: The carbamate and organophosphate inhibitors are effective insecticides and have much shorter environmental half-lives than do the chlorinated hydrocarbons. The cholinesterase inhibitors are inexpensive and, unlike DDT and its analogues, are heavily used in agriculture.

1. **Effects:** As described in Chapter 7, these agents produce increased muscarinic and nicotinic stimulation: pinpoint pupils; sweating; salivation; bronchoconstriction; vomiting and diarrhea; CNS stimulation followed by depression; and muscle fasciculations, weakness, and paralysis. The most common cause of death in mammals is respiratory failure. Chronic exposure to some of these agents may result in a delayed neurotoxicity with axonal degeneration.

2. **Treatment:** Atropine is used in large doses to control muscarinic excess; pralidoxime (2-PAM) is used to "regenerate" cholinesterase. Mechanical ventilation may be necessary.

D. Botanical Insecticides:

1. **Nicotine:** Nicotine has the same effects on nicotinic cholinoceptors in insects as in mammals and probably kills by the same mechanism, ie, excitation followed by paralysis of ganglionic, CNS, and neuromuscular transmission. Treatment is supportive.

2. **Rotenone:** This plant alkaloid insecticide causes gastrointestinal distress when ingested, and irritation when applied to the eye. Treatment is symptomatic.

3. **Pyrethrum:** This mixture of plant alkaloids causes excitation of the CNS and peripheral nervous system, including convulsions. Treatment is symptomatic, with anticonvulsants if necessary.

HERBICIDES

A. Classification & Prototypes: Paraquat and phenoxyacetic acids are the two major groups in this class.

B. Paraquat: Paraquat is used extensively on farms and for highway maintenance and is relatively nontoxic unless ingested. After ingestion, the initial effect is gastrointestinal irritation with hematemesis and bloody stools. Within a few days, signs of pulmonary impairment occur and are usually progressive, resulting in severe pulmonary fibrosis and, often, death. No antidote is available; the best supportive treatment, including gastric lavage and dialysis, still results in less than 50% survival after ingestion of as little as 5 mL.

C. Phenoxyacetic Acids: 2,4-Dichlorophenoxyacetic acid (2,4-D) and 2,4,5-trichlorophenoxyacetic acid (2,4,5-T) are the two most important members of this group. During the manufacturing process, a contaminant, 2,3,7,8-tetrachlorodibenzo-p-dioxin (TCDD or dioxin), is produced. Acute exposure to TCDD causes teratogenic and carcinogenic effects in some animals and dermatitis and chloracne in humans. Increasing evidence suggests that dioxin may have carcinogenic effects in humans, but no long-term toxic effects other than acne scarring have been proved.

POLYCHLORINATED BIPHENYLS

The polychlorinated biphenyls (PCBs) were used extensively in manufacturing electrical equipment until their potential for environmental damage was recognized. PCBs constitute a very large group of related compounds that are among the most stable organic compounds known. They are poorly metabolized and lipophilic. They are therefore highly persistent in the environment and accumulate in the food chain. The effects of PCBs are highly species-specific. In humans, the best documented effects involve the skin and include dermatitis and chloracne. Other effects include hepatic enzyme elevation and increased plasma triglycerides.

QUESTIONS

DIRECTIONS: Each of the numbered items or incomplete statements in this section is followed by answers or by completions of the statement. Select the ONE lettered answer or completion that is BEST in each case.

1. The light-brownish color of smog often apparent in the Los Angeles area on a hot summer day is mainly due to
   (A) Sulfur dioxide
   (B) Hydrocarbons
   (C) Ozone
   (D) Nitrogen dioxide
   (E) Carbon monoxide

2. You are stuck in traffic in New York City (in summer) for 3 or 4 hours and you begin to get a headache, a feeling of tightness in the temporal region, and an increased pulse rate. The most likely cause of these effects is inhalation of
   (A) Sulfur dioxide
   (B) Ozone
   (C) Nicotine
   (D) Carbon monoxide
   (E) Nitrogen dioxide

3. An employee works all day in a storage facility that contains agricultural chemicals and solvents. All of the following statements about his possible exposure to toxic substances in the workplace are accurate EXCEPT
   (A) Ambient air concentrations of such chemicals should be regularly monitored
   (B) He may experience fatigue and possibly become ataxic if he is exposed to halogenated hydrocarbon vapors
   (C) He may develop a delayed neuropathy if he is working in areas where organophosphates are stored
   (D) The worker may develop acne from exposure to chlorophenoxy herbicides
   (E) He may develop a delayed pulmonary edema if he is exposed to chlorinated hydrocarbon insecticides

4. Correct pairings of toxic agent with the best method of treatment include all of the following EXCEPT
   (A) Carbon monoxide: 100% or hyperbaric oxygen
   (B) Parathion: atropine and pralidoxime
   (C) Nitrogen dioxide: nonspecific treatment of noncardiogenic pulmonary edema
   (D) Carbon tetrachloride: support of vital signs
   (E) Paraquat: hemodialysis

DIRECTIONS: The following section consists of a list of four to twenty-six lettered options followed by several numbered items. For each numbered item, select the ONE option that is most closely associated with it. Each answer may be used once, more than once, or not at all.

   (A) Parathion
   (B) Pyrethrum
   (C) Dioxin
   (D) Paraquat
   (E) Polychlorinated biphenyl
   (F) Sulfur dioxide
   (G) Benzene
   (H) Aldicarb
   (I) Rotenone
   (J) Tetrachloroethylene

5. Exposure to this agent leads to irritation of the eyes, nose, and throat, with bronchoconstriction and possibly, bronchospasm

6. Acute exposure to this aliphatic hydrocarbon solvent causes CNS depression; chronic exposure has led to impairment of memory and peripheral neuropathy

7. This compound is a contaminant in the manufacture of an herbicide

8. This is an extremely stable compound previously used in the manufacture of electrical devices

9. This agent is derived from a botanical source. The most frequent adverse effect reported is contact dermatitis. Accidental oral ingestion causes CNS stimulation, including seizures

ANSWERS

1. Smog color is derived in part from suspended particulate matter including sulfides. When smog is light brown, the color derives from nitrogen oxides. All of the other air pollutants listed are colorless. The answer is **(D)**.
2. The symptoms described are those of carbon monoxide inhalation. The answer is **(D)**.
3. Although DDT and related compounds are no longer used as insecticides in this country, they continue to be manufactured here for foreign markets. Exposure to such compounds causes CNS excitation, not pulmonary dysfunction. The answer is **(E)**.
4. Hemodialysis is of no value in paraquat poisoning. The answer is **(E)**.
5. Sulfur dioxide forms sulfurous acid on contact with moist surfaces, and this is responsible for its irritant effects on mucous membranes of the eye, oropharyngeal cavity, and the respiratory tract. The answer is **(F)**.
6. Two solvents are listed, benzene and tetrachloroethylene. Both may cause CNS effects such as headache, fatigue, and loss of appetite. Benzene is an *aromatic* hydrocarbon and is thought to be leukemogenic. The answer is **(J)**.
7. Dioxin is a contaminant in the manufacture of 2,4-D and 2,4,5-T. The answer is **(C)**.
8. The polychlorinated biphenyls (PCBs) are extremely stable lipid-soluble organic insulators formerly used in electrical transformers and switches. The answer is **(E)**.
9. Rotenone and pyrethrum alkaloids are both derived from plants. Both agents may cause dermatitis through skin contact. Accidental oral ingestion of rotenone causes gastrointestinal irritation but no neurotoxic effects. The answer is **(B)**.

59   Chelators & Heavy Metals

OBJECTIVES

You should be able to:

- Describe the general mechanism of metal chelation.
- List the important chelator drugs.
- Describe the major clinical features and treatment of acute and chronic lead poisoning.
- Describe the major clinical features and treatment of arsenic poisoning.
- Describe the major clinical features and treatment of inorganic and organic mercury poisoning.
- Describe the major clinical features and treatment of iron intoxication.

Learn the definitions that follow.

Table 59–1. Definitions.

Term	Definition
Chelating agent	A molecule with two or more electronegative groups that can form stable coordinate complexes with multivalent cationic metal atoms
Erethism	Syndrome resulting from mercury poisoning characterized by insomnia, memory loss, excitability, and delirium
Pica	The ingestion of nonfood substances; in the present context, refers to ingestion of lead-based paint fragments by small children
Plumbism	A range of toxic syndromes due to chronic lead poisoning that may vary as a function of blood/tissue levels and patient age

CONCEPTS

The metals discussed in this chapter, especially lead, arsenic, and mercury, frequently cause significant toxicity in humans. The toxicity profiles of metals differ, but most of their effects appear to result from interaction with sulfhydryl groups of enzymes and regulatory proteins. Chelators are organic compounds with two or more electronegative groups that can form stable covalent-coordinate bonds with cationic metal atoms. As emphasized in this chapter, these stable complexes can often be excreted readily, thus reducing the toxicity of the metal.

CHELATORS

The most useful chelators for clinical purposes are dimercaprol (BAL), penicillamine, edetate (EDTA), deferoxamine, and succimer. Variations between the individual agents in their affinities for specific metal atoms is a determinant of their clinical applications.

A.   Dimercaprol: Dimercaprol (2,3-dimercaptopropanol, BAL [British AntiLewisite]) is useful in arsenic, lead, mercury, and cadmium poisoning. The agent is a bidentate chelator, ie, it forms two bonds with the metal ion, preventing the metal's binding to tissue proteins and permitting its rapid excretion. Dimercaprol is an oily liquid that must be given parenterally. The agent causes a high incidence of minor-to-moderate adverse effects, possibly because it is very lipophilic and enters cells readily. These effects include transient hypertension, tachycardia, headache, nausea, vomiting, and paresthesias.

B.   Penicillamine & N-Acetylpenicillamine: Penicillamine (d-penicillamine) is a derivative of penicillin. The agent is water-soluble, well absorbed from the gastrointestinal tract, and excreted unchanged. Penicillamine, a bidentate chelator, forms two bonds with the metal ion. The major uses of the agent are in the treatment of copper poisoning and Wilson's disease. Penicillamine is sometimes used as adjunctive therapy in gold, arsenic, and lead intoxication, and in rheumatoid arthritis. Toxicity may be severe and may include aplastic anemia, lupus erythematosus, and hemolytic anemia.

C.   Edetate: Edetate (EDTA) is a very efficient polydentate chelator of many divalent and trivalent cations (including calcium). To prevent dangerous hypocalcemia, EDTA is given as the calcium disodium salt. Because the agent is very polar, it is poorly absorbed and does not enter cells. The primary use of EDTA is in the treatment of lead poisoning. The most important adverse effect of the agent is nephrotoxicity, including renal tubular necrosis.

D.   Deferoxamine: Deferoxamine is a polydentate bacterial product that has an extremely selective affinity for iron. Fortunately, the drug competes poorly for heme iron (in hemoglobin and cytochromes). This chelator is used parenterally in the treatment of acute iron intoxication. Skin reactions may occur; with long-term use, neurotoxicity (eg, retinal degeneration), hepatic and renal dysfunction, and severe coagulopathies have been reported. Rapid intravenous administration may cause histamine release and hypotensive shock.

E.   Succimer: This newer chelating agent (2,3-dimercaptosuccinic acid, DMSA) is an orally effective congener of dimercaprol. Succimer is currently approved for the treatment of lead toxicity in children, and it also appears to be more effective than dimercaprol in mercury and arsenic poisoning. While succimer appears to be less toxic than dimercaprol, gastrointestinal distress, CNS effects, skin rash, and elevation of liver enzymes may occur. This agent should not be administered with other chelating drugs.

The applications of the chelators are outlined in Table 59–2.

TOXICOLOGY OF THE HEAVY METALS

A.   Lead: Lead serves no useful purpose in the body and may damage the hematopoietic tissues, liver, nervous system, kidneys, gastrointestinal tract, and reproductive system (Table 59–2). Lead represents a major environmental hazard since it is present in the air and water throughout the world.

Table 59–2. Important characteristics of the toxicology of arsenic, iron, lead, and mercury.[1]

Metal	Form Entering Body	Route of Absorption	Target Organs for Toxicity	Treatment
Lead	Inorganic lead oxides and salts	Gastrointestinal, respiratory, skin (minor)	Hematopoietic system, CNS, kidneys	Dimercaprol, edetate, penicillamine, succimer
	Tetraethyl lead	Skin (major), gastrointestinal	CNS	Seizure control, supportive
Arsenic	Inorganic arsenic salts	All mucous surfaces	Capillaries, gastrointestinal tract, hematopoietic system	Dimercaprol, succimer, penicillamine
	Arsine gas	Inhalation	Erythrocytes	Supportive
Mercury	Elemental	Inhalation	CNS, kidneys	Dimercaprol
	Inorganic salts	Gastrointestinal	Kidneys, gastrointestinal tract	Penicillamine, dimercaprol
	Organic mercurials	Gastrointestinal	CNS	Supportive
Iron	Ferrous sulfate	Gastrointestinal	Gastrointestinal, CNS, blood	Deferoxamine

[1] In all cases, removal of the individual from the source of toxicity is the first requirement of management.

1. **Acute lead poisoning:** Acute inorganic lead poisoning is no longer common in the USA, but may occur from industrial exposures (usually via the inhalation of dust) and in children who have ingested a large quantity of chips or flakes from surfaces covered with lead-containing paint. The primary signs of this syndrome are acute abdominal colic and CNS changes. In children, the latter may take the form of acute encephalopathy. The mortality rate is high in lead encephalopathy, and prompt chelation therapy is mandatory.

2. **Chronic lead poisoning:** Chronic inorganic lead poisoning (plumbism) is much more common than the acute form. Signs include peripheral neuropathy (wrist drop is characteristic), anorexia, anemia, tremor, weight loss, and gastrointestinal symptoms. Treatment includes removal from the source of exposure, and chelation therapy, usually with edetate (severe cases), dimercaprol, or penicillamine. In addition to these agents, succimer is also approved for use in children. In workers exposed to lead, prophylaxis by means of oral chelating agents is contraindicated, since some evidence suggests that lead absorption may be enhanced. In contrast, high dietary calcium is indicated, since lead retention is reduced.

3. **Organic lead poisoning:** Poisoning by organic lead is usually due to tetraethyl or tetramethyl antiknock gasoline additives. This form of lead is readily absorbed through the skin and lungs. The primary signs of intoxication occur in the CNS and may include hallucinations, headache, irritability, convulsions, and coma. Treatment consists of decontamination and seizure control.

B. **Arsenic:** This element is widely used in industrial processes and is also an environmental pollutant released during the burning of coal. Although it exists in both trivalent and pentavalent forms, its toxicity is entirely due to the trivalent form.

1. **Acute arsenic poisoning:** Acute arsenic poisoning results in severe gastrointestinal discomfort, vomiting, rice water stools, and capillary damage with dehydration and shock. A sweet, garlicky odor may be detected in the breath and the stools. Treatment consists of supportive therapy to replace water and electrolytes, and chelation therapy with dimercaprol.

2. **Chronic arsenic poisoning:** Chronic arsenic intoxication is manifested by skin changes, hair loss, bone marrow depression and anemia, and chronic nausea and gastrointestinal disturbances. Dimercaprol therapy appears to be of value.

3. **Arsine gas:** Arsine gas (AsH_3) is formed during the refinement and processing of certain metals and is used in the semiconductor industry; it is an occupational hazard. Arsine causes a unique form of toxicity characterized by massive hemolysis. Pigment overload from red cell breakdown may cause renal failure. Treatment is supportive.

C. **Mercury:** The main source of inorganic mercury as a toxic hazard is through the use of materials in dental laboratories and in the manufacture of wood preservatives, insecticides, and batteries. Organic mercury compounds are used as seed dressings and fungicides.

1. **Acute mercury poisoning:** Acute mercury poisoning usually occurs through inhalation of inorganic elemental mercury. It causes chest pain, shortness of breath, nausea and vomiting, kidney damage, gastroenteritis, and CNS damage. Chelation is effected with dimercaprol.

2. **Chronic mercury poisoning:** Chronic mercury poisoning may occur with inorganic or organic mercury. Inorganic mercury poisoning in the chronic form usually presents as a diffuse set of symptoms involving the gums and teeth, gastrointestinal disturbances, and neurologic and behavioral changes. When mercury was used in the hat-making industry, the personality effects (erethism) were so common that they gave rise to the epithet "mad as a hatter." Chronic inorganic mercury intoxication has been treated with penicillamine and dimercaprol.

3. **Organic mercury poisoning:** Intoxication with organic mercury compounds was first recognized in connection with an epidemic of neurologic and psychiatric disease in the village of Minamata in Japan. The outbreak was found to be the result of consumption of fish containing a high content of methylmercury, which was produced by bacteria in seawater from mercury in the effluent of a nearby vinyl plastics manufacturing plant. Similar epidemics have resulted from the consumption of grain intended for use as seed and treated with fungicidal organic mercury compounds. Treatment with chelators has been tried, but the benefits are uncertain.

D. Iron: Acute poisoning from the ingestion of ferrous sulfate tablets occurs almost as frequently as salicylate intoxication in children. The initial symptoms of iron poisoning include vomiting, gastrointestinal bleeding, lethargy, and gray cyanosis. This may be followed by signs of severe gastrointestinal necrosis, pneumonitis, jaundice, seizures, and coma. Deferoxamine is the chelating agent of choice (see Chapter 60). Chronic excessive intake of iron may lead to hemosiderosis or hemochromatosis.

QUESTIONS

DIRECTIONS: Each numbered item or incomplete statement in this section is followed by answers or by completions of the statement. Select the ONE lettered answer or completion that is BEST in each case.

Items 1–2:   A small child is brought to a hospital emergency room suffering from severe gastrointestinal distress, abdominal colic, and neurologic dysfunction.

1. The differential diagnosis will include all of the following EXCEPT
   - **(A)** Appendicitis
   - **(B)** Pancreatitis
   - **(C)** Acute inorganic lead poisoning
   - **(D)** Exposure to arsine gas
   - **(E)** Peptic ulcer

2. If this patient has severe acute lead poisoning, treatment should be instituted immediately with
   - **(A)** Penicillamine
   - **(B)** EDTA
   - **(C)** Deferoxamine
   - **(D)** Succimer
   - **(E)** Acetylcysteine

3. A young woman employed as a dental laboratory technician complains of conjunctivitis, skin irritation, and hair loss. On examination, she has perforation of the nasal septum and a "milk and roses" complexion. These signs and symptoms are most likely to be due to
   - **(A)** Acute mercury poisoning
   - **(B)** Chronic inorganic arsenic poisoning
   - **(C)** Excessive use of supplementary iron tablets
   - **(D)** Chronic mercury poisoning
   - **(E)** Lead poisoning

4. A patient complains of chronic headache, fatigue, loss of appetite, and constipation. He has a slight weakness of the extensor muscle in the upper limbs. The following data is obtained.

Test	Result in Patient	Normal
Hemoglobin	<13 g/dL	>14 g/dL
Urinary coproporphyrin	>80 mcg/100 mg creatinine	<10 mcg/100 mg creatinine
Urinary aminolevulinic acid	>2 mg/100 mg creatinine	<0.5 mg/100 mg creatinine

In the context of toxicology, the most reasonable diagnosis is that this patient is suffering from chronic poisoning due to
(A) Organophosphates
(B) Inorganic lead
(C) Organic mercury
(D) Benzene arsenicals
(E) Hexane

5. In the treatment of arsenic poisoning, removal of the source of arsenic exposure is the primary therapeutic objective, but if the patient is treated with an oral chelating agent the most likely drug to be used is
(A) Penicillamine
(B) Dimercaprol
(C) EDTA
(D) Deferoxamine

DIRECTIONS: The following section consists of a list of four to twenty-six lettered options followed by several numbered items. For each numbered item, select the ONE option that is most closely associated with it. Each answer may be used once, more than once, or not at all.
(A) Trivalent arsenic
(B) Methylmercury
(C) Dimercaprol
(D) Penicillamine
(E) Edetate calcium disodium
(F) Inorganic mercury
(G) Deferoxamine
(H) Tetraethyl lead

6. Gingivitis, discolored gums, and loose teeth are common symptoms of chronic exposure to this agent

7. This compound may be produced in seawater by the action of bacteria and algae. It is also synthesized chemically for commercial use as a fungicide

8. This agent has been reported to cause lupus erythematosus and hemolytic anemia

9. High doses of this agent may cause histamine release and extreme vasodilation

ANSWERS

1. The diagnosis of acute lead poisoning may be difficult, since the symptoms often simulate a number of disorders of the gastrointestinal system, including acute appendicitis. Exposure to arsine, an industrial gas, is highly unlikely in a small child, and the toxicity of arsine is characterized by massive hemolysis. The answer is **(D)**.

2. In severe lead poisoning, intravenous EDTA is the most effective chelating agent of those listed. Dimercaprol (not listed) may also be used parenterally. Oral succimer is used in children with mild-to-moderate lead poisoning. The answer is **(B)**.

3. The "milk and roses" complexion, which results from vasodilation and anemia, is characteristic of chronic inorganic arsenic poisoning, while patients with lead poisoning often have a gray pallor. Other signs and symptoms include gastrointestinal distress, hyperpigmentation, and white lines on the nails. We hope you were not led astray by her employment. The answer is **(B)**.

4. Of the agents listed, lead is most likely to cause a decrease in heme biosynthesis. Exposure to inorganic arsenic may also cause anemia. The urinary concentrations of lead before and after EDTA treatment may confirm the diagnosis. The answer is **(B)**.

5. Only one of the agents listed is effective orally. Although it is more toxic, penicillamine is more likely to be used at the present time than the newer agent succimer (not listed). The answer is (**A**).

6. Mouth and gastrointestinal complaints are common in chronic mercury poisoning, and tremor, involving the fingers and arms, is often present. The answer is (**F**).

7. Methylmercury continues to be used as a fungicide to prevent mold growth in seed grain. The answer is (**B**).

8. Autoimmune diseases have occurred during the treatment of Wilson's disease with penicillamine. The answer is (**D**).

9. Deferoxamine may cause shock if given by rapid intravenous infusion. The answer is (**G**).

Management of the Poisoned Patient **60**

OBJECTIVES

You should be able to list or describe the following:

- The most common causes of death in the following poisonings: sedative-hypnotics, narcotics, cocaine, paraquat, digitalis, and tricyclic antidepressants.
- Specific antidotes for the following agents: heroin and other opioids, acetaminophen, methanol, ethylene glycol, and parathion.
- The emergency treatment (before laboratory results are available) of a comatose patient.
- The contraindications to the use of emesis for ingestion of a toxin.

CONCEPTS

Toxic agents include drugs usually used for therapeutic purposes, as well as agricultural and industrial chemicals that have no medical applications. Most chemicals are capable of causing toxic effects when given in excessive dosage; even for therapeutic drugs, the difference between obtaining a therapeutic action and a toxic one is a matter of dose. Many toxic effects of therapeutic agents have been discussed in previous chapters of this book. The nontherapeutic chemicals most commonly involved in poisonings are those readily accessible in the environment: solvents, corrosives, insecticides, drugs of abuse, and heavy metals. This unit reviews the general pharmacology of such poisonings.

A. **Toxicokinetics & Toxicodynamics:** Toxicokinetics refers to the pharmacokinetics of poisons. Knowledge of the modes and rates of absorption permits assessment of the value of procedures designed to remove toxins from the skin or gastrointestinal tract. In general, drugs with large volumes of distribution (Vd) are not amenable to dialysis procedures for drug removal in overdosage. In the case of gross overdosage, the capacity of the liver to metabolize the drug may be exceeded, and elimination will change from first-order to zero-order kinetics.

   A knowledge of toxicodynamics (the injurious effects of toxins) can be useful in the diagnosis and management of poisoning. For example, hyperthermia due to reduced sweating (a typical antimuscarinic effect) may assist in the identification of the toxic agent. Similarly, overdoses of agents that are cardiodepressant are likely to affect the functions of all organ systems that are critically dependent on blood flow, including brain, liver, and kidney. Restoration of blood pressure may increase the tissue distribution of a toxin, which can result in a waxing and waning of signs and symptoms.

B. Cause of Death in Intoxicated Patients: The most common causes of death from drug overdose in the USA reflect the drug groups most often selected for abuse or for suicide. Sedative-hypnotics and narcotics cause respiratory depression, coma, aspiration of gastric contents, and other respiratory malfunctions. Drugs such as cocaine, PCP, tricyclic antidepressants, and theophylline cause convulsions, which may lead to vomiting and aspiration of gastric contents, and to postictal respiratory depression. Tricyclic antidepressants and cardiac glycosides cause dangerous and frequently lethal arrhythmias. Severe hypotension may occur with any of these drugs. A few intoxicants cause direct liver and kidney damage. These include acetaminophen and mushroom poisons of the *Amanita phalloides* type, certain inhalants, and some heavy metals. The metals are discussed in Chapter 59.

C. Identification of Poisons: Many intoxicants cause a characteristic syndrome of clinical and laboratory changes. A summary of some of these toxic syndromes is given in Table 60–1. When the chemical used in a case of poisoning cannot be directly examined and identified, the clinician must rely on indirect means to identify the type of intoxication and the progress of therapy. In addition to the history and physical examination, certain laboratory examinations of blood may be useful. A few intoxicants can be directly identified in the blood or urine, especially when information in the history helps to narrow the search. In the more common situation (a comatose patient unable to provide a history), general tests for replacement of anions or osmotic equivalents in the blood (anion gap, osmolar gap) may be useful. A few intoxicants can be identified or strongly suspected on the basis of electrocardiographic or radiologic findings.

1. Osmolar gap: The osmolar gap is the difference between the measured osmolarity (measured by the freezing point depression method) and the predicted osmolarity:

$$\text{Gap} = \text{Osm (measured)} - [(2 \times \text{Na}^+ \text{ [meq/L]}) + (\text{Glucose [mg/dL]} \div 18) + (\text{BUN [mg/dL]} \div 3)]$$

This gap is normally zero. A significant gap is produced by high serum levels of intoxicants of low molecular weight such as ethanol, methanol, and ethylene glycol.

2. Anion gap: The anion gap is the difference between the sum of the two primary cations, sodium and potassium, and the sum of the two primary anions, chloride and bicarbonate:

$$\text{Gap} = (\text{Na}^+ + \text{K}^+) - (\text{HCO}_3^- + \text{Cl}^-)$$

This gap is normally 12–16 meq/L. A significant increase may be produced by diabetic ketoacidosis, renal failure, or drug-induced metabolic acidosis (from aspirin, methanol, ethylene glycol, isoniazid, or iron).

3. Serum potassium: Myocardial function is critically dependent on serum potassium level. Drugs that cause hyperkalemia include beta-adrenoceptor blockers, digitalis, fluoride, and lithium. Drugs associated with hypokalemia include barium, beta-adrenoceptor agonists, methylxanthines, most diuretics, and toluene.

D. Treatment of Poisoning: Management of the poisoned patient consists of maintenance of vital functions, decontamination, enhancement of elimination, and, in a very few instances, the use of a specific antidote.

1. Vital functions: The most important aspect of treatment of a poisoned patient is maintenance of vital functions, as indicated by the mnemonic *ABCs*. The most commonly endangered or impaired vital function is respiration. Therefore, an open and protected airway (the "A" of the mnemonic) must be established first and effective ventilation ("B" for breathing) must be ensured. The circulation ("C") should be evaluated and supported as needed. The cardiac rhythm should be determined, and if ventricular fibrillation is present, it must be corrected at once. The blood pressure should be measured, but rarely needs immediate treatment except in cases of traumatic hemorrhage. *Because of the danger of brain damage from hypoglycemia, intravenous glucose (50% solution) should be given to comatose patients immediately after blood has been drawn for laboratory tests and before laboratory results have been obtained.* Similarly, thiamine should be given to prevent Wernicke's syndrome in alcoholics.

Decontamination: Decontamination consists of removing any unabsorbed poison from the patient's body. In the case of ingested noncorrosive toxins, this may involve inducing

Table 60–1. Toxic syndromes.[1]

Cause	Manifestations
Acetaminophen	Mild anorexia, nausea, vomiting, delayed jaundice, hepatic and renal failure
Amphetamines	Toxic psychosis, hyperthermia, flushing, hypertension, dilated pupils, hallucinations, seizures, tachycardia, rhabdomyolysis
Antifreeze (ethylene glycol)	Renal failure, crystals in urine, anion and osmolar gap, initial CNS excitation; but eye examination normal
Arsenic	Early: garlicky breath, vomiting, profuse bloody diarrhea, burning tears; delayed: hair loss, lines on nails, neuropathy, increased skin pigmentation. Arsine gas: hemolysis
Botulism	Dysphagia, dysarthria, ptosis, ophthalmoplegia, muscle weakness; incubation period 12–36 h
Bromide	Increased skin pigmentation, acne, dementia, psychosis, hyperchloremia
Cadmium	Metallic taste, delayed pulmonary edema; late: kidney and lung disease
Carbon monoxide	Coma, metabolic acidosis, normal PaO_2, retinal hemorrhages
Cocaine	Perforated nasal septum, dilated pupils, psychosis, tachycardia, seizures
Cyanide	Bitter almond odor, seizures, coma, abnormal ECG
Gasoline	Distinctive odor, coughing, pulmonary infiltrates
Heroin	Coma, hypotension, bradycardia, hypoventilation, miosis, needle marks, rapid response to naloxone
Hydrocarbons	Pneumonia, tinnitus, seizures, ventricular fibrillation, unique odor
Hydrogen sulfide	Rotten egg odor, loss of sense of smell, sudden collapse and death
Iron	Bloody diarrhea, coma, radiopaque material in gut (seen on X-ray), high leucocyte count, hyperglycemia
Isopropyl alcohol	Gastritis, ketonemia with normoglycemia, osmolar gap
Lead	Abdominal pain, hypertension, seizures, muscle weakness, metallic taste, anorexia, encephalopathy, delayed motor neuropathy, changes in renal and reproductive function
LSD	Hallucinations, dilated pupils, hypertension
Mercury	Acute renal failure, tremor, salivation, gingivitis, colitis, erethism (fits of crying, irrational behavior), nephrotic syndrome
Methanol	Rapid respiration, visual symptoms, osmolar gap, severe metabolic acidosis
Methylene chloride	History of paint-stripping exposure; confusion, increased carbon monoxide level
Mushrooms (*Amanita phalloides* type)	Severe nausea and vomiting 8 hours after ingestion; delayed hepatic and renal failure
Nitrogen oxides	History of silo or cave exposure; delayed pulmonary edema, chronic chemical pneumonitis
Organophosphates or carbamates	Miosis, abdominal cramps, salivation, lacrimation, urination, increased bronchial secretion, muscle fasciculations, bradycardia
Paraquat	Oropharyngeal burning, headache, vomiting, delayed pulmonary fibrosis and death
Phencyclidine (PCP)	Coma with eyes open, horizontal and vertical nystagmus, hyperacusis, myoclonic jerks, violent behavior
Phosgene	History of exposure to burning plastics; pulmonary edema
Plants, poisonous Nightshade family, Jimson weed	Hallucinations, mydriasis, seizures (these plants contain atropine-like alkaloids)
Oleander and foxglove	Digitalis poisoning
Predatory bean (rosary pea)	Delayed severe gastrointestinal distress, seizures, hemolytic anemia, death
Strychnine	Stiff neck, status epilepticus, hyperacusis
Thallium (rat poison)	Alopecia, gastrointestinal distress, motor and sensory neuropathy, hematologic examination normal
Vacor (rat poison)	Ketoacidosis, postural hypotension
Vanadium	Green tongue, severe pulmonary irritation

[1] Modified and reproduced, with permission, from Katzung BG (editor): *Basic & Clinical Pharmacology,* 6th ed. Appleton & Lange, 1995.

vomiting (emesis) by means of syrup of ipecac if the patient is conscious. Apomorphine and *extract* of ipecac are dangerous emetics and should not be used. In unconscious patients, emesis will lead to aspiration into the respiratory tree and must be avoided. Gastric lavage with a large-bore tube may be used to remove noncorrosive drugs from the stomach of a comatose patient if the airway has been protected with a cuffed endotracheal tube. Corrosives (strong acids and bases) may cause severe esophageal damage during emesis and should be diluted (not neutralized) in the stomach. Activated charcoal, given orally or by stomach tube, may be very effective in adsorbing any remaining drug. Cathartics may be useful to enhance the removal of unabsorbed drug from the intestine. In the case of topical exposure (insecticides, solvents), the clothing should be removed and the patient washed to remove any chemical still present on the skin. Medical personnel must be careful not to contaminate themselves during this procedure.

3. **Enhancement of elimination:** Enhancement of elimination is possible for a number of intoxicants. These methods include manipulation of urine pH to accelerate urinary excretion of weak acids and bases. Hemodialysis or hemoperfusion enhances the elimination of certain compounds including ethylene glycol, methanol, salicylates, lithium, and procainamide.

4. **Antidotes:** Specific antidotes exist for only a few poisons (Table 60–2). Consideration must be given to the fact that the duration of action of most antidotes is shorter than that of the intoxicant, and the antidotes may need to be given repeatedly. The use of chelating agents for metal poisoning is discussed in Chapter 59. "Universal antidote" (burnt toast, magnesium oxide, tannic acid) is of no value and may be harmful.

E. **Snake Bite:** The most common dangerous snake in the USA is the rattlesnake. Although snake bites are common (several thousand per year in the USA), severe envenomation is infrequent.

1. **Effects:** Snake venom contains a large number of enzymes and tissue toxins. The most common effects of envenomation include local tissue necrosis, vascular damage, thrombosis, hemorrhage, and neural injury.

2. **Treatment:** It is now well documented that once-popular remedies such as incision and suction, ice packs, and tourniquets are usually more dangerous than helpful. The most important prehospital therapy is to minimize movement of the bitten part to reduce the spread

Table 60–2. Specific antidotes.[1]

Antidote	Poison(s)
Acetylcysteine	Acetaminophen
Atropine	Cholinesterase inhibitors
Bicarbonate, sodium	Membrane depressant cardiotoxic drugs, eg, quinidine, TCAs
Deferoxamine	Iron salts
Digoxin-specific FAB antibodies	Digoxin and related cardiac glycosides
Esmolol	Caffeine, theophylline, metaproterenol
Ethanol	Methanol, ethylene glycol
Flumazenil	Benzodiazepines
Glucagon	Beta-adrenoceptor blockers
Edetate (EDTA)	Lead
Dimercaprol	Lead, gold, arsenic
Penicillamine	Copper, lead, arsenic, gold
Naloxone	Opioid analgesics
Oxygen	Carbon monoxide
Physostigmine	Suggested for muscarinic receptor blockers, NOT for tricyclics
Pralidoxime (2-PAM)	Cholinesterase inhibitors

[1] Modified and reproduced, with permission, from Katzung BG (editor): *Basic & Clinical Pharmacology,* 6th ed. Appleton & Lange, 1995.

of the venom in the tissues. Effective therapy consists of adequate dosage with antivenin. Since antivenins are prepared in horses, serum sickness frequently follows and may also require therapy.

QUESTIONS

DIRECTIONS: Each of the numbered items or incomplete statements in this section is followed by answers or by completions of the statement. Select the ONE lettered answer or completion that is BEST in each case.

Items 1–2: A patient has taken an overdose of aspirin that has caused metabolic acidosis. Serum electrolyte concentrations are: Na^+, 147 mEq/L; K^+, 6 mEq/L; Cl^-, 100 mEq/L; HCO_3^-, 15 mEq/L.

1. The anion gap in this patient
   (A) Cannot be calculated from the data given
   (B) Is unchanged from normal
   (C) Is increased above normal
   (D) Is decreased below normal
   (E) Is reversed

2. Which of the following agents may cause an INCREASE in anion gap?
   (A) Isoniazid
   (B) Methanol
   (C) Iron
   (D) Ethylene glycol
   (E) All of the above

3. All of the following drugs or toxins are likely to cause hyperthermia in overdosage EXCEPT
   (A) Amphetamine
   (B) Heroin
   (C) Jimson weed
   (D) Aspirin
   (E) Phencyclidine

4. A patient is brought to an emergency room suffering from nausea, vomiting, and abdominal pain. He has muscle weakness, which seems to be progressing downwards from the head and neck. The patient has difficulty talking clearly and has ptosis and ophthalmoplegia. The most likely cause of these symptoms is
   (A) Excessive consumption of ethanol
   (B) An overdose of phenobarbital
   (C) Food poisoning
   (D) Accidental ingestion of thallium (rat poison)
   (E) Organophosphate poisoning

5. All of the following may cause an osmolar gap EXCEPT
   (A) Ethylene glycol
   (B) Ethanol
   (C) Digoxin
   (D) Methanol
   (E) Isopropanol

6. Regarding snake bite,
   (A) Rattlesnake bite is almost always associated with significant tissue injury
   (B) A snake bite should be treated in the field with incision, suction, and a tourniquet before the victim is moved
   (C) The most common manifestation of serious envenomation is convulsions
   (D) When a victim of a serious envenomation reaches the hospital, the most effective therapy is prompt administration of snake antivenin
   (E) All of the above are correct

7. Intoxicants correctly associated with their effects include
   (A) Carbon monoxide: carboxyhemoglobinemia
   (B) Paraquat: pulmonary fibrosis
   (C) Cyanide: cytochrome oxidase inactivation

(D) Sodium nitrite: methemoglobinemia

(E) All of the above

DIRECTIONS: The following section consists of a list of four to twenty-six lettered options followed by several numbered items. For each numbered item, select the ONE option that is most closely associated with it. Each answer may be used once, more than once, or not at all.

(A) Heroin

(B) Methanol

(C) Theophylline

(D) Carbon monoxide

(E) Hydrogen cyanide

(F) Acetaminophen

(G) Parathion

(H) Iron

(I) Acetylsalicylic acid

(J) Hydrogen sulfide

8. The best antidote for this substance is atropine

9. The best antidote for this substance is an anticonvulsant, but beta-blockers are sometimes appropriate

10. The best antidote for this substance is acetylcysteine

11. The best antidote for this substance is ethanol

12. The standard antidote for this substance is sodium nitrite followed by sodium thiosulfate

ANSWERS

1. Anion gap is calculated by subtracting measured serum anions (bicarbonate + chloride) from cations (potassium + sodium). Increases in anion gap above normal are due to the presence of unmeasured anions that accompany acidosis. The answer is **(C).**

2. Toxic levels of all of the agents listed lead to acidosis. The answer is **(E).**

3. Aspirin, sympathomimetics, agents with muscarinic blocking actions, and drugs that cause muscle rigidity or seizures are all likely to cause hyperthermia at toxic doses. Hypothermia is more typical of opioids and the sedative-hypnotics. The answer is **(B).**

4. Food-borne botulism (due to *C botulinum*) may lead to a symmetric descending paralysis that results in respiratory failure. Patients are initially alert, but may suffer from dysarthria and dysphagia. Ptosis and ophthalmoplegia are also characteristic symptoms. The answer is **(C).**

5. Digoxin is lethal at levels much too low to be detected by the osmolar gap method. This method is useful only for poisonings with less potent substances of low molecular weight, eg, methanol and ethylene glycol. The answer is **(C).**

6. Only about 20% of rattlesnake bites involve significant envenomation. Incision, suction, and tourniquets are usually more damaging than helpful. Ice packs are contraindicated. Serious envenomation causes primarily local tissue damage. Antivenin is by far the most effective therapy for serious envenomation. The answer is **(D).**

7. All are correct. The answer is **(E).**

8. Atropine is the primary antidote for poisoning due to organophosphate (or carbamate) inhibition of acetylcholinesterase. Pralidoxime may be administered to regenerate inactivated enzyme. The answer is **(G),** parathion (see Table 60–2).

9. The most dangerous toxic effect of theophylline is convulsions. Cardiovascular toxicity (arrhythmias, hypotension) often responds to beta-blockers. The answer is **(C).**

10. The answer is **(F),** acetaminophen (see Table 60–2).

11. The answer is **(B),** methanol (see Table 60–2).

12. Mitochondrial cytochrome oxidase is inactivated by the binding of cyanide to the iron in heme. Sodium nitrite converts hemoglobin to methemoglobin, which competes favorably for the cyanide ion to form cyanomethemoglobin. Administration of sodium thiosulfate releases cyanide and causes formation of thiocyanate. The answer is **(E).**

Part X. Special Topics

Drugs Used in Gastrointestinal Disorders

61

OBJECTIVES

You should be able to:

- List five different drug groups used in the treatment of peptic ulcer and describe their mechanisms.
- List four drugs used in the prevention of chemotherapy-induced vomiting.
- List three laxative drugs and describe their mechanisms.
- List the two most important antidiarrheal drugs.

CONCEPTS

The gastrointestinal (GI) tract serves several functions: digestive, excretory, endocrine, exocrine, etc. These functions provide numerous important drug targets, and many of the drugs used in GI disease have been discussed in earlier chapters of this book. However, several important drugs used in common GI diseases do not fall into the drug groups discussed earlier; these drugs are described in this chapter.

A. Drugs Used in Acid-Peptic Disease: Ulceration and erosion of the lining of the GI tract are common problems, and several drug groups used in these diseases have been discussed (H_2 blockers, antimuscarinic drugs, mifepristone). Other drugs used in peptic disease include the antacids, sucralfate, omeprazole, and antibiotics.

    1. Antacids: Antacids are simple physical agents that react with protons in the lumen of the gut. Some antacids (eg, aluminum antacids) may also stimulate the protective functions of the gastric mucosa. The antacids effectively reduce the recurrence rate of peptic ulcers when used regularly in doses that significantly raise the stomach pH.

    The antacids differ mainly in their absorption and effects on stool consistency. The most popular antacids in use in the USA are **magnesium hydroxide** ($Mg(OH)_2$) and **aluminum hydroxide** ($Al(OH)_3$). Neither of these weak bases is absorbed from the bowel. Magnesium hydroxide has strong laxative effects, while aluminum hydroxide has constipating actions. These drugs are available as single-ingredient products and as combined preparations. Calcium carbonate and sodium bicarbonate are also weak bases, but they differ from aluminum and magnesium hydroxides in being absorbed from the gut. Because of their systemic effects, calcium and bicarbonate salts are less popular as antacids than magnesium and aluminum salts.

    2. Sucralfate: Sucralfate is aluminum sucrose sulfate, a small, poorly soluble molecule that polymerizes in the acid environment of the stomach. This polymer binds to injured tissue and forms a protective coating over ulcer beds. The drug has been shown to accelerate the healing of peptic ulcers and to reduce the recurrence rate. Sucralfate is too insoluble to have significant systemic effects when taken by the oral route.

    3. Omeprazole: Omeprazole is the first of a class of inhibitors of the proton pump of gastric parietal cells. This pump, a H^+/K^+ ATPase located in the luminal membrane of parietal

405

cells, binds omeprazole irreversibly and remains inhibited for 48 hours or longer. Omeprazole is particularly useful in the treatment of Zollinger-Ellison syndrome (usually associated with a gastrin-secreting tumor), and gastroesophageal reflux.

4. **Antibiotics:** Chronic infection with *Helicobacter pylori* occurs in a large fraction of patients with recurrent peptic ulcers, and eradication of this organism reduces the rate of recurrence of ulcer in these patients. The antibiotic regimen of choice consists of a 14-day course of bismuth (Pepto-Bismol), tetracycline, and metronidazole.

B. **Drugs That Promote Upper GI Motility:** Diabetes and other diseases that damage nerves to the viscera frequently cause a marked loss of motility in the esophagus and stomach (gastric paralysis or gastroparesis). This loss of motility is often associated with delayed emptying, nausea, and severe bloating. **Metoclopramide** and **cisapride** are able to stimulate motility in this condition, probably by acting as acetylcholine facilitators or as dopamine antagonists in the enteric nervous system.

This "prokinetic" action is also of some value in preventing emesis from surgical anesthesia and emesis induced by cancer chemotherapeutic drugs. Adverse effects include induction of parkinsonism and other extrapyramidal effects.

C. **Drugs With Antiemetic Actions:** A variety of drugs have been found to be of some value in the prevention and treatment of vomiting, especially cancer chemotherapy-induced vomiting. In addition to **metoclopramide** and **cisapride,** useful antiemetic drugs include **dexamethasone;** some **H_1 antihistamines;** several **phenothiazines;** the 5-HT_3 inhibitors, eg, **ondansetron;** and **dronabinol,** the active ingredient in marijuana.

D. **Pancreatic Enzyme Replacements:** Steatorrhea, a condition of decreased fat absorption coupled with an increase in stool fat excretion, results from inadequate pancreatic secretion of lipase. The abnormality of fat absorption can be significantly relieved by oral administration of pancreatic lipase **(pancrelipase)** obtained from pigs. Pancreatic lipase is inactivated at a pH below 4.0; thus up to 90% of an administered dose will be destroyed in the stomach, unless the pH is raised with antacids or drugs that reduce acid secretion.

E. **Laxatives:** Laxatives increase the probability of a bowel movement by several mechanisms: an irritant or stimulant action on the bowel wall; a bulk-forming action on the stool that evokes reflex contraction of the bowel; a softening action on hard or impacted stool; and a lubricating action that eases passage of stool through the rectum. Examples of drugs that act by these mechanisms are set forth in Table 61–1.

Table 61–1. The major laxative mechanisms and some representative drugs.

Mechanism	Examples
Irritant	Castor oil, cascara, senna, phenolphthalein
Bulk-forming	Saline cathartics [eg, Mg(OH)$_2$], psyllium
Stool-softening	Dioctyl sodium sulfosuccinate (docusate)
Lubricating	Mineral oil, glycerin

F. **Antidiarrheal Agents:** The most effective antidiarrheal drugs are the opioids and derivatives of opioids that have been selected for maximal antidiarrheal and minimal CNS effect. Of the latter group, the most important are **diphenoxylate** and **loperamide,** meperidine analogues with very weak analgesic effects. Diphenoxylate is formulated with antimuscarinic alkaloids to reduce the likelihood of abuse; loperamide is formulated alone and sold as such.

QUESTIONS

DIRECTIONS: Each numbered item or incomplete statement in this section is followed by answers or by completions of the statement. Select the ONE lettered answer or completion that is BEST in each case.

1. A 55-year-old woman with insulin-dependent diabetes of 40 years duration complains of severe bloating and abdominal distress, especially after meals. Evaluation is consistent with diabetic gastroparesis. The drug you would be most likely to recommend is
   (A) Docusate
   (B) Dopamine
   (C) Loperamide
   (D) Metoclopramide
   (E) Sucralfate

2. A patient who must take verapamil for hypertension and angina has become severely constipated. Which of the following drugs would be most suitable as a cathartic?
   (A) Aluminum hydroxide
   (B) Diphenoxylate
   (C) Magnesium hydroxide
   (D) Metoclopramide
   (E) Mineral oil

3. Your cousin is planning a three-week trip overseas and asks your advice regarding medications for traveler's diarrhea. A suitable drug would be
   (A) Aluminum hydroxide
   (B) Diphenoxylate
   (C) Magnesium hydroxide
   (D) Metoclopramide
   (E) Mineral oil

DIRECTIONS: The following section consists of a list of four to twenty-six lettered options followed by several numbered items. For each numbered item, select the ONE option that is most closely associated with it. Each answer may be selected once, more than once, or not at all.
   (A) Aluminum hydroxide
   (B) Castor oil
   (C) Dexamethasone
   (D) Diphenoxylate
   (E) Loperamide
   (F) Magnesium hydroxide
   (G) Metoclopramide
   (H) Mineral oil
   (I) Omeprazole
   (J) Sucralfate
   (K) Metronidazole

4. A drug that irreversibly inhibits the H^+/K^+ ATPase in gastric parietal cells
5. A drug with antacid and laxative properties
6. An antidiarrheal drug related to meperidine; it is formulated without any admixed drug
7. An antibiotic used in the treatment of recurrent peptic ulcer
8. A glucocorticoid used in preventing chemotherapy-induced vomiting
9. A lubricating laxative; not very effective if bowel tone is absent or severely reduced

ANSWERS

1. Of the drugs listed, only metoclopramide is considered a "prokinetic" agent, ie, one that increases propulsive motility in the gut. The answer is **(D)**.
2. A cathartic that mildly stimulates the gut would be most suitable in a patient taking a smooth muscle relaxant drug such as verapamil. Magnesium hydroxide, by holding water in the intestine, provides additional bulk and stimulates increased contractions. The answer is **(C)**.
3. Diphenoxylate and loperamide are the traditional traveler's antidiarrheal drugs. Diphenoxylate requires a prescription in the USA but is much less expensive than loperamide. The answer is **(B)**.
4. Omeprazole irreversibly inhibits the proton pump. The answer is **(I)**.
5. Magnesium hydroxide has both antacid and laxative effects. The answer is **(F)**.

6. Loperamide is formulated alone; diphenoxylate is mixed with atropine alkaloids. The answer is **(E)**.
7. Metronidazole is part of the antibiotic therapy used to eradicate *H pylori*. The answer is **(K)**.
8. Dexamethasone is a useful antiemetic in cancer chemotherapy. The answer is **(C)**.
9. Mineral oil is a lubricant. It has no irritant or bulk-forming properties. The answer is **(H)**.

62

Drug Interactions

OBJECTIVES

You should be able to:

- Describe the mechanisms of the acute interaction between alcohol and barbiturates and between alcohol and disulfiram.
- Describe the mechanism of the interaction between barbiturates and warfarin.
- Describe the interaction between quinidine and digoxin.
- Describe the interaction between clavulanic acid and amoxicillin, and categorize it as addition, synergism, or potentiation.

Learn the definitions that follow.

Table 62–1. Definitions.

Term	Definition
Pharmacokinetic interaction	A change in the pharmacokinetics of one drug caused by the interacting drug, eg, an inducer of hepatic enzymes
Pharmacodynamic interaction	A change in the pharmacodynamics of one drug caused by the interacting drug, eg, a receptor blocker
Addition	The effect of two drugs given together is equal to the sum of the responses to the same doses given separately
Antagonism	The effect of two drugs given together is less than the sum of the responses to the same doses given separately
Synergism	The effect of two drugs given together is greater than the sum of the responses to the same doses given separately
Potentiation	The ability of one drug with no effect on a particular function to greatly increase the effect of another drug on that function

CONCEPTS

A. **Classification:**
   1. **Drug interactions:** Drug interactions refer to actions of a drug in the body that are the result of, or affect the actions of, another drug. Usually such actions are quantitative—ie, an increase or a decrease in the size of an expected response. Drug interactions may be the result of pharmacokinetic alterations, pharmacodynamic changes, or a combination of both.
   2. **Drug incompatibilities:** Interactions between drugs in vitro (eg, precipitation when mixed in solutions for intravenous administration) are usually classified as drug incompatibilities.

B. Pharmacokinetic Interactions:

1. **Interactions based on absorption:** Absorption from the gut may be influenced by agents that bind the drug (eg, resins, antacids, calcium-containing foods) and by agents that increase or decrease gastrointestinal motility (metoclopramide or antimuscarinics, respectively). Problems caused by slowed gastric emptying may be unexpected, because the antimuscarinic action is often an unwanted effect from, eg, an antihistamine or antidepressant agent. Absorption from subcutaneous sites may be slowed predictably by vasoconstrictors given simultaneously (eg, local anesthetics and epinephrine) and by cardiac depressants that decrease tissue perfusion (eg, beta-blockers).

2. **Interactions based on distribution and binding:** Distribution of a drug may, in theory, be altered by other drugs that compete for binding sites (eg, sulfonamides can displace warfarin). However, it is difficult to document clinically significant interactions of this type. The ability of quinidine to raise the blood levels of digoxin, which was originally attributed to displacement from tissue binding sites, appears to be due mainly to reduced clearance of digoxin. Alteration of the size of the physical compartment in which another drug distributes can cause significant interactions, eg, diuretics can reduce the total body water in which aminoglycosides distribute.

3. **Interactions based on clearance:** Metabolism may be increased by drugs (eg, barbiturates) that cause induction of hepatic drug-metabolizing enzymes; conversely, metabolism may be decreased by a variety of drugs (eg, cimetidine, MAO inhibitors) that inhibit enzymes. Many interactions of this type have been documented. Drugs that reduce hepatic blood flow, eg, propranolol, may reduce the clearance of drugs metabolized in the liver, eg, theophylline.

   A modified form of this interaction results from the ability of some drugs to increase the stores of endogenous substances by blocking their metabolism. These endogenous drugs may subsequently be released by other exogenous drugs, resulting in an unexpected action. The best documented reaction of this type is the sensitization of patients taking MAO inhibitors to indirectly acting sympathomimetics (amphetamine, phenylpropanolamine, etc). Such patients may suffer a severe hypertensive reaction in response to ordinary doses of cold remedies, decongestants, and appetite suppressants.

4. **Interactions based on renal function:** Excretion of drugs by the kidney may be changed by drugs that reduce renal blood flow (eg, beta-blockers) or inhibit specific renal transport mechanisms (eg, aspirin's action on uric acid secretion).

C. Pharmacodynamic Interactions:

1. **Interactions based on opposing actions or effects:** Antagonism, the simplest type of drug interaction, is often predictable (eg, block of beta$_2$-mediated bronchodilation by beta-blockers given for another condition). Antagonism by mixed agonist-antagonist drugs (eg, nalbuphine) or by partial agonists (eg, pindolol) is not as easily predicted but should be expected when such drugs are used with pure agonists. The interaction of a partial agonist with a pure agonist is described quantitatively by the antagonism curve in Fig. 62–1.

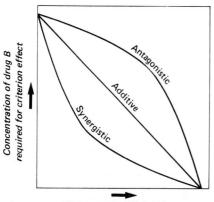

Figure 62–1. Isobologram showing possible interactions between two antimicrobials. The criterion effect is defined in setting up the assay and may be a specific bacteriostatic or bactericidal end point. The lines cross the ordinate at the concentration of drug B that is required to achieve the criterion effect when drug B is used alone. Similarly, the lines cross the abscissa at the concentration required for drug A alone to achieve the same effect. (Reproduced, with permission, from Katzung BG [editor]: *Basic & Clinical Pharmacology*, 5th ed. Appleton & Lange, 1992.)

Table 62–2. Some important interactions.

Drug Causing the Interaction	Drugs Affected	Comment
Alcohol	Other sedative-hypnotic drugs, antihistamines	Additive CNS depression, sedation, ataxia, risk of accidents
Aminoglycosides	Loop diuretics	Enhanced ototoxicity
Antacids	Iron supplements, tetracyclines	Reaction with the drug affected, leading to reduced absorption
Antacids	Ketoconazole	Reduced absorption of ketoconazole (ketoconazole requires acid for dissolution)
Antibiotics	Estrogens, including oral contraceptives	Reduced estrogen levels and reduced contraceptive effectiveness due to reduced enterohepatic cycling of estrogen
Antidepressants	Antimuscarinics	Additive ANS effects
Antihistamines (H$_1$ blockers)	Antimuscarinics, sedatives	Additive sedative effects with the drugs affected
Antimuscarinic drugs	Drugs absorbed from the small intestine	Slowed onset of effect because stomach emptying is delayed
Barbiturates, especially phenobarbital	Other sedative-hypnotics	Additive CNS depression
Barbiturates, especially phenobarbital	Other drugs metabolized in the liver	Increased clearance of the affected drugs because of enzyme induction
Beta-blockers	Drugs metabolized in the liver	Increased effect because hepatic blood flow is reduced
Bile acid-binding resins	Digitalis, thyroid, acetaminophen	Reduced absorption of the affected drug because of binding in the intestine
Carbamazepine	Doxycycline, estrogen	Reduced effect because of induction of metabolism
Cimetidine	Benzodiazepines, lidocaine, phenytoin, quinidine, theophylline, warfarin	Increased effect because of inhibition of metabolism
Cimetidine, other H$_2$ blockers	Ketoconazole	Reduced ketoconazole absorption
Disulfiram, metronidazole, certain cephalosporins	Ethanol	Increased hangover effect of ethanol because aldehyde dehydrogenase is blocked
Ketoconazole	Nonsedating antihistamines	Risk of cardiac arrhythmia because ketoconazole inhibits metabolism of these drugs
MAO inhibitors	Catecholamine releasers (amphetamine, etc)	MAO inhibitors increase the store of norepinephrine in sympathetic nerve endings; these stores are released by the interacting drugs
Nonsteroidal anti-inflammatory drugs	Anticoagulants	Increased bleeding tendency because of reduced platelet aggregation
Nonsteroidal anti-inflammatory drugs	Angiotensin-converting enzyme inhibitors	Decreased efficacy of ACE inhibitor
Nonsteroidal anti-inflammatory drugs	Furosemide	Reduced diuretic efficacy
Phenytoin	Drugs metabolized in the liver	Increased metabolism because of enzyme induction
Quinidine	Digoxin	Increased digoxin levels due to decreased clearance; displacement may play a role
Rifampin	Drugs metabolized in the liver	Decreased efficacy of the other drugs, because rifampin is a potent inducer of hepatic P450 isozymes
Sucralfate	Fluoroquinolone antibiotics	Reduced absorption of the antibiotics
Thiazides	Digitalis	Increased risk of digitalis toxicity because thiazides diminish potassium stores
Thiazides	Lithium	Increased risk of lithium toxicity because thiazides reduce lithium clearance

2. **Interactions based on additive effects:** Additive interaction describes the result of algebraic summing of the effects of two drugs. It is most often seen when two or more drugs that act on the same receptor are used (eg, three sulfonamides in triple sulfas) (Figure 62–1).

3. **Interactions based on greater-than-additive effects:** Synergism ("working together") is a term usually used to describe interactions that are more than additive; ie, they are "super-additive;" (Figure 62–1). Such interactions are more likely to result if the two drugs act on different receptors in a sequence or cascade (eg, sulfonamide and trimethoprim actions on folate synthesis in bacteria).

4. **Interactions based on amplification of effect:** Potentiation is often confused with, or used as a synonym for, synergism. However, potentiation is probably best reserved for situations in which a drug that has little or no effect on a given variable greatly amplifies the effect of another drug on the variable. An example is the dramatic effect of clavulanic acid (which has minimal antimicrobial activity) on the efficacy of penicillins against penicillinase-producing organisms.

D. **Clinical Importance of Drug Interactions:** Although hundreds of drug interactions have been documented, only a few are of clinical significance and constitute a contraindication to simultaneous use or require a change in dosage. Some of these are listed in Table 62–2. In patients taking many drugs, however, the likelihood of significant drug interactions is increased. This is especially true in elderly patients, because they often have age-related changes in drug clearance.

QUESTIONS

DIRECTIONS: Each of the numbered items or incomplete statements in this section is followed by answers or by completions of the statement. Select the ONE lettered answer or completion that is BEST in each case.

1. The risk of digitalis toxicity may be significantly increased by
   (A) Triamterene
   (B) Lidocaine
   (C) Captopril
   (D) Hydrochlorothiazide
   (E) Propranolol

2. Thiazides often reduce the excretion of
   (A) Phenothiazine antipsychotics
   (B) Tricyclic antidepressants
   (C) Second-generation antidepressants
   (D) Lithium ion
   (E) Potassium ion

3. Pharmacokinetic interactions include
   (A) Interaction of cimetidine with phenytoin
   (B) Interaction of antidepressants with antimuscarinics
   (C) Interaction of antacids with calcium
   (D) Interaction of benzodiazepines with alcohol
   (E) Interaction of beta-blockers with aerosol antiasthmatic medications

DIRECTIONS: The following section consists of a list of four to twenty-six lettered options followed by several numbered items. For each numbered item, select the ONE option that is most closely associated with it. Each answer may be selected once, more than once, or not at all.
   (A) Ibuprofen
   (B) Warfarin
   (C) Tetracycline
   (D) Trimethoprim
   (E) Rifampin
   (F) Cholestyramine

      (G) Phenelzine
      (H) Ephedrine
      (I) Carbamazepine
      (J) Terfenadine

4. This antibiotic is a potent inducer of hepatic drug-metabolizing enzymes

5. This drug interferes with the antihypertensive action of captopril and enalapril

6. This drug has a useful synergistic interaction with sulfonamides

7. This agent is absorbed poorly if given with antacids or dairy products

8. This drug has no effect on platelets but is most likely to cause bleeding in patients who are also taking aspirin

9. This agent reduces the absorption of digoxin from the intestine

10. This drug may precipitate a hypertensive crisis in a patient taking an MAO inhibitor

11. A meal with a high content of fermented foods would be dangerous in a person taking this drug

12. This drug is an antihistamine that may cause arrhythmias in a patient who begins taking ketoconazole

ANSWERS

1. The risk of digitalis toxicity is increased by thiazides because these diuretics reduce extracellular potassium. The answer is **(D)**.

2. Thiazides reduce the clearance of lithium by about 25%. They do not alter the clearance of the other agents mentioned, except for potassium, whose clearance is increased. The answer is **(D)**.

3. Cimetidine inhibits the enzymatic clearance of phenytoin. Antacids may contain calcium; they do not interfere with its absorption. The other interactions listed are pharmacodynamic interactions. The answer is **(A)**.

4. Rifampin is an effective inducer of hepatic P450 isozymes. Tetracycline, the other antibiotic listed, has no such effect. The answer is **(E)**.

5. NSAIDs interfere with the antihypertensive action of angiotensin-converting enzyme inhibitors. The answer is **(A)**.

6. In bacterial folate synthesis, trimethoprim inhibits dihydrofolate reductase, the enzyme that follows the step inhibited by sulfonamides. The answer is **(D)**.

7. Tetracyclines form insoluble complexes with calcium and other divalent and trivalent cations. The answer is **(C)**.

8. Warfarin, the oral anticoagulant, reduces synthesis of prothrombin and several other clotting factors. An interaction occurs with antiplatelet drugs such as aspirin. The answer is **(B)**.

9. Cholestyramine binds several drugs, as well as bile acids, in the intestine. The answer is **(F)**.

10. Ephedrine, an indirect sympathomimetic, will cause increased effects in a patient who has increased stores of norepinephrine. The answer is **(H)**.

11. This is the opposite of question 10. MAO inhibitors, eg, phenelzine, increase the stores of norepinephrine, and fermented foods contain a high concentration of tyramine, an indirect sympathomimetic. The answer is **(G)**.

12. Terfenadine is metabolized by P450 enzymes that are inhibited by ketoconazole. The answer is **(J)**.

Vaccines, Immune Globulins, & Other Complex Biologic Products

63

OBJECTIVES

You should be able to:

- Describe the principles of active and passive immunization, and list the differences between them.
- List the types of materials available for passive immunization and the special uses of immune globulin (ISG).
- List the types of materials available for active immunization, and describe the relative merits and disadvantages of live versus dead immunogens.

CONCEPTS

A. Passive Immunization: In passive immunization, **preformed antibodies** of human or animal origin are used to transfer immunity to the host. Such materials, usually **immunoglobulins,** may contain high titers of specific or relatively nonspecific antibodies (eg, **immune globulin, ISG**). Their clinical uses include prevention or amelioration of diseases after exposure (eg, hepatitis, measles, poliomyelitis), treatment of certain snake and insect bites, and management of hypogammaglobulinemias. The most commonly used preparation is ISG, a 25-fold concentration of gamma globulins (95% IgG) from human plasma, available in formulations for intramuscular and intravenous use. The biologic half-life of ISG is about 23 days, and hypersensitivity reactions are rare. ISG is used for passive immunization to hepatitis A, hypogammaglobulinemia, measles, poliomyelitis, and rubella. More specific products include diphtheria antitoxin, snake and spider antivenins, $Rh_o(D)$ immune globulin, and immune globulins for hepatitis B, pertussis, rabies, tetanus, vaccinia, and varicella. Such antibodies usually have a half-life of only 5–7 days. Because animal antibodies can act as antigens in humans, allergic reactions to antibodies from nonhuman sources are more common and severe than those from human sources. Examples of materials used in passive immunization are shown in Table 63–1.

B. Active Immunization: In active immunization, **antigens** are used to stimulate antibody formation and host cell-mediated immunity, giving protection against disease vectors. The major advantage of active over passive immunization is that it confers stronger host resistance by stimulating higher antibody levels. Immunization can be produced by live (attenuated) or dead (inactivated) immunogens. Live attenuated products stimulate natural resistance and confer longer-lasting immunity than dead immunogens; however, the risk of disease is greater. Examples of the use of live attenuated immunogens include the vaccines for measles, mumps, rubella, and poliovirus. Materials utilizing dead immunogens include diphtheria and tetanus toxoids, rabies vaccine, and hepatitis B virus and surface antigen. Polysaccharide vaccines are also available for active immunization of selected individuals at high risk of infection from *Haemophilus influenzae,* meningococci, and pneumococci. Selected examples of products used in active immunization are shown in Table 63–2.

C. Active Immunization of Children: Recommended schedules for active immunization of children include hepatitis B vaccine, DTP (toxoids of diphtheria and tetanus with pertussis antigen), oral poliovaccine, and vaccines for measles, mumps, and rubella (Table 63–3).

Table 63–1. Materials for passive immunization.[1]

Indication	Product	Comments
Black widow spider (BWS) bite	BWS antivenin (equine)	Treatment; use only in children <15 kg
Botulism	ABE polyvalent antitoxin (equine)	Treatment
Hepatitis A (infectious)	Immune globulin (ISG)	Prophylaxis; postexposure & chronic exposure
Hepatitis B (serum)	Hepatitis B immune globulin (HBIG)	Prophylaxis; postexposure
Hepatitis non-A, non-B	Immune globulin (ISG)	Prophylaxis
Hypogamma-globulinemia	Immune globulin (ISG)	Treatment
Organ transplant	Lymphocyte immune globulin (equine)	Adjunctive immunosuppressant
Rabies	Rabies immune globulin (equine)	Give as soon as possible; also need rabies vaccine
Snake bite	Coral snake antivenin; crotalid antivenin (equine)	Treatment; also need antitetanus Rx
Tetanus	Tetanus immune globulin	Only for major or contaminated wounds
Vaccinia	Vaccinia immune globulin	Treatment; generalized, ocular, skin infections
Varicella	Varicella-zoster immune globulin	Immunosuppressed children in contact with the index case

[1] Adapted, with permission, from Katzung BG (editor): *Basic & Clinical Pharmacology*, 6th ed. Appleton & Lange, 1995.

Table 63–2. Materials for active immunization.[1]

Pathogen or Disease	Product	Comments
Hepatitis B	Hepatitis B virus and surface antigen (human)	Give preexposure to infants and high risk individuals (>90% effective); duration, years
Influenza	Influenza virus vaccine (chick embryo)	Annually for the elderly, those with chronic disease, and other high risk individuals
Meningococcal meningitis	Meningococcal polysaccharide vaccine	Epidemic situations
Pneumococci	Pneumococcal polysaccharide vaccine	High risk individuals (asplenia, hemoglobinopathies, cardiovascular disease)
Rabies	Rabies vaccine (human)	Prophylaxis for individuals at risk; post exposure after bites (plus rabies immune globulin)
Rubella	Rubella virus vaccine (human)	Avoid during pregnancy; duration, permanent
Tetanus	DTP (diphtheria and tetanus toxoids, pertussis antigen)	Recommended every 7–10 years
Typhoid	Typhoid vaccine	Exposure from travel, epidemic, or household contact (>70% effective); duration, 3 years

[1] Adapted, with permission, from Katzung BG (editor): *Basic & Clinical Pharmacology*, 6th ed. Appleton & Lange, 1995.

Table 63–3. Recommended schedule for active immunization of children.[1]

Age	Product Administered
Birth–4 days	HBV (hepatitis B vaccine)
2 months	DTP (toxoids of diphtheria & tetanus, pertussis bacterial antigen); HBV; oral polio vaccine
4 months	DTP; oral polio vaccine
6 months	DTP; HBV; oral polio vaccine
15–19 months	DTP; measles vaccine; mumps vaccine; rubella vaccine; oral polio vaccine
18–24 months	*Haemophilus influenzae* type b vaccine
4–6 years	DTP; oral polio vaccine
14–16 years	Rubella vaccine; TD (tetanus & diphtheria toxoids)

[1] Adapted, with permission, from Katzung BG (editor): *Basic & Clinical Pharmacology*, 6th ed. Appleton & Lange, 1995.

QUESTIONS

DIRECTIONS: Each of the numbered items or incomplete statements in this section is followed by answers or by completions of the statement. Select the ONE lettered answer or completion that is BEST in each case.

1. All of the following statements about immunization are accurate EXCEPT
    (A) Passive immunization involves use of preformed immunogens such as human gamma globulin
    (B) Immune globulin is not usually effective in preventing viral upper respiratory tract infections
    (C) The use of black widow spider antivenin should be restricted to small children, the only group with significant morbidity or mortality
    (D) Antibodies from human serum have a shorter half-life than those of animal origin
2. All of the following statements about active immunization are accurate EXCEPT
    (A) Immunization against hepatitis B involves the use of a purified and inactivated virus coat protein
    (B) Poliovirus vaccine containing live virus can be administered orally
    (C) Active immunization results in permanent protection
    (D) Some protective factors may not be stimulated with the use of inactivated (killed) products
3. All of the following statements about passive immunization are accurate EXCEPT
    (A) Patients with IgA deficiency may develop hypersensitivity reactions to ISG
    (B) Rabies immune globulin is recommended only in patients who demonstrate an antibody response from preexposure prophylaxis
    (C) Equine-derived antivenins are used in the treatment of snake bite
    (D) Passive immunization is useful in the treatment of certain diseases that are normally prevented by active immunization (eg, tetanus)
4. Which of the following is used in active immunization of children, and combines bacterial toxoids with a bacterial antigen?
    (A) BSA
    (B) ISG
    (C) DTP
    (D) $Rh_o(D)$
    (E) BCG
5. Which of the following is a polysaccharide used for active immunization in patients with chronic cardiorespiratory ailments?
    (A) Mumps virus vaccine
    (B) BCG vaccine
    (C) Pertussis immune globulin

       (D) Pneumococcal vaccine
       (E) Antilymphocyte immune serum

6. All of the following statements about administration of $Rh_o(D)$ immune globulin are accurate EXCEPT

       (A) It provides Rh isoimmunization from fetal-maternal transfusion
       (B) It is ineffective if administered more than 48 hours after exposure
       (C) It is used for nonimmune females only
       (D) It is categorized as passive immunization

ANSWERS

1. Antibodies derived from human serum not only diminish the risk of hypersensitivity, but also have a much longer half-life than those from animal sources. For example, human IgG antibodies have a half-life of >20 days, compared to 5–7 days for the antibodies derived from animals. Smaller doses of human antibodies can be administered to provide therapeutic levels for several weeks. The answer is **(D)**.

2. Active immunization does not always result in permanent protection. Primary immunization against measles, mumps, poliomyelitis, and rubella appears to be permanent, and in each case live viruses are used. However, the duration of effect of active immunization with killed virus products is about 6 months for cholera, 1–3 years for influenza, and more than 3 years for tetanus. The answer is **(C)**.

3. Rabies immune globulin should be given as soon as possible after exposure and must be combined with immunization using human diploid cell-derived rabies vaccine. Passive immunization is not recommended for individuals with demonstrated antibody response to preexposure prophylaxis with rabies vaccine. The answer is **(B)**.

4. DTP contains diphtheria and tetanus toxoids and pertussis antigen. The answer is **(C)**.

5. The pertussis and antilymphocyte preparations are used in passive immunization. Both the mumps vaccine and BCG (used for tuberculosis) are used in active immunization, but they are live viruses. Pneumococcal vaccine is a polysaccharide recommended for individuals at high risk for pneumococcal disease. The *Haemophilus* and meningococcal vaccines (not listed) are also polysaccharides. The answer is **(D)**.

6. Ideally, $Rh_o(D)$ should be administered to an Rh(D)-negative woman within 72 hours of abortion, amniocentesis, obstetric delivery of an Rh-positive child, or transfusion of Rh-positive blood. However, the product may be effective at much greater postexposure intervals, and should be given even if more than 72 hours has elapsed. The answer is **(B)**.

Appendix I

Key Words for Key Drugs

The following list is a compilation of the drugs that are most likely to appear on examinations. The brief descriptions serve as a rapid review. Use the list in two ways: first, cover the column of properties and test your ability to provide some descriptive information about drugs picked at random from the left column; second, cover the left column and attempt to name a drug that fits the properties described.

Abbreviations: ACE, angiotensin-converting enzyme; ANS, autonomic nervous system; AV, atrioventricular; BP, blood pressure; BPH, benign prostatic hypertrophy; CHF, congestive heart failure; CNS, central nervous system; CV, cardiovascular system; ECG, electrocardiogram; ENS, enteric nervous system; EPS, extrapyramidal system; GI, gastrointestinal; HR, heart rate; HTN, hypertension; MI, myocardial infarction; NM, neuromuscular; PANS, parasympathetic autonomic nervous system; SANS, sympathetic autonomic nervous system; Tox, toxicity; WBC, white blood cells.

Drug	Properties
Acetaminophen	Antipyretic analgesic: very weak cyclooxygenase inhibitor; not anti-inflammatory. Less toxic than aspirin but more dangerous in overdose (causes hepatic necrosis)
Acetazolamide	Carbonic anhydrase inhibitor diuretic: produces a $NaHCO_3$ diuresis, results in bicarbonate depletion, and therefore has self-limited action. Used in glaucoma and mountain sickness
Acetylcholine	Cholinomimetic prototype: transmitter in CNS, ENS, all ANS ganglia, parasympathetic postganglionic synapses, sympathetic postganglionic fibers to sweat glands, and some skeletal muscle vasodilator synapses
Acyclovir	Antiviral: inhibits DNA synthesis in herpes simplex and varicella zoster. Requires activation by viral thymidine kinase (TK^- strains are resistant). Tox: behavioral effects and nephrotoxicity (crystalluria), but not myelosuppression
Adenosine	Antiarrhythmic: unclassified ("Group V"); parenteral only. Hyperpolarizes AV nodal tissue, blocks conduction for 10–15 sec. Used for nodal reentry arrhythmias
Allopurinol	Antigout: inhibitor of xanthine oxidase; reduces production of uric acid
Alprazolam	Benzodiazepine sedative-hypnotic: widely used in anxiety states, selectivity for panic attacks and phobias; possible antidepressant actions. Tox: psychologic and physical dependence, additive effects with other CNS depressants
Alteplase (t-PA)	Thrombolytic: human recombinant tissue plasminogen activator. Used in acute MI to recanalize the occluded coronary. Occasionally used in pulmonary embolism. Tox: bleeding
Amiloride	K-sparing diuretic: blocks Na channels in cortical collecting tubules
Aminoglutethimide	Nonsteroid inhibitor of steroid synthesis: reduces conversion of cholesterol to the hormone precursor, pregnenolone
Amiodarone	Group IA and III antiarrhythmic: broad spectrum, blocks sodium, potassium, calcium channels, beta receptors. High efficacy and very long half-life

(weeks–months). Tox: deposits in tissues; hypo- or hyperthyroidism; pulmonary fibrosis

Amitriptyline	Tricyclic antidepressant: blocks reuptake of norepinephrine and serotonin. Tox: atropine-like, postural hypotension, sedation; cardiac arrhythmias in overdose, additive effects with other CNS depressants
Amoxicillin	Penicillin: wider-spectrum with activity similar to ampicillin but greater oral bioavailability; less adverse effects on GI tract than ampicillin. Susceptible to penicillinases unless used with clavulanic acid. Tox: penicillin allergy
Amphetamine	Indirectly acting sympathomimetic: displaces stored catecholamines in nerve endings. Marked CNS stimulant actions; high abuse liability. Tox: psychosis, seizures, hypertension
Amphotericin B	Antifungal: polyene drug of choice for most systemic mycoses; binds to ergosterol to disrupt fungal cell membrane permeability. Tox: chills and fever, hypokalemia, hypotension, nephrotoxicity (dose-limiting)
Ampicillin	Penicillin: wider-spectrum, susceptible to penicillinases unless used with sulbactam. Activity similar to pen G, plus *E coli, H influenzae, P mirabilis, Shigella* spp. Tox: penicillin allergy; more adverse effects on GI tract than other penicillins; maculopapular skin rash
Anistreplase (APSAC)	Thrombolytic: bacterial streptokinase complexed with human plasminogen. Longer acting in body than other thrombolytics (t-PA, streptokinase, urokinase). Tox: bleeding
Aspirin	NSAID prototype: inhibits cyclooxygenase (COX) I and II irreversibly. Potent antiplatelet agent as well as antipyretic analgesic anti-inflammatory drug
Astemizole	Antihistamine H_1 blocker: newer, less sedating, used in hayfever. Tox: arrhythmias, especially with ketoconazole (which inhibits its metabolism)
Atenolol	Beta$_1$-selective blocker: low lipid solubility, less CNS effect; used for HTN. (Note mnemonic for beta$_1$-selective blockers: their names start with A through M. [Exceptions: carteolol & labetalol are not selective])
Atropine	Muscarinic cholinoceptor blocker prototype: lipid soluble, CNS effects. Tox: "red as a beet, dry as a bone, mad as a hatter"
Benztropine	Centrally acting antimuscarinic prototype for parkinsonism
Bethanechol	Muscarinic agonist: choline ester with good resistance to cholinesterase; used for atonic bowel or bladder
Botulinum	Toxin: produced by *Clostridium botulinum;* interacts with synaptobrevin to block release of acetylcholine vesicles
Bromocriptine	Ergot derivative: dopamine agonist in CNS; inhibits prolactin release. Used in parkinsonism and amenorrhea-galactorrhea syndrome
Bupivacaine	Long-acting amide local anesthetic prototype: greater CV toxicity than most local anesthetics
Buspirone	Anxiolytic: atypical drug that interacts with serotonin receptors; slow onset. Minimal potentiation of CNS depressants including ethanol; low abuse liability
Captopril	ACE inhibitor prototype: used in HTN, diabetic renal disease, and CHF. Tox: hyperkalemia, fetal renal damage, cough ("sore throat")
Carbachol	Nonselective direct muscarinic and nicotinic agonist: choline ester with good resistance to cholinesterase; used for glaucoma (not a first-line drug)
Carbamazepine	Antiepileptic: tricyclic derivative used for grand mal and partial seizures; blocks Na^+ channels in neuronal membranes. Drug of choice for trigeminal neuralgia; back-up drug in mania. Tox: CNS depression, hematotoxic, induces liver drug-metabolizing enzymes

Cefazolin	First-generation cephalosporin prototype: bactericidal beta-lactam inhibitor of cell wall synthesis. Active against gram-positive cocci, *E coli, K pneumoniae,* but does not enter CSF. Tox: potential allergy, partial cross-reactivity with penicillins
Cefoxitin	Second-generation cephalosporin: active against a wide spectrum of gram-negative bacteria including anaerobes *(B fragilis).* Does not enter the CNS
Ceftriaxone	Third-generation cephalosporin: active against resistant bacteria including gonococci, *H influenzae* and other gram-negative organisms. Crosses the blood-brain barrier
Chloramphenicol	Antibiotic: broad spectrum agent; inhibits protein synthesis (50S); uses restricted to back-up drug for bacterial meningitis; infections due to anaerobes and *Salmonella* spp. Tox: reversible myelosuppression, aplastic anemia, gray baby syndrome
Chloroquine	Antimalarial: blood schizonticide used for treatment and as a chemosuppressant where *P falciparum* is susceptible. Tox: GI distress and skin rash at low doses; peripheral neuropathy, skin lesions, auditory and visual impairment, myocardial depression at high doses
Chlorpheniramine	Antihistamine H_1 blocker prototype: Tox: sedation, antimuscarinic
Chlorpromazine	Phenothiazine antipsychotic drug prototype: blocks most dopamine receptors in the CNS. Tox: atropine-like, EPS dysfunction, hyperprolactinemia, postural hypotension, sedation, seizures (in overdose), additive effects with other CNS depressants
Cholestyramine, colestipol	Bile acid-binding resins: sequester bile acids in gut and divert more cholesterol from the liver to bile acids instead of circulating lipoproteins. Tox: constipation, bloating; interfere with absorption of some drugs
Cimetidine	H_2 blocker prototype: used in acid-peptic disease. Tox: inhibits hepatic drug metabolism; antiandrogen effects
Ciprofloxacin	Fluoroquinolone antibiotic: inhibits bacterial DNA gyrase; active against many gram-negative rods including *E coli, H influenzae, Campylobacter, Enterobacter, Pseudomonas, Shigella.* Tox: CNS dysfunction, GI distress, superinfection, collagen damage (avoid in children and pregnant women). Interactions: caffeine, theophylline, warfarin
Clindamycin	Lincosamide antibiotic: bacteriostatic inhibitor of protein synthesis (50S); active against gram-positive cocci, *B fragilis.* Tox: GI distress, pseudomembranous colitis
Clomiphene	Estrogen partial agonist: synthetic used in infertility to induce ovulation
Clonidine	Alpha$_2$ agonist: acts centrally to reduce SANS outflow, lowers BP. Tox: rebound HTN if stopped suddenly
Clozapine	Atypical antipsychotic: low affinity for dopamine D_2 receptors, higher for D_4 and 5-HT receptors; less EPS adverse effects than other antipsychotic drugs. Tox: ANS effects, agranulocytosis (infrequent but significant)
Cocaine	Indirectly acting sympathomimetic; local anesthetic actions: blocks amine reuptake into nerve endings. Marked CNS stimulatory effects; high abuse liability. Tox: psychosis, seizures, cardiac arrhythmias
Colchicine	Microtubule assembly inhibitor: reduces mobility and phagocytosis by WBCs in gout-inflamed joints; useful in acute, not chronic gout. Tox: GI, hepatic, renal damage
Cyclopentolate, tropicamide	Antimuscarinics for ophthalmology: duration a few hours or less; cause cycloplegia and mydriasis

Cyclophosphamide	Antineoplastic, immunosuppressive: cell cycle-nonspecific alkylating agent. Tox: alopecia, gastrointestinal distress, hemorrhagic cystitis, myelosuppression
Cyclosporine	Immunosuppressant: antibiotic; inhibits interleukin-2 synthesis, suppresses T cells. Tox: HTN, hirsutism, nephrotoxicity (dose-limiting), seizures (in overdose). Not a myelosuppressant
DDAVP	ADH analogue: synthetic peptide used for pituitary diabetes insipidus
DDT	Insecticide: prevents inactivation of sodium channels, causes uncontrolled neuronal activity. Stored for years in body fat in mammals, birds, fish
Deferoxamine	Chelator: bacterial product; chelates iron very avidly, aluminum less so
Dexamethasone	Glucocorticoid: very potent, long-acting; no mineralocorticoid activity
Diazepam	Benzodiazepine prototype: binds to BDZ receptors of the $GABA_A$ receptor-chloride ion channel complex; facilitates the inhibitory actions of GABA. Uses: anxiety states, ethanol detoxication, muscle spasticity, status epilepticus. Tox: psychologic and physical dependence, additive effects with other CNS depressants
Digitoxin	Cardiac glycoside: half-life 168 h, excreted in the bile (partially as digoxin); subject to enterohepatic circulation. See digoxin
Digoxin	Cardiac glycoside prototype: positive inotropic drug for CHF, half-life 40 h; renal excretion; inhibits Na/K ATPase, also a cardiac parasympathomimetic. Tox: calcium overload arrhythmias, GI upset
Diltiazem	Calcium channel blocker prototype: like verapamil, has more depressant effect on heart than dihydropyridines (eg, nifedipine). Tox: AV block, CHF, edema, constipation
Dimercaprol (BAL)	Chelator (British AntiLewisite): used for arsenic, lead, and mercury poisoning
Dioxin (TCDD)	Toxin: byproduct of the manufacture of herbicides 2,4-D and 2,4,5-T. Tox: extremely potent carcinogen in guinea pigs; poorly understood in humans except for chloracne, a skin disorder that occurs acutely upon exposure
Diphenhydramine	Antihistamine H_1 blocker prototype: used in hayfever, motion sickness, dystonias. Tox: antimuscarinic, anti-alpha; sedative
Disopyramide	Group IA antiarrhythmic: used for ventricular arrhythmias. Tox: strong antimuscarinic; may cause CHF
Dopamine	Neurotransmitter and agonist drug at dopamine receptors: used in shock to increase renal blood flow, stimulate heart
Doxorubicin	Antineoplastic: anthracycline drug (cell cycle-nonspecific); intercalates between base pairs to disrupt DNA functions and forms cytotoxic free radicals. Tox: cardiotoxicity, myelosuppression
Doxycycline	Tetracycline antibiotic: protein synthesis inhibitor (30S), more effective than other tetracyclines against bacillary dysentery. Unlike other tetracyclines, it is eliminated mainly in the feces. Tox: see tetracycline
Echothiophate	Organophosphate cholinesterase inhibitor: less lipid soluble than most organophosphates; used in glaucoma
Edetate (EDTA)	Chelating agent: used in lead poisoning. Tox: renal tubular necrosis
Edrophonium	Cholinesterase inhibitor: very short duration of action (15 min). Used to reverse NM blockade and as diagnostic test in myasthenia gravis
Ephedrine	Indirectly acting sympathomimetic: like amphetamine but less CNS stimulation, more vascular effect
Epinephrine	Adrenoceptor agonist prototype: product of adrenal medulla, some CNS neurons. Affinity for all alpha and all beta receptors. Used in asthma; as hemostatic and adjunct with local anesthetics; drug of choice in anaphylaxis

Ergonovine	Ergot alkaloid (uterine) prototype: causes prolonged uterine contraction. Used in post-partum bleeding
Ergotamine	Ergot alkaloid (vascular) prototype: causes prolonged vasoconstriction, uterine contraction. Used in migraine, obstetrics
Erythromycin	Macrolide antibiotic: inhibitor of protein synthesis (50S); activity includes gram-positive cocci and bacilli, *M pneumoniae, Legionella pneumophila, C trachomatis.* Tox: cholestatic jaundice, inhibits liver drug-metabolizing enzymes, interactions with astemizole, theophylline, terfenadine, warfarin
Ethacrynic acid	Loop diuretic: not a sulfa derivative. Tox: like furosemide but does not increase serum uric acid.
Ethanol	Sedative-hypnotic: acute actions include impaired judgment, ataxia, loss of consciousness, vasodilation, and cardiovascular and respiratory depression. The most widely used and abused sedative-hypnotic. Chronic use leads to dependence, and liver, cardiovascular, endocrine, gastrointestinal, hepatic, and nervous system pathology. Note: zero-order elimination kinetics
Ethosuximide	Antiepileptic: may block T-type Ca^{2+} channels in thalamic neurons. Used for petit mal. Tox: GI distress but safe in pregnancy
Etidronate, pamidronate	Bisphosphonates: reduce turnover of bone calcium. Used in Paget's disease, osteoporosis
Finasteride	Steroid inhibitor of 5α-reductase: inhibits synthesis of dihydrotestosterone, the active androgen in prostate. Used in BPH
Flecainide	Group IC antiarrhythmic prototype: used in ventricular tachycardia, rapid atrial arrhythmias with Wolff-Parkinson-White syndrome. Tox: arrhythmogenic, CNS excitation
Fludrocortisone	Corticosteroid: synthetic with high mineralocorticoid and moderate glucocorticoid activity
Fluorouracil	Antineoplastic: pyrimidine antimetabolite (cell cycle-specific) used mainly for solid or superficial tumors. Tox: GI distress, myelosuppression
Fluoxetine	Antidepressant: serotonin selective reuptake inhibitor (SSRI) prototype. Less ANS adverse effects and cardiotoxic potential than tricyclics. Tox: CNS stimulation, seizures in overdose
Flutamide	Androgen receptor inhibitor: nonsteroid used in prostatic carcinoma
Furosemide	Loop diuretic prototype: blocks Na/K/2Cl transporter; high efficacy; used in acute pulmonary edema, refractory edematous states, hypercalcemia. Tox: ototoxicity, K^+ wasting, hypovolemia, increased serum uric acid
Gemfibrozil, clofibrate	Antilipemics: stimulate lipoprotein lipase in peripheral tissues. Used in hypertriglyceridemias and mixed triglyceridemia/hypercholesterolemia
Gentamicin	Aminoglycoside prototype: bactericidal inhibitor of protein synthesis (30S); active against many aerobic gram-negative bacteria. Narrow therapeutic window; dose reduction required in renal impairment. Tox: renal dysfunction, ototoxicity
Glipizide, glyburide	Oral hypoglycemics: second generation, very potent. Like other sulfonylureas, act by closing K channels in pancreatic B cells, causing depolarization and release of insulin. Tox: hypoglycemia
Guanethidine	Postganglionic sympathetic neuron blocker: must enter nerve ending by means of uptake-1 and be stored in the ending (effect reversed by TCAs, cocaine). Tox: severe orthostatic hypotension, sexual dysfunction
Haloperidol	Antipsychotic butyrophenone: blocks brain dopamine D_2 receptors. Tox: marked EPS dysfunction, hyperprolactinemia; less ANS adverse effects than phenothiazines

Halothane	General anesthetic prototype: inhaled halogenated hydrocarbon. Causes cardiovascular and respiratory depression and relaxes skeletal and smooth muscle. Use has decreased due to sensitization of heart to catecholamines, and occurrence (rare) of hepatitis and malignant hyperthermia
Hydralazine	Antihypertensive: arteriolar vasodilator, orally active; used in HTN, CHF. Tox: Tachycardia, salt and water retention, lupus
Hydrochlorothiazide	Thiazide diuretic prototype: acts in distal convoluted tubule; blocks Na/Cl transporter; used in HTN, CHF, chronic stone formers. Tox: increased serum lipids, uric acid, glucose; K^+ wasting
Ibuprofen	NSAID prototype: short duration. Inhibits cyclooxygenase (both I and II) reversibly. Used in arthritis, dysmenorrhea, muscle inflammation. Tox: peptic ulcer, renal damage
Imipenem	Antibiotic: carbapenem beta lactam active against many aerobic and anaerobic bacteria including penicillinase-producing organisms; a bactericidal inhibitor of cell wall synthesis. Used with cilastatin (which inhibits metabolism by renal dihydropeptidases). Tox: allergy (partial cross-reactivity with penicillins), seizures (overdose)
Imipramine	Tricyclic antidepressant prototype: blocks reuptake of norepinephrine and serotonin. Tox: ANS (alpha and muscarinic) blockade, cardiac arrhythmias
Indomethacin	NSAID prototype: highly potent. Usually reserved for acute inflammation (eg, acute gout), not chronic; neonatal patent ductus arteriosus. Tox: GI (bleeding), renal damage
Insulin	Hypoglycemic peptide hormone of B (beta) cells of the pancreas: stimulates transport of glucose into cells and glycogen formation; inhibits lipolysis and protein catabolism
Ipodate	Antithyroid: iodine-containing radiocontrast medium used in thyrotoxicosis. Reduces peripheral conversion of T_4 to T_3; may also reduce release of hormone from thyroid
Ipratropium	Antimuscarinic agent: aerosol for asthma, COPD. Good bronchodilator in 20–30% of patients. Not as effective as β_2 agonists
Isoniazid	Antimycobacterial: primary drug in combination regimens for tuberculosis; used as sole agent in prophylaxis. Metabolic clearance via N-acetylases (genetic variability). Tox: hepatotoxicity (age-dependent), peripheral neuropathy (reversed by pyridoxine), hemolysis (in G6PD deficiency)
Isoproterenol	$Beta_1$, $beta_2$ agonist catecholamine prototype: bronchodilator, cardiac stimulant. Always causes tachycardia because both direct and reflex actions increase HR. Tox: arrhythmias, angina
Ketoconazole	Antifungal azole prototype: active systemically; inhibits the synthesis of ergosterol. Used for *C albicans* and for non-life-threatening systemic mycoses. Tox: hepatic dysfunction, inhibits steroid synthesis and other P450-dependent processes
Labetalol	Alpha- and beta-blocker: used in HTN. Tox: AV block, hypotension
Leuprolide	GnRH analogue: synthetic peptide used in pulse therapy to stimulate gonadal steroid synthesis (infertility); used in continuous or depot therapy to shut off steroid synthesis, especially in prostate carcinoma
Levodopa	Dopamine precursor: used in parkinsonism, usually with carbidopa, a peripheral inhibitor of dopamine metabolism. Tox: dyskinesias, hypotension, on-off phenomena, behavioral changes
Lidocaine	Local anesthetic, medium duration amide prototype: highly selective use-dependent Group IB antiarrhythmic; used for nerve block and post MI ischemic ventricular arrhythmias. Tox: CNS excitation

Lithium	Antimanic prototype: drug of choice in mania and bipolar affective disorders; blocks recycling of the phosphatidyl inositol second messenger system. Tox: tremor, diabetes insipidus, goiter, seizures (in overdose), teratogenic potential
Lovastatin	Antilipemic HMG-CoA reductase inhibitor prototype: acts in liver to reduce synthesis of cholesterol. Tox: hepatitis, muscle damage
LSD	"Acid," lysergic acid diethylamide: semisynthetic ergot derivative; orally active; hallucinogen
Malathion	Organophosphate insecticide cholinesterase inhibitor: pro-drug converted to malaoxon. Less toxic in mammals and birds because metabolized to inactive products
Meperidine	Opioid analgesic: synthetic, equivalent to morphine in efficacy, but orally bioavailable. Strong agonist at mu opioid receptors. Effects: see morphine
Mestranol	Synthetic estrogen: used in many oral contraceptives
Methadone	Opioid analgesic: synthetic mu agonist, equivalent to morphine in efficacy, but orally bioavailable with longer half-life (useful in maintenance programs). Effects: see morphine
Methotrexate	Antineoplastic, immunosuppressant: cell cycle-specific drug that inhibits dihydrofolate reductase. Major dose reduction required in renal impairment. Tox: gastrointestinal distress, myelosuppression. Leucovorin rescue used to reduce toxicity after very high doses
Methyldopa	Antihypertensive: pro-drug of methylnorepinephrine, a CNS-active α_2 agonist. Reduces SANS outflow from vasomotor center. Tox: positive Coombs test, hemolysis
Methysergide	Ergot alkaloid: used as prophylactic in migraine. Tox: retroperitoneal and subendocardial fibroplasia
Metoprolol	Beta$_1$-selective blocker: used in HTN and for prevention of post-MI sudden death arrhythmias
Metronidazole	Antiprotozoal antibiotic: drug of choice in extraluminal amebiasis and trichomoniasis; active against bacterial anaerobes including *B fragilis* and useful orally in antibiotic-induced colitis due to *C difficile*. Tox: peripheral neuropathy, gastrointestinal distress, ethanol intolerance, mutagenic potential
Mexiletine	Group IB antiarrhythmic drug: like lidocaine but orally active
Mifepristone (RU 486)	Progesterone, glucocorticoid inhibitor: abortifacient, antineoplastic
Minoxidil	Antihypertensive: pro-drug of minoxidil sulfate, a high efficacy arteriolar vasodilator. Used in HTN; topically for baldness. Tox: tachycardia, salt and water retention, pericardial effusion
Misoprostol	PGE$_1$ derivative: orally active prostaglandin used to prevent peptic ulcers in patients taking NSAIDs for arthritis. Tox: diarrhea
Morphine	Opioid analgesic prototype: strong mu receptor agonist. Poor oral bioavailability. Effects include analgesia, constipation, emesis, sedation, respiratory depression, miosis, and urinary retention. Tolerance may be marked; high potential for psychologic and physical dependence. Additive effects with other CNS depressants
Nafcillin	Penicillinase-resistant penicillin prototype: used for suspected or known staphylococcal infections; not active against methicillin-resistant staphylococci. Tox: penicillin allergy
Nalbuphine	Opioid: mixed agonist-antagonist analgesic that activates kappa and weakly blocks mu receptors. Effective analgesic, but with lower abuse liability and less respiratory depressant effects than most strong opioid analgesics

Naloxone	Opioid mu receptor antagonist: used to reverse CNS depressant effects of opioid analgesics (overdose or when used in anesthesia)
Neostigmine	Cholinesterase inhibitor prototype: quaternary nitrogen carbamate with little CNS effect
Niacin	Antilipemic: reduces release of VLDL from liver into circulation. Tox: flushing
Nifedipine	Calcium channel blocker prototype: vasoselective (less cardiac depression); used in angina, HTN. Tox: constipation, headache
Nitroglycerin	Antianginal vasodilator prototype: releases NO in smooth muscle of veins, less in arteries, and causes relaxation. Standard of therapy in angina (both atherosclerotic and variant). Tox: tachycardia, orthostatic hypotension, headache
Norepinephrine	Adrenoceptor agonist prototype: acts at all alpha and at $beta_1$ receptors; used as vasoconstrictor. Causes reflex bradycardia. Tox: ischemia, arrhythmias
Norfloxacin	Fluoroquinolone antibiotic: inhibits bacterial DNA gyrase; active against many gram-negative rods including *E coli, H influenzae, Klebsiella, Enterobacter, Pseudomonas, Serratia.* Tox: see ciprofloxacin
Norgestrel	Progestin: used in many oral contraceptives and Norplant implantable contraceptive
Omeprazole	Antiulcer: irreversible blocker of H^+/K^+ ATPase proton pump in parietal cells of stomach. Used in Zollinger-Ellison syndrome, gastroesophageal reflux disease (GERD)
Ondansetron	$5\text{-}HT_3$ receptor blocker: used as antiemetic during chemotherapy
Paraquat	Toxic herbicide: very small oral (but not inhaled) doses cause lethal pulmonary fibrosis
Parathion	Organophosphate acetylcholinesterase inhibitor prototype: used as insecticide. Pro-drug: converted in body to paraoxon. Other organophosphates: DFP, soman, tabun, dichlorvos, malathion, echothiophate. Tox: "DUMBELS" mnemonic (Chapter 7)
Penicillamine	Chelator, immunomodulator: copper and sometimes lead, mercury, arsenic. Used in Wilson's disease and rheumatoid arthritis
Penicillin G	Penicillin prototype: active against common streptococci, gram-positive bacilli, gram-negative cocci, spirochetes, and enterococci (if used with an aminoglycoside); penicillinase-susceptible. Tox: penicillin allergy
Phenformin, metformin	Oral biguanide hypoglycemics: different mechanism from sulfonylurea oral hypoglycemics. Some efficacy in the *absence* of functioning pancreatic B cells
Phenobarbital	Long-acting barbiturate prototype: used as a sedative and anticonvulsant (eg, grand mal). Facilitates GABA-mediated neuronal inhibition and may block excitatory neurotransmitters. Partial renal clearance that can be increased by urinary alkalinization in overdose. Chronic use leads to induction of liver drug-metabolizing enzymes and ALA synthase. Tox: psychologic and physical dependence liability; additive effects with other CNS depressants
Phenoxybenzamine	Alpha-blocker prototype: irreversible action. Used in pheochromocytoma
Phentolamine	Alpha-blocker prototype: reversible action. Used in pheochromocytoma
Phenytoin	Antiepileptic hydantoin: used for grand mal and partial seizures; blocks Na^+ channels in neuronal membranes. Serum levels variable due to first-pass metabolism and dose-dependent nonlinear elimination kinetics. Tox: sedation, diplopia, gingival hyperplasia, hirsutism, respiratory depression in overdose. Many drug interactions via effects on plasma protein binding or hepatic metabolism

Physostigmine	Cholinesterase inhibitor prototype: alkaloid tertiary amine carbamate, enters eye and CNS readily. Used in glaucoma
Pilocarpine	Muscarinic agonist prototype: tertiary amine alkaloid. Causes paradoxical hypertension by activating excitatory muscarinic EPSP receptors in postganglionic sympathetic neurons. Used in glaucoma. Tox: muscarinic excess
Piroxicam	NSAID: long-acting ($t_{1/2}$ about 40 h)
Pralidoxime	Acetylcholinesterase regenerator: very high affinity for phosphorus in organophosphates
Prazosin, terazosin, doxazosin	Alpha$_1$-selective blockers: used in HTN. Tox: first-dose orthostatic hypotension
Prednisone	Glucocorticoid prototype: potent, short-acting; much less mineralocorticoid activity than cortisol but more than dexamethasone or triamcinolone
Probenecid	Uricosuric: inhibitor of renal weak acid secretion and reabsorption; prolongs half-life of penicillin, accelerates clearance of uric acid. Used in gout
Probucol	Antilipemic: unknown mechanism; used in patients with hyperlipidemia caused by homozygous LDL receptor deficiency. Tox: causes arrhythmias
Procainamide	Group IA antiarrhythmic drug: short half-life; similar to quinidine but may cause reversible lupus erythematosus
Propranolol	Nonselective beta-blocker prototype: local anesthetic action but no partial agonist effect. Used in HTN, angina, arrhythmias, migraine, hyperthyroidism, tremor. Tox: asthma, AV block, CHF
Propylthiouracil	Antithyroid drug prototype: reduces iodination of tyrosine and coupling of MIT and DIT in the thyroid; orally active. Tox: rash, agranulocytosis (rare)
Prostacyclin	PGI$_2$: prostaglandin vasodilator and inhibitor of platelet aggregation
Pyridostigmine	Cholinesterase inhibitor: long-acting (8 h) quaternary carbamate; used in myasthenia gravis
Quinidine	Group IA antiarrhythmic prototype: used in atrial and ventricular arrhythmias. Tox: cinchonism, GI upset, thrombocytopenic purpura, arrhythmogenic
Quinine	Antimalarial: blood schizonticide; no effect on liver stages. Isomer of quinidine, same toxicity
Ranitidine	H$_2$ blocker: like cimetidine but less inhibition of hepatic drug metabolism; no antiandrogenic effects
Reserpine	Antihypertensive: selective inhibitor of vesicle catecholamine/H$^+$ antiporter; used in HTN, causes depletion of catecholamines and 5-HT from their stores. Tox: severe depression, suicide, ulcers, diarrhea
Rifampin	Antimicrobial: inhibitor of DNA-dependent RNA polymerase, used in the meningococcal carrier state and in drug regimens for tuberculosis. Tox: hepatic dysfunction, induction of liver drug-metabolizing enzymes (drug interactions), flu-like syndrome with intermittent dosing
Selegiline	MAO-B inhibitor: selective inhibitor of the enzyme that metabolizes dopamine (no tyramine interactions). Used in parkinsonism as adjunct
Succimer (DMSA)	Chelator: dimercaptosuccinic acid; used to chelate lead and arsenic
Succinylcholine	Depolarizing neuromuscular relaxant prototype: short duration (5 min) if patient has normal plasma cholinesterase (genetically determined). No antidote (compare with tubocurarine)
Sumatriptan	5-HT$_{1d}$ receptor agonist: used to abort migraine attacks
Tamoxifen	Estrogen partial agonist: used in breast carcinoma

Terbutaline, albuterol, metaproterenol	Beta$_2$-selective agonists: mainstays of acute therapy of bronchospasm in asthma
Terfenadine	Antihistamine (H$_1$ blocker) newer, less sedating drug. Used in hayfever. Tox: like astemizole
Tetracaine	Local anesthetic: long-acting ester prototype
Tetracycline	Antibiotic: tetracycline prototype; bacteriostatic inhibitor of protein synthesis (30S). Broad spectrum, but many resistant organisms. Used for Lyme disease, mycoplasmal, chlamydial, rickettsial infections, chronic bronchitis, acne, cholera; a back-up drug in syphilis. Tox: GI upset and superinfections (*Candida,* staphylococci), antianabolic actions, Fanconi syndrome (outdated drug), photosensitivity, potential hepatotoxicity (overdose), dental enamel dysplasia
Tetrodotoxin	Toxin: very potent sodium channel blocker; blocks action potential propagation in nerve, heart, and skeletal muscle. From puffer fish, California newt. Tox: paresthesias, paralysis
Thiazides	Diuretic prototype: block Na/Cl transporter in distal convoluted tubule; used in HTN, CHF, chronic stone formers. Tox: K$^+$ wasting; increased serum lipids, uric acid, and glucose
Thioridazine	Antipsychotic phenothiazine: blocks most dopamine receptors in the CNS. Tox: atropine-like effects (marked), ECG abnormalities, postural hypotension, retinal pigmentation, sedation, additive effects with other CNS depressants (but less EPS dysfunction than other phenothiazines)
Thyroxine, triiodothyronine	Major hormones produced by the thyroid: stimulate metabolism, growth, and development
Ticarcillin	Penicillin: widely used extended spectrum agent active against selected gram-negative bacteria including *Pseudomonas aeruginosa* (synergistic with aminoglycosides). Susceptible to penicillinases unless used with clavulanic acid. Tox: penicillin allergy
Tolbutamide, tolazamide, chlorpropamide, acetohexamide	Oral hypoglycemics: older sulfonylurea group. (See glipizide.) Chlorpropamide has longest duration of action and potential for hypoglycemia. Interactions through plasma protein binding
Trimethaphan	Ganglion blocker (antinicotinic agent) prototype: last remaining clinically useful ganglion blocker. Used in malignant HTN and for controlled hypotension (in neurosurgery)
Trimethoprim-sulfamethoxazole	Antimicrobial drug combination: causes synergistic sequential blockade of folic acid synthesis. Active against many gram-negative bacteria including *Aeromonas, Enterobacter, H influenzae, Klebsiella, Moraxella, Salmonella, Serratia, Shigella* spp. Possible back-up agent for methicillin-resistant staphylococci. Tox: mainly due to sulfonamide; includes hypersensitivity, hematotoxicity, kernicterus, and drug interactions due to competition for plasma protein binding
Tubocurarine	Nondepolarizing neuromuscular blocking agent prototype: competitive nicotinic blocker. Releases histamine and may cause hypotension. Analogues: pancuronium, atracurium, vecuronium, and other "-curiums" and "-curoniums." Antidote: cholinesterase inhibitor, eg, neostigmine
Tyramine	Indirectly acting sympathomimetic prototype: releases or displaces norepinephrine from stores in nerve endings. Usually inactive by the oral route because of high first-pass effect but will cause potentially lethal hypertensive responses in patients taking MAO inhibitors

Valproic acid	Anticonvulsant: used mainly in petit mal but also effective in clonic-tonic and myoclonic seizure states. Tox: GI distress, hepatic necrosis (rare), teratogenic (spina bifida)
Vancomycin	Glycopeptide bactericidal antibiotic: inhibits synthesis of cell wall precursor molecules. Drug of choice for methicillin-resistant staphylococci and effective in antibiotic-induced colitis. Dose reduction required in renal impairment (or hemodialysis). Tox: ototoxicity, hypersensitivity, renal dysfunction (rare)
Verapamil	Calcium channel blocker prototype: cardiac depressant and vasodilator; used in HTN, angina, and arrhythmias. Tox: AV block, CHF, constipation
Vesamicol	Inhibitor of vesicle ACh/H^+ antiporter in cholinergic nerve endings: prevents storage of ACh. No clinical applications
Vincristine	Antineoplastic plant alkaloid: cell cycle (M phase)-specific agent; inhibits mitotic spindle formation. Tox: peripheral neuropathy. Compare with vinblastine, a congener that causes myelosuppression
Zidovudine (AZT)	Antiviral: major drug for HIV infections; inhibits HIV reverse transcriptase. Tox: severe myelosuppression

Appendix II

Examination 1

DIRECTIONS: Each numbered item or incomplete statement in this section is followed by answers or by completions of the statement. Select the ONE lettered answer or completion that is BEST in each case.

1. Phase II clinical trials typically involve
   (A) Measurement of the pharmacokinetics of the new drug in normal volunteers
   (B) Double blind evaluation of the new drug in thousands of patients with the target disease
   (C) Evaluation of late effects of depolarizing neuromuscular blockers in humans
   (D) Evaluation of the new drug in fifty to several hundred patients with the target disease
   (E) Collection of late toxicity data from patients previously studied in phase I trials

2. A patient is admitted to the emergency department for treatment of an overdose of a drug. The identity of the drug is unknown, but it is observed that when the urine pH is acidic, the renal clearance of the drug is less than the glomerular filtration rate, and that when the urine pH is alkaline, the clearance is greater than the glomerular filtration rate. The drug is probably a
   (A) Strong acid
   (B) Weak acid
   (C) Nonelectrolyte
   (D) Weak base
   (E) Strong base

3. The amide-type local anesthetic with the longest duration of action is
   (A) Cocaine
   (B) Procaine
   (C) Lidocaine
   (D) Bupivacaine
   (E) Tetracaine

4. Aminophylline, dobutamine, and digoxin can each
   (A) Increase the amount of cAMP
   (B) Increase cardiac contractile force
   (C) Decrease conduction velocity in the atrioventricular node
   (D) Increase peripheral vascular resistance
   (E) Decrease venous return

5. The polypeptide agent with the strongest vasodilator properties is
   (A) Bradykinin
   (B) Glucagon
   (C) Nitroprusside
   (D) Prostacyclin
   (E) Angiotensin II

6. A frequent adverse effect of cimetidine is
   (A) Agranulocytosis
   (B) Systemic lupus erythematosus
   (C) Inhibition of hepatic metabolism of other drugs
   (D) Antiestrogenic effects
   (E) Hypertension

7. One property of quinidine that is not associated with procainamide is its
   (A) Ability to control atrial arrhythmias
   (B) Tendency to produce cinchonism

(C) Activity by the oral route

(D) Prolongation of the PR interval

(E) Prolongation of the QRS interval

8. A patient discharged from the hospital after a myocardial infarction has been receiving small doses of quinidine to suppress a ventricular tachycardia. One month later, his local physician prescribes high-dose hydrochlorothiazide therapy for ankle edema, which is ascribed to congestive heart failure. Three weeks after beginning thiazide therapy, the patient is readmitted to the hospital with a rapid multifocal ventricular tachycardia. The most probable cause of this arrhythmia is

(A) Quinidine toxicity caused by inhibition of quinidine metabolism by the thiazide

(B) Direct effects of hydrochlorothiazide on the pacemaker of the heart

(C) Thiazide toxicity caused by the effects of quinidine on the kidneys

(D) Accumulation of quinidine caused by the renal action of hydrochlorothiazide

(E) Reduction of serum potassium caused by the diuretic action of hydrochlorothiazide

9. An important therapeutic or toxic effect of loop diuretics is

(A) Decreased heart rate

(B) Decreased blood volume

(C) Increased total body potassium

(D) Metabolic acidosis

(E) Increased serum sodium

10. The most useful drug for reversing the effects of myasthenic crisis in a patient who is experiencing diplopia, dysarthria, and difficulty swallowing is

(A) Neostigmine

(B) Pilocarpine

(C) Physostigmine

(D) Succinylcholine

(E) Tubocurarine

11. Soon after being put to bed for a nap, a 4-year-old child is found convulsing. Diarrhea and a warm moist skin are apparent. The heart rate is 70/min, and the pupils are markedly constricted. Drug intoxication is suspected. The most probable cause is

(A) An organophosphate-containing insecticide

(B) A nicotine-containing insecticide

(C) Amphetamine-containing diet pills

(D) Phenylephrine-containing eye drops

(E) An atropine-containing medication

12. A patient is admitted to the emergency room 2 hours after taking an overdose of phenobarbital. The plasma level of the drug at time of admission is 100 mg/L, and the apparent volume of distribution, half-life, and clearance of phenobarbital are 35 L, 4 days, and 6.1 L/d, respectively. The ingested dose was approximately

(A) 1 g

(B) 3.5 g

(C) 6.1 g

(D) 40 g

(E) 70 g

13. Most weak-acid drugs as well as weak-base drugs are absorbed primarily from the small intestine after oral administration because

(A) Both types are more ionized in the small intestine

(B) Both types are less ionized in the small intestine

(C) The blood flow is greater in the small intestine than in other parts of the gut

(D) The surface area of the small intestine is greater than most other parts of the gut

(E) The small intestine has nonspecific carriers for most drugs

14. The primary site of action of tyramine is

(A) Preganglionic sympathetic nerve terminals

(B) Ganglionic receptors

(C) Postganglionic sympathetic nerve terminals

(D) Vascular smooth muscle cell receptors

(E) Gut and liver catechol-O-methyltransferase

15. A semiconscious patient in the intensive care unit is being artificially ventilated. Random spontaneous respiratory movements are rendering the mechanical ventilation ineffective. A useful drug to reduce the patient's ineffective spontaneous respiratory activity is

    (A) Pancuronium
    (B) Succinylcholine
    (C) Pyridostigmine
    (D) Baclofen
    (E) Dantrolene

16. A drug suitable for producing mydriasis and cycloplegia lasting more than 24 hours is
    (A) Atropine
    (B) Tropicamide
    (C) Echothiophate
    (D) Edrophonium
    (E) Ephedrine

17. Neostigmine and physostigmine differ in that
    (A) Neostigmine is inactive when given orally
    (B) Physostigmine is inactive when given orally
    (C) The effects of neostigmine are irreversible
    (D) Physostigmine has more effect on the central nervous system
    (E) Neostigmine has less effect on skeletal muscle

18. A 59-year-old woman with a 60 pack-year smoking history was diagnosed with lung cancer 2 months ago. She now enters the hospital in coma. Her serum calcium is 16 mg/dL. Which of the following would be most useful to reduce serum calcium in this patient rapidly?
    (A) Furosemide
    (B) Spironolactone
    (C) Hydrochlorothiazide
    (D) Mannitol
    (E) Acetazolamide

19. A 50-year-old man has macrocytic anemia and early signs of neurologic abnormality. The drug that will probably be required in this case is
    (A) Folic acid
    (B) Vitamin B_{12}
    (C) Iron dextran
    (D) Erythropoietin
    (E) Filgrastim

20. A patient who has been receiving warfarin for 2 weeks will probably have
    (A) Reduced plasma Factor II
    (B) Reduced plasma Factor VIII
    (C) Reduced plasma plasminogen
    (D) Increased tissue plasminogen activator
    (E) Increased platelet adenosine stores

21. The antihypertensive drug most likely to aggravate angina pectoris is
    (A) Hydralazine
    (B) Guanethidine
    (C) Propranolol
    (D) Clonidine
    (E) Methyldopa

22. A drug lacking vasodilator properties that is useful in angina is
    (A) Nitroglycerin
    (B) Nifedipine
    (C) Metoprolol
    (D) Isosorbide dinitrate
    (E) Verapamil

23. A drug that reduces arterial clotting of blood (thrombi) is
    (A) Prostaglandin E_2
    (B) Prostaglandin F_2
    (C) Prostacyclin
    (D) Thromboxane A_2
    (E) Leukotriene B_4

24. A potent facilitator of platelet aggregation is
    (A) Prostaglandin E_2
    (B) Prostaglandin F_2

      (C) Prostacyclin
      (D) Thromboxane A_2
      (E) Leukotriene B_4

25. A drug useful in the treatment of asthma, although it lacks bronchodilator action, is
      (A) Metoprolol
      (B) Isoproterenol
      (C) Ephedrine
      (D) Metaproterenol
      (E) Cromolyn

26. The toxicity of aspirin involves all of the following EXCEPT
      (A) Increased prothrombin levels
      (B) Metabolic acidosis
      (C) Respiratory alkalosis
      (D) Increased risk of peptic ulcers
      (E) Increased risk of hepatic damage and encephalopathy in children with viral infections

27. Although it does not act at the histamine receptor, epinephrine reverses many effects of histamine. Epinephrine is a
      (A) Competitive inhibitor of histamine
      (B) Noncompetitive antagonist of histamine
      (C) Physiologic antagonist of histamine
      (D) Chemical antagonist of histamine
      (E) Metabolic inhibitor of histamine

28. Most drug receptors are
      (A) Small molecules with a molecular weight between 100 and 1000
      (B) Lipids arranged in a bilayer configuration
      (C) Proteins located on cell membranes or in the cytosol
      (D) DNA molecules
      (E) RNA molecules

29. After intravenous bolus administration of lidocaine, the major factors determining the initial plasma concentration are
      (A) Dose and clearance
      (B) Dose and apparent volume of distribution
      (C) Apparent volume of distribution and clearance
      (D) Clearance and half-life
      (E) Half-life and dose

30. The longest-acting insulin preparation is
      (A) Bovine semilente
      (B) Porcine lente
      (C) Bovine ultralente
      (D) Human lente
      (E) Porcine NPH

31. Intravenous administration of norepinephrine in a patient already taking an effective dose of atropine will often
      (A) Increase heart rate
      (B) Decrease total peripheral resistance
      (C) Decrease blood sugar
      (D) Increase skin temperature
      (E) Reduce pupil size

32. A drug that will produce mydriasis without cycloplegia is
      (A) Tropicamide
      (B) Phenylephrine
      (C) Isoproterenol
      (D) Atropine
      (E) Cyclopentolate

33. Which of the following statements is most correct?
      (A) Maximum efficacy of a drug is directly correlated with its potency
      (B) The therapeutic index is the LD50 (or TD50) divided by the ED50
      (C) A partial agonist has no effect on its receptors unless another drug is present

    (D) Graded dose-response data provide information about the standard deviation of sensitivity to the drug in the population studied

34. The heart rate response to the infusion of a moderate dose of phenylephrine in conscious patients is NOT blocked by

    (A) Hexamethonium

    (B) Atropine

    (C) Phenoxybenzamine

    (D) Reserpine

35. All of the following statements about scopolamine are correct EXCEPT

    (A) It has depressant actions on the CNS

    (B) It may cause hallucinations

    (C) It is poorly distributed across the placenta to the fetus

    (D) It may prevent motion sickness when applied as a patch to the skin

    (E) It is similar to atropine in reducing gastrointestinal motility

36. All of the following statements about propranolol and timolol are correct EXCEPT

    (A) Timolol is a nonselective β_1- and β_2-blocker

    (B) Propranolol cannot be given orally

    (C) Timolol has useful cardiac effects after myocardial infarction

    (D) Propranolol has more local anesthetic action than timolol

37. A drug that blocks 5α-reductase in the prostate gland is

    (A) Flutamide

    (B) Finasteride

    (C) Cyproterone

    (D) Leuprolide

    (E) Ketoconazole

38. The increase in heart rate and force of cardiac contraction normally induced by electrical stimulation of sympathetic nerves can be blocked by which of the following?

    (A) Hydralazine

    (B) Atropine

    (C) Clonidine

    (D) Neostigmine

    (E) Propranolol

39. A treatment for angina that consistently increases the product of heart rate and blood pressure (double product) at which anginal symptoms occur is

    (A) Nitroglycerin

    (B) Propranolol

    (C) Nifedipine

    (D) Coronary bypass surgery

    (E) Verapamil

40. Verapamil and diltiazem diminish the symptoms of angina pectoris by causing all of the following EXCEPT

    (A) Reduction in blood pressure

    (B) Reduction in heart rate

    (C) Reduction in cardiac contractile force

    (D) Increase in heart size

    (E) Increase in diastolic interval

41. Which of the following has a self-limited diuretic action even when blood volume is maintained?

    (A) Hydrochlorothiazide

    (B) Triamterene

    (C) Acetazolamide

    (D) Furosemide

    (E) Mannitol

42. Diuretics that increase the delivery of poorly absorbed solute to the thick ascending limb of the nephron include

    (A) Spironolactone

    (B) Mannitol

    (C) Indapamide

       (D) Furosemide

       (E) All of the above

43. In a patient receiving digoxin for congestive heart failure, conditions that may facilitate the appearance of toxicity include

       (A) Hypocalcemia

       (B) Hypomagnesemia

       (C) Hyperkalemia

       (D) Hypernatremia

       (E) All of the above

44. Causes of digitalis toxicity include

       (A) Intracellular calcium overload

       (B) Intracellular potassium overload

       (C) Increased parasympathetic activity

       (D) Increased adrenocorticosteroid levels

       (E) All of the above

45. Methylxanthine drugs such as aminophylline cause all of the following EXCEPT

       (A) Vasodilation in many vascular beds

       (B) Increase in the amount of cAMP in mast cells

       (C) Bronchodilation

       (D) Activation of the enzyme phosphodiesterase

46. Drugs used in asthma that often cause tachycardia and tremor include

       (A) Terbutaline

       (B) Cromolyn sodium

       (C) Ipratropium

       (D) Beclomethasone

       (E) All of the above

47. Drugs with potentially useful effects in the treatment of inoperable metastatic pheochromocytoma include all of the following EXCEPT

       (A) Phenoxybenzamine

       (B) Reserpine

       (C) Phentolamine

       (D) Metyrosine

       (E) Propranolol

48. Agents that can readily cause edema if released or injected near capillaries include

       (A) Norepinephrine

       (B) Serotonin

       (C) Histamine

       (D) Angiotensin II

49. Typical results of beta-receptor activation include all of the following EXCEPT

       (A) Hyperglycemia

       (B) Lipolysis

       (C) Glycogenolysis

       (D) Decreased skeletal muscle strength

       (E) Increased renin secretion

50. Drugs that may be useful for preventing recurrences of atrial fibrillation include

       (A) Quinidine

       (B) Mexiletine

       (C) Bretylium

       (D) Lidocaine

       (E) All of the above

51. A neuronal cell body is located in the locus ceruleus, with fine axonal projections to most brain levels. The neurotransmitter that it releases, which can be either excitatory or inhibitory, is most likely to be

       (A) Acetylcholine

       (B) Dopamine

       (C) Glutamic acid

       (D) Norepinephrine

       (E) Serotonin

Items 52–53: A 40-year-old man had been consuming alcoholic beverages at lunch and in the evenings all his adult life. During the last two years, his alcohol consumption had steadily increased, continuing throughout the day. Due to family pressures, the man abruptly stopped drinking alcohol. Within a few hours he became increasingly anxious and agitated and had symptoms of autonomic hyperexcitability. He developed a hand tremor and the following day had delusions and visual hallucinations. At this point the man was brought to the hospital.

52. All of the following statements about the chronic consumption of alcohol in this patient are true EXCEPT
    (A) Psychologic dependence is an important component of alcohol abuse
    (B) The man has probably been experiencing gastrointestinal distress for some time, and he is likely to have liver dysfunction
    (C) The rate of his metabolism of ethanol is not dependent on its blood level across most of the pharmacologic range
    (D) An increase in the activity of liver alcohol dehydrogenase has caused tolerance
    (E) He may have developed gynecomastia and testicular atrophy

53. All of the following statements about the hospitalization of this patient are accurate EXCEPT
    (A) A preliminary diagnosis of delirium tremens is appropriate in this case
    (B) An intravenous benzodiazepine is likely to be administered
    (C) Since he has delusions and hallucinations, a phenothiazine should be given
    (D) The occurrence of cardiac arrhythmias is a distinct possibility
    (E) Clonidine or beta adrenoceptor-blocking drugs may also be useful in alleviating his symptoms

54. In the use of most modern general anesthetics
    (A) The state of surgical anesthesia is associated with complete muscle paralysis
    (B) Anesthetic potency is quantitated by the minimum alveolar concentration (MAC) that causes 50% of subjects to lose reflex response to a painful stimulus
    (C) Anesthesia is associated with increased blood pressure and total peripheral resistance
    (D) Gaseous agents are used for long procedures because intravenous anesthetics are too toxic to use for more than a few minutes
    (E) Agents that are very insoluble in the blood have a relatively slow onset of anesthetic action

55. A patient is to undergo day surgery for a short procedure, and intravenous anesthesia will be used. All of the following statements about the agents that may be used are accurate EXCEPT
    (A) Thiopental is likely to increase cerebral blood flow
    (B) Recovery from propofol is very rapid
    (C) Ketamine may cause postoperative excitation and delusions
    (D) Fentanyl will provide significant analgesia
    (E) Midazolam is likely to cause postoperative respiratory depression

56. A patient with terminal cancer is suffering from pain that is gradually increasing in intensity. In the management of pain in such a patient
    (A) The placebo effect is absent
    (B) Nonsteroidal anti-inflammatory drugs may control symptoms during a significant portion of the course of the disease
    (C) In order to delay the development of addiction, opioid analgesics should never be given for initial management of chronic pain
    (D) Addiction occurs universally in the later stages of the disease because of the very large opioid doses required
    (E) Meperidine is documentably more effective than morphine in chronic pain states

57. Effects of the opioid analgesics include all of the following EXCEPT
    (A) Anticonvulsant action
    (B) Cough suppressant action
    (C) Constipation
    (D) Sedation
    (E) Reduction of heart rate

58. Which of the following drugs is LEAST likely to cause psychologic or physical dependence?
    (A) Amphetamine
    (B) Fentanyl
    (C) Cocaine

(D) Nicotine

(E) LSD

59. In a patient with status epilepticus, all of the following drugs given intravenously will be effective EXCEPT

(A) Diazepam

(B) Fluphenazine

(C) Lorazepam

(D) Phenytoin

(E) Thiopental

60. Plasma levels of phenytoin are usually monitored in patients with grand mal epilepsy. All of the following factors contribute to interpatient variability in the plasma level of the drug EXCEPT

(A) Oral absorption of the drug is highly variable

(B) The drug undergoes variable first-pass metabolism

(C) Elimination of phenytoin follows first-order kinetics at high doses

(D) Phenytoin competes with other drugs for plasma protein binding sites

(E) The metabolism of phenytoin may be affected by concomitant use of other drugs

61. If one patient is taking amitriptyline and another patient is taking chlorpromazine, they are **both** likely to experience all of the following adverse effects EXCEPT

(A) Sedation

(B) Visual dysfunction

(C) Postural hypotension

(D) Gynecomastia

(E) Urinary retention

62. A patient suffering from a severe depressive disorder was treated first with imipramine and then with an MAO inhibitor. His symptoms did not improve significantly with either drug. A drug that is most likely to be effective in this patient is

(A) Haloperidol

(B) Phenelzine

(C) Amitriptyline

(D) Buspirone

(E) Sertraline

63. The pharmacodynamic effects of the phenothiazines result from the blockade of all of the following receptors EXCEPT

(A) Peripheral adrenoceptors

(B) Histamine receptors

(C) Dopamine receptors

(D) Nicotinic receptors

(E) Muscarinic receptors

64. All of the following statements about tardive dyskinesias are accurate EXCEPT

(A) They are likely to occur during chronic treatment with haloperidol

(B) Their severity can be reduced by muscarinic receptor blocking drugs

(C) Symptoms may be temporarily alleviated by increasing antipsychotic drug dosage

(D) Levodopa is likely to exacerbate the symptoms

(E) They are choreoathetoid-like movement disorders

65. A psychiatric patient on medications develops a tremor, thyroid enlargement, and leukocytosis. The drug that he is taking is MOST likely to be

(A) Chlorpromazine

(B) Desipramine

(C) Haloperidol

(D) Lithium

(E) Fluoxetine

66. The mechanism of action of benzodiazepines is

(A) Blockade of the action of excitatory neurotransmitters

(B) Activation of $GABA_B$ receptors

(C) Facilitation of the actions of the primary inhibitory neurotransmitter in the brain

(D) Inhibition of GABA transaminase

(E) Blockade of glycine receptors in the spinal cord

67. Drugs useful in the treatment of parkinsonism include all of the following EXCEPT
   (A) Amantadine
   (B) Selegiline
   (C) Thioridazine
   (D) Benztropine
   (E) Bromocriptine

68. A patient has taken a very large overdose of a benzodiazepine. Management will include all of the following EXCEPT
   (A) Establishment of a patent airway
   (B) Administration of flumazenil
   (C) Ventilatory support
   (D) Gastric lavage if an endotracheal tube is in place
   (E) Administration of physostigmine

Items 69–71: A 65-year-old man (weight 70 kg) is to be treated with amikacin for a gram-negative sepsis. His renal function is approximately 50% of normal. Pharmacokinetic parameters of the drug (in an individual with normal renal function) include: Vd = 0.3 L/kg; CL = 80 mL/min; half-life = 3 hr.

69. If you wish to establish an optimal plasma drug level of 20 mg/L rapidly, the loading dose should be approximately
   (A) 6 mg
   (B) 60 mg
   (C) 200 mg
   (D) 400 mg
   (E) 600 mg

70. In this patient, amikacin is LEAST likely to be effective for the treatment of bacterial sepsis due to
   (A) *B fragilis*
   (B) *E coli*
   (C) *Enterobacter* species
   (D) *Pseudomonas* species
   (E) *Serratia marcescens*

71. If the organism proves to be resistant to amikacin, the mechanism of resistance is MOST likely
   (A) Bacterial production of beta-lactamases
   (B) Decreased accumulation of the drug in bacteria
   (C) Inactivation of the drug by bacterial group transferases
   (D) A changed pathway of bacterial folate synthesis
   (E) Production of drug-trapping thiols by the bacteria

72. Assuming that a patient is not allergic, penicillin G would be an appropriate drug to use in all of the following situations EXCEPT
   (A) A patient with syphilis of more than 1 year's duration
   (B) Endocarditis prophylaxis for dental surgery
   (C) Community-acquired pneumococcal pneumonia
   (D) Hospital-acquired staphylococcal osteomyelitis
   (E) Meningococcal meningitis acquired on a military base

Items 73–74: A 19-year-old woman with recurrent sinusitis has been treated with different antibiotics on several occasions. During the course of one such treatment she developed a severe diarrhea and was hospitalized. Sigmoidoscopy revealed colitis, and pseudomembranes were confirmed histologically. The colitis was then treated successfully with another antibiotic, administered orally.

73. Which of the following antibiotics has been reported to cause gastrointestinal superinfections with pseudomembrane formation?
   (A) Ampicillin
   (B) Clindamycin
   (C) Tetracycline
   (D) Erythromycin
   (E) All of the above

74. Which of the following drugs, administered orally, is LEAST likely to be effective in the treatment of a colitis due to *C difficile*?
    (A) Bacitracin
    (B) Cefotetan
    (C) Metronidazole
    (D) Vancomycin
    (E) None of the above drugs will be effective

75. Characteristics of the cephalosporin drug group include all of the following EXCEPT
    (A) Bacterial resistance occurs through the production of beta-lactamases
    (B) First-generation drugs have activity against gram-positive cocci, *E coli,* and *K pneumoniae*
    (C) Cefoxitin is an appropriate drug for the treatment of pelvic inflammatory disease
    (D) Since they do not cross the blood-brain barrier, third-generation drugs are ineffective in bacterial meningitis
    (E) Ceftriaxone will eradicate most strains of *N gonorrhoeae* in a single dose

76. Appropriate clinical uses of the tetracyclines include the treatment of all of the following EXCEPT
    (A) Syphilis in a patient allergic to penicillins
    (B) Enterococcal endocarditis
    (C) Chlamydial urinogenital infections
    (D) Traveler's diarrhea
    (E) Prophylaxis in patients with chronic bronchitis

77. A 24-year-old woman is to be treated with ciprofloxacin for a bacterial urinary tract infection. The patient should be instructed about all of the following EXCEPT
    (A) The drug will also be effective against a yeast infection
    (B) She should be aware that theophylline toxicity may be enhanced by the drug
    (C) The drug may make her lightheaded, dizzy, or drowsy
    (D) If she is breast-feeding, she should stop while taking the drug
    (E) Antacids, taken concomitantly, may interfere with oral absorption of the drug

78. In the management of AIDS, the sulfonamides are often used in combination with inhibitors of folate reductase. Such combinations have activity against all of the following organisms EXCEPT
    (A) Methicillin-resistant staphylococcal species
    (B) *Nocardia* species
    (C) *Pneumocystis carinii*
    (D) *Toxoplasma gondii*
    (E) *Treponema pallidum*

Items 79–80: A patient with metastatic choriocarcinoma was treated first with methotrexate and subsequently with a combination of cisplatin and etoposide. In both regimens, drug dosage was maximized to a toxicity limit of a 2-log decrease in blood platelets. The effects of chemotherapy were monitored by urinary chorionic gonadotropin (MU/24 hr), as shown in the data below.

	Urinary Chorionic Gonadotropin Titer (MU/24 hr)	
Drug Regimen	**Initial**	**After Treatment**
Methotrexate	10^8	10^5
Cisplatin plus etoposide	10^7	10^3

79. Which of the following statements about the data is MOST correct?
    (A) The maximal effect of methotrexate was a 2-log decrease in UCG titer
    (B) The drug-induced changes in UCG titer are directly proportional to decreases in platelet count
    (C) The maximal effect of the drug combination regimen was a 4-log decrease in UCG titer
    (D) The effects of the drugs on UCG titer have a direct relationship to cell kill
    (E) The final UCG titer demonstrates that the patient was cured

80. All of the following statements about the drugs used in this case are accurate EXCEPT
   (A) Leucovorin rescue will probably be employed during or after treatment with methotrexate
   (B) Sulfonamide treatment should be avoided in a patient taking methotrexate
   (C) A major advantage of etoposide is its lack of hematotoxicity
   (D) Cisplatin is a cell cycle nonspecific drug
   (E) Saline hydration will be employed during treatment with cisplatin to reduce its nephrotoxicity

81. A 20-year-old Native American college student is treated for pulmonary tuberculosis with isoniazid, rifampin, and ethambutol. All of the following statements about this drug regimen are accurate EXCEPT
   (A) He will probably need higher doses of isoniazid than normal
   (B) He is likely to develop hyperuricemia
   (C) The drug combination is expected to delay the emergence of resistance
   (D) He should have periodic tests for liver function
   (E) If rifampin is not administered more frequently than twice a week, he may experience flu-like symptoms

82. The mechanisms of action of antifungal drugs include all of the following EXCEPT
   (A) Amphotericin B binds to ergosterol to form artificial pores in fungal cell membranes
   (B) Flucytosine is activated to an antimetabolite that inhibits thymidylate synthase
   (C) Griseofulvin inhibits mitochondrial cytochrome oxidase
   (D) Ketoconazole blocks the conversion of lanosterol to ergosterol

83. Acyclovir is effective in all of the following situations EXCEPT
   (A) Suppression of reactivated herpes simplex virus infections in bone marrow recipients
   (B) Treatment of chicken pox in the leukemic patient
   (C) Prophylaxis against herpes zoster infections in the immunocompromised patient
   (D) Treatment of cytomegalovirus retinitis in AIDS patients
   (E) Therapy of a first episode of herpes simplex genitalis

84. All of the following statements about drugs active against the human immunodeficiency virus (HIV) are accurate EXCEPT
   (A) Zidovudine (ZDV) is an inhibitor of viral reverse transcriptase
   (B) Dose reductions of ZDV may be required in both hepatic and renal dysfunction
   (C) Myelosuppressant effects are increased if ganciclovir is administered to a patient on ZDV
   (D) Although it may act on ZDV-resistant strains of HIV, didanosine is more likely to cause hematotoxicity
   (E) Foscarnet has been used to treat cytomegalovirus infections in patients on ZDV

85. This antimalarial is a blood schizonticide active against all four types of malaria, but resistant strains of *Plasmodium falciparum* occur. The drug may cause dose-dependent retinal damage.
   (A) Chloroquine
   (B) Quinine
   (C) Primaquine
   (D) Pyrimethamine
   (E) Amodiaquine

86. All of the following statements about mebendazole are accurate EXCEPT
   (A) It is the drug of choice for hookworm and pinworm infections
   (B) It causes the Mazzotti reaction, which is due to toxic products from dying worms
   (C) It should be avoided in pregnancy
   (D) It inhibits microtubule aggregation
   (E) It has a high therapeutic index

87. This immunosuppressive agent causes selective destruction of T lymphoid cells, resulting in decreased cellular immunity with minor effects on humoral antibody formation.
   (A) Prednisone
   (B) Azathioprine
   (C) Cyclophosphamide
   (D) Lymphocyte immune globulin
   (E) $Rh_0(D)$ immune globulin

88. After initial hospitalization, a 16-year-old boy is treated at home for tuberculosis. The drugs he is receiving include isoniazid, rifampin, and pyrazinamide. All of the following statements about this case are accurate EXCEPT

(A) Household members should receive isoniazid for prophylaxis
(B) Rifampin may increase the activity of liver drug-metabolizing enzymes
(C) The risk of hepatotoxicity due to isoniazid is higher in children than in adults
(D) He should receive supplementary vitamin B6
(E) Exposure to ultraviolet light may cause photosensitivity

89. A farmer is brought to an emergency room after working in a silage storage facility. He has dyspnea, chest pain, frothy sputum, and eye irritation. A few hours later he develops pulmonary edema. The most likely cause of his problems is exposure to
(A) Carbon monoxide
(B) DDT
(C) Nitrogen dioxide
(D) Nicotine
(E) Trichloroethylene

90. A 3-year-old child who has ingested an insecticide becomes nauseous and develops diarrhea with "rice water" stools. His breath has a "sweet, garlicky" odor. Other signs and symptoms include vasodilation and hypotension. The child has no obvious signs of neurotoxicity. The agent MOST likely to cause these effects is
(A) Malathion
(B) Inorganic arsenic
(C) Dieldrin
(D) Rotenone
(E) Nicotine

Items 91–92: A 20-year-old college student is brought to the emergency room after taking an overdose of a non-prescription drug. The patient is confused and lethargic. He has been hyperventilating and is now dehydrated with an elevated temperature. Serum analyses demonstrate that the patient has an anion gap metabolic acidosis.

91. The most likely cause of these signs and symptoms is overdosage of
(A) Acetaminophen
(B) Diphenhydramine
(C) Loperamide
(D) Acetylsalicylic acid
(E) Dextromethorphan

92. In the management of this patient, all of the following procedures are appropriate EXCEPT
(A) Administration of universal antidote
(B) Correction of metabolic acidosis and electrolyte imbalance
(C) Gastric lavage with endotracheal tube in place
(D) Alkalinization of the urine
(E) Hemodialysis, if pH or CNS signs are not readily controlled

DIRECTIONS: The following section consists of lists of four to twenty-six lettered options followed by several numbered items. For each numbered item, select the ONE option that is most closely associated with it. Each answer may be selected once, more than once, or not at all.

Items 93–96:
(A) Prazosin
(B) Guanethidine
(C) Reserpine
(D) Methyldopa
(E) Captopril

93. A drug that appears to block postsynaptic receptors more effectively than presynaptic receptors
94. A drug that blocks a carrier mechanism located in the membrane of synaptic transmitter storage vesicles
95. A drug that inhibits a peptidase enzyme in the vascular system
96. A drug that is converted into the active form in the brain

Items 97–100:

    (A) Botulinus toxin
    (B) Tetrodotoxin
    (C) Saxitoxin
    (D) Cocaine
    (E) 3-Methoxy-4-hydroxy mandelic acid

97. A substance that inhibits reuptake of norepinephrine into sympathetic nerve terminals

98. A toxic substance that is synthesized in protozoans and concentrated in shellfish

99. A substance that prevents release of transmitter from cholinergic nerve endings

100. A substance that is excreted in large amounts by patients with increased catecholamine synthesis

Items 101–104:

(A) Triazolam	(J) Selegiline	(S) Thioridazine
(B) Morphine	(K) Alprazolam	(T) Naloxone
(C) Bromocriptine	(L) Mescaline	(U) Midazolam
(D) Chlorpromazine	(M) Isoflurane	(V) Dronabinol
(E) Valproic acid	(N) Phenytoin	(W) Benztropine
(F) Amitriptyline	(O) Phenobarbital	(X) Clozapine
(G) Phenelzine	(P) Fluoxetine	(Y) Lithium
(H) Ketamine	(Q) Levodopa	(Z) Nalbuphine
(I) MPTP	(R) Carbamazepine	

101. This drug causes marked sedation and many side effects due to its blocking actions at central and peripheral muscarinic receptors; its clinical applications include the treatment of enuresis, phobic disorders, and the adjunctive management of chronic pain states of neurogenic origin

102. When used as a sleeping pill, this drug may cause early-morning awakening; if abruptly withdrawn after just a few days of use, it may cause a rebound increase in rapid eye movement sleep stages

103. Commonly used in the management of generalized tonic-clonic and partial seizures, this agent has also proved effective in the control of mania

104. An inhibitor of monoamine oxidase, this drug does not cause hypertensive crisis if patients ingest tyramine-containing foods

Items 105–108:

(A) Ampicillin	(J) Busulfan	(S) Cefoperazone
(B) Doxycycline	(K) Vinblastine	(T) Bleomycin
(C) Isoniazid	(L) Cyclosporine	(U) Azathioprine
(D) Sulfasalazine	(M) Praziquantel	(V) Sulfadiazine
(E) Streptomycin	(N) Chloroquine	(W) Ethambutol
(F) Imipenem	(O) Erythromycin	(X) Ticarcillin
(G) Amphotericin B	(P) Daunorubicin	(Y) Foscarnet
(H) Acyclovir	(Q) Clarithromycin	(Z) Metronidazole
(I) Methotrexate	(R) Ganciclovir	

105. Although it is not used in the treatment of tuberculosis, this drug is used for prophylaxis against other mycobacteria that cause infections in the immunocompromised patient

106. This agent is the drug of choice for the treatment of a patient with both intestinal and hepatic amebiasis

107. Use of this antibacterial agent is associated with a high incidence of diarrhea; maculopapular skin rashes are common, especially in patients with viral infections

108. This agent is used in the treatment of acute leukemias; it generates free radicals that may be toxic to myocardial cells

Items 109–110:

    (A) Norgestrel
    (B) Etidronate
    (C) Tamoxifen
    (D) Oxandrolone
    (E) Glyburide

109. A drug that is used for Paget's disease and is under investigation for osteoporosis
110. A drug that closes potassium channels, depolarizing its target cells and causing the release of a peptide hormone

Items 111–113:

(A) Angiotensin II	**(G)** Epinephrine	**(L)** Phenylephrine
(B) Atropine	**(H)** Histamine	**(M)** Physostigmine
(C) Bethanechol	**(I)** Isoproterenol	**(N)** Propranolol
(D) Diphenhydramine	**(J)** Norepinephrine	**(O)** Quinidine
(E) Echothiophate	**(K)** Phentolamine	**(P)** Tropicamide
(F) Endothelin		

111–112: An anesthetized subject was given an IV bolus dose of a drug (**Drug 1**) while blood pressure (color) and heart rate were recorded, as shown on the left side of the graph below. While the recorder was stopped, **Drug 2** was given (center). Drug 1 was then administered again, as shown on the right side of the graph.

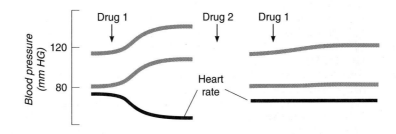

111. Identify Drug 1 from the above list
112. Identify Drug 2 from the above list
113. A drug was administered into the conjunctival sac of a patient, and pupil diameter was measured over a period of days as shown in the graph below. Using the above list, identify the drug placed in the conjunctival sac on day zero.

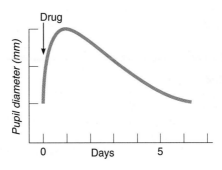

Item 114:

(A) Atropine	**(F)** Lidocaine
(B) Bretylium	**(G)** Nitroglycerin
(C) Epinephrine	**(H)** Prazosin
(D) Flecainide	**(I)** Propranolol
(E) Fluoxetine	**(J)** Quinine

114. A cardiac Purkinje fiber was isolated from an animal heart and placed in a recording chamber. One of the Purkinje cells was impaled with a microelectrode, and action potentials were recorded while the preparation was stimulated at 1 stimulus per second. A representative control action potential is shown in black in the graph below. After equilibration, a drug was added to the perfusate while recording continued. A representative action potential obtained at the peak of drug action is shown as the superimposed action potential. Identify the drug from the above list.

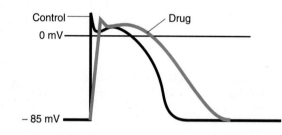

Answer Key for Examination 1.[1]

1. D	(5)		**40.** D	(12)		
2. B	(1)		**41.** C	(15)		
3. D	(25)		**42.** B	(15)		
4. B	(9, 13, 19)		**43.** B	(13)		
5. A	(17)		**44.** A	(13)		
6. C	(16)		**45.** D	(19)		
7. B	(14)		**46.** A	(9, 19)		
8. E	(14, 15)		**47.** B	(10, 11)		
9. B	(11, 15)		**48.** C	(16)		
10. A	(7)		**49.** D	(9)		
11. A	(7)		**50.** A	(14)		
12. B	(3)		**51.** D	(20)		
13. D	(1)		**52.** D	(22)		
14. C	(6, 9)		**53.** C	(31, 60)		
15. A	(25)		**54.** B	(24)		
16. A	(8)		**55.** A	(24)		
17. D	(7)		**56.** B	(30)		
18. A	(15)		**57.** A	(30)		
19. B	(32)		**58.** E	(31)		
20. A	(33)		**59.** B	(23, 28)		
21. A	(11, 12)		**60.** C	(23)		
22. C	(12)		**61.** D	(28, 29)		
23. C	(18)		**62.** E	(29)		
24. D	(18)		**63.** D	(28)		
25. E	(19)		**64.** B	(28)		
26. A	(35)		**65.** D	(28)		
27. C	(2)		**66.** C	(21)		
28. C	(1)		**67.** C	(27)		
29. B	(3)		**68.** E	(21, 60)		
30. C	(40)		**69.** D	(3, 45)		
31. A	(6, 8, 9)		**70.** A	(45)		
32. B	(8, 9)		**71.** C	(45)		
33. B	(2)		**72.** D	(43)		
34. D	(9)		**73.** E	(52)		
35. C	(8)		**74.** B	(43)		
36. B	(10)		**75.** D	(43)		
37. B	(39)		**76.** B	(44)		
38. E	(10)		**77.** A	(50)		
39. D	(12)		**78.** E	(47)		
			79. C	(56)		
			80. C	(56)		
			81. B	(46)		
			82. C	(48)		
			83. D	(49)		

---

[1] Numbers in parentheses are chapters in which answers may be found.

84. D	(49)	
85. A	(54)	
86. B	(55)	
87. D	(57)	
88. C	(46)	
89. C	(58)	
90. B	(59)	
91. D	(60)	
92. A	(35, 60)	
93. A	(10)	
94. C	(6, 11)	
95. E	(11)	
96. D	(11)	
97. D	(6)	
98. C	(6)	
99. A	(6)	

100. E	(6)	
101. F	(29)	
102. A	(21)	
103. R	(23)	
104. J	(27)	
105. Q	(50)	
106. Z	(54)	
107. A	(43)	
108. P	(56)	
109. B	(41)	
110. E	(40)	
111. L	(6, 9, 10)	
112. K	(6, 9, 10)	
113. B	(8)	
114. J	(14)	

Appendix III

Examination 2

DIRECTIONS: Each numbered item or incomplete statement in this section is followed by answers or by completions of the statement. Select the ONE lettered answer or completion that is BEST in each case.

1. Common effects of muscarinic stimulant drugs include all of the following EXCEPT
   (A) Tachycardia
   (B) Increased peristalsis
   (C) Mydriasis
   (D) Stimulation of sweat glands
   (E) Increased secretion by salivary glands

2. Most drugs given by the oral route are
   (A) Proteins with high lipid solubility
   (B) Amino acids with high lipid solubility
   (C) Metabolized in the lumen of the gut to active metabolites
   (D) Freely reabsorbed from the renal tubule
   (E) Molecules between 100 and 1000 molecular weight

3. With regard to distribution of a drug from the blood into tissues
   (A) Blood flow to the tissue is an important determinant
   (B) Solubility of the drug in the tissue is an important determinant
   (C) Concentration of the drug in the blood is an important determinant
   (D) Size (volume) of the tissue is an important determinant
   (E) All of the above are important determinants

4. Receptors that communicate their activation by turning on an integral intracellular tyrosine kinase are typically
   (A) G protein-coupled
   (B) Insulin or epidermal growth factor receptors
   (C) Acetylcholine or GABA channels
   (D) Steroid receptors
   (E) Vitamin D receptors

5. A patient with an arrhythmia is to receive lidocaine by constant IV infusion. The target plasma concentration is 3 mg/L. The pharmacokinetic parameters for lidocaine in the general population are: Vd 70 L, CL 35 L/h, and $t_{1/2}$ 1.4 hours. An infusion of 105 mg/h is begun. The plasma concentration of lidocaine is measured 2.8 hours later and reported to be 1.5 mg/L. This indicates that the final steady-state plasma concentration in this patient will be
   (A) 1.5 mg/L
   (B) 2.0 mg/L
   (C) 2.25 mg/L
   (D) 3.0 mg/L
   (E) 6.0 mg/L

6. A new antihypertensive drug is to be evaluated. Before human trials are begun, FDA regulations require that
   (A) The drug be studied in three mammalian species
   (B) All acute and chronic animal toxicity data be submitted to the FDA

    (C) The drug must be shown to be effective as well as safe in animals with the target disease

    (D) The drug must be shown to be free of carcinogenic effects

    (E) The effect of the drug on reproduction must be studied in at least two animal species

7. A drug that blocks the heart rate effect of a slow IV infusion of phenylephrine is

    (A) Atropine

    (B) Propranolol

    (C) Physostigmine

    (D) Haloperidol

    (E) Pilocarpine

8. A patient is admitted to the emergency room with orthostatic hypotension and evidence of marked GI bleeding. Which of the following most accurately describes the probable autonomic response to this bleeding?

    (A) Slow heart rate, dilated pupils, damp skin

    (B) Rapid heart rate, dilated pupils, damp skin

    (C) Slow heart rate, dry skin, increased bowel sounds

    (D) Rapid heart rate, dry skin, constricted pupils, increased bowel sounds

    (E) Rapid heart rate, constricted pupils, warm skin

9. A patient has open angle glaucoma. The LEAST likely drug for this condition is

    (A) Epinephrine

    (B) Timolol

    (C) Acetazolamide

    (D) Pilocarpine

    (E) Isoproterenol

10. Valid clinical applications of glycopyrrolate include the treatment of

    (A) Hypertension

    (B) Bladder spasm

    (C) Fever of viral infection

    (D) Muscle sprain

    (E) Amphetamine overdose

11. Probable effects of an IM injection of epinephrine include all of the following EXCEPT

    (A) Hypoglycemia

    (B) Leukocytosis

    (C) Hyperkalemia

    (D) Tachycardia

    (E) Bronchodilation

12. Infusion of phentolamine into the cerebrospinal fluid of an experimental animal will prevent the antihypertensive action of

    (A) Guanethidine

    (B) Reserpine

    (C) Trimethaphan

    (D) Enalapril

    (E) Clonidine

13. Which of the following correctly describes the action of nitroglycerin in angina?

    (A) Dilation of systemic veins results in decreased diastolic cardiac size

    (B) Dilation of coronary arterioles reduces resistance and increases coronary flow through ischemic tissue

    (C) Increased sympathetic outflow increases coronary flow

    (D) Dilation of peripheral arterioles increases cardiac work

    (E) Tachycardia increases diastolic coronary flow

14. A drug that is used in angina but causes constipation, edema, and increased cardiac size is

    (A) Diltiazem

    (B) Nitroglycerin

    (C) Isosorbide dinitrate

    (D) Propranolol

    (E) Hydralazine

15. A drug suitable for producing a brief (5- to 15-minute) increase in cardiac vagal tone is

    (A) Pyridostigmine

    (B) Pralidoxime

    (C) Digoxin

    (D) Edrophonium

    (E) Ergotamine

16. Contraindications to the use of oral propranolol include

    (A) Glaucoma

    (B) Migraine

    (C) Benign prostatic hypertrophy

    (D) Asthma

    (E) Hypertension

17. Drugs that block the alpha receptor on effector cells at adrenergic synapses cause

    (A) Reversal of the effects of isoproterenol on the heart rate

    (B) Reversal of the effects of epinephrine on the blood pressure

    (C) Reversal of the effects of epinephrine on adenylyl cyclase

    (D) A decrease in blood glucose levels

    (E) Mydriasis

18. The most accurate description of digitalis' mechanism of action is

    (A) Reduction of the inward sodium gradient results in increased calcium stores in sarcoplasmic reticulum

    (B) Blockade of the sodium pump results in increased calcium entry through calcium channels

    (C) Blockade of potassium transport results in increased intracellular potassium

    (D) Sensitization of actin-myosin filaments to calcium

    (E) Increased inward trigger calcium influx causes increased release of calcium from the sarcoplasmic reticulum

19. Toxicity caused by suicidal digitoxin overdose should be treated by

    (A) Administration of phenytoin IV

    (B) Raising the serum potassium to 7 meq/L

    (C) Lowering serum magnesium

    (D) Administration of digoxin antibodies

    (E) Administration of sodium bicarbonate

20. When treating hypertension, orthostatic hypotension is greatest with

    (A) Hydralazine

    (B) Guanethidine

    (C) Propranolol

    (D) Clonidine

    (E) Methyldopa

21. Valid differences between hydralazine and nitroglycerin include which one of the following?

    (A) Nitroglycerin cannot be given orally

    (B) Hydralazine has a much longer half-life

    (C) Hydralazine causes methemoglobinemia

    (D) Nitroglycerin causes methemoglobinemia

22. Agents that have been shown to protect the upper gastrointestinal tract from ulcer formation include all of the following EXCEPT

    (A) Certain PGE derivatives

    (B) Sucralfate

    (C) Atropine

    (D) Aspirin

    (E) Cimetidine

Items 23–24: A 52-year-old woman is admitted to the emergency room with a history of drug treatment for several conditions. Her serum electrolytes are found to be as follows:

Na^+:	140 meq/L	K^+:	3.0 meq/L
Cl^-:	100 meq/L	pH:	7.50

23. This patient probably has been taking

    (A) Acetazolamide

    (B) Amiloride

    (C) Digoxin

    (D) Furosemide

    (E) Quinidine

24. In view of the electrolyte panel shown (and regardless of its cause), which of the following is MOST correct?
    (A) The patient will be more sensitive to the toxic actions of quinidine
    (B) The patient will be more sensitive to the toxic actions of digoxin
    (C) The patient will be more sensitive to the toxic actions of warfarin
    (D) The patient will be more sensitive to the toxic actions of imipramine
    (E) The patient will be more sensitive to the toxic actions of propranolol

25. A drug that decreases blood pressure by a CNS action is
    (A) Guanethidine
    (B) Trimethaphan
    (C) Nitroprusside
    (D) Prazosin
    (E) Clonidine

26. The most common route of drug entry into cells is
    (A) Uptake by special carrier
    (B) Diffusion through the lipid phase
    (C) Pinocytosis after combining with coated pit receptors
    (D) Aqueous diffusion
    (E) Transport by amino acid carriers

27. Propranolol and hydralazine have which of the following effects in common?
    (A) Tachycardia
    (B) Bradycardia
    (C) Increased vascular resistance
    (D) Decreased mean arterial blood pressure
    (E) Decreased cardiac output

28. A 54-year-old farmer has a 5-year history of frequent, recurrent, and very painful kidney stones. Appropriate chronic therapy for this man is
    (A) Furosemide
    (B) Triamterene
    (C) Spironolactone
    (D) Hydrochlorothiazide
    (E) Morphine

29. The mechanism of action of furosemide is best described as
    (A) Interference with H^+/HCO_3^- exchange
    (B) Blockade of a Na/K/2Cl transporter
    (C) Blockade of a Na/Cl cotransporter
    (D) Blockade of carbonic anhydrase
    (E) Inhibition of genetic expression of DNA in the kidney

30. An 18-year-old patient is admitted to the Emergency Department with a history of depression of 8 months' duration and ingestion 4 hours earlier of a suicidal overdose of his antidepressant medication. He is hypotensive and his ECG is notable for ventricular tachycardia with very broad QRS complexes. The most appropriate therapy for this patient is
    (A) Epinephrine
    (B) $NaHCO_3$
    (C) Atropine
    (D) KCl
    (E) Digoxin

31. All of the following are signs and symptoms of chronic alcohol use EXCEPT
    (A) The Wernicke-Korsakoff syndrome due to thiamine deficiency
    (B) Distal paresthesias
    (C) Salt retention
    (D) Hyperglycemia through increased gluconeogenesis
    (E) Cirrhosis of the liver

32. An individual has ingested an antifreeze solution containing ethylene glycol and comes to a hospital emergency room. All of the following statements about his presentation are accurate EXCEPT
    (A) Metabolic acidosis is likely to occur
    (B) Visual function of the patient will be impaired by flickering white spots "like a snow-storm"

    (C) Ethanol is likely to be administered in management

    (D) Oxalate crystals may be present in the urine

    (E) Dialysis is indicated in the treatment

33. Examine the data in the following table of new anesthetics.

Properties of inhalational anesthetics		
Anesthetic	Blood-Gas Partition Coefficient	Minimal Alveolar Anesthetic Concentration (%)
A	0.8	9.7
B	1.4	1.4
C	9.8	0.6
D	2.3	0.8
E	1.8	1.7

Of the above experimental anesthetics, the agent most likely to have the shortest duration of anesthetic action is

    (A) Anesthetic A

    (B) Anesthetic B

    (C) Anesthetic C

    (D) Anesthetic D

    (E) Anesthetic E

34. This anesthetic agent has been implicated in the rare occurrence of malignant hyperthermia, and it may also sensitize the myocardium to endogenous catecholamines.

    (A) Nitrous oxide

    (B) Midazolam

    (C) Propofol

    (D) Halothane

    (E) Fentanyl

35. Which ONE of the following properties is characteristic of opioid analgesics?

    (A) The ratio of maximal efficacy to addiction liability is a constant

    (B) Tolerance to ocular and gastrointestinal effects develops rapidly during chronic use

    (C) Mixed agonist-antagonists are less effective analgesics than the pure agonist agents in this group

    (D) They have many effects in common with a group of endogenous polypeptides

    (E) All opioid analgesics have good oral bioavailability

36. Naloxone is LEAST likely to be effective in reversing

    (A) Heroin overdose in an addict

    (B) Meperidine analgesia in a cancer patient

    (C) Respiratory depression caused by nalbuphine overdose

    (D) Miosis that occurs during treatment with morphine

    (E) The effects of methadone

37. A patient is brought to an emergency room suffering from an overdose of an illicitly obtained drug. She is agitated, has disordered thought processes, suffers from paranoia, and "hears voices." The drug most likely to be responsible for her condition is

    (A) Heroin

    (B) Ethanol

    (C) Methamphetamine

    (D) Hashish

    (E) Secobarbital

Items 38–39: A woman with long-standing petit mal epilepsy was receiving effective drug therapy for it. However, she developed gastrointestinal problems with nausea and heartburn. The *first* medication was therefore changed to a *second* drug that is also effective, but she is now extremely drowsy at the dose level required for effective seizure control.

38. The *first* drug she was taking was probably

     (A) Diazepam
     (B) Ethosuximide
     (C) Carbamazepine
     (D) Phenytoin
     (E) Valproic acid

39. The *second* drug she received (the one that caused drowsiness) is
     (A) Clonazepam
     (B) Carbamazepine
     (C) Phenobarbital
     (D) Acetazolamide
     (E) Phenytoin

40. All of the following statements concerning the actions of drugs used to treat severe depressive disorders are accurate EXCEPT
     (A) Imipramine blocks reuptake of both norepinephrine and serotonin
     (B) Fluoxetine is a selective serotonin reuptake inhibitor
     (C) Tranylcypromine is a selective inhibitor of monoamine oxidase type B
     (D) Amoxapine appears to block dopamine receptors
     (E) Both amitriptyline and doxepin are antagonists at muscarinic receptors

41. Following the ingestion of a meal that included sardines, cheese, and red wine, a patient under treatment for depression experiences a hypertensive crisis. The antidepressant drug most likely to be responsible is
     (A) Imipramine
     (B) Fluoxetine
     (C) Isocarboxazid
     (D) Selegiline
     (E) Bupropion

Items 42–43: A woman taking antipsychotic medication develops a spectrum of adverse effects that include akathisia, dystonias, hyperprolactinemia, muscle rigidity, and tremor at rest. After several months, her medication is changed to a drug less likely to cause these problems.

42. All of the following statements about the adverse effects are accurate EXCEPT
     (A) They may be reduced if the drug dose is lowered
     (B) They all result from dopamine receptor blockade
     (C) Most of them will be alleviated by treatment with benztropine
     (D) All of them will be alleviated by treatment with levodopa
     (E) The patient is more likely to be taking haloperidol than thioridazine

43. Regular weekly blood counts are ordered for this patient when she starts her new medication. The new drug is probably
     (A) Lithium
     (B) Molindone
     (C) Clozapine
     (D) Thioridazine
     (E) Chlorpromazine

44. An effective dosage regimen of lithium has been established by monitoring the plasma levels of the drug in a 48-year-old musician. This man's plasma levels of lithium are likely to be elevated in all of the following situations EXCEPT
     (A) Restriction of sodium chloride intake
     (B) The concomitant use of thiazide diuretics
     (C) Development of ascites
     (D) The use of NSAIDs
     (E) Severe dehydration

45. Established clinical uses of benzodiazepines include all of the following EXCEPT
     (A) Treatment of a sleep disorder in an elderly patient
     (B) Use as a component of a balanced anesthesia protocol
     (C) Management of the alcohol withdrawal syndrome
     (D) Treatment of enuresis
     (E) Initial management of the behavioral toxicity of phencyclidine

46. All of the following statements about the use of carbidopa with levodopa are accurate EXCEPT

(A) Carbidopa inhibits DOPA decarboxylase
(B) Lower doses of levodopa can be used in the treatment of parkinsonism
(C) Peripheral side effects are reduced when the drugs are used in combination
(D) Carbidopa does not cross the blood-brain barrier
(E) There is a decreased incidence of CNS side effects when the drugs are used together

47. This neurotransmitter, which is located in neurons of hierarchical neuronal systems in the brain, is inhibitory to postsynaptic neurons via an increase in chloride ion conductance.
(A) Acetylcholine
(B) Dopamine
(C) GABA
(D) Glutamic acid
(E) Serotonin

48. Which ONE of the following drugs is LEAST likely to be effective in alleviating withdrawal symptoms in a patient physically dependent on a barbiturate?
(A) Buspirone
(B) Chloral hydrate
(C) Diazepam
(D) Meprobamate
(E) Phenobarbital

49. All of the following statements about the aminoglycoside antibiotics are accurate EXCEPT
(A) In terms of their levels in the blood, the drugs have a narrow therapeutic window
(B) Aminoglycosides interfere with bacterial protein synthesis by inhibiting peptidyl transferase
(C) Although ototoxicity may occur, it is not the most common adverse effect
(D) Synergistic effects may be achieved when aminoglycosides are used with penicillins in the treatment of enterococcal infections
(E) The drugs are polar compounds that are eliminated mainly by renal glomerular filtration

Items 50–51: A young man comes to a community clinic with a urogenital infection that, based on gram stain, appears to be due to gonococcus. The physician is also concerned about the possibility of non-gonococcal urethritis in this patient. He notes that the patient had an anaphylactic reaction to ampicillin plus sulbactam a few months earlier.

50. The physician would like to treat the gonococcal infection and cover for nongonococcal urethritis with a *single drug*. Which ONE of the following agents should be used in this patient?
(A) Metronidazole
(B) Ciprofloxacin
(C) Procaine penicillin G
(D) Spectinomycin
(E) Tetracycline

51. Which ONE of the following agents is likely to be effective (and safe in this patient) if the physician attempts to treat an associated urogenital infection due to *C trachomatis* by giving a *single dose* of a drug?
(A) Azithromycin
(B) Doxycycline
(C) Ceftriaxone
(D) Trimethoprim-sulfamethoxazole
(E) Spectinomycin

52. All of the following statements about the penicillin group of antibiotics are accurate EXCEPT
(A) They are inhibitors of bacterial transpeptidases involved in the cross-linking of linear peptidoglycans
(B) In the case of most penicillins, urinary drug levels are considerably higher than those in the plasma
(C) Use of methicillin is associated with the development of an allergic-based nephritis
(D) Amoxicillin is not effective against organisms that produce penicillinases
(E) The incidence of cross-allergenicity between penicillins and cephalosporins is greater than 30%

Items 53–54: A 52-year-old insurance agent receiving chemotherapy for leukemia is given intramuscular cefazolin (500 mg) for treatment of pneumococcal pneumonia. Within a few minutes, he is wheezing, he develops an urticarial rash, and his systolic blood pressure falls markedly. The patient recovers following the administration of epinephrine, dexamethasone, and fluids.

53. Which ONE of the following statements regarding the use of cefazolin in this case is MOST accurate?
    (A) A first-generation cephalosporin should not be used in a patient who is likely to be immunosuppressed
    (B) The reaction could have been avoided with a lower dose of the drug
    (C) Erythromycin is a more appropriate drug to use in an immunosuppressed patient
    (D) It would have been preferable to use oral ampicillin in this patient
    (E) Penicillin G is usually considered to be the drug of choice for pneumococcal pneumonia

54. Regarding the drug reaction in this case, all of the following statements are accurate EXCEPT
    (A) It was a type I allergic reaction
    (B) Reactions of this type are more frequent after use of the penicillins than with the cephalosporins
    (C) Skin testing with a dilute solution of cefazolin is routinely used to detect hypersensitivity
    (D) The reaction was IgE mediated
    (E) It is likely that the reaction would have been less severe if a test dose (50 mg) of cefazolin was administered initially

55. All of the following statements about the macrolide group of antibiotics are accurate EXCEPT
    (A) They inhibit translocase reactions in bacterial protein synthesis
    (B) Organisms sensitive to erythromycin include gram-positive cocci, *Mycoplasma,* and *Chlamydia*
    (C) The ability of erythromycin to stimulate the activity of hepatic drug-metabolizing enzymes has led to drug interactions
    (D) Clarithromycin has activity against *M avium-intracellulare*
    (E) Cholestatic hepatitis that may occur with the use of erythromycin is age-dependent

56. All of the following statements about the tetracycline group of antibiotics are accurate EXCEPT
    (A) Oral or vaginal candidiasis may occur during the use of tetracyclines
    (B) Tetracyclines block the attachment of aminoacyl-tRNA to the bacterial ribosome
    (C) The intracellular accumulation of tetracyclines in resistant bacterial strains is less than that in sensitive organisms
    (D) A high incidence of kernicterus precludes the use of tetracyclines in the neonate
    (E) Oral absorption of tetracyclines may be decreased by milk products

57. All of the following statements about the fluoroquinolone group of antibiotics are accurate EXCEPT
    (A) Their antibacterial spectrum includes common pathogens of the urogenital system and the gastrointestinal tract
    (B) They are inhibitors of DNA-dependent RNA polymerase
    (C) Resistance may occur though decreases in bacterial accumulation of the drugs
    (D) Their renal elimination is decreased by probenecid
    (E) Animal studies have shown that fluoroquinolones may interfere with collagen metabolism

58. Regarding trimethoprim-sulfamethoxazole (TMP-SMZ), all of the following statements are accurate EXCEPT
    (A) TMP-SMZ is bactericidal against some susceptible organisms
    (B) Synergistic actions may occur through sequential blockade of folic acid synthesis
    (C) Since TMP-SMZ has activity against pneumococci, *H influenzae*, and *M catarrhalis*, it is commonly used for respiratory tract infections
    (D) The trimethoprim component of TMP-SMZ is responsible for the enhanced hypoglycemia seen with the sulfonylureas used in diabetes
    (E) The administration of folinic acid will reduce hematologic side effects of TMP-SMZ

Items 59–60: A patient with diffuse non-Hodgkin's lymphoma is treated with a combination drug regimen that includes cyclophosphamide, vincristine, doxorubicin, and prednisone

59. The drugs used in this patient are likely to cause all of the following adverse effects EXCEPT
    (A) Myelosuppression
    (B) Pulmonary fibrosis

    (C) Cardiotoxicity
    (D) Peripheral neuropathy
    (E) Osteoporosis

60. Which of the drugs employed in this case is cell cycle-specific?
    (A) Cyclophosphamide
    (B) Doxorubicin
    (C) Prednisone
    (D) Vincristine
    (E) None of the above

61. This drug is active against common bacterial pathogens that cause meningitis, is effective in typhoid fever, and has activity against anaerobic gram-negative bacilli. However, it is usually considered to be a "back-up drug" because of its potential hematotoxicity.
    (A) Tobramycin
    (B) Clindamycin
    (C) Chloramphenicol
    (D) Imipenem
    (E) Tetracycline

62. All of the following statements about the toxic effects of antifungal drugs are accurate EXCEPT
    (A) Nephrotoxicity due to amphotericin B is dose-limiting
    (B) If given orally, nystatin causes severe ototoxicity
    (C) Ketoconazole may impair the adrenocortical response to stress
    (D) The most characteristic toxicity of flucytosine is myelosuppression
    (E) Griseofulvin is mutagenic in animals

63. All of the following statements about the clinical use of acyclovir are accurate EXCEPT
    (A) The drug is not effective in infections caused by herpes virus that is deficient in thymidine kinase
    (B) In dehydrated patients crystalluria may occur
    (C) Acyclovir enhances the hematotoxicity of other antiviral agents
    (D) Topical administration of the drug in herpes labialis is ineffective
    (E) The drug is secreted in breast milk

64. This antiparasitic drug is activated to toxic intermediates by the pyruvate-ferredoxin oxido-reductase enzyme system that is present in anaerobes.
    (A) Metronidazole
    (B) Pyrimethamine
    (C) Chloroquine
    (D) Emetine
    (E) Quinine

65. Praziquantel is the drug of choice for *Schistosoma* spp. Its mechanism of action involves
    (A) Inhibition of microtubule synthesis
    (B) Muscle contraction and paralysis via increased Ca^{2+} entry
    (C) Stimulation of the inhibitory effects of GABA
    (D) Inhibition of thiamine uptake
    (E) Activation of nicotinic receptors

66. This anticancer drug is a component of regimens effective in testicular carcinoma. Its distinctive toxicity includes hyperkeratosis, fever with dehydration, pulmonary dysfunction, and anaphylactoid reactions.
    (A) Dactinomycin
    (B) Vinblastine
    (C) Cyclophosphamide
    (D) Bleomycin
    (E) Mercaptopurine

67. All of the following statements about cyclosporine are accurate EXCEPT
    (A) The drug is an effective immunosuppressant in organ and bone marrow transplantations
    (B) Cyclosporine interferes with the action of a T cell transcription factor involved in leukotriene synthesis
    (C) Myelosuppression is dose-limiting
    (D) Cyclosporine is a lipophilic peptide antibiotic
    (E) Nephrotoxicity may be reduced by mannitol diuresis

68. This agent is used commonly for passive immunization (eg, in hepatitis A, hypogammaglobulinemia, and measles)

(A) Lymphocytic immune globulin
(B) BCG vaccine
(C) $Rh_o(D)$ immune globulin
(D) DTP
(E) Human immune globulin

69. Which ONE of the following chemicals is likely to lead to delayed respiratory distress and
pulmonary fibrosis?

(A) Sulfur dioxide
(B) Parathion
(C) Carbon tetrachloride
(D) Paraquat
(E) Ozone

70. Penicillamine has effectiveness in all of the following clinical situations EXCEPT

(A) Wilson's disease
(B) Chronic mercury poisoning
(C) Poisoning due to inorganic arsenic
(D) Acute organic lead poisoning
(E) Rheumatoid arthritis

71. All of the following signs and symptoms are characteristic of poisoning due to ingestion of
the mushroom species *Amanita muscaria* EXCEPT

(A) Hyperthermia with hot dry skin
(B) Decreased bowel sounds
(C) Delayed hepatic and renal failure
(D) Mydriasis
(E) Delirium and hallucinations

72. All of the following signs and symptoms are characteristic of overdosage of tricyclic antidepressants EXCEPT

(A) Hypotension
(B) Increased bowel sounds
(C) Coma
(D) Widening of the QRS complex on the ECG
(E) Seizures

73. All of the following are vasodilator peptides EXCEPT

(A) Atrionatriuretic factor (ANF)
(B) Calcitonin gene-related peptide
(C) Substance P
(D) Vasoactive intestinal peptide
(E) Endothelin

74. Cyclooxygenase I and II are responsible for

(A) The synthesis of prostaglandins from arachidonate
(B) The synthesis of leukotrienes from arachidonate
(C) The synthesis of cyclic AMP
(D) The metabolic degradation of cyclic AMP
(E) The conversion of GTP to cGMP

75. Bronchodilators include all of the following EXCEPT

(A) Albuterol
(B) Ipratropium
(C) Metaproterenol
(D) Nedocromil
(E) Theophylline

76. Toxicities of theophylline in asthma include all of the following EXCEPT

(A) Tachycardia
(B) Tremor
(C) Hypertension
(D) Insomnia
(E) Convulsions

77. Local anesthetic toxicities include all of the following EXCEPT

(A) Cardiovascular arrhythmias and collapse (bupivacaine)
(B) Convulsions (lidocaine)
(C) Methemoglobinemia (prilocaine)
(D) Hypertensive emergencies, strokes (procaine)

78. Muscle spasm of cerebral palsy can be effectively treated with all of the following EXCEPT
    (A) Cyclobenzaprine
    (B) Dantrolene
    (C) Baclofen
    (D) Diazepam

79. A patient undergoing surgery is given a neuromuscular blocker. The anesthesiologist notes a marked drop in blood pressure and an increase in airway resistance immediately after the injection. Intravenous administration of diphenhydramine quickly restores the patient's blood pressure and airway diameter. The neuromuscular blocker used was probably
    (A) Atracurium
    (B) Tubocurarine
    (C) Succinylcholine
    (D) Pancuronium
    (E) Vecuronium

80. Which of the following drugs is correctly associated with its clinical application?
    (A) Erythropoietin: macrocytic anemia
    (B) Filgrastim: leukopenia due to cancer chemotherapy
    (C) Iron dextran: severe macrocytic anemia
    (D) Ferrous sulfate: hemochromatosis
    (E) Folic acid: microcytic anemia of pregnancy

DIRECTIONS: The following section consists of lists of lettered options followed by several numbered items. For each numbered item, select the ONE option that is most closely associated with it. Each answer may be used once, more than once, or not at all.

Items 81–84:

(A) Triazolam	(J) Selegiline	(S) Thioridazine
(B) Morphine	(K) Alprazolam	(T) Naloxone
(C) Bromocriptine	(L) Mescaline	(U) Midazolam
(D) Chlorpromazine	(M) Isoflurane	(V) Dronabinol
(E) Valproic acid	(N) Phenytoin	(W) Benztropine
(F) Amitriptyline	(O) Phenobarbital	(X) Ethosuximide
(G) Phenelzine	(P) Fluoxetine	(Y) Lithium
(H) Ketamine	(Q) Levodopa	(Z) Nalbuphine
(I) Methadone	(R) Carbamazepine	

81. In overdosage, the urinary clearance of this antiepileptic drug can be accelerated by urinary alkalinization

82. The actions of this drug on the central nervous system, plus its effects on peripheral hemodynamics, are responsible for its usefulness—in the past—in the management of patients with pulmonary edema

83. This drug activates kappa (κ) opioid receptors and is an antagonist at mu (μ) opioid receptors

84. The actions of this drug on the central nervous system are enhanced if it is used with an inhibitor of peripheral L-aromatic amino acid decarboxylase

Items 85–88:

(A) Ampicillin	(J) Busulfan	(S) Quinine
(B) Doxycycline	(K) Neomycin	(T) Bleomycin
(C) Isoniazid	(L) Cyclosporine	(U) Azathioprine
(D) Sulfasalazine	(M) Praziquantel	(V) Sulfadiazine
(E) Vidarabine	(N) Chloroquine	(W) Ethambutol
(F) Imipenem	(O) Erythromycin	(X) Zidovudine
(G) Amphotericin B	(P) Trimethoprim	(Y) Foscarnet
(H) Acyclovir	(Q) Clarithromycin	(Z) Metronidazole
(I) Methotrexate	(R) Ganciclovir	

85. Bacterial dihydrofolate reductases may be as much as 10^4 times more sensitive to inhibition by this drug than mammalian forms of the enzyme
86. This polyene antibiotic is given intravenously and causes "shake and bake" chills and fever, electrolyte imbalance, and nephrotoxicity
87. Adverse effects of this antiprotozoal drug include flushed sweaty skin, tinnitus, impaired vision and hearing, gastrointestinal upset, and disturbances in cardiac rhythm and conduction
88. Of the antiviral drugs listed, this agent is LEAST likely to cause myelosuppression

Items 89–91:
   - (A) Diphenhydramine
   - (B) Ergotamine tartrate
   - (C) Terfenadine
   - (D) Cimetidine
   - (E) Ranitidine
89. A drug with significant efficacy against motion sickness
90. A drug that decreases gastric acid secretion and has antiandrogenic effects
91. A drug with partial agonist effects at serotonin receptors and alpha receptors

Items 92–95:
   - (A) Quinidine
   - (B) Digoxin
   - (C) Verapamil
   - (D) Lidocaine
   - (E) Propranolol
92. A drug that predictably prolongs the PR interval and increases cardiac contractility
93. A drug that is useful in supraventricular tachycardias and angina pectoris and is not contraindicated in asthma
94. A drug that is useful in ventricular and atrial arrhythmias and may cause tinnitus
95. A drug that is very useful in early post-myocardial infarction ventricular arrhythmias but not very effective in atrial arrhythmias

Items 96-98:
   - (A) Neostigmine
   - (B) Nicotine
   - (C) Bethanechol
   - (D) Acetylcholine
   - (E) Malathion
96. Converted to active form by substitution of oxygen for sulfur; rapidly detoxified in mammals
97. Direct-acting muscarinic agonist with minimal susceptibility to cholinesterase
98. Cholinoceptor agonist that causes vasoconstriction

Items 99–102:
   - (A) Warfarin
   - (B) Heparin
   - (C) Alteplase
   - (D) Ticlopidine
   - (E) Aspirin
99. A drug that acts immediately in vitro to prevent blood from clotting
100. This drug is manufactured by recombinant DNA technology and must be used in the first few hours after a myocardial infarction
101. A new drug that prevents platelet aggregation without altering prostaglandin synthesis
102. The anticoagulant of choice in pregnant women

Items 103–106:
   - (A) Aspirin
   - (B) Ibuprofen
   - (C) Gold salts
   - (D) Indomethacin
   - (E) Methotrexate
   - (F) Penicillamine
   - (G) Misoprostol

103. Used exclusively in rheumatoid arthritis; has a very slow onset of action (months); efficacy is disputed
104. Used in all forms of arthritis except gouty arthritis; onset of maximum effect is hours to days, but GI toxicity is limiting
105. A drug used in cancer chemotherapy and in rheumatoid arthritis
106. Nonsteroidal anti-inflammatory drug with less GI toxicity and short duration of action; good efficacy in dysmenorrhea

Items 107–112:

(A)	Potassium iodide solution	**(F)**	Ultralente insulin
(B)	Triiodothyronine	**(G)**	Mestranol
(C)	Thyroxine	**(H)**	Norgestrel
(D)	Propylthiouracil	**(I)**	Danazol
(E)	Ipodate	**(J)**	Norethindrone

107. Drug of choice for maintenance therapy of hypothyroid patients
108. Blocks the synthesis of thyroid hormone by preventing coupling of iodotyrosine molecules; agranulocytosis is a rare toxicity
109. Inhibits iodination of tyrosine in the thyroid gland; also reduces size and vascularity of a hyperplastic thyroid gland
110. A partial agonist progestin and androgen; used in endometriosis
111. Major application is as a progestin in oral contraceptives
112. Major application is in the treatment of thyroid storm (severe thyrotoxicosis)

Items 113–115:

(A)	Angiotensin	**(F)**	Isoproterenol
(B)	Endothelin	**(G)**	Norepinephrine
(C)	Epinephrine	**(H)**	Phenylephrine
(D)	Guanethidine	**(I)**	Prazosin
(E)	Hexamethonium	**(J)**	Propranolol

113. A drug was given as an IV bolus to an anesthetized subject while the blood pressure was recorded. The changes in systolic and diastolic pressures in response to the injection of Drug X are shown in the graph below. Identify drug X from the above list.

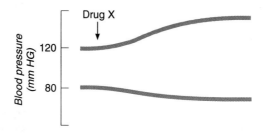

114–115. A drug **(Drug 1)** was given as an IV bolus to another anesthetized subject while blood pressure (color) and heart rate were recorded as shown on the left side of the graph below. After recovery from the effects of Drug 1, a long-acting dose of **Drug 2** was given. After the recorder was turned back on, Drug 1 was repeated with the results shown on the right side of the graph.

114. Identify Drug 1 from the above list.
115. Identify Drug 2 from the above list.

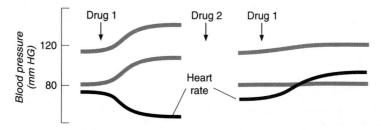

Answer Key for Examination II[1].

1. C	(7)		**57.** B	(50)
2. E	(1)		**58.** D	(47)
3. E	(1)		**59.** B	(56)
4. B	(2)		**60.** D	(56)
5. B	(3)		**61.** C	(44)
6. E	(5)		**62.** B	(48)
7. A	(6, 8, 9)		**63.** C	(49)
8. B	(6)		**64.** A	(53, 54)
9. E	(10)		**65.** B	(53, 55)
10. B	(8)		**66.** D	(56)
11. A	(9)		**67.** C	(57)
12. E	(11)		**68.** E	(57)
13. A	(12)		**69.** D	(58, 60)
14. A	(12)		**70.** D	(59, 60)
15. D	(8)		**71.** C	(60)
16. D	(10)		**72.** B	(29, 60)
17. B	(10)		**73.** E	(17)
18. A	(13)		**74.** A	(18)
19. D	(13)		**75.** D	(19)
20. B	(11)		**76.** C	(19)
21. B	(11, 12)		**77.** D	(25)
22. D	(35, 61)		**78.** A	(25)
23. D	(15)		**79.** B	(26)
24. B	(13)		**80.** B	(32)
25. E	(11)		**81.** O	(3, 21, 60)
26. B	(1, 3)		**82.** B	(30)
27. D	(10, 11)		**83.** Z	(30)
28. D	(15)		**84.** Q	(27)
29. B	(15)		**85.** P	(42, 47)
30. B	(14, 29)		**86.** G	(48)
31. D	(22)		**87.** S	(54)
32. B	(22, 60)		**88.** H	(49)
33. A	(24)		**89.** A	(16)
34. D	(24)		**90.** D	(16)
35. D	(30)		**91.** B	(16)
36. C	(30)		**92.** B	(13)
37. C	(31)		**93.** C	(12)
38. B	(23)		**94.** A	(14)
39. A	(23)		**95.** D	(14)
40. C	(29)		**96.** E	(7)
41. C	(29)		**97.** C	(7)
42. D	(27, 28)		**98.** B	(7)
43. C	(28)		**99.** B	(33)
44. C	(28)		**100.** C	(33)
45. D	(21)		**101.** D	(33)
46. E	(27)		**102.** B	(33)
47. C	(20)		**103.** C	(35)
48. A	(21)		**104.** A	(35)
49. B	(45)		**105.** E	(35, 56)
50. E	(44)		**106.** B	(35)
51. A	(50)		**107.** C	(37)
52. E	(43)		**108.** D	(37)
53. E	(43)		**109.** A	(37)
54. C	(57)		**110.** I	(39)
55. C	(50)		**111.** H	(39)
56. D	(44)		**112.** E	(37)
			113. C	(6, 9, 10)
			114. G	(6, 9, 10)
			115. I	(6, 9, 10)

[1] Numbers in parentheses are chapters in which answers may be found.

Appendix IV

Case Histories

This Appendix contains case histories that illustrate selected aspects of pharmacologic management of clinical problems.* Each case is followed by general self-evaluation questions. Answers will be found at the end of Appendix IV.

Note: Ranges of numbers in parentheses or brackets are the ranges of normal values at the institution where the patient was studied.

CASE 1. THE GARDENER†

A 55-year-old man was found unconscious by his wife in the greenhouse behind their home. During the past week, he had been complaining of abdominal discomfort and frequent stools. His medical history consisted of mild hypertension controlled by salt restriction (about 5 years) and non-insulin-dependent diabetes controlled by diet (about 10 years). He had no history of mental illness or of alcohol or tobacco use, and he was not taking any medication. His last trip outside the country had been to Mexico 5 years earlier. He and his wife operated a small flower shop, and he was an enthusiastic home gardener.

Upon arrival at the emergency room, the patient was unconscious, salivating profusely, and breathing shallowly. His skin was warm and moist. Blood pressure was 140/90 mm Hg, pulse 72/min and regular, respirations 30/min, and temperature normal. There was no evidence of trauma. Both pupils were constricted and did not respond to light. Auscultation of the chest revealed moderate wheezing and numerous rhonchi. The heart was normal. Examination of the abdomen revealed no abnormalities other than hyperactive bowel sounds. The extremities showed subcutaneous muscle fasciculations at the time of admission. These disappeared during the course of the examination, but muscle tone decreased and breathing became shallower during this time. The neurologic examination revealed coma with no response to painful stimuli, no localizing signs, and no abnormal reflexes.

Questions, Case 1
1. What are the possible toxicologic causes of the patient's signs and symptoms?
2. What immediate steps must be taken?
3. What drugs may be considered for the treatment of this patient? What are the risks and benefits of their use?

CASE 2. THE SUICIDAL CARDIAC PATIENT‡

A 39-year-old man with a long-standing history of mitral stenosis had ingested 90 digoxin tablets (0.25 mg each) in a suicide attempt approximately 2 hours before admission. Upon admission, the

---

* These case histories are *not* meant to typify the "clinical vignette" questions found in Step I of the USMLE examination. (Such questions are to be found at the end of each chapter.) Rather, the cases in this Appendix can be used to test one's preparation for pharmacologic questions that occur in Steps 2 and 3 of the USMLE.

† Modified and reproduced, with permission, from Goldfrank L, Kirstein R: SLUD. Hosp Physician 1976;12:20.

‡ Modified and reproduced, with permission, from Smith TW et al: Reversal of advanced digoxin intoxication with Fab fragments of digoxin-specific antibodies. N Engl J Med 1976;294:797.

blood pressure was 110/70 mm Hg, and pulse 40–60/min and irregular. The rest of the examination was normal.

Initial laboratory data included a blood ethanol of 190 mg/dL, but electrolytes were normal. An electrocardiogram revealed atrial fibrillation with a high degree of atrioventricular block and periods of atrioventricular junctional and atrial tachycardias. Ventricular rate did not exceed 50/min. Atropine had no effect on ventricular rate; therefore, a transvenous pacing catheter was inserted, with ventricular pacing instituted at 60/min.

During the next 8 hours, the spontaneous ventricular rate progressively decreased to 33 and then to 13/min. No atrial activity could be detected on the ECG. The QRS duration reached a maximum of 0.33 s (0.08—0.1). Serum potassium increased to 8.7 meq/L (3.5–5). An antidote was administered. The patient made a complete recovery from this episode of poisoning.

Questions, Case 2

1. Assuming 70% bioavailability and a volume of distribution of 440 L, what is the maximum predicted serum concentration?
2. What was the cause and the primary source of the elevated serum potassium?
3. Describe the probable basis for the cardiac rhythm and electrocardiographic abnormalities.
4. Outline the conventional therapy for less severe digitalis intoxication, and explain why it was not used in this case. What antidote was used?
5. What treatment is available for severe intoxication with digitoxin?

CASE 3.   A SEED EATER*

A 15-year-old boy was brought to the emergency room by the police because he "had a flushed face and was acting crazy." He had been found nude, incoherent, and wandering about aimlessly.

Physical examination showed blood pressure 170/100 mm Hg, respirations 44/min, and pulse 144/min. He was comatose, unresponsive to verbal stimuli, and minimally responsive to deep painful stimuli. Occasional decerebrate posturing was noted. The skin was flushed, dry, and hot to the touch. The pupils were widely dilated and equal, with a minimal response to light. Rectal temperature was 39.8 °C.

At this time, physostigmine salicylate, 2 mg, was given intravenously under electrocardiographic, electroencephalographic, and temperature monitoring. Within 15 minutes, the rectal temperature had fallen to 38.8 °C, while blood pressure, respirations, and pulse were 160/68 mm Hg, 40/min, and 112/min, respectively. The patient became more alert and responsive to verbal commands but remained agitated. When questioned about ingestion of a toxic agent, the patient said that he had eaten "loco seeds," small black seeds of a weed that grew freely in the area. Remote memory was intact, but recent memory was grossly impaired.

Six hours later, the rectal temperature was 37 °C, and other vital signs were stable. The patient was talking spontaneously in a rapid and garbled manner. Although completely oriented, he continued to speak of imaginary objects and voices.

The patient improved rapidly and was discharged on the eighth hospital day without neurologic deficit.

Questions, Case 3

1. What drug or drug group do "loco seeds" contain?
2. What is the most life-threatening effect of the intoxicant in this case?
3. What are the dangers of physostigmine therapy? What are the risks of other treatments?

CASE 4.   IATROGENIC SHOCK†

A 61-year-old patient had suffered from severe chronic asthmatic bronchitis with episodes of respiratory failure in the past and was admitted on this occasion with bronchopneumonia. In spite of therapy with antibiotics and bronchodilators, he deteriorated and became confused. His arterial blood pH

---

* Modified and reproduced, with permission, from Mikolich JR, Paulson GW, Cross CJ: Acute anticholinergic syndrome due to Jimson seed ingestion: Clinical and laboratory observation in six cases. Ann Intern Med 1975;83:231.

† Modified and reproduced, with permission, from Spoerel WE, Seleny FL, Williamson RD: Shock caused by continuous infusion of metaraminol bitartrate (Aramine). Can Med Assoc J 1964;90:349.

was 7.29 (7.35–7.45), and the P_{CO_2} was 73 mm Hg (35–45). A tracheostomy was performed under general anesthesia, and he was admitted to the intensive care unit.

Thirty minutes later, his pH was 7.41 and his P_{CO_2} was 59 mm Hg, but his O_2 saturation remained very low (64% [94–100]). Intermittent positive-pressure breathing was begun, and his condition transiently improved. Two hours later, however, his systolic blood pressure had fallen to 60 mm Hg, and an infusion of metaraminol (a vasoconstrictor sympathomimetic drug) was started. His blood pressure rose, and the heart rate promptly decreased from 120 to 75/min. During the next 36 hours, he received an average of 7 mg of metaraminol per hour, but he steadily developed the manifestations of shock, with a falling urine output. His heart rate gradually increased to 90/min. An attempt to overcome these changes by increasing the dosage of metaraminol (up to 50 mg/h) did not influence the progressive deterioration. He had cold extremities and peripheral cyanosis in spite of adequate respiratory exchange on 100% oxygen. His arterial hematocrit was markedly elevated to 70% (40–52).

In an attempt to correct the severe hemoconcentration, the patient was given 1500 mL of dextran solution over the next 18 hours, and the blood pressure was maintained with norepinephrine infusion. With this treatment, his urine output rose, his extremities became warmer, and his color improved. His blood pressure was stable for about 48 hours, requiring only occasional support with norepinephrine in small doses. Two days after initiation of this treatment, his hematocrit was 47%.

Questions, Case 4
1. What is the mechanism by which metaraminol reduced the heart rate?
2. Why did the patient's hematocrit rise?
3. What was the cause of the patient's deteriorating renal function, cold extremities, and cyanosis?
4. What were the effects of the dextran infusion and of the norepinephrine infusion in improving the patient's condition?

CASE 5.   AN ASTHMATIC BUSINESSWOMAN*

A businesswoman with a history of mild asthmatic attacks had onset of symptoms of bronchoconstriction in a restaurant during a business luncheon. Repeated self-administration of a drug from an inhaler did not provide relief, and symptoms progressed until she became cyanotic. Paramedics were called, and they administered a subcutaneous drug upon arrival. She was admitted to the hospital emergency room in severe respiratory distress. Her pulse was 100/min, respiratory rate 32/min, and blood pressure 140/90 mm Hg. Severe wheezing was audible.

After this evaluation, she was given another dose of the subcutaneous medication that had been previously administered by the paramedics. Fifteen minutes later, her symptoms had decreased markedly, but she still had respiratory wheezing. Use of a bronchodilator administered by hand-held nebulizer abolished the wheezing, and she was discharged 3 hours later.

Questions, Case 5
1. What are the probable mediators of the bronchoconstriction evidenced in this woman's asthmatic attack?
2. What medications are commonly used for the outpatient treatment of mild and moderate asthma?
3. What drug was administered subcutaneously by the paramedics and later in the emergency room? Which agents are suitable for nebulizer use?

CASE 6.   ERGOTAMINE TOXICITY†

A 44-year-old woman with a history of moderate intake of ergotamine for migraine was admitted to hospital because of 3 days of increasingly cold and painful legs. Upon examination, the legs were

---

* Modified and reproduced, with permission, from Simon RA: Management of severe asthma in relapse: Case discussion. Chap 28, p 241 in: *The Practical Management of Asthma.* Dawson A, Simon RA (editors). Grune & Stratton, 1984.

† Modified and reproduced, with permission, from Christensen KN et al: Sodium nitroprusside and epidural blockade in the treatment of ergotism. N Engl J Med 1977;296:1271.

found to be cyanotic and cold, with no detectable pulses distal to the femoral arteries. Transfemoral aortography showed normal aortic and pelvic vessels. However, the external iliac and femoral arteries were severely constricted, as were the smaller arteries of both legs.

A continuous epidural blockade with bupivacaine was started, but it had no effect. A continuous infusion of nitroprusside was then begun, starting at 25 mcg/min and increasing by 25 mcg/min every 15 minutes. When the infusion rate reached 100 mcg/min, the skin temperature of the great toe suddenly rose from 21.8 to 31.0 °C, the cyanosis cleared, and a normal pulse was felt in the peripheral vessels. Over a period of several hours, the skin temperature of the toe rose to 36 °C. Thirty-six hours after admission, the infusion could be withdrawn without recurrence of vasoconstriction.

Questions, Case 6
1. What is the mechanism of ergot-induced vasospasm?
2. What is the safe limit of ergot consumption?
3. What is the mechanism of action of nitroprusside?
4. What medications should this patient receive to reduce her dependence on ergotamine for migraine relief?

CASE 7. ABSENCE SEIZURES*

An 18-year-old woman was admitted for evaluation of therapy for frequent epileptic absence attacks associated with minor automatisms. The patient had a history of unsuccessful treatment with ethosuximide. The electroencephalograph showed generalized 3/s spike-and-wave complexes and intermittent left temporal discharges.

Therapy was restarted using sodium valproate, carbamazepine, and primidone. A 24-hour electroencephalographic study revealed 71 absence attacks. Increasing the valproate dosage from 1200 to 2400 mg/d was associated with a significant but transient decline in absence frequency. Serum levels of valproic acid at that time were 81 mg/L mean, 109 mg/L maximum, and 36 mg/L minimum on a twice-daily dosage regimen. Carbamazepine and primidone were slowly withdrawn with no change in the number of clinical or electroencephalographic attacks. Addition of ethosuximide, 1000 mg/d, resulted in disappearance of all seizure activity. Mean serum ethosuximide level was 70 mg/L.

Six months later, an attempt was made to reduce the dosage of valproate. On a twice-daily dose of 300 mg (600 mg/d total), serum levels dropped to 34 mg/L mean, 57 mg/L maximum, and 23 mg/L minimum. There was a prompt recurrence of seizures, but they declined again when valproate dosage was returned to 2400 mg/d. A follow-up study 8 months later demonstrated a continuing favorable response.

Questions, Case 7
1. Why were carbamazepine and primidone used at the beginning of the study?
2. Why were blood levels of the drugs measured several times during the day?
3. What are the hazards of therapy with ethosuximide? With sodium valproate?

CASE 8. THE TIRED PATIENT†

A 37-year-old man visited the outpatient clinic with a chief complaint of chronic tiredness. He reported that over the previous 6 months he had experienced frequent bouts of stomach upset, a weight loss of 5 kg, and occasional headaches.

Physical examination and laboratory studies were within normal limits. A complete history revealed that he had come to the clinic at the request of his wife. He reported having early morning insomnia, loss of appetite, loss of interest in his work, and difficulty in remembering details related to his job. He also admitted a loss of interest in sex.

A diagnosis of major depression was made. Amitriptyline, 50 mg, was prescribed, to be taken at bedtime daily for 3 nights, followed by 100 mg daily thereafter, also taken at bedtime.

---

* Modified and reproduced, with permission, from Rowan AJ et al: Valproate-ethosuximide combination therapy for refractory absence seizures. Arch Neurol 1983;40:797.

† Modified and reproduced, with permission, from Coleman JH, Johnston JA: Affective disorders. Page 1021 in: *Applied Therapeutics,* 3rd ed. Katcher BS, Young LY, Koda-Kimble MA (editors). Applied Therapeutics, 1983.

Two weeks later, a blood sample was taken to determine the plasma amitriptyline level. An interview at that time indicated that the patient was sleeping better, but that his memory and appetite remained poor. The blood level was reported to be 100 ng/mL. The dose of drug was increased to 150 mg/d.

Two weeks later (5 weeks after the initial visit) the patient was feeling much better, with improved interest in his job, family life, and food. He had regained most of his lost weight and no longer had insomnia.

Questions, Case 8
1. What are the major drug groups used in the treatment of endogenous depression?
2. What are the adverse effects associated with each group?

CASE 9. THYROID DISEASE*

A 27-year-old woman was referred for evaluation of thyroid disease. She had a 3-month history of intermittent heat intolerance, sweats, tremor, tachycardia, and muscle weakness. She had lost weight in spite of a marked increase in appetite. She denied taking any medications before seeing her family physician. She had been taking iodide drops since seeing her doctor and initially noted a decrease in symptoms. For the past month, however, they had worsened.

Physical examination revealed blood pressure 180/90 mm Hg, heart rate 110/min, minimal proptosis, and an enlarged thyroid gland. Laboratory tests showed elevated thyroxine, resin T_3 uptake, radioactive iodine uptake, and antimicrosomal antibodies. A diagnosis of hyperimmune hyperthyroidism (Graves' disease) was made.

Questions, Case 9
1. What therapeutic measures should be considered in this case? Why did the iodide drops the patient was taking reduce symptoms at first and then lose their effectiveness?
2. What are the benefits and hazards of pharmacologic therapy in hyperthyroidism?
3. What therapy should be considered if thyrotoxic crisis (thyroid storm) occurs?

CASE 10. A DIABETIC STUDENT†

An 18-year-old woman was referred to the endocrine clinic at her student health service because a routine urinalysis revealed glycosuria and a random plasma glucose measured subsequently was 250 mg/dL.

The history disclosed that this was the student's first time away from home and that she had had a number of symptoms she attributed to anxiety associated with the move to college. These symptoms included weight loss (5 kg), polydipsia, nocturia, fatigue, and three episodes of vaginal yeast infections in the past 3 months. Before moving, she had a long series of recurrent upper respiratory infections. The family history was negative for diabetes, and she was taking no medications.

The physical examination was within normal limits. Her weight was 50 kg, which is in the 20th percentile for her height. The laboratory results were as follows: fasting plasma glucose 280 mg/dL (≤115), urine glucose and ketones strongly positive. On the basis of these and other findings, a diagnosis of type I diabetes was made.

Questions, Case 10
1. What are the primary therapeutic strategies available in this case?
2. What are the complications and hazards of the major therapies for diabetes?
3. What methods of monitoring and adjusting therapy are available to the patient?

---

* Modified and reproduced, with permission, from Dong BJ: Thyroid diseases. Page 1313 in: *Applied Therapeutics,* 3rd ed. Katcher BS, Young LY, Koda-Kimble MA (editors). Applied Therapeutics, 1983.

† Modified and reproduced, with permission, from Koda-Kimble MA, Rotblatt MD: Diabetes mellitus. Page 1357 in: *Applied Therapeutics,* 3rd ed. Katcher BS, Young LY, Koda-Kimble MA (editors). Applied Therapeutics, 1983.

CASE 11. SEVERE RHEUMATOID ARTHRITIS*

A 60-year-old woman was referred for management of severe rheumatoid arthritis. She had had the disease for 15 years and had been managed until age 55 with aspirin. She was then switched to ibuprofen, which diminished the gastrointestinal adverse effects she had developed from aspirin. One year before referral, she started to complain of increased joint pain and stiffness, and laboratory studies confirmed that the disease had become more active. Several attempts to control her symptoms with increased dosage of ibuprofen and with a trial of another NSAID were not effective, and the decision was made to add corticosteroids to the regimen.

Prednisone was started in a dosage of 5 mg daily, given in the morning. After a period of evaluation, the dose was increased to 10 mg and then to 15 mg daily. At this dosage, the patient's symptoms were reduced to a bearable degree.

Questions, Case 11
1. What are the relative advantages and disadvantages of corticosteroids versus NSAIDs in the treatment of inflammatory disease?
2. Why was prednisone given to this patient in the morning?
3. What is the advantage of alternate-day therapy with corticosteroids? Which steroids are unsuitable for alternate-day therapy?

CASE 12. AN INFANT WITH FEVER†

A 19-month-old girl was hospitalized with fever and signs suggestive of bacterial meningitis. She was treated with ampicillin and chloramphenicol for 72 hours and then placed on chloramphenicol alone on the basis of the results of microbiologic laboratory examinations.

After 12 days of antibiotic treatment, the patient was afebrile and cerebrospinal fluid was sterile, with normal protein and glucose levels. Drug treatment was discontinued, but after 3 days she developed vomiting and fever to 40.5 °C. Cerebrospinal fluid culture was sterile, but counterimmunoelectrophoresis was positive for *Haemophilus influenzae* type b polyribosylribitol phosphate antigen.

The patient was treated for 12 days with moxalactam and remained afebrile after the second day. At completion of therapy, cerebrospinal fluid was sterile, counterimmunoelectrophoresis was negative, and the white cell count and protein levels were returning toward the normal range.

Questions, Case 12
1. Why was antibiotic treatment started before microbiologic laboratory examinations were completed?
2. What was the basis for the initial choice of ampicillin and chloramphenicol?
3. Why was ampicillin therapy stopped after 3 days?
4. What is the most likely cause of the apparent relapse after discontinuance of chloramphenicol?
5. What was the basis for the use of moxalactam?

CASE 13. A DRUG REACTION‡

A 64-year-old man was hospitalized for evaluation and treatment of carcinoma of the tongue. Following a course of chemotherapy, the patient was brought to the operating room for radical neck dissection. He was intubated and given 2 g of cefoxitin intravenously. Ten minutes later, he developed severe hypotension with a systolic blood pressure of 40–50 mm Hg, wheezing over both lung fields, and urticaria.

The operation was postponed, and the patient was given intravenous epinephrine, dexamethasone,

---

* Modified and reproduced, with permission, from Kishi DT: Disorders of the adrenals. Page 1279 in: *Applied Therapeutics,* 3rd ed. Katcher BS, Young LY, Koda-Kimble MA (editors). Applied Therapeutics, 1983.

† Adapted from Centers for Disease Control: Ampicillin and chloramphenicol resistance in systemic *Haemophilus influenzae* disease. MMWR 1984;33:35.

‡ Adapted and reproduced, with permission, from Austin SM, Barooah B, Chung SK: Reversible acute cardiac injury during cefoxitin-induced anaphylaxis in a patient with normal coronary arteries. Am J Med 1984;77:729.

diphenhydramine, and fluids over the next 2 hours. Blood pressure was restored and maintained by intravenous infusion of dopamine. In the intensive care unit, electrocardiography suggested acute cardiac injury; the patient had no history of angina pectoris or heart disease. Subsequent chest x-ray revealed a normal heart size with bilateral pulmonary edema.

Questions, Case 13

1. Why was cefoxitin given at the time of surgery?
2. What type of drug allergy did the patient experience?
3. Why were epinephrine, diphenhydramine, and a corticosteroid administered?

CASE 14. DIARRHEA FOLLOWING ANTIBIOTICS*

A 10-year-old girl received erythromycin for a prolonged respiratory tract infection. She continued to have headaches and a stuffy nose; a facial x-ray suggested maxillary sinusitis, which could not be confirmed following sinus puncture. Erythromycin was stopped and she was given amoxicillin (250 mg 3 times a day) for 10 days.

On the last day of amoxicillin treatment, she developed diarrhea with some abdominal pain but no vomiting. Initially the stools were alternately watery and solid, but later they became mucoid with some blood. After 11 days of these symptoms, she was given loperamide for her diarrhea, and a stool culture was positive for *Clostridium difficile*.

She was hospitalized, and sigmoidoscopy revealed colitis with pseudomembranes, confirmed histologically. Stool culture was positive for *C difficile* and negative for *Salmonella, Shigella, Yersinia*, and *Campylobacter*. The girl was treated with oral vancomycin, 250 mg 4 times daily for 7 days, and was discharged following rectoscopic examination that proved normal and a negative *C difficile* stool culture.

Questions, Case 14

1. What was the rationale for the treatment of the upper respiratory tract infections with erythromycin?
2. Why was amoxicillin used to treat the suspected sinusitis?
3. What was the most likely cause of the diarrhea and the overgrowth of *C difficile* in the gastrointestinal tract?
4. Why was oral vancomycin used in this case? What alternative drug treatments could have been employed?

CASE 15. DIARRHEA FOLLOWING A TRIP†

After returning from a trip to Mexico, a 41-year-old woman had a week-long bout of diarrhea that resolved spontaneously. She did not feel well for the succeeding 4 months, and then abdominal discomfort became severe and fever (but no bowel symptoms) occurred. There was no history of jaundice, gallstones, or hepatitis, but acute cholecystitis was suspected; the patient was admitted to the hospital for what proved to be an unrewarding oral cholecystogram.

Following the x-ray studies, diarrhea reappeared. She was referred to another institution and was initially treated with metronidazole, ampicillin, and gentamicin for presumed amebic liver abscesses or acute cholecystitis with liver abscesses. Subsequently, a serologic test for amebic infection was positive, and liver and spleen scans confirmed the presence of abscesses. Based on these findings gentamicin and ampicillin were discontinued.

The patient's symptoms improved with a 10-day course of oral metronidazole and tetracycline. She became afebrile, and serologic tests for amebic infection reverted to negative. Oral iodoquinol was given for 3 weeks, and follow-up examinations showed resolution of the abscess cavities and no recurrence of symptoms.

---

* Adapted and reproduced, with permission, from Vesikari T et al: Pseudomembranous colitis with recurring diarrhea and prolonged persistence of *Clostridium difficile* in a 10-year-old girl. Acta Paediatr Scand 1984;73:135.

† Modified and reproduced, with permission, from Strum WB: Persistent pain, fever after a trip to Mexico. Hosp Pract 1984;19:86.

Questions, Case 15
1. What are the most likely causes of diarrhea in a tourist following a trip to Mexico? Should such cases of traveler's diarrhea be routinely treated with antibiotics?
2. What antimicrobial activity is anticipated for ampicillin and gentamicin used in this case?
3. Why was metronidazole treatment continued after discontinuance of the above antibiotics? What does tetracycline add to the therapeutic regimen?
4. What was the rationale for the 3 weeks of oral treatment with iodoquinol?

CASE 16.   THE AFRICAN TRAVELER*

A 20-year-old woman in good health planned to visit Kenya in a travel and study program. She was immunized against tetanus, typhoid, cholera, and yellow fever, received human immune globulin, and in Kenya took chloroquine and Fansidar (pyrimethamine-sulfadoxine) for malarial prophylaxis. After 10 weeks, she was one of 15 (of 18) students to become ill, with fever, abdominal pain, and non-bloody diarrhea. Five days later, she developed severe back pain and then rapidly lost ambulatory ability. Stool examination showed ova of *Schistosoma mansoni,* and she was diagnosed as having schistosomiasis with transverse myelitis.

She was treated with oxamniquine and transported to the USA, where evaluation showed flaccid paralysis and decreased sensation of touch and temperature in the legs. Cerebrospinal fluid examination showed pleocytosis and protein elevation. Serologic tests for *Mycoplasma* and viral agents were negative. A myelogram showed no masses amenable to surgical removal.

The patient was treated with praziquantel and large doses of dexamethasone. The patient's motor function and sensation improved with treatment, and within a month she was ambulating with assistance in a rehabilitation center.

Questions, Case 16
1. Why was this patient taking both chloroquine and pyrimethamine-sulfadoxine for malarial prophylaxis?
2. Why was oxamniquine used for the initial treatment of schistosomiasis in this case? What are its anticipated adverse effects?
3. How does praziquantel differ from other drugs used in schistosomiasis? What is known about its mechanism of action?
4. What are the anticipated adverse effects of praziquantel? Is there any reason to believe that praziquantel (or oxamniquine) might have been contraindicated in this patient?
5. Why was dexamethasone administered?

ANSWERS: CASE HISTORIES

Answers, Case 1
1. The most probable chemical intoxicants in the case of the 55-year-old gardener are insecticides. The most common constituents of currently available insecticides that produce acute poisoning are the cholinesterase inhibitors and nicotine. This patient's signs of muscarinic excess (abdominal discomfort and diarrhea) developed over a week, suggesting that a long-acting drug was gradually accumulating to a toxic level. The symptoms of cholinergic toxicity are described in Chapter 7. Miosis and perspiration are common signs of cholinesterase inhibition. Nicotine rarely produces this pattern of slow onset and usually induces signs of sympathetic as well as parasympathetic discharge. The diagnosis can be confirmed by measuring the patient's blood cholinesterase level and by identifying a carbamate or organophosphate-containing insecticide among the patient's stock of garden supplies.
2. Immediate measures must be taken to maintain vital signs and to ensure that exposure to the intoxicant has ceased. Because the patient is unconscious, induction of emesis is contraindicated, and gastric lavage should not be attempted unless a cuffed endotracheal tube is in place. Since the patient's symptoms developed over a 1-week period, it is unlikely that the present stomach

---

* Adapted from Centers for Disease Control: Acute schistosomiasis with transverse myelitis in American students returning from Kenya. MMWR 1984;33:445.

contents are contributing much to his intoxication. Since the organophosphates can be absorbed across the skin, the clothing should be removed and the skin cleansed (with care to avoid contamination of medical personnel). With the endotracheal tube in place, mechanical respiratory assistance can be applied as required to maintain normal blood gases, and gastric lavage may be done if there is any chance that the intoxicant was ingested. An intravenous line should be placed for the administration of drugs and for the maintenance of good hydration.

3. Drugs to be considered for this patient include the following: (a) atropine for control of muscarinic effects; (b) pralidoxime for regeneration of cholinesterase, especially at the neuromuscular junction; and (c) cardiovascular stimulants, but only if required to maintain normal tissue perfusion. (They are rarely required.)

Answers, Case 2

1. $0.7 \times 90 \times .25$ mg/440L = 36 mcg/L.

2. The cause of the dramatic rise in serum potassium was the poisoning of membrane Na^+/K^+ ATPase (the sodium pump) in the entire body. The serum potassium concentration can be used as an index of the severity of poisoning and may be more accurate as a prognostic tool than the blood level of digoxin. The source of the ion is the intracellular space, particularly that of skeletal muscle (because of the large mass of this tissue).

3. Digitalis has the well-deserved reputation of causing any and all types of cardiac arrhythmias. The most common are junctional tachycardia (originating in the atrioventricular node) and ventricular tachycardia. The patient's atrial fibrillation detected on admission was probably a chronic condition related to his mitral stenosis. The high degree of atrioventricular block, with the slow ventricular rate, could reflect the strong vagal effects of the cardiac glycoside, but in view of the resistance to atropine in this case, the AV block probably represents direct depression by the drug. The widened QRS complex and the very slow spontaneous rate when pacing was interrupted reflect severe depression of Purkinje and ventricular cell automaticity and conduction velocity. Such depression could have been caused by depolarization by the high extracellular potassium level. Under these circumstances, administration of antiarrhythmic agents, which are also cardiac depressants, was clearly contraindicated.

   The effects noted in this patient are unusually severe. At the more common levels of toxicity observed in nonsuicidal patients, automaticity is usually increased, not decreased. In such patients, depressant interventions such as administration of potassium or antiarrhythmic drugs are often successful in controlling arrhythmias.

4. Conventional therapy of mild-to-moderate cardiac glycoside intoxication consists of the following: (a) Normalization of low serum K^+. In the present case and in most cases of gross overdosage, the serum K^+ is high. However, in many cases of mild-to-moderate toxicity, the serum K^+ is low or normal. In some cases (usually involving vomiting or diarrhea), low serum magnesium is found, and correction of this deficiency corrects the arrhythmia. (b) Use of antiarrhythmic drugs. (Lidocaine is usually tried first.) (c) Avoidance of DC cardioversion unless ventricular fibrillation occurs. The first two of these approaches were clearly not suitable for this severely intoxicated patient. The antidote was digoxin antibodies.

5. Fortunately, severe intoxication is less common with digitoxin than with digoxin. Antidigoxin Fab fragments cross-react sufficiently to be useful in reversing digitoxin effects. Lavage of the small intestine with steroid-binding resins (eg, cholestyramine) has been of value in some cases. The success of such treatment reflects the importance of enterohepatic circulation of digitoxin.

Answers, Case 3

1. The case description is typical of antimuscarinic drug poisoning. A common source of such agents in nature is Jimson weed (*Datura stramonium*). The patient had ingested several of the 2- to 3-mm round black seeds from the pods of this plant.

2. The most life-threatening effect of the antimuscarinic agents in many patients, especially small children and infants, is hyperthermia. Unsupervised hallucinating patients may fall and injure themselves. Convulsions and arrhythmias may occur. Other effects of these drugs, though uncomfortable, are not life-threatening.

3. The chief danger of physostigmine is its central stimulant effect, which may lead to convulsions. Because of this hazard, most emergency departments now prefer to treat antimuscarinic poisoning symptomatically. Other anticholinesterase drugs, such as neostigmine, do not enter the CNS

as readily as physostigmine; they are less dangerous but also less effective in reversing the central effects of the intoxicant. Other treatments are symptomatic (cooling fans, cooling blankets).

Answers, Case 4

1. Because metaraminol is an alpha-receptor agonist, it causes marked vasoconstriction, which can be accompanied by reflex bradycardia. This patient rapidly became dependent upon the exogenous stimulant for maintenance of cardiac output, and attempts to stop the infusion resulted in hypotension.
2. The hematocrit increased because of hemoconcentration. Marked vasoconstriction results in increased Starling forces outward across the capillary wall, and increased capillary permeability caused by local ischemia facilitates the movement of plasma water out of the vascular compartment and into the tissues and the urine.
3. The patient went into shock because of the loss of blood volume described in answer 2 and because the increased cardiac work (secondary to vasoconstriction) was causing heart failure. The result was a form of hypotension that responds well to volume replacement and renal vasodilators.
4. As noted in answer 3, volume replacement (eg, with dextran solution) is the most important aspect of therapy in this situation. Because the patient's cardiovascular system had become dependent upon exogenous sympathomimetics, norepinephrine was necessary for a short time. However, rapid removal of this stimulus was indicated and successfully accomplished in this case.

Answers, Case 5

1. The mediators probably most important in causing asthmatic bronchoconstriction are leukotrienes LTC_4 and LTD_4. Another leukotriene (LTB_4), prostaglandins, peptides, and histamine probably also play a role.
2. The most commonly used bronchodilators are the beta-adrenoceptor agonists and the methylxanthines. In some patients, a muscarinic blocking drug (eg, ipratropium) has a useful bronchodilating effect. Cromolyn and nedocromil inhibit the degranulation of mast cells and are useful as prophylactic agents in some patients. They are not useful in an acute attack. Systemic corticosteroids are reserved for patients with severe asthma who do not respond adequately to other agents, but inhaled steroids (eg, beclomethasone) are now accepted as appropriate prophylactic therapy for all individuals with moderate or severe recurrent asthma.
3. The drug administered by the paramedics and by the personnel in the emergency room was epinephrine. This agent is extremely effective and has a rapid onset of action. However, it is probably no more effective than inhaled β_2-selective agonists (albuterol, terbutaline, metaproterenol). The drugs commonly used in nebulizers include epinephrine, isoproterenol, and the β_2-selective agonists.

Answers, Case 6

1. Ergot causes vasoconstriction through the activation of several receptors, including alpha-adrenoceptors and serotonin receptors. Additional receptors may be involved, since blockade of both adrenoceptors and serotonin receptors is often ineffective in reversing ergot-induced vasospasm.
2. The recommended limits of ergotamine consumption are 2–6 mg of ergotamine tartrate per episode of migraine and not more than 10 tablets (10 mg) per week. For severe migraine, intravenous administration of dihydroergotamine mesylate is sometimes effective. A maximum of 2 mg per dose of this drug is recommended, with a limit of 6 mg per week.
3. Nitroprusside breaks down spontaneously to release nitric oxide. Nitric oxide stimulates the production of cGMP in vascular smooth muscle, which causes relaxation.
4. If the patient has frequent attacks of migraine, prophylactic medication is indicated. Ergonovine and methysergide, a semisynthetic ergot derivative, have been used with partial success in many patients. Propranolol, amitriptyline, some calcium channel blockers, and cyproheptadine have also been effective. Note that sumatriptan, a new 5-HT agonist, is useful in treating acute migraine attacks but not in preventing recurrences.

Answers, Case 7

1. Carbamazepine and primidone were probably used at the start of the study to prevent the automatisms (complex partial seizures) that were reportedly part of the patient's seizure repertoire.

Carbamazepine is considered the drug of choice for this seizure type. When it became apparent that such seizures were actually infrequent in this patient, the drugs were withdrawn.

2. Monitoring of blood levels is very important in the management of epilepsy. The effective levels for valproate and ethosuximide are 50–100 mg/L. Thus, the levels measured in this patient while she was receiving the high dose of valproate were within the effective range for both agents. When the dose of valproate was reduced to 600 mg/d, the mean and minimum plasma levels dropped below the effective range, and seizures recurred.

3. Ethosuximide is associated with a very low incidence of serious adverse effects. Gastric irritation, lethargy, fatigue, and other CNS effects are reported. In contrast, valproate carries with it a low but significant risk of serious hepatic injury. It is contraindicated in pregnant women because it has been shown to cause spina bifida in infants born to mothers taking the drug.

Answers, Case 8

1. Several drug groups are available for the treatment of major (endogenous) depression. These include the tricyclic agents (TCA), a group of heterocyclic second-generation antidepressants, selective serotonin reuptake inhibitors (SSRI), and the monoamine oxidase inhibitors (MAOI).

2. The toxicity of antidepressant drugs is very important, because these drugs are often taken for long periods of time and because depressed patients often use medications close at hand in attempting suicide.

   The tricyclic drugs have autonomic effects much like those of the phenothiazine antipsychotic agents, which are chemically similar to tricyclic drugs. In addition, they can cause serious cardiac arrhythmias that are very difficult to treat. The second-generation drugs are similar. The selective serotonin reuptake inhibitors are relatively free of life-threatening toxicities. The MAO inhibitors cause serious interactions with catecholamine-releasing agents such as vasoconstrictor drugs (eg, ephedrine) and food constituents (eg, tyramine in fermented foods).

Answers, Case 9

1. The major therapies available for Graves' disease are surgery, thyroid-suppressant drugs, and radioactive iodine in sufficient dosage to destroy the gland. Ipodate, an iodine-containing x-ray contrast material, and beta-blockers are of value in severe thyrotoxicosis.

   Iodide therapy (usually saturated solution of potassium iodide) is useful in reducing thyroid hormone release and in decreasing the vascularity of the gland prior to surgery. However, escape from the inhibitory effect of iodide often occurs in Graves' disease, and the increased iodine substrate made available by the therapy may actually accentuate the disease.

2. Radioactive iodine is often the treatment of choice for young adult patients. This treatment provides a permanent cure (in fact, hypothyroidism is common after treatment and is managed with levothyroxine replacement therapy). Even after 35 years of follow-up, there is no evidence that the exposure to radioactivity causes increased incidence of disease. However, radioactive iodine should not be used in pregnant women, because it crosses the placenta and will damage the fetal thyroid as well as that of the mother. Other antithyroid drugs include iodide (discussed above) and the thioamides. The principal thioamides are propylthiouracil and methimazole. Almost all patients respond promptly to these agents. However, immunologic complications are not rare. Skin rashes are the most common. Agranulocytosis, cholestatic jaundice, hepatocellular damage, and exfoliative dermatitis are uncommon.

   Surgical thyroidectomy is the treatment of choice for patients with very large or multinodular glands. Patients are treated preoperatively with antithyroid drugs until they are euthyroid, and they receive iodine for 2 weeks prior to surgery to reduce vascularity of the gland.

3. Patients in a thyrotoxic crisis usually have multiple system involvement. The cardiovascular system is particularly susceptible, and severe tachycardia, arrhythmias, and heart failure are common. The sympathetic nervous system is hyperactive, and this is one of the major causes of the cardiovascular effects. The CNS is also affected, and signs may include severe agitation, delirium, and coma.

   Ipodate, which inhibits the conversion of thyroxine to triiodothyronine, is very useful in reducing the intensity of symptoms of thyroid storm. Sympathoplegic drugs are also very useful in this syndrome. Propranolol is the most commonly used. Further release of hormone from the gland is blocked by intravenous administration of sodium iodide, supplemented by oral potassium iodide. Synthesis is inhibited by oral or, if necessary, parenteral antithyroid drugs. Corticosteroids are sometimes used.

Answers, Case 10

1. In a young diabetic of low or normal weight with a history of viral infections preceding onset of hyperglycemia, it is likely that the disease is due to loss of functioning pancreatic islet B cells. The diagnosis of insulin deficiency (type I) diabetes was made in this case. The oral hypoglycemic agents are not useful in type I diabetes, but they are used in noninsulin-dependent (type II) diabetes. The strategies available in this case are dietary management and insulin.

2. The most important acute complication of insulin therapy is hypoglycemia. This is an emergency that the patient and his or her family must be prepared to deal with, since it may occur suddenly or insidiously and can be fatal or result in brain damage if not treated promptly and effectively. Treatment is by administration of glucose or glucagon.

   The long-term complications of insulin therapy include immunologic problems, eg, insulin allergy and insulin resistance caused by formation of antibodies to the insulin used. These effects can be minimized by the use of purified preparations that contain lower concentrations of non-insulin protein, or by the use of human insulin preparations.

   Another complication of insulin therapy is lipodystrophy at the site of injection. This consists of atrophy of the subcutaneous lipid tissue. It has become much less common since the advent of improved methods of purifying insulin, and now even the standard preparations are relatively free of the effect. In fact, lipid hypertrophy may occur.

   The complications of the oral hypoglycemic drugs (not suitable in this case) are more varied than those of insulin therapy. Tolbutamide is associated with a low incidence of skin rashes and interactions with other drugs that result in prolonged hypoglycemia. Chlorpropamide causes prolonged hypoglycemia more often than tolbutamide, as well as jaundice and an antidiuretic effect. The latter action may cause dilutional hyponatremia. The second-generation agents (glipizide, glyburide) are so much more potent than the older sulfonylureas that care must be exercised to avoid significant hypoglycemia.

3. Most patients should monitor their blood or urine glucose as an aid to adjustment of insulin dosage. The major reason for daily adjustment of dosage is that insulin requirement is altered by many factors: diet, exercise, disease, etc. Considerable evidence indicates that close control of blood glucose is associated with a lower incidence of long-term complications of diabetes.

   The major adjustments made by most patients are the total number of units of insulin injected and the proportions of rapid-acting and intermediate- or long-acting preparations used.

Answers, Case 11

1. Corticosteroids are more effective than NSAIDs in controlling acute severe flare-ups of joint inflammation. However, the severe disadvantages of corticosteroids (adrenocortical suppression, weight gain, buffalo hump, striae, osteoporosis, diabetes, peptic ulcers, cataracts, glaucoma, and psychoses) preclude their use for chronic therapy in most patients.

2. The normal diurnal variation of glucocorticoid release includes a peak in the morning hours and a trough late at night. Therefore, a single dose of an intermediate-acting (12–24 hours) agent such as prednisone mimics the normal variation and reduces the degree of suppression of the pituitary.

3. Alternate-day therapy permits maintenance of a greater degree of pituitary-adrenal interaction and also allows temporary recovery of peripheral tissues from stimulation by high levels of glucocorticoid. This is particularly valuable in growing children. The longest-acting corticosteroids are not suitable for alternate-day regimens because the duration of pituitary suppression extends over 48 hours, and so nothing is gained. Such long-acting agents include paramethasone, dexamethasone, and betamethasone.

Answers, Case 12

1. The principal justification for empiric, presumptive antimicrobial therapy is that the infection is best treated early to avoid serious morbidity or death. Suspected bacterial meningitis is a classic example of the need to initiate therapy immediately—after relevant samples have been taken for culture and sensitivity determination—on the basis of the clinical diagnosis and the initial microbiologic diagnosis. The latter should include history, physical signs, and Gram stain.

2. *Haemophilus influenzae* type b is by far the most common cause of bacterial meningitis in infants and young children. Because of the emergence of ampicillin-resistant strains, chloramphenicol sometimes has been used (in combination with ampicillin) until microbiologic labora-

tory results identify the infecting organism and document its susceptibility to antimicrobial drugs.

3. The microbiologic laboratory confirmed *H influenzae* type b and demonstrated that the isolate was beta-lactamase-positive. Ampicillin is inactivated by penicillinases, unless used in combination with an inhibitor of such enzymes.

4. Although the cerebrospinal fluid was apparently sterile, the counterimmunoelectrophoresis analysis suggests a relapse due to *H influenzae* type b because of inadequate treatment with chloramphenicol or development of resistance.

5. Resistance of *H influenzae* isolates to both ampicillin and chloramphenicol is no longer rare. Most infectious disease specialists would now **start** treatment of suspected bacterial meningitis in children aged 6 months to 6 years with a third-generation cephalosporin such as ceftriaxone or cefotaxime. Moxalactam has also been used in the past for bacterial meningitis, but it is less effective than several other third-generation drugs and may cause bleeding via hypoprothrombinemia and antiplatelet actions.

Answers, Case 13

1. Chemoprophylaxis is indicated when the wound infection rate for surgical procedures, under optimal conditions, is 5% or more. This patient had been treated for cancer, possibly with immunosuppressive agents, and may have been at particular risk for infection. The cephalosporins are the most commonly used antimicrobial agents for surgical prophylaxis because they have activity against gram-positive cocci and selected gram-negative bacilli that are likely pathogens. Most commonly, a first-generation drug (eg, cefazolin) should be used, but under some circumstances a second-generation cephalosporin, such as cefoxitin, may be appropriate.

2. The patient experienced a classic type I (immediate) IgE-mediated allergic reaction, which often includes anaphylaxis, urticaria, and angioedema. Antimicrobial drugs, particularly the beta-lactams and sulfonamides, can cause type I reactions. The degree of cross-allergenicity between penicillins and cephalosporins is probably less than 10%. Skin testing with a dilute solution of drug may reveal drug sensitivity but often gives false-negative results.

3. Epinephrine and isoproterenol (via cAMP mechanisms) and theophylline (via cAMP or block of adenosine receptors) inhibit the release of mediators from mast cells and basophils and produce bronchodilation. Diphenhydramine competitively blocks histamine actions at H_1 receptors, actions that would otherwise cause bronchoconstriction and increased capillary permeability. Dexamethasone probably has multiple effects, including inhibition of IgE-producing clone proliferation, block of T helper cell function, and anti-inflammatory actions.

Answers, Case 14

1. There is no information in the history of the original upper respiratory tract infection regarding possible (or confirmed) pathogens or their susceptibility to antimicrobial drugs. Erythromycin has activity against common streptococci, staphylococci (including penicillinase-producing strains), and *Mycoplasma pneumoniae;* this presumably underlies the choice of the drug in this case. Erythromycin has few adverse effects, although some gastrointestinal irritation and occasional liver dysfunction (rare in children) may occur. There is no cross-allergenicity with the penicillin group.

2. The suspected sinusitis had not responded to erythromycin. Since attempts to confirm bacterial infection had failed, amoxicillin therapy was started on empiric grounds. Amoxicillin has activity against many streptococci and *H influenzae* strains, as well as selected gram-negative rods. The drug is not active against penicillinase-producing organisms or *M pneumoniae*. However, these organisms should have been eradicated by the prior treatment with erythromycin.

3. Ampicillin is more likely to cause diarrhea than most other penicillins, partly by causing direct gastrointestinal irritant effects and partly by disturbing the normal gut flora. In this case, its close congener, amoxicillin, resulted in diarrhea that persisted more than a week after drug discontinuance, suggesting the possibility of microbial superinfection. This was confirmed by culture of *Clostridium difficile*. This organism causes colitis following therapy with various antibiotics, including clindamycin, the tetracyclines, and beta-lactam agents.

4. When given orally, vancomycin has been effective in the treatment of colitis caused by toxin-producing bacteria, including *C difficile*. Vancomycin is poorly absorbed after oral administration, and there is less risk of causing the ototoxicity and nephrotoxicity that may occur with intravenous administration. Oral metronidazole is equally effective, and oral neomycin and bacitracin have also been used.

Answers, Case 15

1. The most common causes of traveler's diarrhea are infections due to coliform bacteria and viruses. Most such infections are self-limiting, and fluid and electrolyte replacement is usually adequate treatment. Antibiotics (eg, doxycycline, trimethoprim-sulfamethoxazole) are useful prophylactic agents against such organisms but are not effective in gastrointestinal infections due to viruses; these drugs have minimal activity against intestinal protozoan parasites.

2. Ampicillin and gentamicin were included in the drug regimen on the basis of a possible bacterial involvement in acute cholecystitis, a component of the initial clinical diagnosis. Neither drug is active against amebic infection. Ampicillin would provide coverage for streptococci (including enterococci) and selected gram-negative enteric organisms, and gentamicin is active against aerobic gram-negative rods. Neither drug has good activity against gram-negative anaerobes, and anaerobic bacteria are a major cause of bacterial liver abscess.

3. The confirmed diagnosis of amebic disease justified empiric therapy with metronidazole, which is effective in most cases of extraluminal amebiasis, although it is not a luminal amebicide. Metronidazole also has antibacterial actions, including activity against gram-negative anaerobes. Oral tetracycline is an inhibitor of bacteria that associate with *Entamoeba histolytica* in the gut, and the drug may indirectly affect luminal amebas by such an action.

4. Iodoquinol (and diloxanide furoate) are not effective in severe intestinal amebiasis or in amebic hepatic abscess. These drugs are used in asymptomatic intestinal amebiasis, to treat concurrent intestinal infection, and to totally eradicate the protozoan to prevent disease recurrence.

Answers, Case 16

1. Chloroquine-resistant *P falciparum* are endemic in Africa, and the prophylactic use of chloroquine as a sole agent will not prevent infection. While pyrimethamine-sulfadoxine has been used prophylactically, it is not the drug of choice. Weekly doses of mefloquine one week before entering an endemic area, during, and for 4 weeks after leaving, is the preferred method.

2. Oxamniquine is active against mature and immature forms of *Schistosoma mansoni* (but not other *Schistosoma* spp), although resistance can occur. The initial use of the drug was presumably based on identification of the parasite ova in stools, its ease of administration (it is orally effective), and possibly its availability. Adverse effects of oxamniquine include dizziness, headache, drowsiness, gastrointestinal irritation, and pruritus. Effects probably due to dying parasites include eosinophilia, pulmonary infiltrates, and urticaria. At high doses, oxamniquine may cause hallucinations and seizures.

3. Praziquantel is the drug of choice for infections caused by all species of schistosomes. The agent increases the permeability of the parasite cell membrane to calcium, causing initial contraction and then paralysis of its musculature. The tegmen becomes vacuolized and disintegrates, causing parasite death.

4. The most common toxic effects of praziquantel are malaise, headache, dizziness, gastrointestinal irritation, urticaria, and fever. Some of these effects may be caused by dying parasites. Praziquantel is contraindicated in pregnancy, since animal studies show that the drug increases the abortion rate. The drug also acts as a co-mutagen in in vitro test systems. Oxamniquine is also mutagenic and is embryocidal in animal test systems.

5. Corticosteroids are used to suppress host immune responses and inflammation, including reactions to eggs deposited in the venules in and around the spinal cord.

Appendix V

Strategies for Improving Test Performance

There are many strategies for studying and exam taking, and decisions about which ones to use are partly a function of individual habit and preference. However, basic study rules may be applied to any learning exercise; test-taking strategies depend upon the type of examination.

FOUR BASIC STUDY RULES

1. Never read more than a few pages of dense textual material without stopping to write out the gist of it from memory. This is a universal rule for effective study. If necessary, refer to the material just read. After finishing a chapter, make up your own tables of the major drugs, receptor types, mechanisms, etc, and fill in as many of the blanks as you can. Refer to tables and figures in the book as needed to fill in your own notes. This is active learning; just reading is passive and far less effective unless you happen to have a photographic memory. Notes should be legible and saved for ready access when reviewing before exams.
2. Experiment with additional study methods until you find out what works for you. This may involve solo study or group study, flash cards, or text reading. You won't know how effective these techniques are until you have tried them.
3. Don't scorn "cramming," but don't rely on it either. Some steady, day-by-day reading and digestion of conceptual material is usually needed to avoid last-minute indigestion. Similarly, don't substitute memorization of lists (eg, the Key Words list, Appendix I) for more substantive understanding.
4. If you are preparing for a course examination, make every effort to attend all the lectures. The lecturer's view of what is important may be very different from that of the author of the textbook, and the chances are good that exam questions will be based on the instructor's own lecture notes.

STRATEGIES APPLICABLE TO ALL EXAMINATIONS

Two general rules apply to all examinations.

1. When starting the examination, scan the entire question set before answering any. If the examination has several parts, allot time to each part in proportion to its length. Within each part, answer the easy questions first, placing a mark in the margin by the questions to which you will return. Practice saving enough time for the more difficult questions by scheduling one minute or less for each question on practice examinations such as those in Appendices II and III in this book. (The time available in the USMLE examination is approximately 45 seconds per question.)
2. When answering multiple choice questions such as those on the USMLE, don't change your first "guess" unless you find a convincing reason for doing so.

STRATEGIES FOR SPECIFIC QUESTION FORMATS

A certain group of students—often characterized as "good test-takers"—may not know every detail about the subject matter being tested but seem to perform extremely well most of the time. The strategy used by these people is not a secret, though few instructors seem to realize how easy it is to break down their questions into much simpler ones. Lists of these strategies are widely available, eg, in the descriptive material distributed by the National Board of Medical Examiners to its candidates. A paraphrased compendium of this advice is presented below.

A. Strategies for the "Choose the One Best Answer" (of Five Choices) Type Question:

1. If two statements are contradictory (ie, only one can be correct), chances are good that one of the two is the correct answer, ie, the other three choices are distracters. For example, consider the following:

   In treating quinidine overdose, the best strategy would be to
   - **(A)** Alkalinize the urine
   - **(B)** Acidify the urine
   - **(C)** Give procainamide
   - **(D)** Give potassium chloride
   - **(E)** Administer a calcium chelator such as EDTA

   The correct answer is (B), acidify the urine. The instructor revealed what was being tested in the first pair of choices and used the last three as "filler." Therefore, if you don't know the answer, you are better off guessing (A) or (B) (a 50% success probability) than (A) or (B) or (C) or (D) or (E) (a 20% success probability). Note that this strategy is only valid if you *must* guess; many instructors now introduce contradictory pairs as distracters. Another "rule" which should only be used if you must guess is the "longest choice" rule. When all the answers in a multiple choice question are relatively long, the correct answer is often the longest one. Note again that sophisticated question writers may introduce especially long *incorrect* choices to foil this strategy.

2. Statements that contain the words "always," "never," "must," etc are usually false. For example,

   Acetylcholine always increases the heart rate when given intravenously because it lowers blood pressure and evokes a strong baroreceptor-mediated reflex tachycardia.

   The statement is false because although acetylcholine often increases the heart rate, it can also cause bradycardia. (When given as a bolus, it may reach the sinus node in high enough concentration to cause initial bradycardia.) The use of "trigger" words such as "always" and "must" suggests that the instructor had some exception in mind.

3. Choices that do not fit the stem grammatically are usually wrong. For example:

   A drug that acts on a beta receptor and produces a maximal effect that is equal to one-half the effect of a large dose of isoproterenol is called a
   - **(A)** Agonist
   - **(B)** Partial agonist
   - **(C)** Antagonist
   - **(D)** Analogue of isoproterenol

   The use of the article *a* at the end of the stem rather than *an* implies that the answer must start with a consonant, ie, choice **B.** Similar use may be made of disagreements in number. Note that careful question writers will avoid this problem by placing the articles in the choice list, not in the stem.

4. A statement is not false just because changing a few words will make it somewhat more true than you think it is now. "Choose the one best answer" does not mean "Choose the only correct statement."

B. Strategies for Matching Type Questions:
Matching questions usually test name recognition, and the most efficient approach consists of scanning the list of choices from the start and picking the first clear "hit." This is especially important on extended matching questions in which just reading the list can be time-consuming. (It should be noted, however, that the strategy suggested by the National Board of Medical Examiners for the USMLE differs from the above; see their *General Instructions* publication.) Occasionally, the strategies described above for the single best answer type question can be applied to the matching and extended matching type.

C. **Strategies for the "Answer A if 1, 2, and 3 Are Correct" Type Question:** This type of question, known as the "K type," is still used in many local examinations. However, it has been dropped from the USMLE and therefore is no longer represented among the practice questions provided in this Review.

For this type of question, one rarely must know the truth about all four statements to arrive at the correct answer. The instructions are to select

(A) if only (1), (2), and (3) are correct;
(B) if only (1) and (3) are correct;
(C) if only (2) and (4) are correct;
(D) if only (4) is correct;
(E) if all are correct.

Useful strategies include the following:

1. If choice (1) is right and (2) is wrong, the answer must be (B), ie, (1) and (3) are correct. You don't need to know anything about (3) or (4).
2. If statement (1) is wrong, then answers (A), (B), and (E) are automatically excluded. Concentrate on statements (2) and (4).
3. The converse of 1 above: If choice (1) is wrong and (2) is right, the answer must be (C), ie, (2) and (4) are correct.
4. If statement (2) is correct and (4) is wrong, the answer is (A), ie, (1) and (3) must be correct and you need not even look at them. (See example below.)
5. If statements (1), (2), and (4) are correct, the answer must be (E). You need not know anything about (3).
6. Similarly, if statements (2) and (3) are right and (4) is wrong, the answer must be (A), and statement (1) must be correct.
7. If statements (2), (3), and (4) are correct, then the answer must be (E), and statement (1) must be correct.

No doubt more of these rules exist (National Board of Medical Examiners, 1984). In general, if you know whether two or three of the four statements in each question are right or wrong (ie, 50–75% the material), you should achieve a perfect score on this kind of question. The best way to learn these rules is to apply them to practice questions until the principles are firmly ingrained.

Consider the following question. Using the above rules, you should be able to answer it correctly even though there is no reason why you should know anything about the information contained in two of the four statements. The answer follows.

Which of the following statements is (are) correct?

1. The "struck bushel" is equal to 2150.42 cubic inches.
2. Medicine is one of the health sciences.
3. The fresh meat of the Atlantic salmon contains 220 IU of vitamin A per 100 g edible portion.
4. Hippocrates was the founder of modern psychoanalysis.

The answer is (A). Since statement (2) is clearly correct, and (4) is just as patently incorrect (let's give Freud the credit), the answer can only be (A), and statements (1) and (3) must be correct. (The data are from Lentner C (editor): *Geigy Scientific Tables,* 8th ed. Vol. 1. Ciba-Geigy, 1981.)

REFERENCES

Bhushan V, Le T, Amin C: *1995 First Aid For The USMLE STEP 1.* Appleton & Lange, 1995.
1992 Step 1 General Instructions, Content Outline, and Sample Items. National Board of Medical Examiners, 1992.
Part I Examination Guidelines and Sample Items. National Board of Medical Examiners, 1984.

Subject Index

NOTE: Page numbers in bold face type indicate a major discussion. A *t* following a page number indicates tabular material and an *f* following a page number indicates an illustration. Drugs are listed under their generic names.

LANGE
medical books

Available at your local health science bookstore

or by calling

Appleton & Lange toll free

1-800-423-1359 (in CT 1-203-838-4400).

A smart investment
in your medical career

(more on reverse)